Measuring Health

MEASURING HEALTH

A Guide To Rating Scales
and Questionnaires

SECOND EDITION

Ian McDowell

Claire Newell

New York   Oxford
OXFORD UNIVERSITY PRESS
1996

Oxford University Press

Oxford   New York
Athens   Auckland   Bangkok   Bombay
Calcutta   Cape Town   Dar es Salaam   Delhi
Florence   Hong Kong   Istanbul   Karachi
Kuala Lumpur   Madras   Madrid   Melbourne
Mexico City   Nairobi   Paris   Singapore
Taipei   Tokyo   Toronto

and associated companies in
Berlin   Ibadan

McDowell, Ian.
Measuring health: a guide to rating scales and questionnaires /
Ian McDowell, Claire Newell. --2nd ed.
p. cm.
Includes bibliographical references and index.
ISBN 0-19-510371-8
1. Health surveys.   2. Social surveys.
I. Newell, Claire.
II. Title.
[DNLM: 1. Health Surveys.
2. Health Status Indicators.
3. Questionnaires.
WA 900.1 M478m 1996]
RA408.5.M38   1996   614'2--dc20
DNLM/DLC   for Library of Congress   95-20980

9
Printed in the United States of America
on acid-free paper

Dedication

To my family: Carrol, Kris, Wes, Graeme, and Karin.
I am deeply sorry that it only seems possible
to write books during family time:
evenings and weekends.

I. McD.

Immeasurable gratitude to Terrell, Misha, and Stefan
for their enduring patience and understanding.

C. N.

Preface

The first edition of this book argued that no concise source of information on health measurement methods existed; this, we wrote, was a major problem for epidemiological and health care researchers. A number of reviews of measurement methods have since been produced (1–3), confirming this truth. There is now a growing awareness of the range of measures available, but it remains challenging to keep pace with new developments in the field. Descriptions of methods are widely scattered in social science, medical, management, and methodological journals. Furthermore, journal articles seldom compare methods and do not indicate which is the most valid for a particular application. The second edition of our book is intended to fill this gap. The methods we discuss have been termed sociomedical measurements, and they cover a variety of topics, including physical disability, emotional and social well-being, pain, life satisfaction, and quality of life.

We have written this book with two main purposes. First, we review the current status of health measurement, describing its theoretical and methodological bases and indicating areas in which further development is required. This is intended to appeal to students and those who develop measurement methods. Second, and more important, we describe the leading health measurement methods, with the interest of those who intend to use the measures for clinical and research applications in mind. An underlying goal is to try and persuade researchers not to invent their own unique measurement scale until they have carefully reviewed the numerous methods that are already available. Our primary focus is therefore on providing a guide to existing health measurement methods.

The methods we review all use subjective judgments obtained from questionnaires or rating scales; they do not include laboratory measurements of the functioning of body systems or processes. We give full descriptions, including copies of the instruments, of over 80 measurement methods; we summarize the reliability and validity of each and provide the information necessary to allow readers to select the most appropriate measurement for their purposes and then to apply and score the method chosen. As an introduction to health measurement methods, this book should be of value to clinicians who wish to select a measure to record the progress of their patients. It should also serve as a reference work for social scientists, for epidemiologists and other health care researchers, for health planners and evaluators: in short, for all who need to measure health status in research studies.

Ottawa, Canada   I. McD.
March 1995   C. N.

REFERENCES

(1) Wilkin D, Hallam L, Doggett MA. Measures of need and outcome for primary health care. Oxford: Oxford University Press, 1992.
(2) Bowling A. Measuring health: a review of quality of life measurement scales. Milton Keynes: Open University Press, 1991.
(3) Spilker B, ed. Quality of life assessment in clinical trials. New York: Raven Press, 1990.

Acknowledgments

The first edition of this book was written while the principal author was supported by a Career Health Scientist Award from the Ministry of Health in Ontario, Canada. The second edition was prepared with support from the National Center for Health Services Research from the United States Department of Health and Human Services (Grant No. HS 06206). We gratefully acknowledge the support of University of Ottawa.

I. McD.
C. N.

Contents

5. PSYCHOLOGICAL WELL-BEING, 177

6. DEPRESSION, 238

List of Exhibits

Measuring Health

1
Introduction

BACKGROUND

The first edition of this book was written because clinicians and researchers often seemed unaware of the wide variety of measurement techniques available for use in health services research. This was unfortunate, for research funds are wasted when studies do not use the best available techniques, and the accumulation of scientific evidence is delayed if comparable measurement methods are not used in different studies. In addition to serving as a guide to available measures, the book also included several criticisms of the current state of development of health measurement in general.

In the years since the first edition was published, progress has been made in consolidating the field of health measurement. It remains true that the quality of health measurements is somewhat uneven, but several promising signs are visible. In place of the enthusiastic proliferation of hastily constructed measures that typified the 1970s, attention is being paid to consolidating information on a narrower range of quality methods. These methods are being used more consistently in growing numbers of studies, providing genuinely compara-

tive information. It may be time to remove our comment in the first edition that bemoaned the tendency to reinvent Activities of Daily Living scales. Furthermore, methodological studies that test the accuracy of measurements now use more sophisticated approaches, and obvious statistical errors are becoming rare. Finally, several books are available to help the user locate the most suitable measurement scale (1–10). That some of these are modeled closely on our own first edition we take as sincere flattery.

In the chapters that follow we review a selection of the leading health measurement methods. Our descriptions are intended to be sufficiently detailed to permit readers to choose, and then apply, the most suitable instrument. Each chapter includes a critical comparison between the methods examined, and to ensure the accuracy of our descriptions we have contacted the original authors of most of the methods described.

SELECTION OF INDICES FOR REVIEW

We have been selective in the scales we present, in part because there are too many indices to review in a single book, and also because there is little point in reviewing an indifferent method when a clearly superior one is available. This is especially true in areas such as the Activities of Daily Living indices and scales of social functioning. We narrowed our selection in several ways. First, we omitted whole areas of measurement from consideration such as indices of child health, which have been well summarized by Johnson (11). We have also omitted indices designed to assess very specific forms of impairment (scales of hand function, severity indices for particular diseases, etc.). Psychological measurements with a clinical focus were excluded in part because they have already been described (4, 12), but also because they are so numerous that they would fill a volume of their own. We have, however, compromised in the area of psychological health indicators by including depression scales, screening tests for cognitive impairment, and more general indices of "psychological well-being" because these are frequently used in health surveys and as outcome measures in clinical trials. We considered only published methods; unpublished scales have been reviewed elsewhere—for example, by Ward and Lindeman (13) and by Bolton (14). We have also excluded measurements that are in the preliminary stages of development, since any description would rapidly become outdated. We do not include complete survey questionnaires, nor do we cover questions on risk factors such as smoking or alcohol consumption. The scales that we do discuss all measure a specific aspect of health; they may be incorporated within a broader survey questionnaire. They cover the following topics: physical disability and handicap, psychological well-being, social health, depression, mental status, pain, quality of life, and general health measurements.

Within each of these fields we have been highly selective, attempting to review the best methods available. Our definition of "best" relied principally on the evidence for the validity and reliability of each measurement. We therefore considered only

measurements for which published information is available, including evidence of reliability and validity. The very few exceptions to this are scales that hold particular conceptual or methodological interest in the development of the field. Naturally, a different selection could have been made, but the areas of disagreement would apply mainly to the less important methods, and in each chapter there are instruments that are clearly superior and whose inclusion cannot reasonably be disputed.

STRUCTURE OF THE BOOK

As we are writing for a broad audience, including those not familiar with the methodological bases for health measurement, Chapter 2 provides a brief historical review of the origins and development of the field, giving an outline of the theoretical and technical foundations of health measurement methods. This discussion introduces the central themes of validity and reliability and explains the various approaches to assessing the quality of a measurement. The explanations are sufficient to permit the reader to understand our descriptions of the methods, but the chapter is not intended to serve as a text on how to develop a measurement scale.

Chapters 3 through 9 are the heart of the book, presenting detailed reviews of the instruments. Each chapter opens with a brief, historical overview of the measurement techniques in that field. This is intended to illustrate the common themes that link the measurement methods, for these are seldom developed in isolation from each other. The overview is followed by a table that gives a summary comparison of the measures reviewed. These tables are intended to assist the reader in selecting the most suitable scale for a particular application. The actual reviews of the measurements are loosely ordered from the simpler to the more complex within each chapter. This is intended to reflect the general evolution of the methods and corresponds roughly to a chronological ordering;

it is also intended to aid the reader in selecting a method of appropriate length and complexity. The accuracy and completeness of our reviews has been ensured in almost every case by having each checked by the person who originally developed the method or by an acknowledged expert.

Our experience in writing these reviews made it clear that many measurement methods do not come equipped with information on basic matters: precisely for whom is the measurement intended? How valid is it? Exactly how is the measurement to be administered? For the leading instruments, however (see, for example, Goldberg's General Health Questionnaire or the Short-Form-36 Health Survey), detailed information is available on all such points; in this respect the contrast between the more adequate and the less adequate scales is clear. Some guidelines that could be followed by those who develop and publish descriptions of health measurement methods are given in Chapter 10, the concluding chapter.

STYLE AND CONTENT OF THE REVIEWS

Our reviews do more than merely reproduce existing descriptions of the various methods, for it is remarkable how often there are errors in the published descriptions. Where we have found inconsistencies, such as between different versions of a scale, we have sought the guidance of the original author concerning the correct version to use. We have frequently clarified obscure statements in the original publications through discussion with their authors. We have tried to avoid technical terms and jargon, but because some technical terms have to be used, we have defined these in the Glossary of Technical Terms at the end of the book. The reviews provide a factually accurate review of each method, and statements of our own opinions are restricted to the Commentary section of each review. In the same vein, we have

avoided repeating the interpretations of authors concerning the validity of their scales; virtually all authors claim their method to be superior to the average, so it seems simplest to let the statistics speak for themselves. It is also perennially true that the original authors report better reliability and validity results than do subsequent users.

FORMAT FOR THE REVIEWS

A standard format is followed in reviewing each measurement. It should be stressed, again, that while we have written the reviews, each was checked for accuracy and completeness by the person who originally developed the method, or by an acknowledged expert, to ensure that we are providing an authoritative description of each measurement. The following information is given for each measurement.

Title

The title of each method is that given by the original author of the instrument.

Author

The attribution of each method to an author is primarily for convenience; we recognize that most methods are developed by team effort. In certain cases additional authors are cited where they have had a continuing involvement in the development of the method.

Year

This is the year the method was first published, followed by that of any major revisions.

Purpose

The purpose of the measurement is summarized in our own words and based as far as possible on words used by the original author. We have indicated the types of person the method is intended for (specifying age, diagnostic group) where this was stated. All too frequently the precise purpose of a measure is not made clear by its author; occasionally it is restated differently in different publications and we have tried to resolve such inconsistencies.

Conceptual Basis

Where specified by the original author, this indicates what theoretical approach was taken to measuring the topics described in the Purpose section.

Description

The description indicates the origins and development of the instrument and shows the questionnaire or rating scale where space permits. Details of administration and scoring are given. Where there are several versions of the instrument, we have sought the advice of the author of the method, and in general present the most recent version.

Exhibits

Within the Description section, we reproduce a copy of the questionnaire or rating scale. Occasionally, where space does not permit us to show an entire instrument, we include one or two sections of it and indicate where the complete version may be obtained.

Reliability and Validity

For most instruments we have summarized all of the information available when our reviews were being prepared. For a few scales (notably the psychological well-being and the depression scales) there is such extensive data on validity that we have been selective. The majority of our information was taken from published sources, at times supplemented or corrected following correspondence with the original author.

Alternative Forms

Different versions exist for many of the measurements. Where revised versions have come to be widely accepted and used, we include these in the Description section of the method. The Alternative Forms section covers other variants and translations. Again we have been selective: for some

methods there has been a proliferation of infrequently used, minor variants that should not be encouraged. These we ignore.

Reference Standards

Where available, these provide a valuable source of information against which the results of the user's study may be compared.

Commentary

Our descriptions of each measurement are as objective as possible; our own comments have been restricted to the Commentary section. Here we summarize the strengths and weaknesses of the method and outline how it compares to others with a similar focus. In conjunction with the summary tables at the beginning of each chapter, this is intended to help the reader choose between alternative measurements and to suggest where further developmental work may be carried out.

Address

For some scales, we provide the address of a contact person from whom further information may be obtained. We have included an address where permission is required to use a scale, where the user's manual is not published, and where we have not reproduced a copy of the instrument. We do not include an address where the measurement is well established and adequately described in the literature, or where the original author is no longer active in the field.

References

Rather than list all available references to each method, we cite those that provide useful information on the instrument or on its validity or reliability. We have not cited studies that merely used the method but did not report on its quality. If needed, such references can be identified through the *Science Citation Index*.

Summary Tables

The summary table at the end of the introduction to each chapter compares the salient characteristics of the measurements reviewed in that chapter. This serves as a "consumer's guide" to the various methods and gives the following information:

1. The numerical characteristics of the scale: nominal, ordinal, interval, or ratio.
2. The length of the test, as indicated by the number of items it contains.
3. The applications of the method: clinical, research, survey, or as a screening test.
4. The method of administering the scale: self-administered, by an interviewer or trained staff member, or requiring an expert rater (e.g., physician, physiotherapist, or psychologist). Where the length of time needed to administer the scale was given, this is indicated.
5. We have made a rating that indicates how widely the method has been used because, other things being equal, it will be advantageous to select a commonly used measurement technique. The rating refers to the number of separate studies in which the method has been used rather than to the number of publications that describe the method, because one study may give rise to a large number of reports. Three categories indicate how widely the scale has been used: a few (one to four) published studies have used the method, several (five to eight) studies by different groups, or many studies (nine or more different studies).
6. Four ratings summarize evidence of reliability and validity. The first and third summarize the *thoroughness* of reliability and validity testing:

$$0 = \text{no reported evidence of reliability or validity}$$
$$+ = \text{very basic information only}$$
$$+ + = \text{several types of test, or several studies have reported reliability/validity}$$
$$+ + + = \text{all major forms of reliability/validity testing reported.}$$

Because the thoroughness of testing may be independent of the results obtained,

two other ratings summarize the *results* of the reliability and validity testing:

$$0 = \text{no numerical results reported}$$
$$? = \text{results uninterpretable}$$
$$+ = \text{weak reliability/validity}$$
$$+ + = \text{adequate reliability/validity}$$
$$+ + + = \text{excellent reliability/validity.}$$

As the field of health measurement develops over time, more and more scales undergo extensive validity and reliability testing. Compared to our first edition, therefore, the ratings for a few scales have been reduced to reflect their status relative to the current standards of testing.

The conclusion to each chapter gives a brief summary of the current state of the art in that area of measurement and suggests directions for further developmental work. The concluding section also mentions other measurements we consider to have merit but which we did not include as formal reviews because of lack of space or insufficient evidence concerning their quality.

EVALUATING A HEALTH MEASUREMENT: THE USER'S PERSPECTIVE

Finally, we recognize that everyone would like a guide book to make recommendations about the "best buy." This, of course, is a difficult judgment to make without knowing about the study in which the reader intends to use the method. We give several indications of the relative merits of the scales, but all of the methods we review have different strengths, so we can only make suggestions to the reader as to how to use the information in this book to choose an appropriate measurement.

The user must decide exactly what is required of the measurement. For example, will it be used to evaluate a program of care or to study individual patients? What type of person will be assessed (what diagnosis, age group, level of disability)? What time frame must the assessment cover: acute or long-term conditions? How broadranging an assessment must be made, and how detailed does the information need to be? For example, would a single rating of pain level suffice, or is a more extensive description of the type as well as the intensity of the pain needed? Bear in mind that this may require 15 minutes of the patient's time and that a person in pain will be unenthusiastic about answering a lengthy questionnaire. The user must decide, in short, on the appropriate balance to strike between the detail and accuracy required and the effort of collecting it. This information can be gleaned from the "consumer's guide" tables at the beginning of each chapter.

Turning to how the user evaluates the published information on a measurement method, the following characteristics of a method should be considered:

1. Is the purpose of the method fully explained and is it appropriate for the intended use? The method should have been tested on the types of person to whom it will be applied.
2. Is the method broad enough for the application, neither asking too many nor too few questions? Is it capable of identifying levels of positive health where this is relevant?
3. What is the conceptual approach to the measurement topic? For example, which theory of pain does it reflect, and is this approach consonant with the orientation of the study? Is the theory well established (e.g., Maslow's hierarchy of needs) or is it an idiosyncratic notion that may not correspond to a broader body of knowledge?
4. How feasible is the method to administer and how long does this take? Can it be self-administered? Is professional expertise required to apply or interpret the instrument? Does it use readily available data (e.g., information already contained in medical records) and will it be readily acceptable to respondents? What response rates have been achieved using the method? Is the questionnaire readily available and is there a cost in-

volved? Above all, is there a clear instruction manual that specifies how the questions should be asked?
5. Is it clear how the method is scored? Is the numerical quality of the scores suited to the type of statistical analyses planned? If the method uses an overall score, how is this to be interpreted?
6. What degree of change can be detected by the method, and is this adequate for the purpose? Does the method detect qualitative changes only, or does it provide quantitative data? Might it produce a false-negative result due to insensitivity to change (e.g., in a study comparing two types of therapy)? Is it suitable as a screening test only, or can it provide sufficiently detailed information to indicate diagnoses?
7. How strong is the available evidence for reliability and validity? How many different forms of quality testing have been carried out? How many other indices has it been compared with? How many different users have tested the method, and did they obtain similar results? How do these compare to the quality of other scales?

A difficulty is commonly encountered in comparing two indices—one with excellent validity results in one or two studies and another that is more widely tested but shows somewhat less adequate validity. We advise the reader to pay attention to the size of the validation studies: frequently, apparently excellent results obtained from initial, small samples are not repeated in larger studies. Ultimately the selection of a measurement contains an element of art and perhaps even luck; it is often prudent to apply more than one measurement. This has the advantage of reinforcing the conclusions of the study when the results from ostensibly similar methods are in agreement, and it also serves to increase our general understanding of the comparability of the measurements.

The chapter that follows describes the methodological bases for health measurements; it provides sufficient information to permit readers to interpret the reviews in Chapters 3 to 9 and to answer the questions raised here. The chapter is intended primarily as an introduction for those who do not have a grounding in the theory of measurement; those who do may prefer to proceed to Chapter 3.

REFERENCES

(1) Mitchell JV. Mental measurements yearbook. Lincoln, Nebraska: Buros Institute of Mental Measurements, 1985.

(2) Keyser DJ, Sweetland RC. Test critiques. Kansas City, Missouri: Test Corporation of America, 1984.

(3) Corcoran K, Fischer J. Measures for clinical practice: a sourcebook. New York: Free Press, 1987.

(4) Sweetland RC, Keyser DJ. Tests: a comprehensive reference for assessments in psychology, education and business. Kansas City, Missouri: Test Corporation of America, 1983.

(5) Bellamy N. Musculoskeletal clinical metrology. Dordrecht, Holland: Kluwer Academic Publishers, 1993.

(6) Spilker B, ed. Quality of life assessment in clinical trials. New York: Raven Press, 1990.

(7) Wilkin D, Hallam L, Doggett MA. Measures of need and outcome for primary health care. Oxford: Oxford University Press, 1992.

(8) Bowling A. Measuring health: a review of quality of life measurement scales. Milton Keynes, England: Open University Press, 1991.

(9) Lipkin M, ed. Functional status measurement in primary care. New York: Springer-Verlag, 1990.

(10) Bowling A. Measuring disease: a review of disease-specific quality of life measurement scales. Buckingham, England: Open University Press, 1995.

(11) Johnson OG. Tests and measurements in child development: handbook II. San Francisco: Jossey-Bass, 1976.

(12) Mittler P, ed. The psychological assessment of mental and physical handicaps. London: Tavistock, 1974.

(13) Ward MJ, Lindeman CA. Instruments for measuring nursing practice and other health care variables. Vol. 2. Washington, DC: Department of Health, Education and Welfare (DHEW Publication No. HRA 78-54), 1978.

(14) Bolton B. Measurement in rehabilitation. In: Pan EL, Newman SS, Backer TE, Vash CL, eds. Annual review of rehabilitation. Vol. 4. New York: Springer, 1985:115–144.

2

The Theoretical and Technical Foundations
of Health Measurement

For over a hundred years, Western nations have collected statistical data characterizing social conditions. The data, describing birth and death rates, education, crime, housing, employment, and economic output, reflect issues of public concern and have often become the focal point for movements of social reform. Measurements of health have always formed a central component in such public accounting; they are used to indicate the major health problems confronting society, to contribute to the process of setting policy goals, and to monitor the effectiveness of medical and health care. Rosser offers some very early examples of such accounting, drawn from ancient Egyptian and Greek times (1, 2).

Social indicators of this kind are based on aggregated data expressed as regional or national rates; they are intended to give a picture of the health of populations rather than of individual people. In addition, many indicators of the health of individuals have been developed; these are principally used in analyzing differences in health, to diagnose illness, to predict the need for care, and to evaluate the outcomes of treatment (3). Both population and individual health indices are necessary and both will continue to be developed, but this book deals only with indicators at the individual level. Population health statistics such as rates of morbidity and mortality, or the mathematical population health indexes developed by Chen, by Chiang, and by others, are not considered here; a brief review of them is given by Rosser (4).

There will probably always be a debate over how best to measure health, and one reason for the debate lies in the complexity and abstract nature of health itself. Furthermore, as Rosser noted, there is a historical tension in approaches to health between those who prefer to keep the concept somewhat imprecise, so that it can be reformulated to reflect changing social circumstances, and others who define it in operational terms, which often means losing subtle shades of meaning (5). Like attitudes or motivation, health cannot be measured directly, as can length or weight; instead the process of its measurement is indirect and requires several steps. The first, perhaps, is classification: symptoms are recorded, disabilities are listed, or the type of pain is described, thus forming variables. There is no single variable that describes health; instead, its measurement relies on assembling a number of variables as *indicators* of health, each of which represents an element of the overall concept. Measurement then implies the application of a standard scale to each variable, giving numerical scores which then may be combined into an overall score. Reflecting this indirect approach, an often-quoted definition of measurement is "the assignment of numbers to objects or events to represent quantities of attributes, according to rules" (6). The "objects or events" that may be used to indicate a person's health are of many types, ranging from a tumor analyzed in a laboratory to the movement of a limb observed by a physiotherapist, from estimates of working capacity to expressions of personal feelings. Of particular interest to us is the growing range of indicators that have been used to measure health, and this trend will be reviewed here. Following that, we will review the methods that may be used to assign numbers to indicators of health.

THE EVOLUTION OF HEALTH INDICATORS

The earliest population health indices used readily available, numerical indicators such as mortality rates. Mortality is unambiguous and since early times death has been recorded by law, so the data are generally complete. But as societies evolve, health problems alter in salience and new health indicators must be chosen to reflect changing health issues. In part this is because the indicators focus attention on the problem they record, and interventions are developed to resolve the issue. As an example, the infant mortality rate (IMR) is often used as an indicator of health levels in preindustrial societies, where high rates are an important concern, and where reductions can be relatively easily achieved. As infant mortality declines, however, a law of diminishing returns begins to apply, and further reductions require increasingly large expenditures of resources. As the numerator becomes smaller, it also becomes less representative as an indicator of the health of the broader population. In effect,

the sensitivity of the IMR to the success of interventions explains both its value as an indicator of progress, and also its eventual demise. The resolution of one type of health problem reveals a new layer of concerns, a process that Morris has called the onion principle (7). For example, as the IMR declines, growing numbers of those who survive exhibit health problems associated with low birth weight or prematurity, problems rarely encountered with high infant mortality. In a similar way, increased life expectancy in industrial countries raises the prevalence of disability in the population (8, 9). In each case, the resolution of one health problem casts new issues into prominence and reduces the usefulness of the prevailing health indicator, necessitating its replacement by others. Such changes may also increase pressure to modify the prevailing definition of health.

Indicators are deliberately chosen to reflect problems of social concern and ones for which improvement is sought. Just as language molds the way we think, our health measurements influence (and are influenced by) the way we define and think about health. Social reforms are based on the information that is available to us, so the selection and publication of indicators of health both reflect and guide social and political goals. Hence the very choice of indicators tends to affect the health of the population; publication of an indicator focuses attention on that problem, such as infant mortality, and the resulting interventions (if successful) will tend to reduce the prevalence of the problem, in turn reducing the value of the indicator as a marker of current health problems. The identification of new concerns tends to raise a demand for new indices of health to monitor progress toward the new goals, and so the cycle begins again (10). Health indicators are in a continuous state of evolution.

The rising expectations of the past 150 years have led to a shift away from viewing health in terms of survival, through a phase of defining it in terms of freedom from disease, onward to an emphasis on the individual's ability to perform daily activities, and more recently to an emphasis on positive themes of happiness, social and emotional well-being, and quality of life. Only where problems of high premature mortality are no longer a pressing social concern does it become relevant to think of health in the World Health Organization's (WHO) terms of "physical, mental, and social well-being, and not merely the absence of disease and infirmity" (11, p459). But here, again, measurements interact with progress. When it was introduced in the 1950s, the WHO definition of health was criticized as unmeasurable, but the subsequent development of techniques to measure the concepts it includes, such as "well-being," contributed to the current wide acceptance of the definition. Goldsmith reviewed a number of definitions of health and has discussed the implications of these for measuring health (12, 13).

This book is concerned with the adequacy of health measures: do the methods successfully reflect an explicit and accepted definition of health? This is the theme of validity, the assessment of what a measurement measures, and hence of how it can be interpreted. A valid health index provides information about health status, not about some other variable, such as personality (3). There has long been concern over the interpretation of many of the statistical indicators, and this concern stimulated the development of individual health measures. For example, consultation rates with physicians can only be interpreted as indicators of health if we can determine how the numbers of services provided are related to health status. Do more consultations imply better health in a population, or that there is more illness that needs treatment? Consultation rates may form more valid indicators of health expenditures than of health. Similar problems arise in interpreting indicators such as rates of bed days or work-loss days: these may reflect a blend of health and the provision of care, for improved access to care may result in activity restrictions ordered by physicians. Without

the care there might have been less activity restriction but a greater risk of long-term damage to the individual's health (14). Studies have, indeed, shown increases in disability days as the availability of medical services grows (15). One way out of the dilemmas in interpreting population indicators is to ask questions of individuals, providing a more direct reflection of health, rather than of the provision of care. This book is concerned with indicators and measures of individual health, which may be of many kinds.

TYPES OF HEALTH MEASUREMENTS

Classifications of health measurements are of several types. *Functional classifications* focus on the purpose or application of the method; *descriptive classifications* focus on their scope; *methodological classifications* consider technical aspects, such as the methods used to record information.

An example of a functional classification is Bombardier and Tugwell's distinction between three purposes for measuring health: diagnostic, prognostic, and evaluative (16). Diagnostic indices include measurements of blood pressure or sedimentation rates and are judged for their correspondence with a clinical diagnosis. Prognostic measures include screening tests, scales such as the Apgar score (17), and measures such as those that predict the likelihood that a patient will be able to live independently in the community following rehabilitation. Kirshner and Guyatt also gave a functional classification. Discriminative indices are designed to classify people when no external criterion exists, as with IQ tests. Predictive indices classify people according to some criterion, which may exist now (hence equivalent to Bombardier's diagnostic measures) or in the future (equivalent to the prognostic measures). Finally, evaluative indices measure change over time (18). A simpler functional classification was proposed by Kind and Carr-Hill (19). Measurements monitor either health status or change in health status, and they may do this for individuals or for groups. Measuring the health status of individuals is the domain of the clinical interview; measuring change in the individual is the purpose of a clinical evaluation. Measuring health status in a group is the aim of a survey instrument, while measuring group change is the domain of a macro health index (19, Table 1).

Health measurements may also be classified descriptively according to their scope or the range of topics they cover. The spectrum of measures ranges from those that focus on a particular organ system (vision, hearing), to methods concerned with a diagnosis (anxiety or depression scales), to those that measure broader syndromes (emotional well-being), to measurements of overall health, and, broadest of all, to measures of overall quality of life. The diagnostic instruments described by Bombardier tend to lie at the narrow end of this spectrum; evaluative measures may be drawn from any point on the continuum. Another commonly drawn distinction is that between broad-spectrum, generic health measures and specific instruments. The latter are often specific to a disease (such as a quality of life scale for cancer), but can also be specific to a particular type of person (women's health measures, patient satisfaction scales) or to an age group (child health indicators). Specific instruments are generally designed for clinical application and to be sensitive to change following treatment. Generic instruments are commonly developed for descriptive epidemiological or social science research applications. They permit comparisons across disease categories and are used in evaluating types of care or patient management. Elinson termed these broad-spectrum methods "sociomedical" indicators of health (20). By assessing the whole person in his environment, these complement traditional laboratory measurements that focus on body systems or functions.

There are many methodological classifications of health measurements. There is the distinction, for example, used in the subtitle of this book, contrasting rating scales and questionnaires; there is the distinction between health indices (or indexes) and health profiles. Cutting across these categories, there is the more complex distinction between subjective and objective measures. In essence, the contrast between rating scales and questionnaires lies in the flexibility of the measurement process. In a rating scale an expert, normally a clinician, assesses defined aspects of health, but the precise questions can vary from rater to rater and from subject to subject. An example is the Hamilton Rating Scale for Depression: Hamilton gave only general guides to the types of questions to ask. By contrast, in self-completed questionnaires and in interview schedules the questions are preset, and we carefully train interviewers not to alter the wording in any way. The debates over which approach is better generate more heat than light; they also reveal deeper contrasts in how we approach the measurement of subjective phenomena. Briefly, the argument in support of structured questionnaires holds that standardization is essential to ensure that assessments can be compared across individuals; this may be presented as a cornerstone of the scientific method and reflects the nomothetic philosophy of measurement. This assumes that a standard set of measurement dimensions or scales is relevant to every person being measured and that scoring procedures should remain constant. Thus, for example, in measuring social support, this philosophy would not accept the idea that social isolation might be perfectly acceptable, even healthy, for certain people, although undesirable for many. In reaction to this, the idiographic approach is more flexible and allows differences in measurement approach from person to person. It holds, for example, that it is naive to believe that wording a question precisely the same way for every respondent provides standardized information: we cannot assume that the same phrase will be interpreted identically by people of different cultural backgrounds. What is important is to ensure that *equivalent* stimuli are given to each person, and this is the forte of the skilled clinician who can control for differences in use of language by different subjects. Not only may symptoms of depression vary from person to person, but the significance of an identical symptom may vary from one patient to another, so the same sympton should not necessarily receive the same score. This type of approach has, of course, long been used clinically in psychiatry; more formal approaches to developing equivalent measurement approaches for different subjects include the repertory grid technique. Briefly, this classifies people's thoughts on two dimensions: the elements or topics thought about; and constructs, the qualities used to define and think about elements. An interview (for example, rating a person's subjective quality of life) would identify the constructs a person uses in thinking about quality of life and then rate each of these in the person's situation. This permits a more fully subjective assessment of quality of life than is possible using a structured questionnaire. Methods of this type are just beginning to be used in quality of life measurement—for example, in the Smith-Kline Beecham Quality of Life Scale (21) and in the work of Thunedborg et al. (22).

The second methodological classification refers to two contrasting approaches to summarizing the data collected by generic instruments: as a single score (a "health index") or as a profile. Supporters of the profile approach argue that health or quality of life is inherently multidimensional and scores on the different dimensions should be presented separately. If replies to several, contrasting themes are added together, there are so many ways a respondent can attain an intermediate score that such scores do not provide interpretable information. This reflects the philosophy of the Rasch measurement model, which holds that items to be combined should cover one dimension only, and so profile measures are often used by clinicians. Proponents of the index approach agree that mixing apples and oranges may indeed be

hard but argue that making payoffs between dimensions is one of the necessary challenges of making real-life decisions. A single score is often needed to answer questions concerning which of two treatments is better. Thus, index scores are commonly used in economic analyses and in policy decision-making.

The contrast between objective and subjective measures reflects the contrast between methods based on laboratory or diagnostic tests and methods in which a person (a clinician, patient, or family member) makes a judgment that forms the indicator of health. Ratings based on judgments of this type are generally termed "subjective" measurements, and we use the term in this sense here. By contrast, objective measurements involve no judgment in the collection of information (although judgment may be required in its interpretation). This distinction is not simple, however. Mortality statistics are commonly considered "objective," although judgment may be required in coding the cause of death. Similarly, observing behaviors only constitutes an objective measure if the observations are recorded without subjective interpretation. Hence climbing stairs may be considered an objective indicator of disability if it is observed and subjective if it is reported by the person. This distinction reflects the difference between performance (what a person does do) and capacity (what they can do), for observations tend to record performance, while assessments of capacity tend to be subjective. Note that the distinction between "subjective" and "objective" measurements does not refer to *who* makes the rating: objectivity is not bestowed on a measurement merely because it is made by an expert (23). For reasons of simplicity and cost, most health measures rely on subjective verbal report rather than observation, although in the area of gerontology some researchers emphasize the benefits of assessments based on observation of behaviors (24). This has led to a number of recent observational tests of performance (25, 26).

Subjective health measurements hold

several advantages. They extend the information obtainable from morbidity statistics or physical measures by describing the quality rather than merely the quantity of function. They give insights into matters of human concern such as pain, suffering, or depression that could not be inferred solely from physical measurements or laboratory tests. They give information about individuals whether they seek care or not; they can reflect the positive aspects of good health; and they do not require invasive procedures or expensive laboratory analyses. They may also offer a systematic way to record and present "the small, frantic voice of the patient" (20). Subjective measurements are, of course, little different from the data collected for centuries by physicians when taking a medical history. The important difference lies in the standardization of these approaches and the addition of numerical scoring systems.

Despite these potential advantages of subjective indicators, several problems delayed their acceptance. Compared to the inherent accuracy of mortality rates as a source of data, asking questions of a patient seemed to be abundantly susceptible to bias. There was also the issue of completeness: population health indicators are collected routinely from the whole population rather than from a selection of individuals. Applying individual health measurements to whole populations is prohibitively expensive, although questions on health were asked in the Irish census as far back as 1851 (27).

Gradually, however, indices of personal health that relied on subjective judgments came to be accepted. The reasons for this included several methodological advances in survey sampling and data analysis made at the time of World War II. The war brought with it the need to assess the physical and mental fitness of large numbers of recruits for military service, and indicators of the health of individuals applicable on a large scale were accordingly developed and standardized. Wartime screening tests of physical capacity later influenced the design of postwar questionnaires (27, 28), while

the psychological assessment techniques developed by Lazarsfeld, Guttman, Suchman, and others during the war formed the basis for the first generation of psychological well-being measurements in the postwar years (see Chapter 5).

A major contribution of this wartime work concerned the application of numerical scaling techniques to health indices. Because subjective reports of health are not inherently quantitative, some form of rating method was required to translate statements such as "I feel severe pain" into a form suitable for statistical analysis. The scaling techniques originally developed by social psychologists to scale attitudes soon found application in health indices. The use of these (and later of more sophisticated) rating methods permitted subjective health measurements to rival the quantitative strengths of the traditional indicators. After the war, survey sampling techniques were refined by political scientists concerned with predicting voting behavior. This provided the technical basis for using individual measurements to provide data representative of the larger population. Coming somewhat later, technical advances in data processing had a profound effect on the range of statistical analyses that could be applied to data. Computers greatly simplified the application of principal components or factor analysis in refining questionnaires; they also simplified the analysis and presentation of the voluminous information collected in health questionnaires.

THEORETICAL BASES FOR MEASUREMENT: PSYCHOPHYSICS AND PSYCHOMETRICS

Before we review the procedures for evaluating the accuracy of health measurements, a more fundamental question needs to be addressed: what evidence is there that subjective judgments form a sound basis for measuring health? Set against the measurement tradition of the exact sciences, it is by no means self-evident that such "soft" data can be considered anything more than a crude approximation to measurement. Indeed, many health measurements *are* exceedingly crude and merely affix numbers to qualitative subjective judgments. However, this need not be so, as will be seen from some of the more sophisticated instruments reviewed in this book. To introduce the scientific basis for health measurement, we will begin with a brief introduction to psychophysics and psychometrics, describing the procedures used to assign numerical scores to subjective judgments. The following sections presume a familiarity with some basic statistical terms that are, however, defined in the Glossary of Technical Terms (page 499).

The arguments for considering subjective judgments as a valid approach to measurement derive ultimately from the field of psychophysics. Psychophysical principles were later incorporated into psychometrics, from which most of the techniques used to develop subjective measurements of health were derived. Psychophysics is concerned with the way in which people perceive and make judgments about physical phenomena such as the length of a line, the loudness of a sound, or the intensity of a pain: psychophysics investigates the performance of the human being as a measuring instrument.

The early search for a mathematical relationship between the intensity of a stimulus and its perception was illustrated by the work of Gustav Fechner, whose major text was published in 1860. Subjective judgments of any stimulus, Fechner discovered, are not simple reflections of the event. For example, it is easy for us to feel the 4-ounce difference between a 1- and a 5-ounce weight, but distinguishing a 40-pound weight from one 4 ounces heavier is much less certain. To discern the mathematical form of the link between a physical stimulus and our perception of it, Fechner proposed a method of scaling sensations based on "just-noticeable differences"; he recorded the objective magnitude of just-noticeable differences at different levels of the stimulus. A difference of 1 ounce between two weights may be noticeable when the weights are small, but with larger weights the just-noticeable difference increases. In this case our perceptions are more attuned to detecting small differences at lower levels of a stimulus than they are at higher levels. Fechner concluded that a geometric increase in the stimulus as received by the senses produces an arithmetic increase in conscious sensation. This relationship is conveniently expressed as a natural logarithm; details of the derivation of Fechner's law are given by Baird and Noma (29).

Fechner's approach generally agreed with empirical data; it was intuitively appealing; and it also incorporated Weber's earlier law of 1846, which proposed that the magnitude of just-noticeable differences was proportional to the absolute level of the stimulus. Fechner's law became accepted, and psychophysics turned its attention to other issues for more than 70 years. During this time, however, evidence accumulated from various sources that the logarithmic relationship did not fit all types of stimuli. Experimental investigations of how people judge the loudness of sounds, the intensity of an electric shock, or the saltiness of food, for example, showed that the logarithmic relationship between stimulus and response did not always apply, but it proved hard to find a more adequate mathematical formulation.

In 1962 Stevens wrote:

If you shine a faint light in your eye, you have a sensation of brightness—a weak sensation, to be sure. If you turn on a stronger light, the sensation becomes greater. Clearly, then, there is a relation between perceived brightness and the amount of light you put in the eye. . . . But how, precisely, does the output of the system (sensation) vary with the input (stimulus)? Suppose you double the stimulus, does it then look twice as bright?

The answer to this question happens to be no. It takes about nine times as much light to double the apparent brightness, but this specific question, interesting as it may be, is only one instance of a wider problem: what are the input-output characteristics of sensory systems in general? Is there a single, simple, pervasive psychophysical law? (30, p29).

Stevens's answer to this question was that psychophysics had apparently discovered such a law, and it was well substantiated by empirical evidence. The logarithmic approach came to be replaced by the more generally applicable power law he proposed (30). Like Fechner's law, the power law recognized that humans can make consistent, numerically accurate estimates of sensory stimuli. It agreed, also, that the relationship between stimulus and subjective response was not linear, but it differed from Fechner's law in stating that the exact form of the relationship varied from one sensation to another. This was described by an equation with a different power-function exponent for each type of stimulus, of the following general form:

$$R = k \times S^b,$$

where R is the response, k is a constant, S the level of the stimulus, and b is an exponent that typically falls in the range 0.3 to 1.7 (29, p83; 31, p25). When the exponent b is unity, the relationship between stimulus and response is linear, as proposed by Weber's law. Conveniently, the exponent for judging short lengths is unity, so that a line of 2 inches is judged to be twice as long as one of 1 inch. This result justifies the interpretation of the visual analogue response scales used in several health indices. The varying exponents for other judgments imply that subjective perceptions of different types of stimulus grow at different, although characteristic, rates. The size of the exponent is an indicator of psychological sensitivity to the stimulus. The exponent for force of handgrip is 1.7, while that for sound pressure is 0.67. The exponent of 0.67 for loudness means that a doubling of decibels will typically be judged as only two-thirds louder. Sensitivity to electrical stimulation is much greater, with an exponent of 3.5; this has implications for describing responses to pain.

Considerable attention has been paid to validating the power law, and some of the most convincing evidence comes from a complex-sounding technique called cross-modality matching. In the research to establish the power law and to identify the characteristic exponents b, judgments of various stimuli were made by rating responses on numerical scales (29, p82). Knowing the response exponents, in terms of numerical judgments, for different stimuli (loudness, brightness, pressure, and so on), arithmetical manipulation of these exponents can postulate how a person would rate one stimulus by analogy to another. Thus, in theory, a certain loudness of sound should match a predictable brightness of light or pressure of handgrip—the cross-modality matching. Experimental testing of the predicted match could then be used to test the internal consistency of the power law. As it turned out, the experimental fit between observed and predicted values was remarkably close, often within only a 2% margin of error (31, pp27–31). This has important implications for health measurement: people can make numerical estimates of subjective phenomena in a remarkably consistent manner, even when the comparisons are abstract, indeed, more abstract than those involved in subjective health measurements. The validation experiments also confirmed that the exponent for line length was unity, which means that we could use different lengths of lines to represent abstract themes such as intensity of pain; this is the approach used in visual analogue scales. Finally, studies validating the power law suggested that people can make accurate judgments of stimuli on a ratio, rather than merely on an ordinal scale of measurement; that is, people can accurately judge how many times stronger one stimulus is than another. Judgments of this type are termed magnitude estimation and are used in creating ratio-scaled measurements (see page 19).

Traditionally, psychophysics studied subjective judgments of stimuli that may be objectively measured on physical scales such as decibels or millimeters of mercury. In the social or health sciences, by contrast, we often use subjective judgments because there are no objective, physical ways to measure the phenomena under consideration. There are extended discussions of the way that psychophysical methods have been adapted to measure qualities for which there is no physical scale (32–34). This is the field of psychometrics, and the work of psychologists in this area has been applied by those who develop health measurement methods.

The following sections introduce two psychometric issues in making and recording subjective estimates of health. How are numerical values assigned to statements describing levels of health, and how far are subjective judgments influenced by the personal bias of the rater, instead of giving an accurate reflection of the actual level of health?

NUMERICAL ESTIMATES OF HEALTH: SCALING METHODS

The simplest way to quantify estimates of healthiness is to ask directly for a numerical estimation: "On a 0-to-100 scale, how severe is your pain?" This magnitude estimation approach is illustrated by the visual analogue scales reviewed in Chapter 8. However, concerns are commonly expressed that patients are not familiar with using a 100-point scale to rate pain, and so adjectives are often used: mild or severe pain. Measurement requires the assignment of numerical scores to such descriptions, and this is achieved by using any of a number of scaling procedures (33, 35). The logic of doing this holds well for responses that represent severity and reasonably well for frequency (e.g., daily, weekly, or occasional headaches). The scaling procedures may also be applied to qualitative statements such as "Needs help to climb stairs," providing a type of quantified classification that is usually considered a measurement. The scaling procedures assign a numerical

weight to each answer category (e.g., needs help: often, sometimes, never) for each topic covered (e.g., climbing stairs, using public transport); combining the scores for a given pattern of responses provides a numerical indicator of the degree of disability reported. A second application of scaling methods is used in merging scores from different dimensions of a health measurement or health profile (e.g., physical, emotional, social) to form an overall score, or "health index." Different dimensions do not necessarily reflect equivalent severity of disability, and unless a scheme is used to weight the dimensions before they are combined, the numbers of ratings made in each dimension will determine the relative weight of each in the overall score.

Methods to calculate scale weights vary in their complexity, but fundamental to all scaling methods is a distinction between four ways of using numbers in measurement; these lie in a hierarchy of mathematical adequacy. The lowest level is not a measurement, but refers to a classification: *nominal or categorical scales* use numbers simply as labels for categories (such as 1 = male and 2 = female). The assignment of numbers is arbitrary, and no inferences can be drawn from the relative size of the numbers used. The only acceptable mathematical expressions are $A = B$ or $A \neq B$. For the second type, *ordinal scales,* numbers are again used as labels for response categories and their assignment is again arbitrary, except that the numbers reflect the increasing order of the characteristic being measured. The responses are ordered in terms of magnitude and a numerical code is assigned to each. "Mild," "moderate," and "severe" disability might be coded 1, 2, and 3 with the property $A < B < C$. There are many limitations to this approach, and Bradburn and Miles gave a critical review (36). Because people use adjectives in different ways we cannot assume that "mild" implies the same thing to different people, nor that "often" implies the same frequency when referring to common health problems as when referring to rare ones. Thus the actual value of the numbers and the distance between each hold no intrinsic meaning in an ordinal scale: a change from scale point 3 to point 2 is not necessarily equivalent to a change from 2 to 1. Because of this, it is not strictly appropriate to subtract the ordinal scores taken before and after treatment to compare the progress made by different patients. Nor is it appropriate to combine scores by addition: this might imply, for example, that a mild plus a moderate disability is equivalent to a severe disability. This is not to say that adding or subtracting ordinal scales cannot be done—it is frequently done. Purists may criticize (37, 38) but pragmatists argue that the errors produced are small (32, pp12–33). Although many health indices are scored by adding ordinal answer scales, this may lead to incorrect conclusions and is the main motivation for developing more accurate scale weights for answer categories. As a crude approach to this, some ordinal scales deliberately leave gaps between the numerical codes to better represent the presumed distance between categories: see the 6, 5, 3, 0 scoring in the Barthel Index (Exhibit 3.4).

Adding and subtracting scores is, however, permissible with the third type of numerical scale. An *interval scale* is one in which numbers are assigned to the response categories in such a way that a unit change in scale values represents a constant change across the range of the scale. Temperature in degrees Celsius is an example. Here $A - B = C - D$, so it is possible to interpret differences in scores, to add and subtract them, and to calculate averages. It is not, however, possible to state how many times greater one score is than another, which is the distinguishing feature of the fourth type of scale, the *ratio scale*. This may be expressed as $A \times B = C$ and $C / B = A$. The key here is a meaningful zero point, making it possible to state that one score is, for example, twice another; the measurement of pressure is an illustration.

Nonetheless, variables that satisfy the numerical requirements of an interval or ratio scale should not necessarily be considered as such. Age is often treated as an interval scale, but the changing rate of growth around puberty, for example, challenges the interpretation of age as an interval-scale indicator of development. The definition of a scale as ordinal or interval depends more on the way it will be interpreted than on its inherent numerical properties. Rasch analysis (see page 21) provides an approach to assessing whether a measurement constitutes an interval scale; an example is offered by Silverstein et al. (39).

In constructing a health measurement, scaling procedures are often used to improve the numerical characteristics of response scales, typically by converting ordinal responses to interval scales. These provide metric values that are substituted for the arbitrary 1, 2, or 3 codes described above. Most health measurements include a number of questions, each with a response scale. The questions are commonly called items, simply because not all instruments use actual questions: some use rating scales and others use statements with which the respondent agrees or disagrees. The response scale may be a yes/no dichotomy, a series of graded adjectives (mild, moderate, or severe pain, for example), or a numerical rating scale that may have as many as 100 points. Scaling procedures can be classified into (*i*) those that are stimulus centered, that estimate variation due to the items, (*ii*) those that are subject centered and record variation due to the differences between respondents, and (*iii*) approaches such as item response theory that capture both sources. The first category includes procedures such as Thurstone Equal-Appearing Intervals scaling; the response-centered approaches include techniques such as Guttman scaling; and item response approaches include methods such as Rasch analysis. Stimulus-centered scaling procedures involve samples of people who make judgments in one of two broad categories of scaling tasks: psychometric methods or econometric methods (32, pp50–66). Both approaches have been used in developing health indices and are briefly introduced here.

Psychometric Methods

The many psychometric scaling procedures may be grouped into comparative techniques and magnitude estimation methods. Among those in the former category, several of the measurements described in this book have used Thurstone's Equal-Appearing Intervals scaling method to produce what is argued to be an interval scale. There are variants of the approach, but in essence a sample of people is asked to judge the relative severity (or "utility" in the economic term) of each response category. The people making the judgments may be patients or experts or a combination of both. Items such as "Pain prevents me from sleeping," "I have aches and pains that bother me," and "I require prescription medicines to control my pain" are sorted by each judge into categories and rank ordered by severity. There are typically ten or 15 categories. For each item a score is based on the median of the category numbers into which it was placed by the group of judges; this is used as a numerical indicator of the judged severity of that response. Where disagreement between raters is high, the item may be eliminated, as this suggests ambiguity in it. This scaling approach has been used in instruments such as the Sickness Impact Profile. Similar techniques may be used to provide numerical scores for response categories: "strongly agree," "agree," "disagree," and "strongly disagree." A method called summated ratings was described by Likert for doing this, but in practice the correlation between the scaled version and arbitrarily assigned scores of 1, 2, 3, and 4 is very high (40, pp149–152).

Magnitude estimation procedures have been proposed as an improvement on category scaling tasks, which use a fixed number of categories in the scaling procedure. Psychophysical experiments show that people can make much more accurate judgments of the relative magnitude of stimuli than categorical scales permit. Magnitude estimation exploits this, asking people to judge the relative severity implied by each statement on scales without limitations on the values. This has been used, for example, in rating how much more serious one type of crime is compared to another. Proponents argue that this approach produces a ratio scale estimate of the absolute value of the stimulus. The approach has, however, been challenged on the grounds that it is not related to a specific theory of measurement and that the precise meaning of judging one stimulus as twice as desirable as another is not clear. It is not, for example, necessarily linked to a behavior such as being willing to pay twice as much. While magnitude estimation in the form of visual analogue scales is often used as a response mode in health measurements, it has seldom been used in its psychometric form as a way to score categorical responses. This may be because it appears complex, and so the simpler categorical rating methods are most commonly used, despite their technical inferiority. The appeal of the two methods is different: accuracy and theoretical sophistication versus simplicity (29). Magnitude estimation is, however, seeing increasing use in econometric scaling procedures.

Psychometric scaling methods are described in detail in many sources (29, 31, 33, 35, 40–42). They demand more effort during the development of a measurement but provide measurements at the interval level, which may be especially important in scales with few items. However they are calculated, item weights do not necessarily alter the impression gained from unweighted scores. As shown in the chapters that follow, weighted and unweighted scores have been compared for instruments such as the Physical and Mental Impairment-of-Function Evaluation, the

Multilevel Assessment Inventory, the McMaster Health Index Questionnaire, the Nottingham Health Profile, and the Health Opinion Survey, and the correlation is uniformly high: generally between 0.95 and 0.98. Item weights are most likely to exert an effect when a scale includes a small number of items that cover different topics. Where there are more than 20 questions and where these all measure a common theme, weights are unlikely to have a strong effect on the relative ranks established by the scale.

A cautionary note should be sounded about using weighted scores for health measurement instruments. Psychometric scaling techniques were originally intended for attitude measurement, under conditions in which an affirmative answer to an extreme statement would imply affirmative answers to less severe statements on the same dimension as well. The dimension score would be the total of the weights for items answered affirmatively. Items on a health measurement are factual, however, and may have more complex logical connections between them. For example, in a set of items on walking, the statement "I cannot walk at all" logically precludes answering other, less severe items on the same scale. Hence the score on that dimension will be the scale weight of the statement "I cannot walk at all," and this may be less than the sum of weights for two or three less severe items; an empirical example is given by Jenkinson (43). To overcome this, affirmative answers to such items are awarded the scores of all items that were excluded. This introduces the theme of analyzing the scale properties of *sets* of items.

Instead of scoring for a single question, some category scaling procedures analyze the properties of the scale as a whole. These are the response-centered approaches used to provide scale values for individual respondents, rather than for items. A method sometimes used in measuring functional abilities is the Guttman approach to "scalo-gram analysis" (see Glossary). This procedure identifies groups of questions which stand in a hierarchy of severity. Where questions form a Guttman scale, an affirmative reply to a question indicating severe disability will imply an affirmative reply to each question lower on the scale. This provides evidence that the items measure varying levels of a single aspect of health, such as functional disability as opposed to pain. On such a scale a person's status can be described by noting the question at which the replies switch from affirmative to negative. Indices that use Guttman scaling include Meenan's Arthritis Impact Measurement Scale and Lawton and Brody's Physical Self-Maintenance Scale. Guttman scaling is less well suited to the measurement of psychological attributes, which seldom form cumulative scales (32, p75).

Guttman scaling is only one example of several, related approaches to analyzing response patterns. A more extensive approach is item response theory (44) or latent trait analysis (45), within which a measurement model developed by Georg Rasch is now being applied to health measurements (39, 46). Item response theory is a response centered approach to scaling in which both items and subjects are scaled. The "latent trait" refers to the unobservable continuum that the test items are designed to measure. To make this concrete we will use depression as an illustration. In describing the model graphically, the level of depression (the latent trait) is laid along the horizontal axis of a graph, running from no depression at the left to severe at the right. Items that measure different severities of depression will be spaced along this continuum, with items such as "I occasionally feel sad" near the left and such as "I feel so low that I rarely eat anything" nearer the right. The threshold along the depression continuum at which an item is answered positively represents the first parameter of the latent trait model; the Rasch model is a one parameter model. The threshold is the point on the depression scale where the probability of endorsement is 0.5; the greater the threshold value, the greater the depression before a person endorses the item. The purpose of a Rasch analysis is both to identify the threshold for each item in a questionnaire and also to locate respondents on the continuum of depression measured by the items. Thus, it scales the people and the items at the same time. Ideally, a measurement instrument should contain items that are spaced evenly along the continuum being measured. Rasch's method began with a series of postulates: (i) scores on a measure depend on the ability of the person and the level of disability implied by the items. (ii) A good scale should have items that range in difficulty and whose rank order of difficulty does not vary from respondent to respondent. (iii) Good measurement requires that a person's ability be accurately reflected regardless of the scale used. (iv) Where a measurement contains several scales, such as physical, mental, and social, the Rasch model holds that these should each be unidimensional because if diverse questions are combined, the resulting score cannot be clearly interpreted (unless it is an extreme score). Applied to a measurement instrument, a Rasch analysis provides several statistics. Addressing postulate (i), it shows where each patient fits along the measurement scale, and also where items fit along the unidimensional continuum. For postulate (ii), it gives a score to each item that reflects its difficulty on a parametric scale, equivalent to a scaling task that translates ordinal responses into an interval scale (47). The analysis also indicates how consistently the relationships among the items hold in different subgroups of respondents (e.g., classified by age, diagnosis, or overall score on the test). For postulate (iv), an error term and a fit statistic indicate how well each item matches the ideal pattern of the cumulative scale. As with Guttman analyses, these statistics can be used to select the items that best define the continuum being measured. Unlike Guttman analyses, however, the Rasch approach

also indicates how each patient performs on the scale and which patients are giving idiosyncratic responses.

The limitation of the Rasch single parameter model is that it only describes the mean severity of the trait represented by each item; a second parameter is required to indicate how sharply the item demarcates people above and below that level of depression (a notion closely related to sensitivity and specificity). The item discrimination parameter is proportional to the slope of the "item characteristic curve" at its threshold value; items with steeper slopes are more useful in separating subjects into different levels of the trait (depression in our example). Expressed graphically, a vertical axis is added that indicates the cumulative probability of endorsing each item as the level of the trait increases. This produces S-shaped (or normal ogive) item characteristic curves for each item starting at the base of the graph and sloping up to meet the top line. The distance of the curve for each item from the left of the graph indicates the threshold or severity of the trait at which the item will be answered positively; the slope of the curve indicates the discriminability or accuracy of the item. The ideal is a steep slope so that the item sharply demarcates people at higher and lower levels of the trait. Item slopes may, however, vary across the severity range, with severe symptoms often forming more reliable indicators than mild symptoms: it is harder to write a good questionnaire item reflecting mild illness than severe (45, p401). Latent trait analysis provides valuable insight into the structure and quality of measurements and is ideal for selecting a subset of items from an initial item pool when constructing a questionnaire. It helps to explain why a measure may work well for one group of respondents and not for another or be good for one task and poor for another. The use of latent trait analyses in analyzing and in abbreviating health questionnaires was illustrated by Duncan-Jones et al. (45) and by Clark et al.'s study of depressive symptoms (48). General discussions of item response theory are provided by Hambleton and others (49, 50).

Econometric Methods

To allocate medical resources rationally, we need a way to compare the health benefits achieved per unit cost for different medical procedures. A table listing such benefits could guide us in directing resources away from procedures that are relatively expensive in terms of health benefits and toward those that are cheaper. While economists have debated details of assessing both the cost and benefit components, we are concerned here only with the measurement of benefits.

Early economic evaluations approached benefits in terms of whether a treatment reduced the costs associated with disability and lost production. Accounting gains in strictly financial terms, however, encountered philosophical challenges, since this appeared to ignore the inherent value of life; it leads to a preference for treatments that kill if they cannot cure. Just as the WHO had moved physical health measurement from impairment toward disability and handicap, so economists began to develop indices of effectiveness or utility that recorded benefits in terms of physical units, such as life-years gained (51). Utility has been defined differently in different disciplines, but here it refers to subjective valuation (4). The challenge was to develop an indicator of the combined quality and quantity of life which could be applied to patients with any medical condition. This is the field of cost-utility analysis, and the most common unit of measurement of health benefit in this equation is the quality-adjusted life year, or QALY (52). The QALY for a given procedure is calculated as the average number of additional years of life gained from the intervention, multiplied by a judgment of the quality of life in each of those years; this gives a composite indicator of outcome. Thus, for example, survival for a year with a residual disability that prevented a person from working and caused emotional distress

might be deemed equivalent to 0.75 of a healthy life year. The main application of QALYs lies in comparing different interventions, rather than in evaluating the health status of individual patients. They are typically used in policy analysis, for example. A scale will compare, on the one hand, the merit of devoting resources to an intervention that extends life but with high levels of disability, to, on the other, another intervention that does not prolong life as much but offers higher levels of well-being. QALYs may be used, for example, to propose levels of hypertension below which intervention is judged not to be cost-effective (53).

Econometric scaling methods are generally applied to composite health indexes (i.e., complete descriptions of an individual of given age, with specified symptoms, diagnosis, and functional limitations) that lie along a single continuum. They are not commonly used in deriving scale weights for scoring the more complex permutations possible in profile measurement methods such as the Sickness Impact Profile. The scale weights may be derived from expert judgment or from a preference weighting study, and they commonly use a variant of the "standard gamble" approach. Approaches such as willingness to pay or the time tradeoff are alternative ways to present the standard gamble, rather than different methods. As in psychometric scaling, the standard gamble involves a sample of people who make value judgments; in some utility measures the weights are provided by the patient whose health is being evaluated. Most studies that have compared the weights provided by different types of judges show that the weights provided by experts, patients, and well people are very similar (54); most studies now take a sample that includes all three. The standard gamble involves asking subjects to choose between (i) a certain option of intermediate desirability and (ii) a gamble that involves achieving a more desirable outcome with likelihood p, or a less desirable outcome with risk $1-p$. Applied to health states, the weighting procedure asks the rater to imagine that, for the first option, they are suffering from a chronic condition for which the symptoms, functional limitations, and pain are described. They are then asked to imagine that, for the second option, they are offered an operation that, if successful, would result in complete recovery. However, the operation incurs a risk of $1-p$ of death, and the rater is asked how great a risk of operative mortality they would tolerate to avoid remaining in the condition described in the first option. In principle, the more severe their assessment of the condition, the greater the risk $1-p$ of operative mortality (perhaps 5% or 10%) they would accept to escape. The severity of the condition is expressed by subtracting the tolerated risk of operative mortality from 1, to give the utility of the state described in the first option.

Because such judgments are difficult to make, various simplifying procedures may be used in administering the task, including the time tradeoff technique (42, p36). As before, the judges are asked to imagine that they are suffering from the condition whose severity is to be rated. They are asked to choose between remaining in that state for the rest of their natural lifespan (e.g., 30 years for a 40-year-old person), or returning to perfect health for fewer years. The number of years of life expectancy that would be sacrificed (e.g., five or ten) to regain health indicates how severely the condition is rated. The utility for the person with 30 years of life expectancy would be given as

Utility = (30 − Years Traded) / 30.

A third approach is to ask the person how much of their income they would be willing to pay to achieve the hypothetical cure.

Once the utility for a given state has been estimated, QALYs are calculated by multiplying the number of years to be expected in each state by the weight for that state. For example, if a state of "Choice of work or performance at work very severely limited; person is moderately distressed by this" were rated 0.942 (52), and if a person remained in this state for ten years, the QALY would be 9.42 years. Many refinements have been proposed to this basic approach. For example, QALYs may be adjusted to reflect the individual's preference or aversion for risk-taking. This characterizes the "healthy years equivalent" (HYE) indicator, which permits the rate of tradeoff between length and quality of life to depend on the expected lifespan (51).

By providing a common unit for measuring health status, economic methods permit us to compare the impact of different forms of disability and the cost-utility of different treatments; they are being increasingly applied in health policy analysis and in discussions of resource allocation. These methods also allow us to address broader philosophical questions, such as whether there is a social consensus over the valuation of life, whether it is equally valuable to extend the life of a 20-year-old and a 50-year-old, or whether it is equally valuable to extend one life for a thousand days, or a thousand lives for one day (4). LaPuma and Lawlor sketch the history of QALYs and the philosophical and ethical bases for their use and offer a cautionary discussion of potential misuse (53).

IDENTIFYING AND CONTROLLING BIASES IN SUBJECTIVE JUDGMENTS

Psychophysical experiments have shown that people can make accurate and internally consistent judgments of phenomena. This is the case, at least, with laboratory experiments concerned with lights or noises in which the person has no particular stake. Judgments of health may not be as dispassionate: in real life people have a personal stake in the estimation of their health. Bias refers to responses that depart systematically from the true values. We should, however, be careful to distinguish between two influences in the judgment process. There is the underlying and consistent perceptual tendency to exaggerate or underestimate stimuli described by the exponent b of the psychophysical experiments. This may be applicable, also, to health; we do not know. Then there is a tendency to alter response to a stimulus across times or under different situations, and this is termed bias. One person may exaggerate symptoms in order to qualify for sick leave or a pension, while another may show the opposite bias and minimize ailments in the hope of returning to work. Subjective ratings of health blend an estimate of the severity of the health problem with a personal tendency to exaggerate or conceal the problem—a bias that varies among people and over time.

Such uncertainty has led to skepticism about the accuracy of subjective health measurements; indeed, we know relatively little about the process of making subjective health judgments. Research is beginning on this, however; a number of studies have compared subjective responses with physical or laboratory measurements of health status (55), and other studies have identified circumstances under which patient reports may be biased.

Bias in subjective measurements can arise from the respondents' personalities, from the way they perceive questionnaires, or may reflect the particular circumstances of their illnesses. Illustrative examples will be given here, rather than an exhaustive list, for the main question concerns how to reduce the extent of response bias. Personality traits that may lead to response biases include stoicism, defensiveness, hypochondriasis, or a need for attention. The drive to portray oneself in a good light by giving socially desirable responses illustrates a bias that reflects social influences. Goldberg cites the example of a person, regarded by outside observers as fanatically tidy, but who judges himself untidy (56). This is unconscious, rather than a deliberate deception, and is typically more extreme where questions concern socially undesirable acts, such as sexual behavior or the use of drugs. Several scales have been proposed to measure a person's tendency to give socially desirable responses (57, 58),

but these appear to show rather low intercorrelations (42, p57). A correlation of 0.42 between the Crowne-Marlowe and Edwards scales was reported in one study, for example (59, Table 1). Attitudes may also bias responses and this has long been studied, for example, in reports from the National Opinion Research Center in Chicago (60). Biases may also arise from the way people interpret questionnaire response scales: some prefer to use the end-position on response scales, while others more cautiously prefer the middle (56, pp26–34). Other biases may be particular to the health field and reflect the anxiety that surrounds illness. One example is named the "hello–goodbye" effect, in which the patient initially exaggerates symptoms to legitimate the need for treatment (42, p58). Subsequently, the person minimizes any problems that remain, either to please the clinician or out of cognitive dissonance (61). Similarly, in the rebound effect, a patient recovering from a serious illness tends to exaggerate reported well-being (62).

Two general approaches are used to deal with bias in health measurement. The first bypasses the problem and argues that health care should consider symptoms as presented by the patient, bias and all, since this forms a part of the overall complaint: consideration of "the whole patient" is a hallmark of good care. From this viewpoint it can be argued that the biases inherent in subjective judgments do not threaten the validity of the measurement process: health, or quality of life, is inherently subjective and is as the patient perceives it. The second viewpoint argues that this is merely a convenient simplification and that the interests of diagnosis and patient management demand that health measurements should disentangle the objective estimate from any personal response bias. As an example, different forms of treatment are appropriate for the person who objectively reports pain of an organic origin and for the one whose pain is exaggerated by psychological distress; several of the pain scales we review are concerned with this distinction.

Most health indices do not disentangle the subjective and objective components in the measurement and thereby tacitly assume that the admixture of subjective and objective data is inevitable. Among the relatively few indices that do try to separate these components, we may discern several different tactics. The simplest is to try and dissemble the intent of the questions, either by giving them a misleading title, or by phrasing questions to hide their intent. This is commonly done with psychological measurement scales. For example, the Health Opinion Survey (Chapter 5) has nothing to do with opinions; it is designed to identify psychoneurotic disorders. Several of the questions appear to refer to physical symptoms (upset stomach, dizziness) but are intended as markers of psychological problems. A second approach is to have the questionnaire completed by someone who is familiar with the patient. Katz used this technique in rating social adjustment, as did Pfeffer in rating functional disability. A third way of handling response bias is to make an explicit assessment of the patient's emotional response to the condition. This was done in the pain measurements of Pilowsky, Leavitt, and Zung, where separate scores are provided for the two elements.

A fourth approach is a statistical method of analyzing patterns of responses that provides two scores; the first is concerned with perception and indicates the patient's ability to discriminate low levels of the stimulus, a notion akin to estimating the size of just–noticeable differences. The second score is concerned with the decision whether or not to report a stimulus; under conditions of uncertainty this reflects a personal response bias. Where it is difficult to judge whether or not a stimulus is present (e.g., whether or not an x-ray shows a small fracture) two types of error may occur: I may falsely report a fracture, or I may incorrectly exclude one. Where the x-ray is unclear, my decision is influenced by factors such as the frequency of seeing fractures of this type, my clinical conservatism, and the relative importance of avoiding each type of error. The way that I weigh these considerations forms my personal response tendency and involves concepts such as the posterior odds and the likelihood ratio, which are familiar in clinical epidemiology. The statistical approach to distinguishing the roles of perception and decision tendency in reaching the final decision is known as signal detection theory (SDT) or sensory decision theory. This has been applied in a few health indices such as Tursky's pain measurement and so deserves a brief mention here; fuller discussions are available (29, 63–66). It has also been applied to describe the behavior of baseball players in deciding whether or not to swing at the ball and the behavior of drivers in deciding when it is safe to enter a stream of traffic. The problem of distinguishing signals from background noise in radio and radar applications gave rise to SDT. It has formed the basis for the field of statistical decision analysis, which is concerned with how people make judgments under conditions of uncertainty. Their response pattern is assumed to derive from the discriminability of the stimulus and an estimate of the consequences of making each judgment. In an experimental situation, two types of stimulus are presented in random order—noise alone or noise plus low levels of signal—and the ability of an individual to identify the presence of a signal against the noise is recorded. Applied to pain research, the stimulus is usually an electric shock and the "noise" is a low level of fluctuating current. For each trial the respondent judges whether or not the shock was present and from the resulting pattern of true- and false-positive responses two indices are calculated: discriminal ability and response bias. Using some basic assumptions it is possible to estimate these two parameters from a single pair of estimates of a person's rate of correctly identifying a signal and his false-alarm rate; this is well described by Hertzog (66). In pain research, this technique has been used to study whether the use of analgesics influences pain by altering discriminability (i.e., by making the stimulus feel less noxious) or by shifting the response bias (making the respondent less willing to call the feeling "painful"). Studies of this type are further described in Chapter 8. It has also been applied in analyzing the confounding effect of age on test scores: is it possible that the declines in memory scores among elderly people reflect changes in approach to taking a test, rather than real reductions in memory? For example, elderly people may be more cautious or conservative in answering test questions and thereby achieve falsely low scores (66). From signal detection analyses, characteristic graphs known as receiver operating characteristic (or ROC) curves may be drawn showing the probability of the individual correctly reporting the presence of a signal against the probability of reporting a false alarm. In an experiment designed to illustrate the respondent's level of bias, ROC curves show the influence of varying rewards or penalties for making correct or incorrect decisions (63, 67, 68). While this is the original application of ROCs, similar curves are often drawn to summarize the validity of screening tests; this is because the two types of error are equivalent to sensitivity and 1-specificity (see page 32). The area under the ROC curve indicates the discriminal ability of the instrument, ranging from 0.5 (indicating no discrimination) to 1.0 (indicating perfect discrimination). Signal detection analyses are among the most complex methods currently applied to analyze subjective judgment of health. The field is relatively new, and although there is some disagreement over the interpretation of the results (65), the method may come to be more widely used.

CONCEPTUAL BASES FOR HEALTH MEASUREMENTS

It may appear obvious that a health measurement must be based on a specific conceptual approach: if we are measuring

health, what do we mean by "health"? The conceptual definition of an index justifies its content and relates it to a broader body of theory, showing how the results obtained may be interpreted in light of that theory. Yet by no means do all of the methods we review in this book offer a conceptual explanation of what they measure or of the value judgments they incorporate. A basic issue in constructing a health index is how to choose among the virtually unlimited number of questions that could potentially be included. There are two ways of confronting this problem: questions may be chosen from an empirical, or from a theoretical, standpoint. The two approaches are represented among the methods we review, although purely empirically based measures are becoming less common.

The empirical method to index development is typically used when the measurement has a practical purpose—for example, to predict which patients are most likely to be discharged home following a rehabilitation program. After testing a large number of questions, statistical procedures based on correlation methods are used to select those that best predict the eventual outcome. These "item analysis" statistics are described in the next section. Empirical selection of items has a practical appeal. It does, however, suffer the weakness that the user cannot necessarily interpret why those who answer a certain question in a certain manner tend to have better outcomes: the questions were not selected in relation to any particular theory of rehabilitation. Many illustrations exist; the questions in the Health Opinion Survey were selected because they distinguished between mental patients and normal people, and while they succeed in doing this, debates over what exactly they measure have continued for 35 years. A more recent example is Leavitt's Back Pain Classification Scale, which was developed empirically to distinguish between pain of an organic origin and pain related to emotional disorders. It succeeds well, but Leavitt himself commented:

"Why this particular set of questions works as discriminators and others do not is unclear from research to date" (see Chapter 8). Accordingly, the back pain scale may have clinical value, but it does not advance our understanding of the phenomenon of pain as a response to emotional disorders and of how psychological factors modify the pain response.

The alternative strategy to developing a health measurement is to choose questions that are considered relevant from the standpoint of a particular theory of health. As science develops and tests theories, so some indices have been designed to represent particular theories of health, and their use in turn permits the theory to be tested. Melzack's McGill Pain Questionnaire was based on his theory of pain; Bush's Quality of Well-Being Scale was based on an explicit conceptual approach to disability. Basing a measurement on a particular concept has important advantages. Linking the measurement with a body of theory means the method can be used analytically, rather than simply descriptively: studies using these methods may be able to explain, rather than merely to describe, the patient's condition in terms of that theory. The underlying theories also provide a guide to the appropriate procedures to be used in testing the validity of the method. The conceptual approaches used in many indices share common elements that will be introduced here, while finer details of the conceptual basis for each method are given in the reviews of individual indices.

The majority of indices of physical health, and some psychological scales, build their operational definitions of health on the concept of functioning: how far is the individual able to function normally and to carry on his typical daily activities? In this view, someone is healthy if he is physically and mentally able to do the things he wishes and needs to do. The phrase "activities of daily living" epitomizes this principle. There are many discussions of the concept of functional disability, including those by Gallin and Given (69) and Slater et al. (70). As Katz et al. pointed out, functional level may be used as a marker of the existence, severity, and impact of a disease even though knowledge about its etiology and pathogenesis is not advanced enough to permit measurement in these terms (27, p49). Measuring functional level offers a convenient way to compare the impact of different types of disease on different populations at different times. A common approach to measuring health is therefore via the impact of disease on various aspects of function. The notion of impact is contained in the titles of several scales, such as the Arthritis Impact Measurement Scales and the Sickness Impact Profile. Stating that an index of disability will assess functioning, however, does not indicate what questions should be included. At this more detailed level, indices diverge in their conceptual basis; approaches that have been used include psychological theories such as Maslow's hierarchy of human needs, biological models of human development (as in Katz's ADL scale), or sociological theories such as Mechanic's concept of illness behavior.

Alterations in function are commonly assessed at three sequential stages, termed impairment, disability, and handicap by the WHO (71–74). Very similar concepts are unfortunately named differently by other writers (75). In the WHO definitions, "impairment" refers to a reduction in physical or mental capacities. Impairments are generally disturbances at the organ level; they need not be visible and may not have adverse consequences for the individual: impaired vision can normally be corrected by wearing glasses. Where the effects of an impairment are not corrected, a disability may result. "Disability" refers to restriction in a person's ability to perform a function in a manner considered normal for a human being (to walk, to have full use of one's senses, and so forth). In turn, disability may or may not limit the individual's ability to fulfill a normal social role, depending on the severity of disability and on what the person wishes to do. "Handicap" refers to the social disadvantage (e.g., loss of earnings) that may arise from disability. A minor injury can handicap an athlete but may not noticeably restrict someone else; a condition producing mild vertigo may prove handicapping to a construction worker but not to a writer. Although medical care generally concentrates on treating impairment, the patient's "problem" is usually expressed in terms of disability or handicap, and the outcome of treatment may therefore best be assessed using disability or handicap indicators rather than measures of impairment. "Disablement" has been proposed to refer to both disability and handicap: a field normally covered by subjective health indices. These terms and their variants are discussed by Duckworth (72); Patrick and Bergner give a brief overview (76).

Health measurements that record the impact of disease may be viewed as fitting conceptually under the impairment–disability–handicap triad, but cover more than one element. Scales such as the Health Assessment Questionnaire are broad ranging, and cover the impact of sickness on disability and discomfort, but also cover the direct and indirect economic effects of illness—part of handicap.

The positive aspect of health is often mentioned and is linked to resilience and resistance to disease. Here health implies not only current well-being but also the likelihood of future disease. This is relevant because planning health services requires an estimate of what the burden of sickness is likely to be in the future. Nor is it appropriate to consider as equally healthy two people at equal levels of functional capacity if one has a presymptomatic disease that will very seriously affect future functional levels. For this reason, some indices (such as the Functional Assessment Inventory or the Quality of Well-Being Scale) assess prognosis as well as current health status. This prognostic element relates only to health, for there are external factors, such as an accident, which could drastically alter future health levels but which are not an aspect of a person's health.

The conceptual basis for a health index narrows the range of questions that could possibly be asked, but a relatively broad choice remains among, for example, the many questions that could be asked to measure "functional disability." Whether the index reflects a conceptual approach to health or whether it is developed on a purely empirical basis, procedures of item selection and item analysis are used to guide the final stages of selecting and validating the questions to be included in the measurement.

THE QUALITY OF A MEASUREMENT: VALIDITY AND RELIABILITY

Someone learning archery must first learn to hit the center of the target, and then learn to do this consistently. This is analogous to the validity and reliability of a measurement (77). The consistency (or reliability) of a measurement would be represented by how close successive shots fall to each other, wherever they land on the target. Validity would be represented by the aim of the shooting—how close, on average, the shots come to the center of the target. Ideally, a close grouping of shots should lie at the center of the target (reliable and valid), but a close grouping of shots may strike away from the center, representing an archer who is consistently off target, or a test that is reliable but not valid, perhaps due to bias in the measurement.

The core idea in validity concerns the meaning, or interpretation, of scores on a measurement. "Validity" is commonly defined as the extent to which a test measures what it is intended to measure. This approach is commonly used in epidemiology and underlies the notion of sensitivity. This is not a sufficient explanation of validity, however, for valuable interpretations of a measurement may be found that go beyond the original intent of the test. As an example, mortality rates were recorded to indicate levels of health or need for care, but the infant mortality rate may also serve as a convenient indicator of the socioeconomic development of a region or country. Hence, a more general definition holds that validity describes the range of interpretations that can be appropriately placed on a measurement score: What do the results mean? What can we conclude about the person who produced particular scores on the test? By focusing attention on the breadth of a measure, this approach also reflects its specificity (see page 31). The shift in definition is significant, for validity is no longer a property of the measurement, but rather of the interpretation we place on the results. This view holds advantages and disadvantages. It may stimulate a search for other interpretations of an indicator, as illustrated in the development of unobtrusive measures (78). This can lead to discovering links between constructs thought to be independent. An advantage of the broader definition is also seen in the dementia screening tests we review in Chapter 7. Most of these are valid in that they succeed in their purpose of identifying cognitive impairments (i.e., they are sensitive). However, several of the tests show low specificity in that people with low educational attainment also achieve positive scores, suggesting that the scales provide a more general indicator of cognitive functioning. A disadvantage of broadening the definition of validity is that it may foster sloppiness in defining the precise purpose of a measurement. Because of this, immense amounts of time have been wasted over arcane speculation on what certain scales of psychological well-being are actually supposed to measure. This can best be avoided by closely linking the validation process to a conceptual expression of the aims of the measurement and also linking that concept with other, related concepts to

indicate alternative possible interpretations of scores.

The practical concern then becomes how we tell if a measurement is striking close to the center of the target and measuring what it is supposed to. There are many ways of testing validity. The choice depends on the purpose of the method (e.g., screening test or outcome measurement) and on the level of abstraction of the topic to be measured. The following section gives a brief introduction to the methods that will be mentioned in the reviews. More extensive discussions are given in many sources (e.g., references 32, 34, 79–81).

ASSESSING VALIDITY

Most validation studies begin by referring to content validity. Each health measurement represents a sampling of questions from a larger number that could have been included. Similarly, the selection of a particular instrument is a choice among alternatives, and the score obtained at the end of this multistage sampling process is of interest to the extent that it is representative of the universe of relevant questions that could have been asked. "Content validity" refers to comprehensiveness, or to how adequately the sampling of questions reflects the aims of the index that were specified in the conceptual definition of its scope. For example, in a patient satisfaction scale, do all the items appear relevant to the concept being measured, and are all aspects of satisfaction covered? If not, invalid conclusions may be drawn. Feinstein has proposed the notion of sensibility, which includes, but slightly extends, the idea of content validity (82, Chapter 10). "Sensibility" refers to the clinical appropriateness of the measure: is its design, content and ease of use appropriate to the measurement task? Feinstein offered a check list of 21 attributes to be used in judging sensibility; these involve subjective assessments rather than statistical analyses. Indeed, content validity is seldom tested formally; instead, the face validity or clinical credibility of a measure is commonly inferred from the comments of experts who review its clarity and completeness. A common procedure to establish content validity is to ask patients and experts in the field to critically review the content of the scale. It is difficult, perhaps impossible, to prove formally that the items chosen are representative of all relevant items (83). Occasionally, tests of linguistic clarity are used to indicate whether the phrasing of the questions is clear.

Following content validation, more formal, statistical procedures are used to assess the validity of a measurement. These generally begin with "criterion validity," which considers whether the instrument correlates highly with a "gold standard" measure of the same theme. Criterion validity may test the accuracy of the complete measurement, or of each question. The latter involves "item analysis."

Several statistical procedures may be used in testing criterion validity. In the simplest case there is already an accepted way to measure the concept in question, a criterion or gold standard against which the new measurement may be compared. This typically occurs when the new instrument is being developed as a simpler, more convenient alternative to an accepted measurement. The new and the established tests are applied to a suitable sample of people and the results are compared using an appropriate indicator of agreement. Hence, this is sometimes known as correlational validity; typically, the correlation of each question with the criterion score is used to select the best questions and thereby refine draft versions of the questionnaire. Criterion validity is usually divided into "concurrent" and "predictive" validity, depending on whether the criterion refers to a current or future assessment. In the former, a questionnaire on hearing difficulties might be compared with the results of audiometric testing. In predictive validation, the test is applied in a prospective study in which the measurements made at the start of the study are compared to subsequent patient outcomes (mortality, discharge, etc.). Since this may demand a long investigation it is rarely used; there are also logical problems with the method. It is likely that during the course of a prospective study (and perhaps as a result of the prediction) interventions will be applied to selectively treat the individuals at highest risk. If successful, the treatment will alter the predicted outcome (contaminate the criterion) and wrongly make the test appear invalid. To avoid this predictive validity paradox, predictions are more commonly tested over a very brief time interval, making this approach equivalent to concurrent validity.

Our chapter on psychological measurements describes several screening tests, and their validation illustrates a major category of criterion validation studies. Here the criterion takes the form of a diagnosis made by a clinician who does not see the test result. The task is to show how well the test agrees with this classification and also to identify the threshold score on the test that most clearly distinguishes between well and sick respondents. The test is applied to contrasting groups of respondents and the patterns of their responses are compared. Two potential errors are recognized: a test may fail to identify people who have the disease or it may falsely classify people without the disease as being sick. The "sensitivity" of a test refers to the proportion of persons with a particular disease who are correctly classified as diseased by the test, while "specificity" refers to the proportion of people without the disease who are so classified by the test. These terms are quite logical: the sensitivity of the test indicates whether the test can identify the presence of a disease, while specificity indicates the degree to which it responds only to that disease. Specificity hence corresponds to "discriminal validity" in the language of psychometrics. Accordingly, tests of specificity may compare scores for people with the disease to others who have different diseases, rather than to people who are completely healthy; as so often in research, the choice of comparison group is subtle but critical. Several extensions to sensitivity and specificity analyses exist, some of which will be encountered in this book. For example, Goldberg illustrates various ways of combining sensitivity and specificity estimates to give a single estimate of the adequacy of a test. He also gives formulae for calculating the prevalence of a disease using a screening test of imperfect, but known, sensitivity and specificity, correcting for the imperfections in the test (56, p93).

Sensitivity and specificity analyses require that the scores obtained using the test be divided into two categories, indicating presumed sick and presumed well. The threshold score that divides these two categories is known as the cutting point or cutting score; to avoid confusion it is often expressed as two numbers, such as 23/24, indicating that the threshold lies between these. While simple, the division into two categories fails to reflect the notion of disease as a continuum, and so results in a loss of information. Several ways to describe the sensitivity of the test over a range of possible cutting points have been proposed. Changing the cutting point alters the proportions of well and sick people correctly classified by the test such that an increase in sensitivity is generally associated with a decrease in specificity. Because of this, the two parameters may be plotted graphically at different cutting points for the test in a further application of the ROC analyses described earlier. The true-positive probability (sensitivity) is plotted against the false-positive probability (1 − specificity) for various cutting points. The resulting curve illustrates the tradeoff between sensitivity and specificity. The area under the curve (AUC) provides an indicator of the usefulness of the test, indicating the probability that a randomly chosen, healthy person will score higher than a randomly chosen person with the disease (67, 84). AUC

values of 0.5 to 0.7 represent poor accuracy, 0.7 to 0.9 indicate "useful for some purposes," while values over 0.9 indicate high accuracy (85). Likelihood ratios offer another way of summarizing sensitivity and specificity; their use seeks to avoid the undue reliance on a single cutting point implicit in sensitivity analyses. The likelihood ratio for a particular value of a diagnostic test is the probability of the test result in people with the disease, divided by the probability of the same result in people without the disease (86). This is clinically useful, as it indicates how much more likely the test result is to occur in people with the disease than in those without.

Some caveats should be considered in interpreting sensitivity and specificity figures. Sensitivity may be influenced by factors such as age or educational level, and the dementia screening scales described in Chapter 7 illustrate this. It is convenient to report sensitivity for a single cutting point, but optimal detection may demand that the cutting point be varied for different age or educational groups. The reader should also critically review the study design in which sensitivity and specificity were estimated. The ideal is a study in which the gold standard and the test are applied to all persons in a selected population. This is rarely feasible, however, for it implies obtaining gold standard assessments from large numbers of people who do not have the condition; there are often cost or ethical constraints to this. Hence a common alternative is to take samples of those with and those without the condition, selected on the basis of the gold standard; typically these are people in whom the condition was suspected and who are attending hospital for assessment. Sensitivity and specificity are calculated in the normal manner. The problem is that the comparison group typically includes patients with other conditions; this may give misleading validity results if the test is to be used on an unselected population. An alternative approach is often used in validating a screening test in a population sample; here, the screening test is applied, and those who score positively receive the gold standard assessment, along with a random subsample of those scoring negatively. This approach incurs a bias known as diagnostic workup bias, which inflates the estimate of sensitivity and reduces that of specificity. This bias must be corrected, although regrettably often it is not. There are several alternative formulae for this (87).

Construct Validity

For measurements of pain, quality of life, and depression, gold standards do not exist; validity testing is more challenging. It requires assembling multiple indicators of validity in a process known as construct validation. This is akin to assembling evidence to support or refute a complex scientific theory and to show under what circumstances it holds true. Construct validation begins with a conceptual definition of the topic or construct to be measured, indicating the internal structure of its components and the theoretical relationship of scale scores to external criteria. These may be expressed as hypotheses indicating, for example, what correlations should be obtained with other instruments, which respondents should score high or low, or what other findings would be predicted from the scores. None of these challenges alone proves validity and each suffers logical and practical limitations, although when carefully applied they build a composite picture of the adequacy of the measurement. A well-developed theory is required to specify such a detailed pattern of data, a requirement that is not easily met. The main types of evidence used to indicate construct validity are briefly described here; their practical application is illustrated in the reviews of individual measurements.

Correlational Evidence

Hypotheses are formulated which state that the measurement will correlate with other methods that measure the same concept; the hypotheses are tested in the normal way. This is known as a test of "convergent validity" and is equivalent to assessing sensitivity. Where no single criterion exists, the measurement is sometimes compared with several other indices using multivariate procedures. Hypotheses may also state that the measurement will *not* correlate with others which measure different themes. This is termed divergent validity, and is equivalent to the concept of specificity. For example, a test of "Type A behavior patterns" may be expected to measure something distinct from neurotic behavior. Accordingly, a low correlation would be hypothesized between the Type A scale and a neuroticism index and, if obtained, would lend reassurance that the test was not simply measuring neurotic behavior. Naturally, this provides little information on what it *does* measure.

Correlating one method with another would seem straightforward, but there are logical problems. Because a new measurement is often not designed to replicate precisely the existing method against which it is being compared (indeed, it may be intended to be superior), the expected correlation may not be perfect. But how high should it be, given that the two indices are inexact measurements of similar, but not identical, concepts? Here lies a common weakness in reports of construct validation: few studies declare what levels of correlation are to be taken as demonstrating adequate validity. The literature contains many illustrations of authors who seem pleased to arbitrarily interpret virtually any level of correlation as supporting the validity of their measure. Construct validation should begin with a reasoned statement of the types of variable with which the measure should logically be related; the recent studies of the EuroQol illustrate this (88). The expected strength of correlation coefficients (or of the variance to be explained) should be stated prior to the empirical test of validity.

Several guidelines may assist the reader in interpreting reported validity correlations. First, as there is always some error of measurement, the maximum correlation can never reach 1.00. It can only rise to the square root of the reliability of the measurement. Where two measurements are compared, the maximum correlation between them is the square root of the product of their reliabilities (80, p84). Where the reliability coefficients are known, it is possible to compare the observed correlation to the maximum theoretically obtainable; this helps in interpreting the convergent validity coefficients between two scales. For example, a raw correlation between two scales of, say, 0.6 seems modest; but if their reliabilities are 0.7 and 0.75, the maximum correlation between them would only be 0.72, making the 0.6 seem quite high. By extension, we can estimate what the criterion validity correlation would be if both scales were perfectly reliable:

$$r_{xy}' = \frac{r_{xy}}{\sqrt{(r_{xx}r_{yy})}},$$

in our example 0.83. These corrections are only appropriate in large samples, of 300 or more; with smaller samples they can lead to validity coefficients that exceed 1.0; this seems over-optimistic for most of the measurements we review.

The second guideline involves translating a correlation coefficient into more interpretable terms. This assumes that the measurement is being used to predict a criterion, and the purpose is to assess how much the accuracy of prediction is increased by knowing the score on the measurement. The simplest approach is to square the correlation coefficient, showing the reduction in error of prediction that would be achieved by using the measurement compared to not using it. As an example, if a health measurement correlates 0.70 with a criterion, using the test will provide 0.7^2, or almost a 50% reduction in error compared with simply guessing. Applying this indicates that the value of a measurement declines rapidly below a validity coefficient of roughly 0.50. The derivation of this

approach is given by Helmstadter (80, p119), who also describes other ways of interpreting validity coefficients.

The adequacy of validity (and reliability) coefficients may be interpreted in light of the values typically observed. The convergent validity correlations between the tests reviewed in this book are low, typically falling between 0.40 and 0.60, with only occasional correlations falling above 0.70 for very similar instruments (such as the Barthel Index and PULSES Profile). The attenuation of validity coefficients due to unreliability implies that a correlation of 0.60 between two measures represents an extremely strong association.

Pearson correlations are often used in reporting reliability and validity findings, but they should be interpreted with caution. If points are drawn on a graph to plot one rating against another for a series of patients, the correlation coefficient shows how closely the points lie to a straight line. This indicates how accurately one rating can be predicted from another. Coefficients range from −1.0 (indicating an inverse association) through 0.0 (indicating no association at all) to +1.0. Pearson correlations quantify the association between two measurement scales, but do not indicate agreement. This is because a perfect correlation requires only that the pairs of readings fall on a straight line but does not specify which line. For example, if one sphygmomanometer consistently gives blood pressure readings 10 mmHg higher than another, the correlation between them would be 1.0, but the agreement would be zero. Correlations are also influenced by the range of the scale: wider ranges tend to produce higher correlations, even though the agreement remains the same. Bland and Altman discuss these limitations and propose alternative approaches to expressing the agreement between two ratings (89).

Factorial Validity

Factor analysis can be used to describe the underlying conceptual structure of an instrument; it examines how far the items accord in measuring one or more common themes. It can therefore be used in studying content validity: do the items fall into the expected groupings? Using the pattern of intercorrelations among replies to questions, the analysis forms the questions into groups or factors that appear to measure common themes, each factor being distinct from the others. For example, Bradburn selected questions to measure two aspects of psychological well-being which he termed positive and negative affect. Factor analysis of the questions confirmed that they fell into two distinct groups, which were homogeneous and unrelated to each other, and which by inspection appeared to represent positive and negative feelings. This analytic method is therefore commonly used to study the internal structure of a health index that contains separate components, each reflecting a different aspect of health. Typically, these components of the measurement will be scored separately. Factor analysis can also be used in construct validation by indicating the association among several measurements. Scales measuring the same topic would be expected to be grouped by the analysis onto the same factor (a test of convergent validity), while scales measuring different topics would group on different factors (divergent validity).

Factor analysis is widely used, and all too frequently misused, in the studies reported in this book; several principles guide its appropriate use (90, 91). The items to be analyzed should be measured at the interval-scale level; the response distributions should be approximately normal and there should be at least five (some authors say 20) times more respondents in the sample than there are variables to be analyzed. Because so many health indices use categorical response scales (such as "frequently," "sometimes," "rarely," and "never") the first and second of these principles are often contravened. In such cases latent trait analysis can be used to provide a factor analysis applicable to binary (yes/no) responses. In addition, for purposes of scale development, items can be selected on the basis of their association with the trait of interest.

Group Differences or Discriminant Evidence

An index that is intended to distinguish between categories of respondent (e.g., well and sick, before and after treatment) may be tested by applying it to samples of each group and by analyzing the scores for significant differences. Significant differences on the scores would disprove the null hypothesis that the method fails to differentiate between them. This approach is very frequently used, but like all other validation procedures, it suffers logical limitations. Screening tests for emotional disorder may compare psychiatric patients with the general population but they will underestimate the adequacy of the method if some members of the general population have undiagnosed emotional disorders. Many indices are developed for highly selected cases in clinical research centers. Just as it is risky to generalize the results of clinical trials from tertiary-care centers to other settings, so referral patients may score highly on an index, yet high scores in a community survey may not be diagnostic (83). New measurements should be retested in a variety of settings.

When the results of several drug trials are combined in a meta-analysis, the average impact of the treatment may be indicated using the effect size statistic to compare mean scores in treatment and control groups or before and after treatment. Results are expressed in standard deviation units: $(M_t - M_c)/SD_c$. The effect size is comparable to a z score where, assuming a normal distribution of scores, the effect size indicates how far along the percentile range of scores a patient will be expected to move following treatment. With an effect size of $+1.00$, a patient whose initial score lies at the mean of the pretreatment distribution will be expected to rise to about the 84th percentile of the control, or untreated, group after treatment. Meta-analyses are now beginning to summarize the results of several trials in terms of the effect sizes achieved by selected treatments; an example is given by Felson et al. (92).

The idea of effect size for a treatment can be turned on its side and applied to measurement instruments to compare how sensitive they are in indicating change—an example is given by Liang et al. (93). For outcome measurements, sensitivity to change is a crucial characteristic, although there is no clear consensus as to how this should be assessed. Many indicators have been proposed, and careful reading of articles is often needed to identify which statistic has been used. Most indicators agree on the numerator, which is the raw score change; there is little agreement on the appropriate denominator. The basic measure of effect size is the raw score change on the measure divided by the standard deviation of the measure at time 1 (94). Alternatives include a t-test approach which divides the raw score change by its standard error (95), or a responsiveness statistic that divides the raw score change by the standard deviation among stable subjects (95); as an alternative, the standardized response mean divides the mean change in score by the standard deviation of individuals' changes in scores (96). Further alternatives include relative efficiency (97), measurement sensitivity, receiver operating characteristic analyses (in terms of the ratio of signal to noise) (98, 99) and an F-ratio comparison (100, 101). Refinements to the basic formulae correct for the level of test–retest reliability (102). The largest effect size that can be attained for a given measure in a given sample is the baseline mean score divided by its standard deviation. As a general convention, effect sizes of 0.2 to 0.49 are considered small; 0.5 to 0.79 are moderate, and 0.8 or above are large (94). These interpretations give a guide to assessing the clinical importance of an intervention: while large sample sizes may make the comparison between drug and placebo groups significant, the effect size can be used to indicate whether the

difference is clinically important. Knowing the effect size of an instrument is also valuable in calculating the power of a study and the sample size required; as with all sample size calculations, this requires a prior estimate of the likely effect size for a particular comparison (say, of drug and placebo), with a particular measurement instrument. To illustrate, if the effect size is expected to be 0.2, about 400 subjects will be required per group to show the contrast as significant, setting alpha at 0.05 and power at 0.8. To detect a moderate effect size of 0.5, one would need about 64 patients per group (94, pS187). Effect sizes also help in comparing results from studies that used different measurements: an instrument with a large effect size will show a higher mean improvement following treatment than an instrument with a smaller effect size. Information on the effect sizes of various measurement instruments is starting to accumulate; one example is in the depression field (103).

Construct validation of a health measurement is part science and largely art form. Construct validity cannot be proved definitively, but it is a continuing process in which testing often contributes to our understanding of the construct, following which new predictions are made and tested. This is the ideal, but the literature contains examples of inadequate and seemingly arbitrary presentations of construct validity. We still see statements of the type, "Our instrument correlated 0.34 with the Serenity Scale, 0.21 with the Idiosyncrasy Index, and 0.55 with the Turpitude Test and this pattern of associations supports its construct validity." In the absence of *a priori* hypotheses of association, the reader may well wonder what pattern of correlations would have been interpreted as refuting validity. Mercifully, there are several examples of a more systematic approach to construct validation, such as those by McHorney et al. (104) and Kantz et al. (105). Good validation studies state clear hypotheses and test them, with justification for considering those hypotheses the most relevant. Good studies will also try to disprove the hypothesis that the method measures something other than its stated purpose, rather than merely assembling information on what it does measure. A variety of approaches should be used in testing any index, rather than relying on a single validation procedure. Future developments should see greater use of recently developed structural modeling techniques that allow theoretical and unmeasured variables to enter into multivariate analyses of the links among a series of measurements. An example of this approach to construct validation is given by Andrews (106).

ASSESSING RELIABILITY

Reliability, or consistency, is concerned with error in measurement. In the metaphor of the target, reliability was symbolized by the dispersion of shots. This referred to the consistency or stability of the measurement process across time, patients, or observers. Feinstein prefers the term "consistency," feeling that "reliability" carries connotations of trustworthiness, which may not be appropriate if, for example, a measurement repeatedly yields erroneous results (82). Nonetheless, reliability is the most widely accepted term, and is used here. Unreliability can be seen as the discrepancies that would arise if a measurement were repeated many times. Unfortunately, repeating a health measurement to assess its stability is often not as simple as repeating a measurement in the physical sciences: repeating a patient's blood-pressure measurement may not be welcomed and may influence the blood pressure itself. This has led to the development of alternative techniques for assessing the reliability of health measurements based on theoretical assumptions that justify the approach used. There are many sources of measurement error; the different approaches focus on different sources of error, and as with validity, there is no single way to express reliability but most ways share a common ancestry in classical test theory.

Traditional reliability theory views the value obtained from any measurement as a combination of two components: an underlying true score and some degree of error. The true score, of course, is what we are trying to establish; "error" refers to imprecision in the measurement, or "noise" that frustrates our aim of finding the true score. Errors are commonly grouped into two types: random errors and systematic errors or bias (107). Traditional reliability theory considers only errors that occur randomly; systematic errors, or biases, are generally considered under validity testing. Random errors include the numerous mistakes in making a measurement, due to inattention, tiredness, or mechanical inaccuracy that may equally lead to an over- or underestimate of the true quantity. The assumption that such errors are random holds several corollaries. They are as likely to increase the observed score as to decrease it; the magnitude of the error is not related to the magnitude of the true score (error is not greater in extreme scores), and the observed score is the arithmetic sum of the error component and the underlying true score that we are attempting to measure. Random errors cancel each other out if enough observations are made, so the average score a person would obtain if tested repeatedly gives a good estimate of the true score. In traditional test theory, reliability then refers to the extent to which a score is free of random error. More formally, the reliability of a measurement is defined as the proportion of observed variation in scores (e.g., across patients, or across repeated measurements) that reflects actual variation in health levels. This is normally written as the ratio of true score variance to observed score variance, or σ^2_T / σ^2_O. Because the observed score is assumed to be the sum of true and error scores, this formulation is equivalent to $\sigma^2_T / \sigma^2_T + \sigma^2_E$. This provides a number with no units that reaches unity when all of the variance in observed scores reflects true variance and zero when all the observed variance is due to errors of measurement. To illustrate this idea, imagine that two nurses measure the blood pressure of five people. For simplicity, imagine also that each patient's blood pressure remains stable. The true variation refers to the range of blood-pressure readings across patients; error refers to discrepancies between the nurses' ratings for any of the patients assessed. Reliability increases as true variation increases and as error variation is small. Within this traditional approach, two types of reliability are distinguished: whether different raters assessing a respondent obtain the same result (inter-rater agreement or observer variation) and whether the same result is obtained when the same rater makes a second assessment of the patient (variously termed intrarater reliability, stability, test–retest reliability, and repeatability).

Although a mainstay of test development, traditional test theory has frequently been criticized. More detailed approaches to reliability testing, such as Rasch's item response model and generalizability theory, are now being applied in testing health indices (42, p98; 108). The main reason is that the conventional test theory groups many sources of error variance together, whereas we may wish to record these separately to gain a fuller understanding of the performance of a measurement. Generalizability theory uses analysis of variance to separate different sources of variation, distinguishing, for example, the effect of using an interview or a questionnaire, or the sex or age of the interviewer. The results indicate the likely performance of the measurement under different conditions of administration. There will be a different reliability coefficient for each, which underscores the point that there is no single reliability result for a measurement.

Reliability can be translated into a convenient statistic in several ways. Unfortunately the reliability of many health measurements has been reported incorrectly. Several basic points may illustrate this, beginning with the difference between agreement and association introduced on page 34. Agreement assesses whether our two sphygmomanometers provide identical blood-pressure readings for the same person; in estimating error in measurement, this is the relevant idea. One approach to recording agreement examines the distribution of differences in pairs of scores. This can be presented graphically, plotting the difference in the two scores for each person against the mean of the two scores. The graph illustrates whether the error changes across the range of the scale and readily identifies outliers. It is expected that 95% of the differences will lie within two standard deviations of the mean. The standard deviation of the differences is calculated by squaring the differences, summing them, dividing by N, and taking the square root (89). By contrast, association refers to a relationship (typically linear) between two sets of readings and is commonly represented by a Pearson correlation coefficient. The use of Pearson correlations to indicate inter-rater agreement can seriously exaggerate the impression of reliability (109). As an illustration, Siegert et al. obtained a Pearson correlation of 0.95 and a Spearman coefficient of 0.94 between self-and interviewer-administered questionnaires; despite the high correlation, interview and questionnaire agreed precisely in only 65% of cases (110, p307). The central point is that there are many possible types of discrepancy in pairs of ratings: as with the blood-pressure example, the whole distribution may shift for one assessment, or the relative position of certain individuals may change, or one measure may achieve greater precision than the other, or one scale may be stretched compared with the other. Correlation coefficients reflect some types of mismatch between scores but ignore others. Thus, although a simple rule would advise against the Pearson correlation for reporting reliability, a more sophisticated guide would begin by considering what types of variation in scores are considered erroneous. For example, if patients in a test–retest study are recovering and their average scores improve over time, the correlation coefficient will ignore this shift in the distribution of scores and will focus on whether the relative position of each person was maintained. An index of agreement, by contrast, would classify the general improvement as unreliability in the measure and would provide an absolute indicator of stability of the test results. This question of what sources of variation in scores should be considered as part of unreliability introduces the theme of the intraclass correlation (ICC).

For measurements made on a continuous scale, the intraclass correlation is increasingly used to indicate reliability instead of Pearson or rank-order coefficients. Like the Pearson correlation, when two ratings are compared for each subject, the ICC ranges from -1 to $+1$, but it measures the average similarity of the subjects' actual scores on the two ratings, not merely the similarity of their relative standings on the two. Hence, if one set of scores is systematically higher than the other, the ICC will not reach unity (99). Intraclass correlations refer to a family of analysis of variance approaches that express reliability as the ratio of true to total variance in scores (111, 112); the procedure for calculating the ICC is illustrated by Deyo et al. (99). As different sources of variance may be considered in the numerator in different reliability studies, there is no single type of intraclass correlation. Shrout and Fleiss described six forms of ICC, noting that research reports frequently fail to specify the form used (113). Intraclass correlations may also compare agreement among more than two raters; for ordinal measurement scales the equivalent statistic is Kendall's index of concordance *(W)*. A statistical relative of the intraclass correlation is the concordance correlation coefficient, which indicates the agreement between the observed data and a 45° slope (the Pearson correlation indicates agreement between the data and the best-fitting line, wherever this may lie) (99, p151S).

A second mistake, happily now rare, concerns the statistic used to report reliability for nominal or ordinal rating scales.

When the ratings are dichotomous (e.g., agreement over whether or not a chest x-ray shows pneumonia), a simple table can indicate the proportion of agreement. A correction is necessary because chance agreement will inflate the impression of reliability, especially if a majority of cases fall in one category. If most chest x-rays do not show pneumonia, a second rater may produce high agreement merely by guessing that all the films are normal. The kappa coefficient corrects for this by calculating the extent of agreement expected by chance alone and removing this from the estimation (see formula in Glossary). Kappa coefficients can also be applied to ordinal data in several categories, and a weighted kappa formula can be used to discriminate minor from major discrepancies between raters (42, p95).

Internal Consistency

The notion of repeatability is central to reliability, but repeated assessments run the risk of a falsely negative impression where the measurement correctly identifies changes in health between administrations. A sensitive instrument may appear unreliable. To reduce this risk, the delay between assessments should be brief. However, this means that recall by respondent or rater may influence the second application, so the two assessments may not be independent.

Various tricks have been proposed to overcome this and the underlying logic introduces the notions of equivalent forms and of internal consistency. In theory, it is argued, if we could develop two, parallel forms of the test that contain different questions, but that give the same results, this would overcome the problem of memory biasing the second administration. This approach has been used, for example, in the Depression Adjective Check Lists (Chapter 6), which are intended to measure depression before and after treatment. The assessment of reliability then compares the two versions, which are administered after a brief delay or even at the same time. The concept of reliability has thereby shifted from the repeatability of the same instrument over time to comparing two versions. If the two correlate highly, they are reliable; this is, indeed, a more challenging test than comparing the same instrument at two different times. Note that here a correlation is appropriate, for we only wish to show that the two forms give equivalent results— that one could be translated into the other with a simple arithmetic conversion. The next step in the logic builds on the idea that as the forms are different, they might as well be applied at the same time to assess their reliability. Hence a simpler approach has been proposed, in which the alternate versions are merged into one longer instrument, applied in a single session. Reliability is then assessed by using an appropriate statistic to indicate how comparable the results would be if the measurement had been split into two component versions. A simple way is to correlate the odd- and even-numbered questions, but a more general approach is to estimate the correlations between all possible pairs of items, which introduces the theme of internal consistency. The higher the intercorrelations among the items on a measurement, the easier it would be to create two versions that are equivalent and therefore reliable. Thus, the theory holds that the higher the internal consistency, the higher the test–retest reliability will be. Cronbach's coefficient alpha is the most frequently used indicator of internal consistency (34, pp380–385). Several other formulae were proposed by Kuder and Richardson, and their formula 20 is the equivalent of alpha for dichotomous items. Such formulae estimate what the correlation would be between different versions of the same measurement. A related measure of internal consistency derives from Guttman's scalogram analysis. Guttman's coefficient of reproducibility indicates how closely the overall score on a scale will indicate the precise pattern of a person's responses: an indicator of internal consistency.

The true score is viewed as the mean score of repeated measurements; more observations give a more accurate estimate of the mean. In a similar manner, increasing the number of items in an assessment increases its internal consistency and hence reliability, very much in the way that a standard deviation becomes narrower with increasing numbers of observations. It is also clear that the reliability of a composite scale will increase as a function of the reliability of the individual items that compose it. The joint influence of the number of items and the reliability of each item on the reliability of a scale was described in formulae derived independently by Spearman and by Brown in 1910. For example, if one requires a reliability of 0.8, this can be achieved with two items with individual reliabilities of 0.7, or with four of 0.5 or ten of 0.3 (114). With most health measurements, there is a steep increase in reliability up to about ten items and thereafter a gradually diminishing improvement with additional items. Shrout and Yager provide graphs to illustrate this, and also describe how test length affects validity (115). Nonetheless, as with food and other good things, moderation in internal consistency is best. Where items intercorrelate very highly there is redundancy in the measurement and it is narrow in scope; it might be very specific but is not likely to be highly sensitive. If item intercorrelations are kept moderate, each item will add a new piece of information to the measurement (91). Hence it is not reasonable to expect a high internal consistency if the measurement covers several dimensions of health. A broad measurement may also show lower repeatability since there are more ways in which the scores can vary from test to retest. Reliability may also vary according to the topic that is measured. Not all patients with depression or rheumatoid arthritis exhibit consistent patterns of symptoms. While the internal consistency of a depression symptom check list might be improved by deleting questions that are not highly correlated with others, this might compromise content validity. Furthermore, the requirements for reliability differ according to the purpose of the measurement. With an evaluative measure that is intended to be sensitive to changes in health over time, stability is likely to appear low, but the important quality is internal consistency at one time. The link between scale length and reliability does not hold for evaluative measures, although it does hold for discriminative measures (18). If the health index is to be used to predict outcomes, it must be able to predict itself accurately, and so test–retest reliability is crucial. If it is intended mainly to measure current status, the internal structure is the most crucial characteristic. This is especially true when the measurement is designed to reflect a specific concept of health, for greater reliability implies greater validity. Achieving such balances forms the art of test development.

Interpreting Reliability Coefficients

The reliability coefficient shows the ratio of true score variance to observed score variance. Thus, if reliability is calculated from an analysis of variance model as 0.85, this indicates that an estimated 15% of the observed variance is due to error in measurement. For a Pearson correlation the equivalent information is obtained by squaring the coefficient and subtracting the result from 1.0. The reliability also indicates the confidence with which a score for an individual represents his true score or, put another way, the confidence we have that a change in scores represents a change in health status. As reliability increases, the confidence interval around a score narrows, and so we are more confident that the true score would fall close to the observed score. To illustrate, with a standard deviation of 20 for an imaginary measurement, a reliability of 0.5 would give a 95% confidence interval of 28.4, a reliability of 0.7 yields a confidence interval of 22.0, 0.9 translates into 12.8, and a reliability of 0.95 gives a confidence interval of 8.8.

As our book is concerned with evaluating measurement methods, we need to suggest what level of reliability coefficient is adequate. As with most interesting topics, there is no absolute answer; the purpose of the measurement influences the standard of reliability required. Tests used for clinical assessment of individual patients demand higher reliability than those used in population studies. Larger studies can tolerate lower standards of reliability of measurement than can smaller ones, for large sample sizes reduce the error of measurement in estimating mean values. Recommended values also vary from statistic to statistic and are, at best, expressions of opinion. Helmstadter, for example, quotes desirable reliability values for various types of psychological tests intended for individuals, the median for personality tests being 0.85, that for ability tests being 0.90, and for attitude tests, 0.79 (80, p85). A lower reliability, perhaps of >0.50 (80) or >0.70 (32), may be acceptable in comparing groups. Various guidelines for interpreting kappa values have been proposed; one example views values of less than 0.4 as indicating poor agreement, 0.41 to 0.6 as moderate, 0.61 to 0.8 as substantial, and over 0.8 as almost perfect (116). Typical Pearson correlations for inter-rater reliability in the scales reviewed in this book fall in the range 0.65 to 0.95, and values above 0.85 may be considered acceptable. Pearson correlations for repeatability are often high, falling between 0.85 and 0.90. Empirical results help us to interpret the level of agreement implied by a particular correlation coefficient; Andrews obtained a test–retest coefficient of 0.68 when 54% of respondents gave identical answers on retest and a further 38% scored within one point of their previous answer on a seven-point scale (117, p192). Intraclass correlations tend to give slightly lower numerical values than the Pearson equivalent. Articles by Rule et al. (118, Table 2) and by Yesavage et al. (119, Table 2) illustrated alternative indicators of internal consistency for depression scales. The commonly used Cronbach alpha coefficients consistently gave slightly higher values than split-half reliability coefficients for the same scale, but the major contrast lay between these and the mean inter-item correlations and item-total correlations. An alpha of 0.80 corresponded to a mean inter-item correlation of only 0.14 and an item-total correlation of 0.50. An alpha of 0.94 corresponded to a mean inter-item correlation of 0.36 and a median item-total coefficient of 0.56. Similar results have been reported elsewhere: a mean inter-item correlation of 0.15 for 17 items corresponded to an alpha of 0.76 for the Hamilton Rating Scale for Depression (120, pp34–35). Hence, high alpha values are consistent with very modest agreement between individual items. McHorney et al. reported both inter-item correlations and alpha values for eight scales of the SF-36 instrument; the alpha values were typically 0.15 to 0.30 higher than the inter-item correlations, while the correlation between the two statistics was only 0.27 (121, Table 7).

Finally, Wolf and Cornell complicated the issue by warning against lightly dismissing low correlations (122). They described a technique that translates correlations derived from 2×2 tables into the metaphor of the estimated difference in probability of success between treatment and control groups. They show, for example, that a correlation of 0.30 (producing shared variance of only 9%) translates into an increase in success rate from 0.35 to 0.65: clinically speaking, a major improvement!

SUMMARY

Recent years have seen exciting technical advances in the methods used to develop and test health measurement instruments. This has come in part through the importation of techniques from disciplines such as psychometry and educational measurement, but we have also seen home-grown advances in procedures for assessing and expressing validity and reliability results. In past years, many widely used scales were developed by individual clinicians, based mainly on their clinical experience. These days seem to be numbered as we move toward greater technical and statistical sophistication. The process of developing a scale has become a long, complex, and expensive one involving a team of experts, and in most cases the quality of the resulting method is better. We should be careful, however, not to forget the importance of sound clinical insight into the nature of the condition being measured; the ideal is to use statistically correct procedures to refine an instrument whose content is based on clinical wisdom and common sense.

REFERENCES

(1) Rosser R. A history of the development of health indicators. In: Teeling-Smith G, ed. Measuring the social benefits of medicine. London: Office of Health Economics, 1983:50–62.

(2) Rosser R. The history of health related quality of life in 10½ paragraphs. J R Soc Med 1993;86:315–318.

(3) Ware JE, Brook RH, Davies AR, et al. Choosing measures of health status for individuals in general populations. Am J Public Health 1981;71:620–625.

(4) Rosser R. Issues of measurement in the design of health indicators: a review. In: Culyer AJ, ed. Health indicators. Amsterdam: North Holland Biomedical Press, 1983:36–81.

(5) Rosser RM. Recent studies using a global approach to measuring illness. Med Care 1976;14(suppl):138–147.

(6) Chapman CR. Measurement of pain: problems and issues. In: Bonica JJ, Albe-Fessard DG, eds. Advances in pain research and therapy. Vol. I. New York: Raven Press, 1976:345–353.

(7) Morris JN. Uses of epidemiology. 3rd ed. London: Churchill Livingstone, 1975.

(8) Gruenberg EM. The failures of success. Milbank Q 1977;55:1–24.

(9) Wilkins R, Adams OB. Health expectancy in Canada, late 1970s: demographic, regional and social dimensions. Am J Public Health 1983;73:1073–1080.

(10) Moriyama IM. Problems in the measurement of health status. In: Sheldon EB, Moore W, eds. Indicators of social change: concepts and measurements. New York: Russell Sage, 1968:573–599.

(11) World Health Organization. The first ten

years of the World Health Organization. Geneva: World Health Organization, 1958.

(12) Goldsmith SB. The status of health status indicators. Health Serv Rep 1972; 87:212–220.

(13) Goldsmith SB. A reevaluation of health status indicators. Health Serv Rep 1973; 88:937–941.

(14) Wilson RW. Do health indicators indicate health? Am J Public Health 1981;71:461–463.

(15) Colvez A, Blanchet M. Disability trends in the United States population 1966–76: analysis of reported causes. Am J Public Health 1981;71:464–471.

(16) Bombardier C, Tugwell P. A methodological framework to develop and select indices for clinical trials: statistical and judgmental approaches. J Rheumatol 1982;9:753–757.

(17) Apgar V. A proposal for a new method of evaluation of the newborn infant. Anesth Analg 1953;32:260–267.

(18) Kirshner B, Guyatt G. A methodologic framework for assessing health indices. J Chronic Dis 1985;38:27–36.

(19) Kind P, Carr-Hill R. The Nottingham Health Profile: a useful tool for epidemiologists? Soc Sci Med 1987;25:905–910.

(20) Elinson J. Introduction to the theme: sociomedical health indicators. Int J Health Serv 1978;6:385–391.

(21) Stoker MJ, Dunbar GC, Beaumont G. The SmithKline Beecham 'Quality of Life' Scale: a validation and reliability study in patients with affective disorder. Qual Life Res 1992;1:385–395.

(22) Thunedborg K, Allerup P, Bech P, et al. Development of the repertory grid for measurement of individual quality of life in clinical trials. Int J Methods Psychiatr Res 1993;3:45–56.

(23) Mor V, Guadagnoli E. Quality of life measurement: a psychometric Tower of Babel. J Clin Epidemiol 1988;41:1055–1058.

(24) Guralnik JM, Branch LG, Cummings SR, et al. Physical performance measures in aging research. J Gerontol 1989; 44:M141–M146.

(25) Podsiadlo D, Richardson S. The Timed "Up & Go": a test of basic functional mobility for frail elderly persons. J Am Geriatr Soc 1991;39:142–148.

(26) Weiner DK, Duncan PW, Chandler J, et al. Functional reach: a marker of physical frailty. J Am Geriatr Soc 1992;40:203–207.

(27) Katz S, Akpom CA, Papsidero JA, et al. Measuring the health status of populations. In: Berg RL, ed. Health status indexes.

Chicago: Hospital Research and Educational Trust, 1973:39–52.

(28) Moskowitz E, McCann CB. Classification of disability in the chronically ill and aging. J Chronic Dis 1957;5:342–346.

(29) Baird JC, Noma E. Fundamentals of scaling and psychophysics. New York: Wiley, 1978.

(30) Stevens SS. The surprising simplicity of sensory metrics. Am Psychol 1962;17:29–39.

(31) Lodge M. Magnitude scaling: quantitative measurement of opinions. Beverly Hills, California: Sage Publications (Quantitative Applications in the Social Sciences No. 07–001), 1981.

(32) Nunnally JC. Psychometric theory. 2nd ed. New York: McGraw-Hill, 1978.

(33) Torgerson WS. Theory and methods of scaling. New York: Wiley, 1958.

(34) Guilford JP. Psychometric methods. 2nd ed. New York: McGraw-Hill, 1954.

(35) Young FW. Scaling. Annu Rev Psychol 1984;35:55–81.

(36) Bradburn NM, Miles C. Vague quantifiers. Public Opin Q 1979;43:92–101.

(37) Merbitz C, Morris J, Grip JC. Ordinal scales and foundations of misinference. Arch Phys Med Rehabil 1989;70:308–312.

(38) McClatchie G, Schuld W, Goodwin S. A maximized-ADL index of functional status for stroke patients. Scand J Rehabil Med 1983;15:155–163.

(39) Silverstein B, Fisher WP, Kilgore KM, et al. Applying psychometric criteria to functional assessment in medical rehabilitation: II. Defining interval measures. Arch Phys Med Rehabil 1992;73:507–518.

(40) Edwards AL. Techniques of attitude scale construction. New York: Appleton-Century-Crofts, 1975.

(41) Stevens SS. Measurement, psychophysics and utility. In: Churchman CW, Ratoosh P, eds. Measurement, definitions and theories. New York: Wiley, 1959:18–63.

(42) Streiner DL, Norman GR. Health measurement scales: a practical guide to their development and use. New York: Oxford, 1989.

(43) Jenkinson C. Why are we weighting? A critical examination of the use of item weights in a health status measure. Soc Sci Med 1991;32:1413–1416.

(44) Lord FM. Applications of item response theory to practical testing problems. Hillsdale, New Jersey: Lawrence Erlbaum Associates, 1980.

(45) Duncan-Jones P, Grayson DA, Moran PAP. The utility of latent trait models in

psychiatric epidemiology. Psychol Med 1986;16:391–405.

(46) McArthur DL, Cohen MJ, Schandler SL. Rasch analysis of functional assessment scales: an example using pain behaviors. Arch Phys Med Rehabil 1991;72:296–304.

(47) Wright BD, Masters G. Rating scale analysis. Chicago: MESA Press, 1982.

(48) Clark DC, Cavanaugh SA, Gibbons RD. The core symptoms of depression in medical and psychiatric patients. J Nerv Ment Dis 1983;171:705–713.

(49) Hambleton RK, Jones RW. Comparison of classical test theory and item response theory and their applications to test development. Educ Meas Issues Practice 1993; Fall:38–47.

(50) Hambleton RK, Swaminathan H, Rogers HJ. Fundamentals of item response theory. Newbury Park, California: Sage, 1991.

(51) Johannesson M, Pliskin JS, Weinstein MC. Are healthy-years equivalents an improvement over quality-adjusted life years? Med Decis Making 1993;13:281–286.

(52) Robinson R. Cost-utility analysis. Br Med J 1993;307:859–862.

(53) LaPuma J, Lawlor EF. Quality-adjusted life years: ethical implications for physicians and policymakers. JAMA 1990; 263:2917–2921.

(54) Kaplan RM. Application of a General Health Policy Model in the American health care crisis. J R Soc Med 1993; 86:277–281.

(55) Kaplan SH. Patient reports of health status as predictors of physiologic health measures in chronic disease. J Chronic Dis 1987;40(suppl):S27–S35.

(56) Goldberg DP. The detection of psychiatric illness by questionnaire. London: Oxford University Press (Maudsley Monograph No. 21), 1972.

(57) Crowne DP, Marlowe D. A new scale of social desirability independent of psychopathology. J Consult Psychol 1960;24:349–354.

(58) Edwards AL. The social desirability variable in personality assessment and research. New York: Dryden, 1957.

(59) Kozma A, Stones MJ. Social desirability in measures of subjective well-being: a systematic evaluation. J Gerontol 1987;42:56–59.

(60) Bradburn NM, Sudman S, Blair E, et al. Question threat and response bias. Public Opin Q 1978;42:221–234.

(61) Totman R. Social causes of illness. London: Souvenir Press, 1979.

(62) Sechrest L, Pitz D. Commentary: measuring the effectiveness of heart transplant pro-grammes. J Chronic Dis 1987;40:S155–S158.

(63) Swets JA. The relative operating characteristic in psychology. Science 1973; 182:990–1000.

(64) Clark WC. Pain sensitivity and the report of pain: an introduction to sensory decision theory. In: Weisenberg M, Tursky B, eds. Pain: new perspectives in therapy and research. New York: Plenum Press, 1976:195–222.

(65) Rollman GB. Signal detection theory assessment of pain modulation: a critique. In: Bonica JJ, Albe-Fessard DG, eds. Advances in pain research and therapy. Vol. I. New York: Raven Press, 1976:355–362.

(66) Hertzog C. Applications of signal detection theory to the study of psychological aging: a theoretical review. In: Poon LW, ed. Aging in the 1980s: psychological issues. Washington, DC: American Psychological Association, 1980:568–591.

(67) McNeil BJ, Keeler E, Adelstein SJ. Primer on certain elements of medical decision making. N Engl J Med 1975;293:211–215.

(68) Yaremko RM, Harari H, Harrison RC, et al. Reference handbook of research and statistical methods in psychology. New York: Harper & Row, 1982.

(69) Gallin RS, Given CW. The concept and classification of disability in health interview surveys. Inquiry 1976;13:395–407.

(70) Slater SB, Vukmanovic C, Macukanovic P, et al. The definition and measurement of disability. Soc Sci Med 1974;8:305–308.

(71) World Health Organization. International classification of impairments, disabilities, and handicaps. A manual of classification relating to the consequences of disease. Geneva: World Health Organization, 1980.

(72) Duckworth D. The need for a standard terminology and classification of disablement. In: Granger CV, Gresham GE, eds. Functional assessment in rehabilitation medicine. Baltimore, Maryland: Williams & Wilkins, 1984:1–13.

(73) Harris A. Handicapped and impaired in Great Britain. London: HMSO, 1971.

(74) Haber LD. Identifying the disabled: concepts and methods in the measurement of disability. Soc Secur Bull 1967;December:17–34.

(75) Nagi SZ. The concept and measurement of disability. In: Berkowitz ED, ed. Disability policies and government programs. New York: Praeger, 1979:1–15.

(76) Patrick DL, Bergner M. Measurement of health status in the 1990s. Annu Rev Public Health 1990;11:165–183.

(77) Ahlbom A, Norell S. Introduction to modern epidemiology. Chestnut Hill, Montana: Epidemiology Resources, 1984.

(78) Webb EJ, Campbell DT, Schwartz RD, et al. Unobtrusive measures: nonreactive research in the social sciences. Chicago: Rand McNally, 1966.

(79) Anastasi A. Psychological testing. New York: Macmillan, 1968.

(80) Helmstadter GC. Principles of psychological measurement. London: Methuen, 1966.

(81) American Psychological Association. Standards for educational and psychological testing. Washington DC: American Psychological Association, 1985.

(82) Feinstein AR. Clinimetrics. New Haven, Connecticut: Yale University Press, 1987.

(83) Seiler LH. The 22-item scale used in field studies of mental illness: a question of method, a question of substance, and a question of theory. J Health Soc Behav 1973;14:252–264.

(84) Hanley JA, McNeil BJ. The meaning and use of the area under a receiver operating characteristic (ROC) curve. Radiology 1982;143:29–36.

(85) Swets JA. Measuring the accuracy of diagnostic systems. Science 1988;240:1285–1293.

(86) Fletcher RH, Fletcher SW, Wagner EH. Clinical epidemiology: the essentials. Baltimore, Maryland: Williams & Wilkins, 1988.

(87) Choi BCK. Sensitivity and specificity of a single diagnostic test in the presence of work-up bias. J Clin Epidemiol 1992; 45:581–586.

(88) Brazier J, Jones N, Kind P. Testing the validity of the Euroqol and comparing it with the SF-36 Health Survey questionnaire. Qual Life Res 1993;2:169–180.

(89) Bland JM, Altman DG. Statistical methods for assessing agreement between two methods of clinical measurement. Lancet 1986;1:307–310.

(90) Comrey AL. Common methodological problems in factor analytic studies. J Consult Clin Psychol 1978;46:648–659.

(91) Boyle GJ. Self-report measures of depression: some psychometric considerations. Br J Clin Psychol 1985;24:45–59.

(92) Felson DT, Anderson JJ, Meenan RF. The comparative efficacy and toxicity of second-line drugs in rheumatoid arthritis. Arthritis Rheum 1990;33:330–338.

(93) Liang MH, Fossel AH, Larson MG. Comparisons of five health status instruments for orthopedic evaluation. Med Care 1990;28:632–642.

(94) Kazis LE, Anderson JJ, Meenan RF. Effect sizes for interpreting changes in health status. Med Care 1989;27(suppl):S178–S189.

(95) Siu AL, Ouslander JG, Osterweil D, et al. Change in self-reported functioning in older persons entering a residential care facility. J Clin Epidemiol 1993;46:1093–1101.

(96) Katz JN, Larson MG, Phillips CB, et al. Comparative measurement sensitivity of short and longer health status instruments. Med Care 1992;30:917–925.

(97) Liang MH, Larson MG, Cullen KE, et al. Comparative measurement efficiency and sensitivity of five health status instruments for arthritis research. Arthritis Rheum 1985;28:542–547.

(98) Deyo RA, Centor RM. Assessing the responsiveness of functional scales to clinical change: an analogy to diagnostic test performance. J Chronic Dis 1986;39:897–906.

(99) Deyo RA, Diehr P, Patrick DL. Reproducibility and responsiveness of health status measures. Statistics and strategies for evaluation. Controlled Clin Trials 1991; 12:142S-158S.

(100) MacKenzie CR, Charlson ME, DiGioia D, et al. Can the Sickness Impact Profile measure change? An example of scale assessment. J Chronic Dis 1986;39:429–438.

(101) MacKenzie CR, Charlson ME, DiGioia D, et al. A patient-specific measure of change in maximal function. Arch Intern Med 1986;146:1325–1329.

(102) Lambert MJ, Hatch DR, Kingston MD, et al. Zung, Beck, and Hamilton rating scales as measures of treatment outcome: a meta-analytic comparison. J Consult Clin Psychol 1986;54:54–59.

(103) Edwards BC, Lambert MJ, Moran PW, et al. A meta-analytic comparison of the Beck Depression Inventory and the Hamilton Rating Scale for Depression as measures of treatment outcome. Br J Clin Psychol 1984;23:93–99.

(104) McHorney CA, Ware JE Jr, Raczek AE. The MOS 36–Item Short-Form Health Survey (SF-36): II. Psychometric and clinical tests of validity in measuring physical and mental health constructs. Med Care 1993;31:247–263.

(105) Kantz ME, Harris WJ, Levitsky K, et al. Methods for assessing condition-specific and generic functional status outcomes after total knee replacement. Med Care 1992;30(suppl):MS240–MS252.

(106) Andrews FM. Construct validity and error components of survey measures: a

structural modelling approach. Public Opin Q 1984;48:409–442.

(107) Wittenborn JR. Reliability, validity, and objectivity of symptom-rating scales. J Nerv Ment Dis 1972;154:79–87.

(108) Evans WJ, Cayten CG, Green PA. Determining the generalizability of rating scales in clinical settings. Med Care 1981;19:1211–1220.

(109) Bartko JJ. Measurement and reliability: statistical thinking considerations. Schizophr Bull 1991;17:483–489.

(110) Siegert CEH, Vleming L-J, Van Den Broucke JP, et al. Measurement of disability in Dutch rheumatoid arthritis patients. Clin Rheumatol 1984;3:305–309.

(111) Bartko JJ. The intraclass correlation as a measure of reliability. Psychol Rep 1966;19:3–11.

(112) Bartko JJ. On various intraclass correlation reliability coefficients. Psychol Bull 1976;83:762–765.

(113) Shrout PE, Fleiss JL. Intraclass correlations: uses in assessing rater reliability. Psychol Bull 1979;86:420–428.

(114) Bohrnstedt GW. Measurement. In: Rossi PH, Wright JD, Anderson AB, eds. Handbook of survey research. New York: Academic Press, 1983:69–95.

(115) Shrout PE, Yager TJ. Reliability and validity of screening scales: effect of reducing scale length. J Clin Epidemiol 1989; 42:69–78.

(116) Landis JR, Koch GG. The measurement of observer agreement for categorical data. Biometrics 1977;33:159–174.

(117) Andrews FM, Withey SB. Social indicators of well-being: Americans' perceptions of life quality. New York: Plenum, 1976.

(118) Rule BG, Harvey HZ, Dobbs AR. Reliability of the Geriatric Depression Scale for younger adults. Clin Gerontol 1989;9:37–43.

(119) Yesavage JA, Brink TL, Rose TL, et al. Development and validation of a geriatric depression screening scale: a preliminary report. J Psychiatr Res 1983;17:37–49.

(120) Rehm LP, O'Hara MW. Item characteristics of the Hamilton Rating Scale for Depression. J Psychiatr Res 1985;19:31–41.

(121) McHorney CA, Ware JE Jr, Lu JFR, et al. The MOS 36-item Short-Form Health Survey (SF-36): III. Tests of data quality, scaling assumptions, and reliability across diverse patient groups. Med Care 1994;32:40–66.

(122) Wolf FM, Cornell RG. Interpreting behavioral, biomedical, and psychological relationships in chronic disease from 2 × 2 tables using correlation. J Chronic Dis 1986;39:605–608.

3

Physical Disability and Handicap

Because they cover an area of such fundamental concern in health care, there has been a proliferation of scales designed to measure physical disability and handicap. The available measurement methods serve a variety of purposes: some apply to particular diseases while others are broadly applicable; some assess impairments, others cover disability, handicap, or the social environment; there are research instruments, screening tests, and clinical rating scales; some methods are designed for severely ill inpatients, while others are for outpatients with lower levels of disability. In this chapter we have reviewed the best methods available and have omitted little-used scales, those that have not stood the test of time, and those which lack published evidence for validity and reliability. Thus, of more than 50 activities of daily living scales described in the literature (1–8), we review only seven. As it turns out, our selection is comparable to that made quite independently in another review article (9). The main surprise, perhaps, will be the inclusion of several older scales in our selection. Many of the newer methods lack the information on reliability and validity that has been accumulated for the older instruments, and we have not included

methods simply because they are new. To introduce the basis for our selection, we begin with a brief historical overview of the development of the field. This identifies the main categories of physical and functional disability measurement, and the chapter will review examples from each category.

THE EVOLUTION OF PHYSICAL DISABILITY MEASUREMENTS

The concepts of impairment, disability, and handicap were introduced in Chapter 2. This conceptual framework has been reflected in the evolution of measurements of physical functioning. Measurement began with the early impairment scales (covering physical capacities such as balance, sensory abilities, and range of motion); attention then shifted toward measuring disability (gross body movements and self-care), and later moved to assessments of handicap (fulfillment of social roles, working ability, and household activities).

Formal measurements of physical impairments began with diagnostic tests and standardized medical summaries of a patient's condition typically used with elderly or chronically ill patients. These were mostly rating scales applied by a clinician; they are represented in this chapter by the PULSES Profile. These measurements were often used in assessing fitness for work or in reviewing claims for accident and injury compensation; the emphasis was on rigorous, standardized ratings that could withstand legal examination. It was later recognized that although impairment may be accurately assessed, it is by no means the only factor that predicts a patient's need for care: environmental factors, the availability of social support, and the patient's determination all affect how far an impairment will be translated into disability or handicap. As the scope of rehabilitation expanded to include the return of patients to an independent existence, the assessment of physical impairment was no longer sufficient and it became important to measure disability and handicap as well. Assessment methods were enlarged to consider the activities a patient could or did perform at his level of physical capacity. Assessments of this type are generally termed functional disability indicators. Most of the scales we review are measures of functional disability; the chapter title refers to "physical disability" to distinguish physical, rather than mental, problems as the source of the functional limitations. The activities of daily living (ADL) scales are typical; an early example is Katz's index. This was developed in 1957 to study the effects of treatment on the elderly and chronically ill. It summarizes the patient's degree of independence in bathing, dressing, using the toilet, moving around the house, and eating—topics that Katz selected to represent "primary biological functions." Katz's scale is one of the few instruments to provide a theoretical justification for the topics it includes. Unfortunately, most other ADL scales are not built on any conceptual approach to disability, and there is little systematic effort to specify what topics should be covered in such scales. In part because of this, progress in the field was uncoordinated, and scales proliferated apparently at the whim of their creators. Furthermore,

scant attention was paid to formal testing of the ADL methods and we know little about their comparative validity and reliability.

The ADL scales are concerned with more severe levels of disability, relevant mainly to institutionalized patients and to the elderly. During the 1970s, the ADL concept was extended to consider problems more typically experienced by those living in the community: mobility, difficulty in shopping, cooking, or managing money, a field that has come to be termed Instrumental Activities of Daily Living (IADL) or Performance Activities of Daily Living. By broadening the scope of ADL scales, the IADL methods offer indicators of "applied" problems that extend the disability theme of ADL scales to include some elements of the handicap concept. This forms the second major category of measurements described in this chapter. Although the IADL scales are newer and have been somewhat better tested than the ADL instruments, there is often little conceptual justification or theory to guide their content.

The development of IADL scales was stimulated in part by the movement toward community care for the elderly. While ADL scales tend to be universal in content, IADL scales may vary from culture to culture. For example, a British IADL scale included items on making tea and carrying a tray, a Dutch scale included making a bed, and a New Zealand scale covered gardening ability (10, p704). Rehabilitation medicine has increasingly stressed the need to restore patients to meaningful social roles, and this has inspired measurement scales that cover social adjustment as well as physical abilities. To assess a patient's ability to live in the community requires information on the level of disability, on the environment in which the patient has to live, on the amount of social support that may be available, and on some of the compensating factors that determine whether or not a disability becomes a handicap. The IADL scales cover one part of this area, but other, more extensive scales have been developed to record factors that may explain different levels of handicap for a given disability such as the type of work the patient does, his housing, his personality, and the social support available. Such extensions to the original theme of functional disability produce measurements that are conceptually close to the indices of social functioning described in Chapter 4.

Some general issues inherent in the design of ADL and IADL scales should be borne in mind by those who are choosing a scale for a particular application. As noted earlier, most ADL questions reflect relatively severe levels of disability and so are insensitive to variations at the upper levels of functioning, where most people score. Care has to be taken, therefore, in selecting a measure for use in surveys or with relatively healthy patients. Those selecting a measure for such applications may prefer instruments such as the Medical Outcomes Study (MOS) Physical Functioning Measure, which includes items on more strenuous physical activities, while still retaining items on basic abilities such as dressing or walking. The other approach is to rely on IADL items to reflect higher levels of function. However, IADL scales are not pure measures of physical function: activities such as cooking, shopping, and cleaning reflect social roles as well as physical capacity. For example, however much their wives may complain, there are reasons other than physical limitations why some men may not cook or clean house. By comparison, ADL items on walking or bathing are more likely to offer pure measures of physical function. A further consideration is that assessing the extent of difficulty, or the need for help in performing an activity, as opposed to merely asking about performance, may improve sensitivity. Jette used separate measures of pain, difficulty, and dependency in the Functional Status Index.

The distinction between a person's physical capacity and his actual performance in managing his life in the face of physical limitations has been mentioned. Reflecting this contrast, there are two ways of phrasing questions on functional disability. One can ask what a person *can* do (the "capacity" wording) or what she *does* do ("performance" wording). Both are common and both hold advantages and disadvantages. Asking a patient what she can do may provide a hypothetical answer that records what the patient thinks she can do even though she does not normally attempt it. An index using such questions may exaggerate the healthiness of the respondent—perhaps by as much as 15% to 20% (11, p70). While the performance wording may overcome this, it can run the opposite risk. As factors other than ill health may restrict behavior, such questions may not be very specific. Performance wording must select only the health reasons why a person did not do an activity, but this is difficult to judge as health interacts with other factors such as the weather. It may become very difficult, therefore, to determine whether something that a person did not do was due to health reasons. For example, for reasons of safety, hospitals may require nurses to supervise patients, and hospital patients may be kept in bed. For these reasons performance questions may give a lower score than capacity questions, which provide rather more discretion in accounting for nonperformance of a task. Capacity wording is therefore often used in IADL questions, which are more susceptible to such bias than ADL questions. Most recent ADL indices favor the performance approach for ADL items, although an intermediate phrasing can be used, such as "Do you have difficulty with . . . ?" as used in the Lambeth Disability Screening Questionnaire and the Organization for Economic Cooperation and Development (OECD) Disability Questionnaire.

It would be misleading to present the general evolution of functional disability measurements in a way that suggests the field is well established, for the actual quality of the measurements is, regrettably, not yet impressive. In the first edition of this book, we noted that this field of measurement is in its infancy in terms of the psychometric properties of the measurements—reliability, validity, and conceptual clarity (12). Since then, considerable progress has been made, and we have added new psychometric evidence for virtually all of the measurements. Nonetheless, the field remains less well established than the others we review. Items are commonly selected on the basis of clinical judgment without broader reference to a body of theory. Scoring is often rudimentary, and reliability and validity are inadequately assessed. The resulting uncertainty leaves the potential user with a wide choice of scales but an inadequate basis from which to choose among them (13).

The uncertain quality of many of the available scales did, however, provide an approach to narrowing our selection. Because our emphasis is on instruments that can be used in research studies, we stress the importance of reliability and validity results in their selection. As very few disability measurements have been thoroughly tested, we compromised between describing large numbers of measurement methods that we could not really recommend because their quality remains unknown, and the opposite extreme of reviewing an exceedingly small number of scales of proven quality. Because so little is known about many methods, we have described several scales that appear to hold potential, although this is not fully established. We have classified the available measurements into those that cover physical functioning alone (ADL scales) and those that are broader in scope (IADL scales). Within each category we included only those measurements for which the questionnaire is available, for which there is some evidence on reliability or validity, and which have been used in published studies. We have sought to keep the scope of the chapter broad and have included methods whose purpose is primarily clinical as well as those intended for survey research. Readers should note that many of the general health measures reviewed in Chapter 9 also include sections on physical functioning and disability. Examples include the Multidimensional Functional Assessment Questionnaire and the Sickness Impact Profile, both of which contain ADL and IADL sections that may prove suitable for use as stand-alone scales.

Before describing individual scales, we provide a summary table designed to help the reader review the alternative measurements and select at a glance those that may be of particular interest. Table 3.1 summarizes the format, length, and use of each scale and published evidence on its reliability and validity.

REFERENCES

(1) Berg RL, ed. Health status indexes. Chicago: Hospital Research and Educational Trust, 1973.

(2) Bruett TL, Overs RP. A critical review of 12 ADL scales. Phys Ther 1969;49:857–862.

(3) Donaldson SW, Wagner CC, Gresham GE. A unified ADL evaluation form. Arch Phys Med Rehabil 1973;54:175–179, 185.

(4) Forer SK. Functional assessment instruments in medical rehabilitation. J Organization Rehabil Evaluators 1982;2:29–41.

(5) Linn MW, Linn BS. Problems in assessing response to treatment in the elderly by physical and social function. Psychopharmacol Bull 1981;17:74–81.

(6) Liang MH, Jette AM. Measuring functional disability in chronic arthritis: a critical review. Arthritis Rheum 1981;24:80–86.

(7) Brown M, Gordon WA, Diller L. Functional assessment and outcome measurement: an integrative view. In: Pan EL, Backer TE, Vasch CL, eds. Annual review of rehabilitation. Vol. 3. New York: Springer, 1983:93–120.

(8) Katz S, Hedrick SC, Henderson NS. The measurement of long-term care needs and impact. Health Med Care Serv Rev 1979;2:1–21.

(9) Gresham GE, Labi MLC. Functional assessment instruments currently available for documenting outcomes in rehabilitation medicine. In: Granger CV, Gresham GE, eds. Functional assessment in rehabilitation medicine. Baltimore, Maryland: Williams & Wilkins, 1984:65–85.

(10) Fillenbaum GG. Screening the elderly: a brief instrumental activities of daily living

Table 3.1 Comparison of the Quality of Physical Disability Indices*

ADL Scales	Scale	Number of items	Application	Administered by (time)	Studies using method	Reliability		Validity	
						Thoroughness	Results	Thoroughness	Results
PULSES Profile (Moskowitz, 1957)	ordinal	6	clinical	staff	many	+	++	+	++
Barthel Index (Mahoney, 1955)	ordinal	10	clinical	staff (2–5 min), self (10 min)	many	+++	+++	+++	++
Index of ADL (Katz, 1959)	ordinal	6	clinical	staff	many	+	+	++	++
Kenny Self-Care Evaluation (Schoening, 1965)	ordinal	85	clinical	staff	several	+	+	+	++
Physical Self-Maintenance Scale (Lawton, 1969)	Guttman	6	survey	self-, staff	few	+	++	+	++
Functional Status Rating System (Forer, 1981)	ordinal	30	clinical	staff (15–20 min)	few	+	++	+	0
Medical Outcomes Study Physical Functioning Measures (Stewart, 1992)	ordinal	14	survey	self	few	+	+	+	++
IADL Scales									
Rapid Disability Rating Scale (Linn, 1982)	ordinal	18	research	staff (2 min)	several	++	++	++	+
Functional Status Index (Jette, 1980)	ordinal	45	clinical	interviewer (60–90 min)	several	+++	++	++	++
Patient Evaluation Conference System (Harvey, 1981)	ordinal	79	clinical	staff	few	+	+	+	+
Functional Activities Questionnaire (Pfeffer, 1982)	ordinal	10	survey	lay informant	few	+	+	++	++
Lambeth Disability Screening Questionnaire (Patrick, 1981)	ordinal	25	survey	self	few	+	?	++	++
Disability Interview Schedule (Bennett, 1970)	ordinal	17	survey	interviewer	few	+	+	+	+
OECD Disability Questionnaire (OECD, 1981)	ordinal	16	survey	self	many	++	+	++	+
Health Assessment Questionnaire (Fries, 1980)	ordinal	20	clinical, research	self, staff (5–8 min)	many	+++	+++	+++	+++
Functional Independence Measure (Granger, 1987)	ordinal	18	clinical	expert, interviewer	many	++	+++	++	++

* For an explanation of the categories used, see Chapter 1, pages 6–7

measure. J Am Geriatr Soc 1985;33:698–706.

(11) Patrick DL, Darby SC, Green S, et al. Screening for disability in the inner city. J Epidemiol Community Health 1981;35: 65–70.

(12) Frey WD. Functional assessment in the '80s: a conceptual enigma, a technical challenge. In: Halpern AS, Fuhrer MJ, eds. Functional assessment in rehabilitation. Baltimore, Maryland: Paul H. Brookes, 1984.

(13) Keith RA. Functional assessment measures in medical rehabilitation: current status. Arch Phys Med Rehabil 1984;65:74–78.

ADL SCALES

This section provides descriptions of seven ADL scales: the PULSES, Barthel, Katz, and Kenny scales, a less widely known scale by Lawton and Brody, one by Forer, and the most recent, the Medical Outcomes Study instrument. It was not originally our intention to include so many older scales but in general they have been more fully tested than the newer methods. Testing, of course, does not guarantee quality, but at least we have information on their performance, information that is sorely lacking for several dozen other ADL scales that we also considered for inclusion. Some of the scales that we considered but did not include are described briefly in the Conclusion to this section, page 81.

The first of the ADL scales we review, the PULSES Profile, is an example of the physical impairment and disability assessment methods from which the subsequent functional disability scales were derived. As mentioned in Chapter 2, the need to assess the physical fitness of recruits in World War II led to the development of a number of assessment scales, mostly known by acronyms that indicate their content. Thus, the PULSES Profile was developed from the Canadian Army's "Physical Standards and Instructions" for the medical examination of soldiers and army recruits (1943), known as the PULHEMS Profile. In this acronym, P = physique, U = upper extremity, L = lower extremity, H = hearing and ears, E = eyes and vision, M = mental capacity, and S = emotional stability, with ratings in each category ranging from normal to totally unfit. A subsequent revision was known as PLUMSHEAF. The United States Army later adapted the PULHEMS system and merged the mental and emotional categories under the acronym PULHES. Moskowitz and McCann made further modifications to produce the PULSES Profile described here. Although the PULSES Profile is old and is included primarily for its historical significance, it continues to be used (often in conjunction with other ADL scales such as the Barthel) and is also used occasionally as a validation criterion scale. The PULSES Profile and the Barthel Index have both influenced the design of the other scales we review here.

THE PULSES PROFILE
Eugene Moskowitz and
Cairbre B. McCann, 1957

Purpose

The PULSES Profile was designed to evaluate functional independence in activities of daily living of chronically ill and elderly institutionalized populations (1, 2). It expresses "the ability of an aged, infirm individual to perform routine physical activities within the limitations imposed by various physical disorders" (2, p2009). The profile is commonly used to predict rehabilitation potential, to evaluate patient progress, and to assist in program planning (3).

Conceptual Basis

No information is available.

Description

The PULSES Profile was modified from earlier assessments of fitness for military duty. The components of the acronym are:

P = physical condition
U = upper limb functions
L = lower limb functions

S = sensory components (speech, vision, hearing)

E = excretory functions

S = mental and emotional status

The profile may be completed retrospectively from medical records, or from interviews and observations of the patient (4, p146). In this vein, Moskowitz saw the profile "as a vehicle for consolidation of fragments of clinical information gathered in a rehabilitation setting by various staff members involved in the patient's daily care" (5, p647).

Four levels of impairment were originally specified for each component (1, Table 1) and the six scores were presented separately, as a profile. Thus, "L-3" describes a person who can walk under supervision and "E-3" indicates frequent incontinence (5). The original PULSES Profile was reproduced in our first edition, page 46; a summary of it is shown in Exhibit 3.1, and the revised version is shown in Exhibit 3.2. Moskowitz argued against calculating an overall score, which may obscure changes in one category that are balanced by opposite changes in another. For clinical applications, Moskowitz later summarized the categories (see Exhibit 3.1) and presented them in a color-coded chart (reproduced in reference 5).

Granger proposed a revised version of the PULSES Profile with slight modifications to the classification levels and an expanded scope for three categories. Exhibit 3.2 shows that the upper limb category was extended to include self-care activities, the lower limb category was extended to include mobility, and the social and mental category was extended to include emotional adaptability, family support, and finances (4, p153). This version provides an overall score, with equal weighting for each category to give a scale from 6, indicating unimpaired independence, to 24, indicating full dependence. Granger suggested that a score of 12 distinguishes lesser from more marked disability and that 16 or above indicates very severe disability (4, p152).

Reliability

For the revised version, Granger et al. reported a test–retest reliability of 0.87 and an inter-rater reliability exceeding 0.95, comparable to their results for the Barthel Index (4, p150).

Validity

In a study of 307 severely disabled adults in ten rehabilitation centers across the United States, Granger et al. showed the PULSES Profile to be capable of reflecting changes between admission and discharge. Scores at discharge corresponded to the disposition of patients: those returning home were rated significantly higher than those sent to long-term institutions, who in turn scored significantly higher than those referred for acute care (3, 4, 7). Pearson correlation coefficients between PULSES and Barthel scores ranged from -0.74 to -0.80 ($p < 0.001$; the negative correlations reflect the inverse scoring of the scales) (4, pp146–147).

Alternative Forms

Granger's modifications to the PULSES have been outlined earlier. Warren developed a modified version called PULHEEMS to screen for disability in the general population (6).

Commentary

The PULSES scale is the last of the physical measurement scales developed during World War II that still sees some use. Although it is often compared with the Barthel Index, the two are not strictly equivalent. Granger et al. noted that the Barthel measures discrete functions (e.g., eating and ambulation), which may be relevant to clinical staff; PULSES cannot do this. However, the PULSES Profile is broader than the Barthel, tapping communication as well as social and mental factors (4, p146).

As reflected in Table 3.1 in the introduction to this chapter, the reliability and validity of the PULSES have been less well

Exhibit 3.1 Summary Chart from the Original PULSES Profile

	P Physical Condition	U Upper Extremities	L Lower Extremities	S Sensory Function	E Excretory Functions	S Social and Mental Status
	cardiovascular pulmonary and other visceral disorders	shoulder girdles, cervical and upper dorsal spine	pelvis, lower dorsal and lumbosacral spine	vision, hearing, speech	bowel and bladder	emotional and psychiatric disorders
NORMAL	1 Health maintenance	1 Complete function	1 Complete function	1 Complete function	1 Continent	1 Compatible with age
MILD	2 Occasional medical supervision	2 No assistance required	2 Fully ambulatory despite some loss of function	2 No appreciable functional impairment	2 Occasional stress incontinence or nocturia	2 No supervision required
MODERATELY SEVERE	3 Frequent medical supervision	3 Some assistance necessary	3 Limited ambulation	3 Appreciable bilateral loss or complete unilateral loss of vision or hearing. Incomplete aphasia	3 Periodic incontinence or retention	3 Some supervision necessary
SEVERE	4 Total care Bed or chair confined	4 Nursing care	4 Confined to wheelchair or bed	4 Total blindness Total deafness Global aphasia or aphonia	4 Total incontinence or retention (including catheter and colostomy)	4 Complete care in psychiatric facility

Adapted from Moskowitz E. PULSES Profile in retrospect. Arch Phys Med Rehabil 1985;66:648.

Exhibit 3.2 The PULSES Profile: Revised Version

P - Physical condition: Includes diseases of the viscera (cardiovascular, gastrointestinal, urologic, and endocrine) and neurologic disorders:

1. Medical problems sufficiently stable that medical or nursing monitoring is not required more often than 3-month intervals.
2. Medical or nurse monitoring is needed more often than 3-month intervals but not each week.
3. Medical problems are sufficiently unstable as to require regular medical and/or nursing attention at least weekly.
4. Medical problems require intensive medical and/or nursing attention at least daily (excluding personal care assistance only).

U - Upper limb functions: Self-care activities (drink/feed, dress upper/lower, brace/prosthesis, groom, wash, perineal care) dependent mainly upon upper limb function:

1. Independent in self-care without impairment of upper limbs.
2. Independent in self-care with some impairment of upper limbs.
3. Dependent upon assistance or supervision in self-care with or without impairment of upper limbs.
4. Dependent totally in self-care with marked impairment of upper limbs.

L - Lower limb functions: Mobility (transfer chair/toilet/tub or shower, walk, stairs, wheelchair) dependent mainly upon lower limb function:

1. Independent in mobility without impairment of lower limbs.
2. Independent in mobility with some impairment in lower limbs; such as needing ambulatory aids, a brace or prosthesis, or else fully independent in a wheelchair without significant architectural or environmental barriers.
3. Dependent upon assistance or supervision in mobility with or without impairment of lower limbs, or partly independent in a wheelchair, or there are significant architectural or environmental barriers.
4. Dependent totally in mobility with marked impairment of lower limbs.

S - Sensory components: Relating to communication (speech and hearing) and vision:

1. Independent in communication and vision without impairment.
2. Independent in communication and vision with some impairment such as mild dysarthria, mild aphasia, or need for eyeglasses or hearing aid, or needing regular eye medication.
3. Dependent upon assistance, an interpreter, or supervision in communication or vision.
4. Dependent totally in communication or vision.

E - Excretory functions: (bladder and bowel):

1. Complete voluntary control of bladder and bowel sphincters.
2. Control of sphincters allows normal social activities despite urgency or need for catheter, appliance, suppositories, etc. Able to care for needs without assistance.
3. Dependent upon assistance in sphincter management or else has accidents occasionally.
4. Frequent wetting or soiling from incontinence of bladder or bowel sphincters.

S - Support factors: Consider intellectual and emotional adaptability, support from family unit, and financial ability:

1. Able to fulfill usual roles and perform customary tasks.
2. Must make some modification in usual roles and performance of customary tasks.
3. Dependent upon assistance, supervision, encouragement or assistance from a public or private agency due to any of the above considerations.
4. Dependent upon long-term institutional care (chronic hospitalization, nursing home, etc.) excluding time-limited hospital for specific evaluation, treatment, or active rehabilitation.

Reproduced from Granger CV, Albrecht GL, Hamilton BB. Outcome of comprehensive medical rehabilitation: measurement by PULSES Profile and the Barthel Index. Arch Phys Med Rehabil 1979;60:153. With permission.

tested than those of alternative scales such as the Barthel Index. In recent years the PULSES Profile has seen less use than other scales and eventually it may be superseded. Nonetheless, as a brief rating method it appears adequate.

REFERENCES

(1) Moskowitz E, McCann CB. Classification of disability in the chronically ill and aging. J Chronic Dis 1957;5:342–346.
(2) Moskowitz E, Fuhn ER, Peters ME, et al. Aged infirm residents in a custodial institu-

tion: two-year medical and social study. JAMA 1959;169:2009–2012.

(3) Granger CV, Greer DS. Functional status measurement and medical rehabilitation outcomes. Arch Phys Med Rehabil 1976;57:103–109.

(4) Granger CV, Albrecht GL, Hamilton BB. Outcome of comprehensive medical rehabilitation: measurement by PULSES Profile and the Barthel Index. Arch Phys Med Rehabil 1979;60:145–154.

(5) Moskowitz E. PULSES Profile in retrospect. Arch Phys Med Rehabil 1985; 66:647–648.

(6) Warren MD. The use of the PULHEEMS system of medical classification in civilian practice. Br J Ind Med 1956;13:202–209.

(7) Granger CV, Sherwood CC, Greer DS. Functional status measures in a comprehensive stroke care program. Arch Phys Med Rehabil 1977;58:555–561.

THE BARTHEL INDEX
(Formerly The Maryland Disability Index)
(Florence I. Mahoney and
Dorothea W. Barthel; In Use Since 1955,
First Published by Originators in 1958)

Purpose

The Barthel Index measures functional independence in personal care and mobility; it was developed to monitor performance in chronic patients before and after treatment and to indicate the amount of nursing care needed (1). It was intended for long-term hospital patients with paralytic conditions and has been used with rehabilitation patients to predict length of stay, estimate prognosis, anticipate discharge outcomes, and as an evaluative instrument.

Conceptual Basis

Items were chosen to indicate the level of nursing care required by a patient. A weighting system for each item reflects the relative importance of each type of disability in terms of nursing care needed and social acceptability (1, p606). Reflecting this orientation, Granger has placed the Barthel Index conceptually within the WHO impairment, disability, and handicap framework (2).

Description

The Barthel Index is a rating scale completed by a health professional from medical records or from direct observation (3). It takes two to five minutes to complete (4, p62), or it can be self-administered in about ten minutes (5, p125). Two main versions exist: the original ten-item form and an expanded 15-item version. The original ten activities cover personal care and mobility. Each item is rated in terms of whether the patient can perform the task independently, with some assistance, or is dependent on help. An overall score is formed by adding scores on each rating and suggests the amount of time and assistance a patient will require (6, p61). Scores range from 0 to 100, in steps of 5, with higher scores indicating greater independence. The items and scoring system are shown in Exhibit 3.3; rating guidelines are shown in Exhibit 3.4. The "with help" category is used if any degree of supervision or assistance is required. Wylie and White also published detailed scoring instructions (7, Appendix).

Many modifications have been made to the Barthel scale, of which two have been commonly used: a variant of the ten-item version proposed by Collin and Wade in England (4), and 15-item versions proposed by Granger (3, 8, 9). Collin and Wade's version, shown in Exhibit 3.5, reordered the original ten items, clarified the rating instructions, and modified the scores for each item. Total scores range from 0 to 20. This version also moves from the capacity orientation of the original to a performance rating, indicating what the patient actually does rather than what she could do. Shah et al. retained the original ten items but proposed five-point rating scales for each item to improve sensitivity in detecting change (10). At present there seems little consensus over which should be viewed as the definitive version if the ten-item Barthel is chosen.

Granger extended the Barthel Index to cover 15 topics in an instrument sometimes called the Modified Barthel Index. Two versions exist: a 1979 variant that includes eating and drinking as separate items (3) and a 1981 form that merges eating and drinking and adds an item on dressing after using the toilet (9, Table 1). The latter version is recommended; it uses four-point response scales for most items, with overall scores ranging from 0 to 100 (8, Table 12–2; 9, Table 1). This version is outlined in Exhibit 3.6.

Several authors have proposed guidelines for interpreting Barthel scores. Shah et al. suggested that scores of 0–20 (on either ten- or 15-item versions) indicate total dependency, 21–60 indicate severe dependency, 61–90 moderate dependency, and 91–99 indicate slight dependency (10, p704). Lazar et al. proposed the following interpretation for 15-item scores: 0–19: dependent; 20–59: self-care assisted; 60–79: wheelchair assisted; 80–89: wheelchair independent; 90–99: ambulatory assisted; 100 indicates independence (11, p820). For the 15-item version Granger commonly takes a score of 60 as the threshold between more marked dependence and independence (12). Forty or below indicates severe dependence, with markedly diminished likelihood of living in the community (2,

p48). Twenty or below reflects total dependence in self-care and mobility (3, p152). Later studies continue to apply the 60/61 cutting point, with the recognition that the Barthel Index should not be used alone for predicting outcomes (13, p102; 14, p508).

Reliability

Ten-Item Version. Shah reported alpha internal consistency coefficients of 0.87 to 0.92 (at admission and discharge) for the original scoring system and 0.90 to 0.93 for her revised scoring method (10, p706).

Wartski and Green retested 41 patients after a 3-week delay. For 35 patients, scores fell within ten points; of the six cases with more discrepant scores, two could be explained (15, pp357–358).

Collin et al. studied agreement among four ways of administering the scale to 25 patients: self-report, report by a nurse, based on clinical impressions, testing by a nurse, and testing by a physiotherapist (4). Kendall's coefficient of concordance among the four rating methods was 0.93 (4, p61). This figure somewhat obscures the extent of disagreement, however. There was no major disagreement for 60% of patients and disagreement on one rating for 28%;

Exhibit 3.3 The Barthel Index

Note: A score of zero is given when the patient cannot meet the defined criterion.

	With help	Independent
1. Feeding (if food needs to be cut up = help)	5	10
2. Moving from wheelchair to bed and return (includes sitting up in bed)	5–10	15
3. Personal toilet (wash face, comb hair, shave, clean teeth)	0	5
4. Getting on and off toilet (handling clothes, wipe, flush)	5	10
5. Bathing self	0	5
6. Walking on level surface	10	15
(or if unable to walk, propel wheelchair)	0*	5*
* score only if unable to walk		
7. Ascend and descend stairs	5	10
8. Dressing (includes tying shoes, fastening fasteners)	5	10
9. Controlling bowels	5	10
10. Controlling bladder	5	10

Reproduced from Mahoney FI, Barthel DW. Functional evaluation: the Barthel Index. Maryland State Med J 1965;14:62. With permission.

Exhibit 3.4 Instructions for Scoring the Barthel Index

Note: A score of zero is given when the patient cannot meet the defined criterion.

1. Feeding
    10 = Independent. The patient can feed himself a meal from a tray or table when someone puts the food within his reach. He must put on an assistive device if this is needed, cut up the food, use salt and pepper, spread butter, etc. He must accomplish this in a reasonable time.
    5 = Some help is necessary (when cutting up food, etc., as listed above).
2. Moving from wheelchair to bed and return
    15 = Independent in all phases of this activity. Patient can safely approach the bed in his wheelchair, lock brakes, lift footrests, move safely to bed, lie down, come to a sitting position on the side of the bed, change the position of the wheelchair, if necessary, to transfer back into it safely, and return to the wheelchair.
    10 = Either some minimal help is needed in some step of this activity or the patient needs to be reminded or supervised for safety of one or more parts of this activity.
    5 = Patient can come to sitting position without the help of a second person but needs to be lifted out of bed, or if he transfers, with a great deal of help.
3. Doing personal toilet
    5 = Patient can wash hands and face, comb hair, clean teeth, and shave. He may use any kind of razor but must put in blade or plug in razor without help as well as get it from drawer or cabinet. Female patients must put on own make-up, if used, but need not braid or style hair.
4. Getting on and off toilet
    10 = Patient is able to get on and off toilet, fasten and unfasten clothes, prevent soiling of clothes, and use toilet paper without help. He may use a wall bar or other stable object of support if needed. If it is necessary to use a bed pan instead of a toilet, he must be able to place it on a chair, empty it, and clean it.
    5 = Patient needs help because of imbalance or in handling clothes or in using toilet paper.
5. Bathing self
    5 = Patient may use a bathtub, a shower, or take a complete sponge bath. He must be able to do all the steps involved in whichever method is employed without another person being present.
6. Walking on a level surface
    15 = Patient can walk at least 50 yards without help or supervision. He may wear braces or prostheses and use crutches, canes, or a walkerette but not a rolling walker. He must be able to lock and unlock braces if used, assume the standing position and sit down, get the necessary mechanical aids into position for use, and dispose of them when he sits. (Putting on and taking off braces is scored under dressing.)
    10 = Patient needs help or supervision in any of the above but can walk at least 50 yards with a little help.
6a. Propelling a wheelchair
    5 = If a patient cannot ambulate but can propel a wheelchair independently. He must be able to go around corners, turn around, maneuver the chair to a table, bed, toilet, etc. He must be able to push a chair a least 50 yards. Do not score this item if the patient gets score for walking.
7. Ascending and descending stairs
    10 = Patient is able to go up and down a flight of stairs safely without help or supervision. He may and should use handrails, canes, or crutches when needed. He must be able to carry canes or crutches as he ascends or descends stairs.
    5 = Patient needs help with or supervision of any one of the above items.
8. Dressing and undressing
    10 = Patient is able to put on and remove and fasten all clothing, and tie shoe laces (unless it is necessary to use adaptations for this). The activity includes putting on and removing and fastening corset or braces when these are prescribed. Such special clothing as suspenders, loafer shoes, dresses that open down the front may be used when necessary.
    5 = Patient needs help in putting on and removing or fastening any clothing. He must do at least half the work himself. He must accomplish this in a reasonable time.
       Women need not be scored on use of a brassiere or girdle unless these are prescribed garments.
9. Continence of bowels
    10 = Patient is able to control his bowels and have no accidents. He can use a suppository or take an enema when necessary (as for spinal cord injury patients who have had bowel training).
    5 = Patient needs help in using a suppository or taking an enema or has occasional accidents.
10. Controlling bladder
    10 = Patient is able to control his bladder day and night. Spinal cord injury patients who wear an external device and leg bag must put them on independently, clean and empty bag, and stay dry day and night.
    5 = Patient has occasional accidents or cannot wait for the bed pan or get to the toilet in time or needs help with an external device.

Reproduced form Mahoney FI, Barthel DW. Functional evaluation: the Barthel Index. Maryland State Med J 1965;14:62–65. With permission.

Exhibit 3.5 Scoring and Guidelines for the 10-Item Modified Barthel Index

General

The Index should be used as a record of *what a patient does*, NOT as a record of *what a patient could do*.

The main aim is to establish *degree of independence from any help*, physical or verbal, however minor and for whatever reason.

The need for *supervision* renders the patient, NOT *independent*.

A patient's performance should be established *using the best available evidence*. Asking the patient, friends/relatives and nurses will be the usual source, but direct observation and common sense are also important. However, *direct testing is not needed*.

Usually the performance over the *preceding 24–48 hours* is important, but occasionally longer periods will be relevant.

Unconscious patients should score "0" throughout, even if not yet incontinent.

Middle categories imply that patient supplies *over 50% of the effort*.

Use of aids to be independent is *allowed*.

Bowels (preceding week)

0 = incontinent (or needs to be given enemata)
1 = occasional accident (once/week)
2 = continent
   If needs enema from nurse, then 'incontinent.'
   Occasional = once a week.

Bladder (preceding week)

0 = incontinent, or catheterized and unable to manage
1 = occasional accident (max. once per 24 hours)
2 = continent (for over 7 days)
   Occasional = less than once a day.
   A catheterized patient who can completely manage the catheter alone is registered as 'continent.'

Grooming (preceding 24–48 hours)

0 = needs help with personal care
1 = independent face/hair/teeth/shaving (implements provided)
   Refers to personal hygiene: doing teeth, fitting false teeth, doing hair, shaving, washing face. Implements can be provided by helper.

Toilet use

0 = dependent
1 = needs some help, but can do something alone
2 = independent (on and off, dressing, wiping). Should be able to reach toilet/commode, undress sufficiently, clean self, dress and leave
   With help = can wipe self, and do some other of above.

Feeding

0 = unable
1 = needs help cutting, spreading butter etc.
2 = independent (food provided in reach). Able to eat any normal food (not only soft food). Food cooked and served by others. But not cut up.
   Help = food cut up, patient feeds self.

Transfer (from bed to chair and back)

0 = unable—no sitting balance
1 = major help (one or two people, physical), can sit
2 = minor help (verbal or physical)
3 = independent
   Dependent = no sitting balance (unable to sit); two people to lift.
   Major help = one strong/skilled, or two normal people. Can sit up.
   Minor help = one person easily, OR needs any supervision for safety.

Mobility

0 = immobile
1 = wheelchair independent including corners etc.
2 = walks with help of one person (verbal or physical)
3 = independent (but may use any aid, e.g. stick)

Exhibit 3.5 *(Continued)*

Exhibit 3.5 *(Continued)*

Refers to mobility about the house or ward, indoors. May use aid. If in wheelchair, must negotiate corners/doors unaided.

Help = by one, untrained person, including supervision/moral support.

Dressing

0 = dependent

1 = needs help, but can do about half unaided

2 = independent (including buttons, zips, laces, etc.)

Should be able to select and put on all clothes, which may be adapted.

Half = help with buttons, zips, etc. (check!), but can put on some garments alone.

Stairs

0 = unable

1 = needs help (verbal, physical, carrying aid)

2 = independent up and down

Must carry any walking aid used to be independent.

Bathing

0 = dependent

1 = independent (or in shower)

Usually the most difficult activity.

Must get in and out unsupervised, and wash self.

Independent in shower = 'independent' if unsupervised/unaided.

Total (0–20)

Adapted from Collin C, Wade DT, Davies S, Horne V. The Barthel ADL Index: a reliability study. Int Disabil Stud 1988;10:63.

Exhibit 3.6 Scoring for the 15-Item Modified Barthel Index

Independent		Dependent		
I Intact	II Limited	III Helper	IV Null	
10	5	0	0	Drink from cup/feed from dish
5	5	3	0	Dress upper body
5	5	2	0	Dress lower body
0	0	−2		Don brace or prosthesis
5	5	0	0	Grooming
4	4	0	0	Wash or bathe
10	10	5	0	Bladder continence
10	10	5	0	Bowel continence
4	4	2	0	Care of perineum/clothing at toilet
15	15	7	0	Transfer, chair
6	5	3	0	Transfer, toilet
1	1	0	0	Transfer, tub or shower
15	15	10	0	Walk on level 50 yards or more
10	10	5	0	Up and down stairs for one flight or more
15	5	0	0	Wheelchair/50 yards—only if not walking

Reproduced from Fortinsky RH, Granger CV, Seltzer GB. The use of functional assessment in understanding home care needs. Med Care 1981;19:489, Table 1. With permission.

12% had more discrepancies (16, p357). Self-report accorded least well with the other methods; agreement was lowest for items on transfers, feeding, dressing, grooming, and toileting. Roy et al. found an inter-rater correlation of 0.99. The correlation between ratings and patient self-report was 0.88 (17, Table 2).

Fifteen-Item Version. Granger et al. reported a test–retest reliability of 0.89 with severely disabled adults; the inter-rater agreement exceeded 0.95 (3, p150).

Shinar et al. obtained an inter-rater agreement of 0.99 and a Cronbach's alpha of 0.98 for 18 patients (18, pp724, 726). They also compared administration by telephone interview and by observation for 72 outpatients. Total scores correlated 0.97, and rho correlations exceeded 0.85 for all but one item (18, Table 3).

Validity

Ten-Item Version. Wade reported validity information for the revised ten-item version shown in Exhibit 3.5. Correlations between 0.73 and 0.77 were obtained with an index of motor ability for 976 stroke patients (19, p178). A factor analysis identified two factors, which approximate the mobility and personal-care groupings of the items. Wade et al. also provided evidence for a hierarchical structure in the scale in terms of the order of recovery of function (19, Table 4).

Several studies have assessed predictive validity. In studies of stroke patients, the percentages of those who died within six months of admission fell significantly ($p < 0.001$) as Barthel scores at admission rose (7, p836; 12, p557; 20, p799; 21, Table 4). Among survivors, admission scores also predicted the length of stay and subsequent progress as rated by a physician. Seventy-seven percent of those scoring 60 to 100 points at admission were later said to have improved compared to 36% of those scoring 0 to 15 (20, p800; 22, p894). Most discrepancies between the change scores and the physician's impression of improve-

ment occurred because of the omission of speech and mental functioning from the index (7, p836).

Fifteen-Item Version. Fortinsky et al. reported correlations between Barthel scores and performance of 72 tasks. The overall correlation was 0.91; the closest agreement was for personal-care tasks (9, p492). Barthel scores also correlated with age, psychological problems, and role performance (9, p495).

Correlations between the Barthel and the PULSES Profile range from -0.74 to -0.80 (3, p146), to -0.83 (2, p48), and -0.90 (12, p556) ($p < 0.001$; the negative sign results from the inverse scoring of the scales). In a study of 45 elderly patients, correlations were calculated with the Functional Independence Measure (0.84), with the Katz Index of ADL (0.78), and with Spitzer's Quality of Life Index (0.52) (23, Table 2). Granger found that four items (bowel and bladder control, grooming, and eating) offered predictions of return to independent community living after six months that were comparable to the entire scale (13, p103).

Alternative Forms

There are many variants of the Barthel Index. Among the less widely used are a 12-item version by Granger (13, 14), a 14-item version (24), a 16-item version (25), and a 17–item version (5). Chino et al. proposed a scoring system for the 15-item version that is slightly different from the method presented in Exhibit 3.6 (26). Because of these differing versions, caution is required when comparing results across studies. Coordination is needed in the further development of the Barthel scale, and we recommend that users select either the Collin version of the ten-item scale or the 15-item version proposed by Granger and his colleagues in 1981. Other variants should be discouraged.

The Barthel Index has been translated for use in Japan (26).

Commentary

In use for decades, the Barthel Index continues to be widely applied and refined and has been incorporated into broader evaluation instruments such as the Long-Range Evaluation System developed by Granger et al. (8, 26, 27). More recently, the latter has been superseded by the Uniform Data System for Medical Rehabilitation, which also incorporates the Barthel items as part of the Functional Independence Measure (described in the IADL section of this chapter).

The Barthel Index is usually applied as a rating scale; self-reports may give results that differ from therapist ratings (4, 5, 17, 18). The direction of the difference, however, is not consistent and in most cases is small.

Several criticisms have been made of the Barthel Index, mainly concerning the scoring method. Indeed, criticisms of the scoring stimulated the development of several different versions. Collin and Wade commented on the difficulty of interpreting the middle categories of the scale and so proposed their more detailed guidelines (4). Shah et al. noted the insensitivity of the crude rating scheme and suggested more detailed intermediate categories (10). The Collin/Wade and Shah approaches improve on the original, but a definitive scoring approach is needed. The Barthel scale is also limited in scope and may not detect low levels of disability, reflecting its origins as a measure for severely ill patients. Thus, while a score of 100 indicates independence in all ten areas, assistance may still be required, for example, with cooking or house cleaning. Other scales that include IADL topics overcome this, and the PULSES Profile also cover a wider range of activities, such as communication, psychosocial, and situational factors.

The Barthel Index is widely respected as a good ADL scale; it also occupies an important place in the development of this field. Validity data are more extensive than those for many other ADL scales, and the results appear superior to others we review. As with most traditional ADL scales, its scope is narrow; broader measurements are described in Chapter 9. Further development should be coordinated and should build on one of the major versions of the scale. Norms by age, sex, and medical condition would be valuable.

REFERENCES

(1) Mahoney FI, Wood OH, Barthel DW. Rehabilitation of chronically ill patients: the influence of complications on the final goal. South Med J 1958;51:605–609.
(2) Granger CV. Outcome of comprehensive medical rehabilitation: an analysis based upon the impairment, disability, and handicap model. Int Rehabil Med 1985;7:45–50.
(3) Granger CV, Albrecht GL, Hamilton BB. Outcome of comprehensive medical rehabilitation: measurement by PULSES Profile and the Barthel Index. Arch Phys Med Rehabil 1979;60:145–154.
(4) Collin C, Wade DT, Davies S, et al. The Barthel ADL Index: a reliability study. Int Disabil Stud 1988;10:61–63.
(5) McGinnis GE, Seward ML, DeJong G, et al. Program evaluation of physical medicine and rehabilitation departments using self-report Barthel. Arch Phys Med Rehabil 1986;67:123–125.
(6) Mahoney FI, Barthel DW. Functional evaluation: the Barthel Index. Md State Med J 1965;14:61–65.
(7) Wylie CM, White BK. A measure of disability. Arch Environ Health 1964;8:834–839.
(8) Granger CV. Health accounting—functional assessment of the long-term patient. In: Kottke FJ, Stillwell GK, Lehmann JF, eds. Krusen's handbook of physical medicine and rehabilitation. 3rd ed. Philadelphia, Pennsylvania: WB Saunders, 1982:253–274.
(9) Fortinsky RH, Granger CV, Seltzer GB. The use of functional assessment in understanding home care needs. Med Care 1981;19:489–497.
(10) Shah S, Vanclay F, Cooper B. Improving the sensitivity of the Barthel Index for stroke rehabilitation. J Clin Epidemiol 1989;42:703–709.
(11) Lazar RB, Yarkony GM, Ortolano D, et al. Prediction of functional outcome by motor capability after spinal cord injury. Arch Phys Med Rehabil 1989;70:819–822.

(12) Granger CV, Sherwood CC, Greer DS. Functional status measures in a comprehensive stroke care program. Arch Phys Med Rehabil 1977;58:555–561.

(13) Granger CV, Hamilton BB, Gresham GE, et al. The stroke rehabilitation outcome study: part II. Relative merits of the total Barthel Index score and a four-item subscore in predicting patient outcomes. Arch Phys Med Rehabil 1989;70:100–103.

(14) Granger CV, Hamilton BB, Gresham GE. The stroke rehabilitation outcome study—part I: general description. Arch Phys Med Rehabil 1988;69:506–509.

(15) Wartski SA, Green DS. Evaluation in a home-care program. Med Care 1971;9:352–364.

(16) Collin C, Davis S, Horne V, et al. Reliability of the Barthel ADL Index. Int J Rehabil Res 1987;10:356–357.

(17) Roy CW, Togneri J, Hay E, et al. An interrater reliability study of the Barthel Index. Int J Rehabil Res 1988;11:67–70.

(18) Shinar D, Gross CR, Bronstein KS, et al. Reliability of the activities of daily living scale and its use in telephone interview. Arch Phys Med Rehabil 1987;68:723–728.

(19) Wade DT, Hewer RL. Functional abilities after stroke: measurement, natural history and prognosis. J Neurol Neurosurg Psychiatry 1987;50:177–182.

(20) Wylie CM. Gauging the response of stroke patients to rehabilitation. J Am Geriatr Soc 1967;15:797–805.

(21) Granger CV, Greer DS, Liset E, et al. Measurement of outcomes of care for stroke patients. Stroke 1975;6:34–41.

(22) Wylie CM. Measuring end results of rehabilitation of patients with stroke. Public Health Rep 1967;82:893–898.

(23) Rockwood K, Stolee P, Fox RA. Use of goal attainment scaling in measuring clinically important change in the frail elderly. J Clin Epidemiol 1993;46:1113–1118.

(24) Yarkony GM, Roth EJ, Heinemann AW, et al. Functional skills after spinal cord injury rehabilitation: three-year longitudinal follow-up. Arch Phys Med Rehabil 1988;69:111–114.

(25) Nosek MA, Parker RM, Larsen S. Psychosocial independence and functional abilities: their relationship in adults with severe musculoskeletal impairments. Arch Phys Med Rehabil 1987;68:840–845.

(26) Chino N, Anderson TP, Granger CV. Stroke rehabilitation outcome studies: comparison of a Japanese facility with 17 U.S. facilities. Int Disabil Stud 1988;10:150–154.

(27) Granger CV, McNamara MA. Functional assessment utilization: the Long-Range Evaluation System (LRES). In: Granger CV, Gresham GE, eds. Functional assessment in rehabilitation medicine. Baltimore, Maryland: Williams & Wilkins, 1984:99–121.

THE INDEX OF INDEPENDENCE IN ACTIVITIES OF DAILY LIVING, OR INDEX OF ADL
(Sidney Katz, 1959, Revised 1976)

Purpose

The Index of ADL was developed to measure the physical functioning of elderly and chronically ill patients. Frequently it has been used to indicate the severity of chronic illness and to evaluate the effectiveness of treatment; it has also been used to provide predictive information on the course of specific illnesses (1–3).

Conceptual Basis

In empirical studies of aging, Katz noted that the loss of functional skills occurs in a particular order, the most complex functions being lost first. Empirically, the six activities included in the index were found to lie in a hierarchical order of this type while other items, such as mobility, walking, or stair climbing, did not fit the pattern and were excluded (4). Katz further suggested that, during rehabilitation, skills are regained in order of ascending complexity, in the same order that they are initially acquired by infants (1, pp917–918). He concluded that the Index of ADL appears to reflect "primary biological and psychosocial function" (1, 4–6).

Description

The Index of ADL was originally developed for elderly and chronically ill patients with strokes or fractured hips. It assesses independence in six activities: bathing, dressing, toileting, transferring from bed to chair, continence, and feeding. Through observation and interview, the therapist rates each activity on a three-point scale of independence, shown in Exhibit 3.7. The

Exhibit 3.7   The Index of Independence in Activities of Daily Living: Evaluation Form

For each area of functioning listed below, check description that applies. (The word "assistance" means supervision, direction, or personal assistance.)

Bathing—either sponge bath; tub bath, or shower

☐   ☐   ☐

Receives no assistance (gets in and out of tub by self if tub is usual means of bathing) | Receives assistance in bathing only one part of the body (such as back or a leg) | Receives assistance in bathing more than one part of the body (or not bathed)

Dressing—gets clothes from closets and drawers—including underclothes, outer garments and using fasteners (including braces if worn)

☐   ☐   ☐

Get clothes and gets completely dressed without assistance | Gets clothes and gets dressed without assistance except for assistance in tying shoes | Receives assistance in getting clothes or in getting dressed, or stays partly or completely undressed

Toileting—going to the "toilet room" for bowel and urine elimination; cleaning self after elimination, and arranging clothes

☐   ☐   ☐

Goes to "toilet room," cleans self, and arranges clothes without assistance (may use object for support such as cane, walker, or wheelchair and may manage night bedpan or commode, emptying same in morning) | Receives assistance in going to "toilet room" or in cleansing self or in arranging clothes after elimination or in use of night bedpan or commode | Doesn't go to room termed "toilet" for the elimination process

Transfer—

☐   ☐   ☐

Moves in and out of bed as well as in and out of chair without assistance (may be using object for support such as cane or walker) | Moves in and out of bed or chair with assistance | Doesn't get out of bed

Continence—

☐   ☐   ☐

Controls urination and bowel movement completely by self | Has occasional "accidents" | Supervision helps keep urine or bowel control; catheter is used, or is incontinent

Feeding—

☐   ☐   ☐

Feeds self without assistance | Feeds self except for getting assistance in cutting meat or buttering bread | Receives assistance in feeding or is fed partly or completely by using tubes or intravenous fluids

most dependent degree of performance during a two-week period is recorded. In applying the index:

The observer asks the subject to show him (1) the bathroom, and (2) medications in another room (or a meaningful substitute object). These requests create test situations for direct observation of transfer, locomotion, and communication and serve as checks on the reliability of information about bathing, dressing, going to toilet, and transfer. (1, p915).

Full definitions of the six items are given by Katz et al. (5, pp22–24).

The first stage in scoring involves translating the three-point scales into a "dependent/independent" classification using the guidelines shown in the lower half of Exhibit 3.8. The middle categories in Exhibit 3.7 are rated as "independent" for bathing, dressing, and feeding but as "dependent" for the others. The patient's overall performance is then summarized on an eight-point scale that considers the numbers of areas of dependency and their relative importance (shown in the upper half of Exhibit 3.8). Alternatively, a simplified scoring system counts the number of activities in which the individual is dependent, on a scale from 0 through 6, where 0 = independent in all six functions and 6 = dependent in all functions (4, p497). This

Exhibit 3.8 The Index of Independence in Activities of Daily Living: Scoring and Definitions

The Index of Independence in Activities of Daily Living is based on an evaluation of the functional independence or dependence of patients in bathing, dressing, going to toilet, transferring, continence, and feeding. Specific definitions of functional independence and dependence appear below the index.

A—Independent in feeding, continence, transferring, going to toilet, dressing and bathing.
B— Independent in all but one of these functions.
C—Independent in all but bathing and one additional function.
D—Independent in all but bathing, dressing, and one additional function.
E— Independent in all but bathing, dressing, going to toilet, and one additional function.
F— Independent in all but bathing, dressing, going to toilet, transferring, and one additional function.
G—Dependent in all six functions.
Other—Dependent in at least two functions, but not classifiable as C, D, E or F.

Independence means without supervision, direction, or active personal assistance, except as specifically noted below. This is based on actual status and not on ability. A patient who refuses to perform a function is considered as not performing the function, even though he is deemed able.

Bathing (sponge, shower or tub)
Independent: assistance only in bathing a single part (as back or disabled extremity) or bathes self completely
Dependent: assistance in bathing more than one part of body; assistance in getting in or out of tub or does not bathe self

Dressing
Independent: gets clothes from closets and drawers; puts on clothes, outer garments, braces; manages fasteners; act of tying shoes is excluded
Dependent: does not dress self or remains partly undressed

Going to toilet
Independent: gets to toilet; gets on and off toilet; arranges clothes; cleans organs of excretion; (may manage own bedpan used at night only and may or may not be using mechanical supports)
Dependent: uses bedpan or commode or receives assistance in getting to and using toilet

Transfer
Independent: moves in and out of bed independently and moves in and out of chair independently (may or may not be using mechanical supports)
Dependent: assistance in moving in or out of bed and/or chair; does not perform one or more transfers

Continence
Independent: urination and defecation entirely self-controlled
Dependent: partial or total incontinence in urination or defecation; partial or total control by enemas, catheters, or regulated use of urinals and/or bedpans

Feeding
Independent: gets food from plate or its equivalent into mouth; (precutting of meat and preparation of food, as buttering bread, are excluded from evaluation)
Dependent: assistance in act of feeding (see above): does not eat at all or parenteral feeding

method obviates the need for the miscellaneous scoring category, "other."

Reliability

Little formal reliability (or validity) testing has been reported. Katz et al. assessed inter-rater reliability, reporting that differences between observers occurred once in 20 evaluations or less frequently (1, p915). Guttman analyses on 100 patients in Sweden yielded coefficients of scalability ranging from 0.74 to 0.88, suggesting that the index forms a successful cumulative scale (7, p128).

Validity

Katz et al. applied the Index of ADL and other indices to 270 patients at discharge from a hospital for the chronically ill. Index scores were found to correlate 0.50 with a mobility scale and 0.39 with a house confinement scale (5, Table 3). At a two-year follow-up, Katz concluded that the Index of ADL predicted long-term outcomes as well as or better than selected measures of physical or mental function (5, p29). Other studies of predictive validity are summarized by Katz and Akpom (4); typical of these findings are the results presented by Brorsson and Åsberg. Thirty-two of 44 patients rated as independent at admission to hospital were living at home one year later while eight had died. By contrast, 23 of 42 patients initially rated as dependent had died while only eight were living in their homes (7, p130).

Åsberg examined the ability of the scale to predict length of hospital stay, likelihood of discharge home, and death (N = 129). In predicting mortality, sensitivity was 73% and specificity, 80%; in predicting discharge, sensitivity was 90% and specificity, 63%. Similar results were obtained from ratings by independent physicians (8, Table IV).

Like all other activities of daily living scales, the Index of ADL encounters a floor effect whereby it is insensitive to variations in low levels of disability. This has been reported many times; one example may suffice. Compared to the Functional Status Questionnaire (FSQ) in a study of polio survivors, the Index of ADL rated 32 patients fully independent, six partly dependent, and one dependent. Using the instrumental ADL questions from the FSQ, only four of the same patients had no difficulty with walking several blocks, six had no difficulty with light housework, and only one patient had no difficulty with more vigorous activities (9, Table II). Even more indicative of the limited sensitivity of the ADL questions to disabilities, 15 of the patients had difficulty or required assistance to stand up, and seven were unable to stand alone; ten of the patients could not go out of doors (9, Table IX).

Commentary

The Index of ADL is very widely used. It has been used with children and with adults, with the mentally retarded and the physically disabled, in the community and in institutions (4, 6). It has been used in studies of many conditions, including cerebral palsy, strokes, multiple sclerosis, paraplegia, quadriplegia, and rheumatoid arthritis (2–4, 10–14). As with all ADL scales, the Index is only appropriate with severely sick respondents; minor illness or disability frequently does not translate into the limitations in basic activities of daily living covered in this scale. ADL scales are therefore unlikely to be suitable for health surveys or in general practice, for they are not sensitive to minor deviations from complete well-being.

Katz's Index of ADL rose to prominence largely because it was the first such scale published. Illustrations exist in several areas of health measurement of acceptance of certain scales by acclaim rather than following clear demonstration of validity and reliability; this commonly applies to the first scale in a field previously lacking in measurement tools. On reviewing the Katz scale, it is surprising to find that so little evidence has been published on its reliability and validity. Considerably more evidence has been accumulated, for example, on the Barthel Index. The work of Brorsson and Åsberg begins to fill this need, although more evidence for validity and reliability is needed before we can fully support its use. Among the various critiques of the scale, potential users should be aware of the criticisms of the scoring system made by Chen and Bryant (15, p261). Other scales should be reviewed closely before the Index of ADL is selected.

REFERENCES

(1) Katz S, Ford AB, Moskowitz RW, et al. Studies of illness in the aged. The Index of ADL: a standardized measure of biological and psychosocial function. JAMA 1963;185:914–919.

(2) Katz S, Ford AB, Chinn AB, et al. Prognosis after strokes: II. Long-term course of 159 patients with stroke. Medicine 1966;45:236–246.

(3) Katz S, Heiple KG, Downs TD, et al. Long-term course of 147 patients with fracture of the hip. Surg Gynecol Obstet 1967;124:1219–1230.

(4) Katz S, Akpom CA. A measure of primary sociobiological functions. Int J Health Serv 1976;6:493–507.

(5) Katz S, Downs TD, Cash HR, et al. Progress in development of the Index of ADL. Gerontologist 1970;10:20–30.

(6) Katz S, Akpom CA. Index of ADL. Med Care 1976;14:116–118.

(7) Brorsson B, Åsberg KH. Katz Index of Independence in ADL: reliability and validity in short-term care. Scand J Rehabil Med 1984;16:125–132.

(8) Åsberg KH. Disability as a predictor of outcome for the elderly in a department of internal medicine. Scand J Soc Med 1987;15:261–265.

(9) Einarsson G, Grimby G. Disability and handicap in late poliomyelitis. Scand J Rehabil Med 1990;22:1–9.

(10) Steinberg FU, Frost M. Rehabilitation of geriatric patients in a general hospital: a follow-up study of 43 cases. Geriatrics 1963;18:158–164.

(11) Katz S, Vignos PJ, Moskowitz RW, et al. Comprehensive outpatient care in rheumatoid arthritis: a controlled study. JAMA 1968;206:1249–1254.

(12) Grotz RT, Henderson ND, Katz S. A comparison of the functional and intellectual performance of phenylketonuric, anoxic, and Down's Syndrome individuals. Am J Ment Defic 1972;76:710–717.

(13) Katz S, Ford AB, Downs TD, et al. Effects of continued care: a study of chronic illness in the home. Washington, DC: U.S. Government Printing Office (DHEW Publication No. (HSM) 73–3010), 1972.

(14) Katz S, Hedrick S, Henderson NS. The measurement of long-term care needs and impact. Health Med Care Serv Rev 1979;2:1–21.

(15) Chen MK, Bryant BE. The measurement of health—a critical and selective overview. Int J Epidemiol 1975;4:257–264.

THE KENNY SELF-CARE EVALUATION
(Herbert A. Schoening and Staff of the Sister Kenny Institute, 1965, Revised 1973)

Purpose

The Kenny Self-Care Evaluation records functional performance to estimate a patient's ability to live independently at home or in a protected environment. Intended for setting treatment goals and evaluating progress, the method is limited to physical activities and was designed to offer a "more precise measuring device than the traditional ADL form" (1, p690).

Conceptual Basis

The topics covered were selected to represent the minimum requirements for independent living (2, p2). The rating system considers all the self-care abilities to be equally important and assigns equal weight to them (3, p222).

Description

The Kenny evaluation is hierarchical. The revised version covers seven aspects of self-care activities: bed activities, transfers, locomotion, dressing, personal hygiene, bowel and bladder, and feeding. Within each category there are between one and four general activities, each of which is in turn divided into component tasks. These comprise the small steps involved in the activity—for example, "legs over side of bed" is one of the steps in "rising and sitting." In all, there are 17 activities and 85 tasks (see Exhibit 3.9). The questionnaire and a 24–page user's manual are available from the Publications Office of the Sister Kenny Institute (2).

Exhibit 3.9   The Sister Kenny Institute Self-Care Evaluation

Activities	Tasks	Evaluation Date:	Progress Rounds:	Progress Rounds:

BED ACTIVITIES

Activities	Tasks					
Moving in Bed	Shift position					
	Turn to left side					
	Turn to right side					
	Turn to prone					
	Turn to supine					

Rising and Sitting	Come to sitting position					
	Maintain sitting balance					
	Legs over side of bed					
	Move to edge of bed					
	Legs back onto bed					

TRANSFERS

Sitting Transfer	Position wheelchair					
	Brakes on/off					
	Arm rests on/off					
	Foot rests on/off					
	Position legs					
	Position sliding board					
	Maintain balance					
	Shift to bed/chair					

Standing Transfer	Position wheelchair					
	Brakes on/off					
	Move feet and pedals					
	Slide forward					
	Position feet					
	Stand					
	Pivot					
	Sit					

Activities	Tasks	Evaluation Date:	Progress Rounds:	Progress Rounds:
Toilet Transfer	Position equipment			
	Manage equipment			
	Manage undressing			
	Transfer to commode/toilet			
	Manage dressing			
	Transfer back			
Bathing Transfer	Tub/shower approach			
	Use of grab bars			
	Tub/shower entry			
	Tub/shower exit			

LOCOMOTION

Activities	Tasks			
Locomotion	Walking			
	Stairs			
	Wheelchair			

DRESSING

Activities	Tasks			
Upper Trunk and Arms	Hearing aid and eyeglasses			
	Front opening on/off			
	Pullover on/off			
	Brassiere on/off			
	Corset/brace on/off			
	Equipment/prostheses on/off			
	Sweater/shawl on/off			
Lower Trunk and Legs	Slacks/skirt on/off			
	Underclothing on/off			
	Belt on/off			
	Braces/prostheses on/off			
	Girdle/garter belt on/off			

Exhibit 3.9 *(Continued)*

Exhibit 3.9 *(Continued)*

Activities	Tasks	Evaluation Date:	Progress Rounds:	Progress Rounds:
Feet	Stockings on/off			
	Shoes/slippers on/off			
	Braces/prostheses on/off			
	Wraps/support hose on/off			

PERSONAL HYGIENE

Activities	Tasks			
Face, Hair and Arms	Wash face			
	Wash hands and arms			
	Brush teeth/dentures			
	Brush/comb hair			
	Shaving/make-up			

Activities	Tasks			
Trunk and Perineum	Wash back			
	Wash buttocks			
	Wash chest			
	Wash abdomen			
	Wash groin			

Activities	Tasks			
Lower Extremities	Wash upper legs			
	Wash lower legs			
	Wash feet			

BOWEL AND BLADDER

Activities	Tasks			
Bowel Program	Suppository insertion			
	Digital stimulation			
	Equipment care			
	Cleansing self			

Activities	Tasks			
Bladder Program	Manage equipment			
	Stimulation			
	Cleansing self			

Activities	Tasks	Evaluation Date:		Progress Rounds:		Progress Rounds:	
Catheter Care	Assemble equipment						
	Fill syringe						
	Inject liquid						
	Connect/disconnect						
	Sterile technique						

FEEDING*

Activities	Tasks						
Feeding	Adaptive equipment						
	Finger feeding						
	Use of utensils						
	Pour from container						
	Drink (cup/glass/straw)						

*If patient cannot swallow, he is to be scored 0 in feeding

Exhibit 3.9   (Continued)

Clinical staff observe the performance of each task and rate it on a three-point scale: "totally independent," "requiring assistance or supervision" (regardless of the amount), or "totally dependent." Every task must be observed; self-report is not accepted. If the rater believes that the performance did not reflect the patient's true ability, special circumstances that may have affected the score can be noted on the score sheet (e.g., acute illness).

The ratings for the tasks within each activity are combined to provide an activity score, as follows:

Four: All tasks rated independent.
Three: One or two tasks required assistance or supervision; all others are done independently.
Two: Other configurations not covered in classes 0, 1, 3, or 4.
One: One or two tasks required assistance or supervision, or one was carried out independently, but in all others the patient was dependent.
Zero: All tasks were rated dependent.

Category scores are calculated as the average of the activity scores within that category (as shown on the scoring sheet at the end of the exhibit). The category scores may be summed to provide a total score in which the seven categories receive equal weights. Equal weights were justified on the basis of empirical observations suggesting that roughly equal nursing time was required for helping the dependent patient with each group of activities (1, pp690–693). No guidelines are given on how to interpret the scores.

Reliability

The inter-rater agreement among 43 raters for the Kenny total score was 0.67 or 0.74, according to whether it was applied before or after another rating scale. The reliability of the locomotion score (0.46 or 0.42) was markedly lower than that of the other scores, which ranged from 0.71 to 0.94 (4, Table 2). Iversen et al. commented that the locomotion category is the most difficult to score (2, p14). Gordon et al. achieved higher inter-rater reliabilities: error was only 2.5% (5, p400).

Exhibit 3.9 *(Continued)*

Self-Care Score

Category	Activities	Activity Scores	Category Total	Category Score	Activity Scores	Category Total	Category Score	Activity Scores	Category Total	Category Score
BED ACTIVITIES	Moving in Bed									
	Rising and Sitting		÷ 2	= .		÷ 2	= .		÷ 2	= .
TRANSFERS	Sitting Transfer									
	Standing Transfer									
	Toilet Transfer									
	Bathing Transfer		÷ 4	= .		÷ 4	= .		÷ 4	= .
LOCOMOTION	Walking									
	Stairs									
	Wheelchair		÷ 3	= .		÷ 3	= .		÷ 3	= .
DRESSING	Upper Trunk and Arms									
	Lower Trunk and Legs									
	Feet		÷ 3	= .		÷ 3	= .		÷ 3	= .
PERSONAL HYGIENE	Face, Hair and Arms									
	Trunk and Perineum									
	Lower Extremities		÷ 3	= .		÷ 3	= .		÷ 3	= .
BOWEL AND BLADDER	Bowel Program									
	Bladder Program									
	Catheter Care		÷ 2	= .		÷ 2	= .		÷ 2	= .
FEEDING	Feeding		=	.0 .		=	.0 .		=	.0 .
TOTAL SELF-CARE SCORE										

Reproduced from Iversen IA, Silberberg NE, Stever RC, Schoening HA. The revised Kenny Self-Care Evaluation: a numerical measure of independence in activities of daily living. Minneapolis, Minnesota: Sister Kenny Institute, 1973. With permission.

Validity

Gresham et al. compared Kenny and Barthel Index ratings of stroke patients, giving a kappa coefficient of 0.42 and a Spearman correlation of 0.73 ($p < 0.001$) (6, Table 3). They found that the Kenny form tends to rate slightly more patients as independent than other indices. Complete independence was designated in 35.1% of 148 stroke patients by the Barthel Index, in 39.2% by the Katz Index of ADL, and in 41.9% using the Kenny instrument (differences not statistically significant) (6, p355).

Commentary

In addition to this self-care scale, the Kenny Institute uses separate rating scales for behavior and for speech (7, p60). While its scope is limited, the Kenny Self-Care Evaluation is distinctive in that its coverage is detailed. Also, it requires direct observation of the patient. The available evidence suggests somewhat greater inter-rater agreement for the Kenny than is obtained using simpler ratings. As the Kenny breaks activities down into their component parts, raters were able to achieve higher levels of agreement because the narrower scope of the task evaluations reduced the number of behavioral components that could be subjectively weighted (4, pp164–165).

However, comparisons of the Kenny with simpler scales suggest that the additional detail does not provide superior discriminative ability (4, p164). The correlation of 0.73 with the Barthel Index is high, and if this were corrected for attenuation due to the imperfect reliability of the two scales, it would imply that the simpler Barthel Index provides results that are virtually identical. The quality of the Kenny scale is also comparable to that of the Katz index; there is little evidence that supports the superiority of the Kenny for research purposes. Its detailed ratings may, however, be advantageous for clinical applications.

Address

J. Kent Canine, PhD, Director, Research and Education, Sister Kenny Institute, 800 East 28th Street at Chicago Avenue, Minneapolis, Minnesota, USA 55407

REFERENCES

(1) Schoening HA, Anderegg L, Bergstrom D, et al. Numerical scoring of self-care status of patients. Arch Phys Med Rehabil 1965;46:689–697.
(2) Iversen IA, Silberberg NE, Stever RC, et al. The revised Kenny Self-Care Evaluation: a numerical measure of independence in activities of daily living. Minneapolis, Minnesota: Sister Kenny Institute, 1973 (Reprinted, 1983).
(3) Schoening HA, Iversen IA. Numerical scoring of self-care status: a study of the Kenny Self-Care Evaluation. Arch Phys Med Rehabil 1968;49:221–229.
(4) Kerner JF, Alexander J. Activities of daily living: reliability and validity of gross vs specific ratings. Arch Phys Med Rehabil 1981;62:161–166.
(5) Gordon EE, Drenth V, Jarvis L, et al. Neurophysiologic syndromes in stroke as predictors of outcome. Arch Phys Med Rehabil 1978;59:399–409.
(6) Gresham GE, Phillips TF, Labi MLC. ADL status in stroke: relative merits of three standard indexes. Arch Phys Med Rehabil 1980;61:355–358.
(7) Ellwood PM Jr. Quantitative measurement of patient care quality. Part 2—a system for identifying meaningful factors. Hospitals 1966;40:59–63.

THE PHYSICAL SELF-MAINTENANCE SCALE
(M. Powell Lawton and Elaine M. Brody, 1969)

Purpose

Lawton and Brody developed the Physical Self-Maintenance Scale (PSMS) as a disability measure for use in planning and evaluating treatment for elderly people living in the community or in institutions.

Conceptual Basis

This scale is based on the theory that human behavior can be ordered in a hierarchy of complexity, an approach similar to that used by Katz for the Index of ADL. The hierarchy runs from physical health through self-maintenance ADL and IADL, to cognition, time use (e.g., participation in hobbies or community activities), and finally to social interaction (1, 2). Within each category a further hierarchy of complexity runs from basic to complex activities (2, Figure 1; 3).

Description

The PSMS is a modification of a scale developed at the Langley-Porter Neuropsychiatric Institute by Lowenthal et al., which is discussed, but not presented, in Lowenthal's book (4). In turn, the PSMS items have been incorporated into subsequent instruments. The PSMS includes both ADL and IADL items (1; 5, Appendix B). The following description concentrates on the six ADL items because Lawton and Brody's original article reports little information on the validity and reliability of the eight IADL items. Rating scale and self-administered versions of both scales exist. Both were designed for people over 60 years of age and concentrate on observable behaviors.

The rating version of the ADL scale may be applied by a variety of staff members. Five-point rating scales ranging from total independence to total dependence are used for all six items, which fall on a Guttman scale. Two scoring methods may be used: a count of the number of items on which any degree of disability is identified, or a severity scale that sums the response codes for each item, resulting in an overall score ranging from 6 to 30. The ADL scale, showing the response codes, is presented in Exhibit 3.10.

Reliability

A Pearson correlation of 0.87 was obtained between pairs of nurses who rated 36 patients; the agreement between two research assistants who independently rated 14 patients was 0.91 (1, p182). The six items fell on a Guttman scale when cutting points were set between independent (code 1 in each item) and all levels of dependency.

The rank order of the items was feeding (77% independent), toilet (66%), dressing (56%), bathing (43%), grooming (42%), and ambulation (27% independent). A Guttman reproducibility coefficient of 0.96 was reported (N = 265) (1, Table 1).

Validity

The PSMS was tested on elderly persons, some in an institution and others living at home. It correlated 0.62 with a physician's rating of functional health (N = 130) and 0.61 with an IADL scale (N = 77) (1, Table 6). As would be expected, it correlated less highly ($r = 0.38$) with the Kahn Mental Status Questionnaire and it also correlated 0.38 with a behavioral rating of social adjustment (1, Table 6).

Commentary

The PSMS appears to be a reliable and valid ADL scale for clinical and survey research applications. On its own, the PSMS has not been widely reported in the literature, but is known mainly as a component of other instruments. Most notably, a self-rating version of the ADL scale that contains eight items was expanded from the original six. These eight items were included in the 1975 OARS Multidimensional Functional Assessment Questionnaire (MFAQ) and later in Lawton's 1982 Multilevel Assessment Instrument (both reviewed in Chapter 9). The self-rating version of the PSMS is shown in Lawton's 1988 article (2, pp795–797) and the items are virtually identical to the physical ADL items in the OARS MFAQ shown in Exhibit 9.18. The IADL scale described by Lawton and Brody (1) was also modified for inclusion in the 1975 OARS instrument and it was then further adapted for the Multilevel Assessment Instrument.

The other noteworthy feature of Lawton and Brody's work is their carefully developed conceptual definition of competence in everyday activities. This hierarchical model of disability extends the scope of Katz's approach in his Index of ADL.

Exhibit 3.10   The Physical Self-Maintenance Scale

Circle one statement in each category A–F that applies to subject.

A. Toilet
   1. Cares for self at toilet completely, no incontinence.
   2. Needs to be reminded, or needs help in cleaning self, or has rare (weekly at most) accidents.
   3. Soiling or wetting while asleep more than once a week.
   4. Soiling or wetting while awake more than once a week.
   5. No control of bowels or bladder.

B. Feeding
   1. Eats without assistance.
   2. Eats with minor assistance at meal times and/or with special preparation of food, or help in cleaning up after meals.
   3. Feeds self with moderate assistance and is untidy.
   4. Requires extensive assistance for all meals.
   5. Does not feed self at all and resists efforts of others to feed him.

C. Dressing
   1. Dresses, undresses and selects clothes from own wardrobe.
   2. Dresses and undresses self, with minor assistance.
   3. Needs moderate assistance in dressing or selection of clothes.
   4. Needs major assistance in dressing, but cooperates with efforts of others to help.
   5. Completely unable to dress self and resists efforts of others to help.

D. Grooming (neatness, hair, nails, hands, face, clothing)
   1. Always neatly dressed, well-groomed, without assistance.
   2. Grooms self adequately with occasional minor assistance, e.g., shaving.
   3. Needs moderate and regular assistance or supervision in grooming.
   4. Needs total grooming care, but can remain well-groomed after help from others.
   5. Actively negates all efforts of others to maintain grooming.

E. Physical Ambulation
   1. Goes about grounds or city.
   2. Ambulates within residence or about one block distant.
   3. Ambulates with assistance of (check one) a ( ) another person, b ( ) railing, c ( ) cane,
      d ( ) walker, e ( ) wheelchair
      1 _____ Gets in and out without help.
      2 _____ Needs help in getting in and out.
   4. Sits unsupported in chair or wheelchair, but cannot propel self without help.
   5. Bedridden more than half the time.

F. Bathing
   1. Bathes self (tub, shower, sponge bath) without help.
   2. Bathes self with help in getting in and out of tub.
   3. Washes face and hands only, but cannot bathe rest of body.
   4. Does not wash self but is cooperative with those who bathe him.
   5. Does not try to wash self and resists efforts to keep him clean.

REFERENCES

(1) Lawton MP, Brody EM. Assessment of older people: Self-maintaining and instrumental activities of daily living. Gerontologist 1969;9:179–186.

(2) Lawton MP. Scales to measure competence in everyday activities. Psychopharmacol Bull 1988;24:609–614.

(3) Lawton MP. Environment and other determinants of well-being in older people. Gerontologist 1983;23:349–357.

(4) Lowenthal MF. Lives in distress: the paths of the elderly to the psychiatric ward. New York: Basic Books, 1964.

(5) Brody EM. Long-term care of older people: a practical guide. New York: Human Sciences Press, 1977.

THE FUNCTIONAL
STATUS RATING SYSTEM
(Stephen K. Forer, 1981)

Purpose

The Functional Status Rating System (FSRS) estimates the assistance required by rehabilitation patients in their daily lives. It covers independence in ADL, ability to communicate, and social adjustment.

Conceptual Basis

No information is available.

Description

This rating scale was based on a method developed by the Hospitalization Utilization Project of Pennsylvania (HUP) initiated in 1974 to provide national statistics on hospital utilization and treatment outcomes (1). A preliminary version of the FSRS covered five ADL topics (2); the revised rating form described here is broader in scope: 30 items cover five topics. The items are summarized in Exhibit 3.11; the scales on which the items are rated are shown at the foot of the exhibit. An instruction manual gives more detailed definitions of each item (3). Ratings are made by the treatment team member with primary responsibility for that aspect of care. Item scores are averaged to form scores for each of the five sections. The scale can be completed in 15 to 20 minutes.

Reliability

Information is available for the preliminary version only. Inter-rater agreement was high, but varied according to the professional background of the rater and the method of administration. Correlations ranged from 0.81 to 0.92 (2, p362).

Validity

Some predictive validity results are presented by Forer and Miller (2). Admission scores on bladder management and cognition were found to predict the eventual placement of the patient in home or institutional care. The instrument was shown capable of reflecting improvement between admission and discharge for a number of diagnostic groups (2, Table 2).

Commentary

Despite its lack of validation we have included this scale because of its broad scope and because, as a clinical instrument, the scale appears relevant in routine patient assessment and in setting rehabilitation goals. The lack of formal reliability and validity testing makes it unsuitable as a research instrument.

A revised version of the scale presented in the exhibit was incorporated into the Functional Independence Measure described at the end of this chapter.

REFERENCES

(1) Breckenridge K. Medical rehabilitation program evaluation. Arch Phys Med Rehabil 1978;59:419–423.
(2) Forer SK, Miller LS. Rehabilitation outcome: comparative analysis of different patient types. Arch Phys Med Rehabil 1980;61:359–365.
(3) Forer SK. Revised functional status rating instrument. Glendale, California: Rehabilitation Institute, Glendale Adventist Medical Center, December 1981.

THE MEDICAL OUTCOMES STUDY
PHYSICAL FUNCTIONING MEASURE
(Anita Stewart, 1992)

Purpose

The Medical Outcomes Study (MOS) measurement of physical functioning offers an extended ADL scale that is sensitive to variations at relatively high levels of physical function. It is suitable for use in health surveys and in outcome assessment for outpatient care.

Conceptual Basis

As part of the comprehensive measurement battery designed for the MOS, several considerations guided the design of the physical functioning scale. First, there was an

Exhibit 3.11 The Functional Status Rating System

Functional Status in Self-care
  A. *Eating/feeding:* Management of all aspects of setting up and eating food (including cutting of meat) with or without adaptive equipment.
  B. *Personal hygiene:* Includes set up, oral care, washing face and hands with a wash cloth, hair grooming, shaving, and makeup.
  C. *Toileting:* Includes management of clothing and cleanliness.
  D. *Bathing:* Includes entire body bathing (tub, shower, or bed bath).
  E. *Bowel management:* Able to insert suppository and/or perform manual evacuation, aware of need to defecate, has sphincter muscle control.
  F. *Bladder management:* Able to manage equipment necessary for bladder evacuation (may include intermittent catheterization).
  G. *Skin management:* Performance of skin care program, regular inspection, prevention of pressure sores, rashes, or irritations.
  H. *Bed activities:* Includes turning, coming to a sitting position, scooting, and maintenance of balance.
  I. *Dressing:* Includes performance of total body dressing except tying shoes, with or without adaptive equipment (also includes application of orthosis & prosthesis).

Functional Status in Mobility
  A. *Transfers:* Includes the management of all aspects of transfers to and from bed, mat, toilet, tub/shower, wheelchair, with or without adaptive equipment.
  B. *Wheelchair skills:* Includes management of brakes, leg rests, maneuvering and propelling through and over doorway thresholds.
  C. *Ambulation:* Includes coming to a standing position and walking short to moderate distances on level surfaces with or without equipment.
  D. *Stairs and environmental surfaces:* Includes climbing stairs, curbs, ramps or environmental terrain.
  E. *Community mobility:* Ability to manage transportation.

Functional Status in Communication
  A. *Understanding spoken language*
  B. *Reading comprehension*
  C. *Language expression (non-speech/alternative methods):* Includes pointing, gestures, manual communication boards, electronic systems.
  D. *Language expression (verbal):* Includes grammer, syntax, and appropriateness of language.
  E. *Speech intelligibility*
  F. *Written communication (motor)*
  G. *Written language expression:* Includes spelling, vocabulary, punctuation, syntax, grammar, and completeness of written response.

Functional Status in Psychosocial Adjustment
  A. *Emotional adjustment:* Includes frequency and severity of depression, anxiety, frustration, lability, unresponsiveness, agitation, interference with progress in therapies, motivation, ability to cope with and take responsibility for emotional behavior.
  B. *Family/significant others/environment:* Includes frequency of chronic problems or conflicts in patient's relationships, interference with progress in therapies, ability and willingness to provide for patient's specific needs after discharge, and to promote patient's recovery and independence.
  C. *Adjustment to limitations:* Includes denial/awareness, acceptance of limitations, willingness to learn new ways of functioning, compensating, taking appropriate safety precautions, and realistic expectations for long-term recovery.
  D. *Social adjustment:* Includes frequency and initiation of social contacts, responsiveness in one to one and group situations, appropriateness of behavior in relationships, and spontaneity of interactions.

Functional Status in Cognitive Function
  A. *Attention span:* includes distractibility, level of alertness and responsiveness, ability to concentrate on a task, ability to follow directions, immediate recall as the structure, difficulty and length of the task vary.
  B. *Orientation*
  C. *Judgment reasoning*
  D. *Memory:* Includes short- and long-term.
  E. *Problem-solving*

Exhibit 3.11 *(Continued)*

Exhibit 3.11   *(Continued)*

Summary of Rating Scales

Self-care and mobility items	Communication, psychosocial and cognitive function items
1.0 = Unable—totally dependent	1.0 = Extremely severe
1.5 = Maximum assistance of 1 of 2 people	1.5 = Severe
2.0 = Moderate assistance	2.0 = Moderately severe
2.5 = Minimal assistance	2.5 = Moderate impairment
3.0 = Standby assistance	3.0 = Mild impairment
3.5 = Supervised	3.5 = Minimal impairment
4.0 = Independent	4.0 = No impairment

Adapted from the Rating Form obtained from Steven K Forer.

attempt to include activities that reflect physical disabilities rather than social roles. Activities of daily living such as shopping or cleaning the house reflect a blend of physical functioning and social roles and there are reasons other than physical limitations why some do not cook or clean house. The MOS team developed separate scales for physical function and role performance (1, 2). A second issue concerned the level of disability implicit in the questions. Most ADL questions reflect relatively severe disabilities and are insensitive to variations at the upper levels of functioning, where most people score. For use with relatively healthy patients, the MOS instrument included items on more strenuous physical activities while still retaining items on basic abilities such as dressing and walking. Finally, the MOS team argued that people's differing values for functional ability should be recognized: some people may not wish to perform activities such as running. Accordingly, the MOS instrument includes a question on satisfaction with performance, which was expected to be somewhat independent of the level of functioning (1, p89).

The instrument described here is an extension of the six-item physical functioning scale included in the Short-Form-20 Health Survey (reviewed in Chapter 9). Pilot studies suggested that a longer battery would have higher sensitivity in detecting disabilities (1, p90).

Description

The MOS Physical Functioning Measure includes ten items on functioning, one on satisfaction with physical activity, and three on mobility (see Exhibit 3.12).

Three scores are derived. A physical function score is formed by averaging nonmissing items from question 1; the score is transformed to a 0-to-100 scale in which a higher score indicates better function. Persons omitting more than five items are awarded a missing score. Stewart and Kamberg tested several approaches to scoring the mobility items and found that the best approach was to sum the responses from items 3 and 4 only (see Exhibit 3.12). A missing score is given if either question was not answered (1, pp97–98). For other analyses, the item on use of transportation is dichotomized so that 0 = unable to use transport for health reasons, and 1 = all other replies (1, pp93–94). A satisfaction score is based on item 2, transformed to a 0-to-100 scale.

Reliability

Eight of the ten function items correlated 0.70 or greater with the physical scale scores; the vigorous activity item correlated 0.62 and the bathing or dressing item showed a lower correlation of 0.48 (1, Table 6-3). Internal consistency for the physical functioning score was 0.92; for the mobility scale it was 0.71 (1, p98).

Exhibit 3.12   The Medical Outcomes Study Physical Functioning Measure

1. The following items are activities you might do during a typical day. *Does your health limit you* in these activities? (Circle One Number on Each Line)

ACTIVITIES	Yes, limited a lot	Yes, limited a little	No, not limited at all
a. *Vigorous activities,* such as running, lifting heavy objects, participating in strenuous sports	1	2	3
b. *Moderate activities,* such as moving a table, pushing a vacuum cleaner, bowling, or playing golf	1	2	3
c. Lifting or carrying groceries	1	2	3
d. Climbing *several* flights of stairs ...	1	2	3
e. Climbing *one* flight of stairs	1	2	3
f. Bending, kneeling or stooping	1	2	3
g. Walking *more than one mile*	1	2	3
h. Walking *several blocks*	1	2	3
i. Walking *one block*	1	2	3
j. Bathing or dressing yourself	1	2	3

2. How satisfied are you with your physical ability to do what you want to do?

(Circle One)

Completely satisfied 1
Very satisfied 2
Somewhat satisfied 3
Somewhat dissatisfied 4
Very dissatisfied 5
Completely dissatisfied 6

3. When you travel around your community, does someone have to assist you because of your health?

(Circle One)

Yes, all of the time 1
Yes, most of the time 2
Yes, some of the time 3
Yes, a little of the time 4
No, none of the time 5

4. Are you in bed or in a chair *most* or *all* of the day because of your health?

(Circle One)

Yes, every day 1
Yes, most days 2
Yes, some days 3
Yes, occasionally 4
No, never 5

5. Are you able to use public transportation?

(Circle One)

No, because of my health. 1
No, for some other reason 2
Yes, able to use public
    transportation 3

From Stewart AL, Ware JE Jr. Measuring functioning and well-being: the Medical Outcomes Study approach. Durham, North Carolina: Duke University Press, 1992:375–376. With permission.

Validity

The physical functioning scale scores correlated 0.58 with the mobility scores and 0.63 with the satisfaction scores (1, Table 6-6). A factor analysis identified a single factor accounting for 70% of the variance.

Alternative Forms

The same ten physical functioning items appear in the Short-Form-36 survey instrument reviewed in Chapter 9.

Commentary

Overlapping with the content of the Short-Form-36, this brief instrument offers a well-established set of ADL and mobility items. It seeks to provide a relatively pure measure of functional ability, independent of role functioning, which was covered in a separate MOS instrument (2). The physical functioning measure has 21 scale levels, all of which were represented in preliminary testing (1, p100). The inclusion of an item covering satisfaction with function serves to extend the scope of the functioning items by identifying people who report no disability on the items listed but are still dissatisfied. Stewart and Kamberg also found the reverse to be significant and noted that 31% of those reporting some level of physical disability nonetheless said they were very or completely satisfied: their level of functioning appeared to allow them to do what they wanted to do (1, p101).

This measure should be considered for use in relatively healthy populations, such as those attending primary care or those included in social surveys.

REFERENCES

(1) Stewart AL, Kamberg CJ. Physical functioning measures. In: Stewart AL, Ware JE Jr, eds. Measuring functioning and well-being: the Medical Outcomes Study approach. Durham, North Carolina: Duke University Press, 1992:86–101.
(2) Sherbourne CD, Stewart AL, Wells KB. Role functioning measures. In: Stewart AL, Ware JE Jr, eds. Measuring functioning and well-being: the Medical Outcomes Study approach. Durham, North Carolina: Duke University Press, 1992:205–219.

CONCLUSION: ADL SCALES

It is unfortunate that the development of ADL scales has been so uncoordinated. Many scales have not been planned on a systematic review of the strengths and weaknesses of previous instruments, and the definition of disability itself is more often assumed than clearly stated. The application of these instruments does not seem to have led to a cumulative understanding of the concept of disability, of its relationship to impairment and handicap, or of the sequence in which changes in disability occur as a patient's condition changes. One exception to this is the conceptual work of Latwon (1). We still know relatively little about the overlap among the various measurement methods, and the few comparative studies that exist mainly review the older scales. For example, Donaldson et al. designed a unified ADL evaluation form that incorporated the Barthel, Katz, and Kenny ratings (2). This was applied to 100 patients at admission and one month later. For 68 of the 100 patients the change (or lack of it) between scores was reflected in all three scales. Of the 32 cases in which a discrepancy occurred, 19 showed no change on the Katz, but change on the other two scales; in five cases the Kenny score had changed and the others had not. These and other results led Donaldson to conclude that the Katz scale is the least sensitive of the three methods, followed by the Barthel, with the Kenny being most sensitive to change. The Kenny's omission of continence explains some of the discrepancies between its results and those of the other scales. Gresham et al. also found that these three indices "are documenting the same basic group of functional skills and classifying the overall degree of independence in ADL in a very similar manner"(3, p357). They noted that the Barthel Index had several practical advantages: continuing widespread use, clarity of scoring system, and completeness. While these three are among the most widely used scales, they are also old and the available validity results are not impressive, although the majority of newer scales contain even less evidence for reliability and validity, and few studies have compared their results.

In preparing this chapter we examined a large number of other ADL scales, most of which we excluded on the grounds of inadequate evidence for validity and reliability. Some of the scales are, however, worthy of mention because of characteristics that may commend them for particular applications. The ADL scale of Pool and Brown, for example, offers considerable coverage in the area of locomotion: 13 of the 23 questions are devoted to walking, managing wheelchairs, and transport. No validity results are available, but an inter-rater concordance of 0.87 was reported (4). A scale that Sainsbury outlined (but did not present in detail) is imaginative in the way that each disability item is explicitly linked with the types of impairment it reflects. For example, doing the shopping and carrying groceries reflect coordination, sustained effort, mobility, and reach (5). Several scales combine questions on ADL with psychosocial factors but lack reliability and validity data (6–8). Susset et al. describe, but do not present, the questions on a scale of this type. The ADL form described by Rinzler et al. pays close attention to objectivity by standardizing the activities: performance is timed and exact distances are specified (9).

Several of the scales described in Chapter 9 include ADL-type questions, usually in the context of a broader-ranging instrument. This makes it questionable whether the ADL sections of the scales can be applied alone. However, the quality of validity results is superior for most of the scales in Chapter 9, and we recommend that readers looking for an ADL scale consider those also.

REFERENCES

(1) Lawton MP. Environment and other determinants of well-being in older people. Gerontologist 1983;23:349–357.
(2) Donaldson SW, Wagner CC, Gresham GE. A unified ADL evaluation form. Arch Phys Med Rehabil 1973;54:175–179, 185.
(3) Gresham GE, Phillips TF, Labi MLC. ADL status in stroke: relative merits of three standard indexes. Arch Phys Med Rehabil 1980;61:355–358.
(4) Pool DA, Brown RA. A functional rating scale for research in physical therapy. Tex Rep Biol Med 1968;26:133–136.
(5) Sainsbury S. Measuring disability. London: G. Bell, 1973.
(6) Gauger AB, Brownell WM, Russell WW, et al. Evaluation of levels of subsistence. Arch Phys Med Rehabil 1964;45:286–292.
(7) Susset V, Vobecky J, Black R. Disability outcome and self-assessment of disabled persons: an analysis of 506 cases. Arch Phys Med Rehabil 1979;60:50–56.
(8) Scranton J, Fogel ML, Erdman WJ. Evaluation of functional levels of patients during and following rehabilitation. Arch Phys Med Rehabil 1970;51:1–21.
(9) Rinzler SH, Brown H, Benton JG. A method for the objective evaluation of physical and drug therapy in the rehabilitation of the hemiplegic patient. Am Heart J 1951;42:710–718.

IADL SCALES

Instrumental Activities of Daily Living scales extend the ADL theme to cover tasks that require a finer level of motor coordination than is necessary for the relatively gross activities covered in ADL scales. IADL scales are commonly used with less severely handicapped populations, often as survey instruments for use in the general population, and cover activities needed for continued community residence. They were intended to improve on the sensitivity of ADL scales that were found not to identify low levels of disability, nor minor changes in level of disability. It should be noted that several scales include both ADL and IADL questions; our classification was based on what appears to be the primary orientation of the scale.

We describe nine IADL scales—three that are used in clinical settings, one used as a clinical or a research scale, one research scale, and four population survey instruments. The survey instruments include Pfeffer's Functional Activities Questionnaire, the questionnaire developed by the international Organization for Economic Cooperation and Development, and two disability screening scales developed in England: the Lambeth scale and Bennett and Garrad's interview schedule. We review Linn's Rapid Disability Rating Scale as a research scale and the Health Assessment Questionnaire, widely used in clinical and research settings. The clinical scales include the Functional Status Index of Jette, the Patient Evaluation Conference System developed by Harvey and Jellinek, and the Functional Independence Measure, which has become the standard instrument in rehabilitation research in North America. In addition to these scales the reader should consult Chapter 9, which presents several scales such as the OARS Multidimensional Functional Activities Questionnaire that include sections with IADL themes.

A RAPID DISABILITY RATING SCALE
(Margaret W. Linn, 1967, Revised 1982)

Purpose

The Rapid Disability Rating Scale (RDRS) was developed as a research tool for summarizing the functional capacity and mental status of elderly chronic patients. It may be used with hospitalized patients and with people living in the community.

Conceptual Basis

No information is available.

Description

The 1967 version of the RDRS contained 16 items covering physical and mental functioning and independence in self-care. A revised scale of 18 items was published by Linn and Linn as the RDRS-2 in 1982 (1, 2). Changes included the addition of

three items covering mobility, toileting, and adaptive tasks (i.e., managing money, telephoning, shopping); the question on safety supervision was dropped (1, p379). Four-point response scales replaced the earlier three-point scales. The RDRS-2 has eight questions on activities of daily living, three on sensory abilities, three on mental capacities, and one question on each of dietary changes, continence, medications, and confinement to bed (see Exhibit 3.13). The following review refers mainly to the revised version.

The rating scale is completed by a nurse or a person familiar with the patient. Because the scale describes performance, the rater must observe the patient carrying out the various tasks rather than rely on self-report. Once the rater has made the observations, it takes about two minutes to complete the scale.

Response categories are phrased in terms of the amount of assistance the patient requires so that the instrument indicates handicap rather than impairment. Each item is weighted equally in calculating an overall score. The scores range from 18 to 72, with higher values indicating greater disability; items may be combined to provide three subscores indicating the degree of assistance required with activities of daily living, physical disabilities, and psychosocial problems (1, p380).

Reliability

Inter-rater reliability of the preliminary version was assessed by comparing ratings of 20 patients made independently by three raters; a coefficient of 0.91 was obtained using Kendall's W index of concordance (3, p213). Test–retest reliability was investigated by repeating ratings of 238 patients before and after admission to nursing homes. With a mean delay of three and a half days, the correlation between ratings was 0.83, and the mean scores of the two sets of ratings were within one point of each other (3, p213). Linn et al. reported a one-week test–retest correlation of 0.89 on 1,000 male patients for the 16-item

Exhibit 3.13 The Rapid Disability Rating Scale-2

Directions: Rate what the person *does* to reflect current behavior. Circle one of the four choices for each item. Consider rating with any aids or prostheses normally used. None = completely independent or normal behavior. Total = that person cannot, will not or may not (because of medical restriction) perform a behavior or has the most severe form of disability or problem.

Assistance with activities of daily living

Eating	None	A little	A lot	Spoon-feed; intravenous tube
Walking (with cane or walker if used)	None	A little	A lot	Does not walk
Mobility (going outside and getting about with wheelchair, etc., if used)	None	A little	A lot	Is housebound
Bathing (include getting supplies, supervising)	None	A little	A lot	Must be bathed
Dressing (include help in selecting clothes)	None	A little	A lot	Must be dressed
Toileting (include help with clothes, cleaning, or help with ostomy, catheter)	None	A little	A lot	Uses bedpan or unable to care for ostomy/catheter
Grooming (shaving for men, hair-dressing for women, nails, teeth)	None	A little	A lot	Must be groomed
Adaptive tasks (managing money/possessions; telephoning, buying newspaper, toilet articles, snacks)	None	A little	A lot	Cannot manage

Degree of disability

Communication (expressing self)	None	A little	A lot	Does not communicate
Hearing (with aid if used)	None	A little	A lot	Does not seem to hear
Sight (with glasses, if used)	None	A little	A lot	Does not see
Diet (deviation from normal)	None	A little	A lot	Fed by intravenous tube
In bed during day (ordered or self-initiated)	None	A little (<3 hrs)	A lot	Most/all of time
Incontinence (urine/feces, with catheter or prosthesis, if used)	None	Sometimes	Frequently (weekly +)	Does not control
Medication	None	Sometimes	Daily, taken orally	Daily; injection; (+ oral if used)

Degree of special problems

Mental confusion	None	A little	A lot	Extreme
Uncooperativeness (combats efforts to help with care)	None	A little	A lot	Extreme
Depression	None	A little	A lot	Extreme

Reprinted with permission from the American Geriatrics Society. The Rapid Disability Rating Scale-2, by Linn MW and Linn BS (Journal of the American Geriatrics Society, Vol 30, p 380, 1982).

version of the RDRS (4, p340). Linn and Linn reported item reliability results for the revised version: two nurses independently rated 100 patients and item correlations ranged from 0.62 to 0.98; the three lowest correlations were for the mental status items (1, Table 2). Test–retest reliability on 50 patients after an interval of three days produced correlations between 0.58 and 0.96 (1, pp380–381).

Validity

A factor analysis of ratings of 120 hospitalized patients provided a three-factor solution (1, p381). Linn and Linn interpreted the factors as reflecting activities of daily living, disability, and psychological problems. The latter were labeled "special problems" by the authors, as shown in Exhibit 3.13.

Ratings of 845 men (mean age, 68 years) were used to predict subsequent mortality using multiple regression and discriminant function analyses. Twenty percent of the variance in mortality was explained, correctly classifying 72% of patients who would die (1, p382).

Correlations of 0.27 were obtained between the RDRS-2 and a physician's 13-item rating scale of impairment of 172 elderly patients living in the community; a correlation of 0.43 was obtained with a six-point self-report scale of health (1, p382).

Alternative Forms

A French version has been used (7).

Reference Standards

No formal reference standards are available, but Linn and Linn noted that for the RDRS-2 scores for elderly community residents with minimal disabilities average 21 to 22. For hospitalized elderly patients the average is about 32, and for those transferred to nursing homes it is about 36 (1, p380).

Commentary

This is a broad-ranging scale that rates the amount of assistance required in 18 activities, broader in scope than the PULSES, Barthel, and most ADL scales. It has been used in several evaluative studies (4–6) and a French version was used by Jenicek et al. (7). Its research orientation is reflected in the reliability and validity testing, which is superior to the clinical scales. Nonetheless, the validity tests could be improved. For example, correlations with physicians' ratings commonly produce low coefficients because the physician is not aware of details of the patient's functioning. The use of predictive validation is imaginative, but as this is rarely attempted with such indices it is hard to judge whether a 20% explanation variance is high or low. It would be advantageous if studies of predictive validity reported findings in a comparable manner: Granger expressed the predictive validity of the Barthel Index in terms of percentages of patients with low scores who died.

Criticisms have been made of the scoring system. For example, the same weight is assigned to different degrees of disability: "permanent confinement to bed" and "following a special diet" both rate three points (7, p345). This limits the validity of the scale in giving absolute indications of disability, although it may be less serious if the scale is used to monitor change over time.

REFERENCES

(1) Linn MW, Linn BS. The Rapid Disability Rating Scale-2. J Am Geriatr Soc 1982;30:378–382.
(2) Linn MW. Rapid Disability Rating Scale-2 (RDRS-2). Psychopharmacol Bull 1988; 24:799–800.
(3) Linn MW. A Rapid Disability Rating Scale. J Am Geriatr Soc 1967;15:211–214.
(4) Linn MW, Gurel L, Linn BS. Patient outcome as a measure of quality of nursing home care. Am J Public Health 1977; 67:337–344.
(5) Ogren EH, Linn MW. Male nursing home patients: relocation and mortality. J Am Geriatr Soc 1971;19:229–239.
(6) Linn MW, Linn BS, Harris R. Effects of counseling for late stage cancer patients. Cancer 1982;49:1048–1055.
(7) Jenicek M, Cléroux R, Lamoureux M. Principal component analysis of four health indicators and construction of a global health index in the aged. Am J Epidemiol 1979;110:343–349.

THE FUNCTIONAL STATUS INDEX
(Pilot Geriatric Arthritis Program, Alan M. Jette, 1978, Revised 1980)

Purpose

The Functional Status Index (FSI) was designed to assess the functional status of adult arthritics living in the community (1). Intended both as a clinical and an evaluative tool, the scale measures the degree of dependence, pain, and difficulty experienced in performing daily activities (2).

Conceptual Basis

The FSI was developed to evaluate a Pilot Geriatric Arthritis Program (PGAP) which sought to improve the quality of life of elderly arthritics (3). The goals of the program were to prevent disability, restore activity, reduce pain, and encourage social and emotional adjustment (3). Previous instruments were criticized "for their use of broad categories of activity (e.g. dressing) which incorporated complex series of activities involving many different joints and muscle groups" (4, p576). Jette also argued that the outcomes of care should not be viewed solely in terms of independence, as is the case in most ADL scales. Sometimes providing assistance to a patient, which increases dependence, may alleviate pain and reduce difficulty. He challenged "the exclusive emphasis on level of dependence in previous work as well as the assumption that assistance in ADL constitutes a loss of health" (4, p576). Accordingly, the FSI was designed to measure pain and difficulty, as well as level of dependence, in performing tasks.

Description

Based on the Barthel, PULSES, and Katz instruments, the FSI was developed as a comprehensive ADL assessment for adults living in the community (2, 3). The original FSI contained 45 ADL items (shown in reference 2, Table 1). Three questions were asked for each activity, yielding separate ratings for dependency, difficulty, and pain. The resulting 135 questions (45 items × three dimensions) took between 60 and 90 minutes to administer (5).

This proved unworkable, and factor analyses guided the abbreviation of the FSI to the current version, which is shown in Exhibit 3.14. The 18 items are grouped under five headings: mobility, hand activi-

ties, personal care, home chores, and social/role activities. The FSI is administered by an interviewer and covers performance over the previous seven days. The questions are asked three times. To assess dependency (or level of assistance used) the respondent is asked: "How much help did you use to do _____, on average, during the past week?" A five-point rating scale runs from independent to unable to do the activity. Four-point scales are used to rate the amount of pain experienced when doing each activity and the amount of difficulty experienced in performing each activity. Alternatively, 0–13 and 0–7 ladder scales have been used, but the four-point rating is the standard approach (Dr. Jette, personal communication, 1993). Cue cards may be used to show the answer categories to the respondent. The 18-item version of the FSI takes 20 to 30 minutes to administer (5).

Reliability

Forty-five-Item Version. Jette and Deniston studied inter-rater reliability in assessing 19 patients and found that as the degree of pain and difficulty increased, agreement between raters decreased (1, Table 3). The agreement among nine raters yielded intraclass correlations averaging 0.78 for the dependence dimension, 0.61 for difficulty, and 0.75, for pain (1, Table 4). Liang and Jette reported equivalent figures of 0.72, 0.75, and 0.78 (6).

Liang and Jette reported test–retest reliability of 0.75 in the dependence dimension, 0.77 in the difficulty dimension, and 0.69 in the pain dimension (6, p83).

Eighteen-Item Version. Jette compared the internal consistency reliability for the five dimensions of this version and he also examined three different response modes: defined response options (of the type listed above), a ladder scale, and a Q-sort technique (5). For 149 patients, the internal consistency of the mobility and personal-care sections ranged from 0.70 to over 0.90 (5, Tables 5–7). Similar reliability results were achieved with each of the three re-

Exhibit 3.14   The Functional Status Index

Functional Dependence

"In this first section of the interview, we are trying to measure the degree to which you used *help* to perform your daily activities, on the average, during the past 7 days. By help, I mean the extent to which you used equipment (such as a cane), whether you used human assistance (such as a friend or relative), and whether you used both equipment and human assistance to do certain activities.

"I would now like you to tell me how much help you used, on the average, during the past week, to do each activity I will read to you. Tell me if you did the activity without help, used equipment, used human assistance, used both equipment and human assistance, or if you were unable or it was unsafe to do it. "Do you have any questions before we begin?

"How much help did you use when _____, on average, during the past week?" (Repeat for each item).

Items:

Gross Mobility
Walking inside
Climbing up stairs
Rising from a chair

Personal Care
Putting on pants
Buttoning a shirt/blouse
Washing all parts of the body
Putting on a shirt/blouse

Social/Role Activities
Performing your job
Driving a car
Attending meetings/appointments
Visiting with friends and relatives

Hand Activities
Writing
Opening a container
Dialing a phone

Home Chores
Vacuuming a rug
Reaching into low cupboards
Doing laundry
Doing yardwork

Functional Pain

"In this section of the interview, we are trying to measure the amount of *pain* you experienced when you performed your daily activities during the past week. For each activity performed during the past 7 days, I would like you to judge the amount of pain you experienced when doing it. For each activity you performed, please judge whether you experienced no, mild, moderate, or severe pain when performing the activity.

"By pain, I mean the discomfort or sensation of hurting you experienced when doing the activity. "Do you have any questions before we start?

"How much pain did you experience, on average, during the past week when _____? Would you say no, mild, moderate or severe pain?" (Repeat for each item, except those that the person has said they did not attempt).

Functional Difficulty

"In this section of the interview, we are trying to measure how *difficult* it was to perform each activity, on average, during the past 7 days. By difficulty, we mean how easy or hard it was to do the activity. For each activity you performed, please tell me whether you experienced no, mild, moderate, or severe difficulty in doing it.

"Do you have any questions?

"How much difficulty did you have in _____, on average, during the previous 7 days? Would you say no, mild, moderate or severe difficulty?" (Repeat for each item, except those that the person has said they did not attempt).

Adapted from an original sent by Dr. AM Jette. With permission.

sponse modes, except that in assessing pain levels the fixed answer categories proved less reliable than the other scaling techniques (5). A subsequent publication repeated the same analyses but added test–retest results (ranging from 0.69 to 0.88) and inter-observer agreement (0.64 to 0.89) (7, Tables 2–4).

Validity

Forty-five-Item Version. Deniston and Jette compared responses to the 45-item FSI with ratings made by hospital staff and with self-ratings made by 95 elderly arthritics. Correlations between the patients' judgments of their "number of good days in the past week" and their FSI scores were 0.14 for the dependence dimension, 0.41 for difficulty, and 0.46 for pain (3, Table 2). Correlations of the FSI scores and a self-rating of ability to deal with disease-related problems averaged 0.24; correlations with a self-rating of joint condition averaged 0.39 (3, Table 1). Correlations with ratings made by the staff were lower, ranging from 0.11 to 0.22 (3, Table 4).

Eighteen-Item Version. A factor analysis identified the five factors shown in Exhibit 3.14 (5). In a different study analyzing 36 items, Jette again obtained five factors, accounting for 58.5% of the variance (2, Table 2). There was some contrast in the factor structure for the pain, difficulty, and dependency items, but Jette concluded that five functional categories are common to the three dimensions (2). These amplify the three categories (mobility, personal care, and work) that were originally proposed.

In a sample of 80 patients with rheumatoid arthritis, Shope et al. obtained correlations ranging from 0.40 to 0.43 with the American Rheumatism Association functional class and from 0.40 to 0.47 with a physician assessment of functional ability (8, Table V). The FSI has been used in evaluating change following treatment; in a small study of 15 arthritics, change in FSI scores correlated 0.49 with improvement in muscle strength, 0.53 with improvement in

endurance, and −0.67 with change in time taken. These variables predicted 77% of the variance in FSI change scores (9). Liang et al. provide a more comprehensive comparison of sensitivity to change of five scales in evaluating change following hip or knee surgery (10). The FSI proved to be the least sensitive of the measures, in some comparisons requiring a sample size three or four times greater than those needed by the Arthritis Impact Measurement Scales to demonstrate a significant improvement (10, Table 3).

Alternative Forms

Jette, Harris, and others have described a different instrument that they also named the Functional Status Index (11, 12). Rudimentary validity data for a 17-item version were reported by Harris et al. for 47 elderly patients with hip fractures (11).

A 12-item modification of the FSI showed an alpha reliability of 0.91 and correlated 0.46 with the Quality of Well-Being Scale (13, p962).

Commentary

This instrument is similar to the Kenny scale in its aim of providing a more detailed disability rating than rival scales. The FSI is well founded on a conceptual analysis of disability; the distinction between difficulty, dependence, and pain is innovative and may prove helpful. These dimensions have received some empirical support through factor analyses and contrasting correlations with other scales. Deniston and Jette noted that the distinction between dependence and the other two dimensions is meaningful, but that between pain and difficulty is still equivocal (3). Jette does not report the correlation between the pain and difficulty dimensions; it is to be hoped that future studies will examine the necessity of keeping these two dimensions separate. Reliability results for the FSI are good.

The existence of different versions (15 items reported by Shope, 17 by Harris, and the standard 18 items) is a problem shared by several other health measures. The suggestion (11, p35; 12, p736) that reliability data for the 18-item version also hold for the very different 17-item version is misleading. Some validity results may cause concern: several of the criterion correlations are lower than for other scales that we review. It is desirable that more evidence on validity be accumulated, including testing on conditions other than arthritis, before this scale can be fully recommended.

REFERENCES

(1) Jette AM, Deniston OL. Inter-observer reliability of a functional status assessment instrument. J Chronic Dis 1978;31:573–580.

(2) Jette AM. Functional capacity evaluation: an empirical approach. Arch Phys Med Rehabil 1980;61:85–89.

(3) Deniston OL, Jette A. A functional status assessment instrument: validation in an elderly population. Health Serv Res 1980; 15:21–34.

(4) Jette AM. Health status indicators: their utility in chronic-disease evaluation research. J Chronic Dis 1980;33:567–579.

(5) Jette AM. Functional Status Index: reliability of a chronic disease evaluation instrument. Arch Phys Med Rehabil 1980; 61:395–401.

(6) Liang MH, Jette AM. Measuring functional ability in chronic arthritis: a critical review. Arthritis Rheum 1981;24:80–86.

(7) Jette AM. The Functional Status Index: reliability and validity of a self-report functional disability measure. J Rheumatol 1987;14(suppl 15):15–19.

(8) Shope JT, Banwell BA, Jette AM, et al. Functional status outcome after treatment of rheumatoid arthritis. Clin Rheumatol Pract 1983;Nov/Dec:243–248.

(9) Fisher NM, Pendergast DR, Gresham GE, et al. Muscle rehabilitation: its effect on muscular and functional performance of patients with knee osteoarthritis. Arch Phys Med Rehabil 1991;72:367–374.

(10) Liang MH, Fossel AH, Larson MG. Comparisons of five health status instruments for orthopedic evaluation. Med Care 1990;28:632–642.

(11) Harris BA, Jette AM, Campion EW, et al. Validity of self-report measures of functional disability. Top Geriatr Rehabil 1986;1:31–41.

(12) Jette AM, Harris BA, Cleary PD, et al. Functional recovery after hip fracture. Arch Phys Med Rehabil 1987;68:735–740.

(13) Ganiats TG, Palinkas LA, Kaplan RM. Comparison of Quality of Well-Being Scale and Functional Status Index in patients with atrial fibrillation. Med Care 1992; 30:958–964.

THE PATIENT EVALUATION CONFERENCE SYSTEM
(Richard F. Harvey and Hollis M. Jellinek, 1981)

Purpose

The Patient Evaluation Conference System (PECS) rates the functional and psychosocial status of rehabilitation patients. It is intended for use in defining treatment goals and in evaluating progress toward them.

Conceptual Basis

Although no formal conceptual basis was given to justify the content of the instrument, Harvey and Jellinek described several principles that guided the design of the PECS. These included its need to be able to reflect minor changes in functional level, its multidisciplinary scope (covering medical, psychological, social, and vocational topics), and its simplicity of application, scoring, and interpretation (1).

Description

The PECS is a broad-ranging instrument containing 79 functional assessment items grouped into 15 sections with an additional three sections pertaining to the results of a case conference. Each section is completed by the staff member who has primary responsibility for that aspect of care. The ratings made by each therapist are collated onto a master form that summarizes the rehabilitation goals. This is used in case conferences to record the patient's progress. The PECS form shown in Exhibit 3.15 was obtained from Dr. Harvey and is a slightly expanded version of that shown in reference 2 (Figure 2).

Eight-point responses are used for most items, with 0 representing unmeasured or unmeasurable function and 7 representing

Exhibit 3.15 The Patient Evaluation Conference System

Scores range from 0 to 7, with 0 being the lowest score, or not assessed, and 7 being the highest score, such as normal or independent. Scores of 1 to 4 indicate dependent function. Scores of 5 or more indicate independent function.

Keys to scores are available in each participating discipline.

<u>Instructions:</u> Circle (0) the goal score   example
X the current status score   0   1   2   3   4 | ⑤   6   7
                                      Dependent | Independent

I. Rehabilitation Medicine (MED)
1. Motor loss (including muscle weakness and limb deficiency)   0 1 2 3 4 5 6 7
2. Spasticity/involuntary movement (including dystonia and ataxia)   0 1 2 3 4 5 6 7
3. Joint limitations   0 1 2 3 4 5 6 7
4. Autonomic disturbance   0 1 2 3 4 5 6 7
5. Sensory deficiency   0 1 2 3 4 5 6 7
6. Perceptual and cognitive deficit   0 1 2 3 4 5 6 7
7. Associated medical problems   0 1 2 3 4 5 6 7

II. Rehabilitation Nursing (NSG)
1. Performance of bowel program   0 1 2 3 4 5 6 7
2. Performance of urinary program   0 1 2 3 4 5 6 7
3. Performance of skin program   0 1 2 3 4 5 6 7
4. Assumes responsibility for self-care   0 1 2 3 4 5 6 7
5. Performs assigned interdisciplinary activities   0 1 2 3 4 5 6 7

III. Physical Mobility (PHY)
1. Performance of transfers   0 1 2 3 4 5 6 7
2. Performance of ambulation   0 1 2 3 4 5 6 7
3. Performance of wheelchair mobility (primary mode)   0 1 2 3 4 5 6 7
4. Ability to handle environmental barriers (e.g., stairs, rugs, elevators)   0 1 2 3 4 5 6 7
5. Performance of car transfer   0 1 2 3 4 5 6 7

6. Driving mobility   0 1 2 3 4 5 6 7
7. Assumes responsibility for mobility   0 1 2 3 4 5 6 7

IV. Activities of Daily Living (ADL)
1. Performance in feeding   0 1 2 3 4 5 6 7
2. Performance in hygiene/grooming   0 1 2 3 4 5 6 7
3. Performance in dressing   0 1 2 3 4 5 6 7
4. Performance in home management   0 1 2 3 4 5 6 7
5. Performance of mobility in home environment (including utilization of environmental adaptations for communication)   0 1 2 3 4 5 6 7

V. Communication (COM)
1. Ability to comprehend spoken language   0 1 2 3 4 5 6 7
2. Ability to produce language   0 1 2 3 4 5 6 7
3. Ability to read   0 1 2 3 4 5 6 7
4. Ability to produce written language   0 1 2 3 4 5 6 7
5. Ability to hear   0 1 2 3 4 5 6 7
6. Ability to comprehend and use gesture   0 1 2 3 4 5 6 7
7. Ability to produce speech   0 1 2 3 4 5 6 7

VI. Medications (DRG)
1. Knowledge of medications   0 1 2 3 4 5 6 7
2. Skill with medications   0 1 2 3 4 5 6 7
3. Utilization of medications   0 1 2 3 4 5 6 7

VII. Nutrition (NUT)
1. Nutritional status—body weight   0 1 2 3 4 5 6 7

Exhibit 3.15 *(Continued)*

Exhibit 3.15 *(Continued)*

2. Nutritional status—lab values · 0 1 2 3 4 5 6 7
3. Knowledge of nutrition and/or modified diet · 0 1 2 3 4 5 6 7
4. Skill with nutrition and diet (adherence to nutritional plan) · 0 1 2 3 4 5 6 7
5. Utilization of nutrition and diet (nutritional health) · 0 1 2 3 4 5 6 7

VIII. **Assistive Devices (DEV)**
1. Knowledge of assistive devices(s) · 0 1 2 3 4 5 6 7
2. Skill with assuming operating position of assistive device(s) · 0 1 2 3 4 5 6 7
3. Utilization of assistive device(s) · 0 1 2 3 4 5 6 7

IX. **Psychology (PSY)**
1. Distress/comfort · 0 1 2 3 4 5 6 7
2. Helplessness/self-efficacy · 0 1 2 3 4 5 6 7
3. Self-directed learning skills · 0 1 2 3 4 5 6 7
4. Skill in self-management of behavior and emotions · 0 1 2 3 4 5 6 7
5. Skill in interpersonal relations · 0 1 2 3 4 5 6 7

X. **Neuropsychology (NP)**
1. Impairment of short-term memory · 0 1 2 3 4 5 6 7
2. Impairment of long-term memory · 0 1 2 3 4 5 6 7
3. Impairment in attention-concentration skills · 0 1 2 3 4 5 6 7
4. Impairment in verbal linguistic processing · 0 1 2 3 4 5 6 7
5. Impairment in visual spatial processing · 0 1 2 3 4 5 6 7
6. Impairment in basic intellectual skills · 0 1 2 3 4 5 6 7

XI. **Social Issues (SOC)**
1. Ability to problem solve and utilize resources · 0 1 2 3 4 5 6 7
2. Family: communication/resource · 0 1 2 3 4 5 6 7
3. Family understanding of disability · 0 1 2 3 4 5 6 7

4. Economic resources · 0 1 2 3 4 5 6 7
5. Ability to live independently · 0 1 2 3 4 5 6 7
6. Living arrangements · 0 1 2 3 4 5 6 7

XII. **Vocational-Educational Activity (V/E)**
1. Active participation in realistic voc/ed planning · 0 1 2 3 4 5 6 7
2. Realistic perception of work-related activity · 0 1 2 3 4 5 6 7
3. Ability to tolerate planned number of hours of voc/ed activity/day · 0 1 2 3 4 5 6 7
4. Vocational/educational placement · 0 1 2 3 4 5 6 7
5. Physical capacity for work · 0 1 2 3 4 5 6 7

XIII. **Recreation (REC)**
1. Participation in group activities · 0 1 2 3 4 5 6 7
2. Participation in community activities · 0 1 2 3 4 5 6 7
3. Interaction with others · 0 1 2 3 4 5 6 7
4. Participation and satisfaction with individual leisure activities · 0 1 2 3 4 5 6 7
5. Active participation in sports · 0 1 2 3 4 5 6 7

XIV. **Pain (consensus) (PAI)**
1. Pain behavior · 0 1 2 3 4 5 6 7
2. Physical inactivity · 0 1 2 3 4 5 6 7
3. Social withdrawal · 0 1 2 3 4 5 6 7
4. Pacing · 0 1 2 3 4 5 6 7
5. Sitting · 0 1 2 3 4 5 6 7
6. Standing tolerance · 0 1 2 3 4 5 6 7
7. Walking endurance · 0 1 2 3 4 5 6 7

XV. **Pulmonary Rehabilitation (PUL)**
1. Knowledge of pulmonary rehabilitation program · 0 1 2 3 4 5 6 7
2. Skill with pulmonary rehabilitation program · 0 1 2 3 4 5 6 7
3. Utilization of pulmonary rehabilitation program · 0 1 2 3 4 5 6 7

XVI. **Patient Participation** 1 2
at Conference
  1. Attended   N   Y
  2. Participated in goal   N   Y
    setting
  3. Family (significant   N   Y
    other) attended

XVII. **Preparation Com-** 1 2
pleted for Pass and/or
Discharge
  1. Recreational Ther-   N   Y
    apy pass
  2. P.R.N. pass   N   Y
  3. T.L.O.A pass   N   Y
  4. Is this the dis-   N   Y
    charge conference?
  5. Equipment ordered   N   Y
  6. Type of assistive   0 1 2 3 4 5 6 7
    device
  7. Phase of device de-   0 1 2 3 4 5 6 7
    velopment
  8. Therapy schedule   N   Y
    set according to
    priority

  9. Rehab. Med. Clinic   N   Y
    standard follow-up
    (1, 3, 6, 12 mo.)

XVIII. **Specialty Program**
(Specify):
  1. _____ 0 1 2 3 4 5 6 7
  2. _____ 0 1 2 3 4 5 6 7
  3. _____ 0 1 2 3 4 5 6 7
  4. _____ 0 1 2 3 4 5 6 7
  5. _____ 0 1 2 3 4 5 6 7
  6. _____ 0 1 2 3 4 5 6 7
  7. _____ 0 1 2 3 4 5 6 7

Summary

_____
_____
_____
_____
_____
_____
_____
_____
_____
_____
_____

Reproduced from the Patient Evaluation Conference System rating form provided by Dr. Richard F Harvey. With permission.

full independence. Scores are comparable across different scales: a cutting point of 5 distinguishes between a need for human assistance and managing independently (with or without aids). A few items use four-point scales.

Reliability

Inter-rater reliability for different sections of the PECS ranged from 0.68 to 0.80 for 125 patients (1, p459).

Validity

An abbreviated, self-administered version of the PECS was compared with the Brief Symptom Inventory, which measured emotional distress, for 22 brain-injured patients. Significant correlations in the range 0.38 to 0.47 were obtained with the self-care, mobility, living arrangements, and communication scales on the PECS (3, Table 2). Two PECS scales, bladder and skin care, were assessed at time of discharge on 28 patients. The results correlated with several depression scores recorded at admission to the rehabilitation program, with

coefficients between 0.37 and 0.39 (4, p361).

A study of 30 head trauma patients compared change in PECS scores between admission and discharge with the results of computerized tomography (CT) scans (5). Three patients found by CT scan to have no lesions achieved complete recovery in four out of five PECS scales; all ten patients with one-hemisphere lesions achieved independence in at least two areas, while for 17 patients with bilateral lesions, there were no areas in which all patients recovered completely (5, Table 2).

In a discriminant analysis, PECS scores correctly categorized 75% of patients in three contrasting levels of rehabilitation program (6).

Commentary

Harvey and associates have been expanding the PECS to include documentation for outpatient evaluation, with reports to referring physicians. Its use of a goal-attainment approach is distinctive, and a graphical presentation of data has been developed (2). Most of the validation studies used very small samples, however, and in some cases (4) it is not clear what the rationale for the study was. Although additional evidence on the quality of this scale is required, it appears to hold considerable potential as a clinical measurement system for rehabilitation settings.

Address

Richard F Harvey, MD, Vice President and Chief of Medical Staff, Marianjoy Hospital, Roosevelt Road, PO Box 795, Wheaton, Illinois, USA 60189

REFERENCES

(1) Harvey RF, Jellinek HM. Functional performance assessment: a program approach. Arch Phys Med Rehabil 1981;62:456–461.
(2) Harvey RF, Jellinek HM. Patient profiles: utilization in functional performance assessment. Arch Phys Med Rehabil 1983; 64:268–271.
(3) Jellinek HM, Torkelson RM, Harvey RF. Functional abilities and distress levels in brain injured patients at long-term follow-up. Arch Phys Med Rehabil 1982; 63:160–162.
(4) Malec J, Neimeyer R. Psychologic prediction of duration of inpatient spinal cord injury rehabilitation and performance of self-care. Arch Phys Med Rehabil 1983; 64:359–363.
(5) Rao N, Jellinek HM, Harvey RF, et al. Computerized tomography head scans as predictors of rehabilitation outcome. Arch Phys Med Rehabil 1984;65:18–20.
(6) Harvey RF, Silverstein B, Venzon MA, et al. Applying psychometric criteria to functional assessment in medical rehabilitation: III. Construct validity and predicting level of care. Arch Phys Med Rehabil 1992;73:887–892.

THE FUNCTIONAL ACTIVITIES QUESTIONNAIRE
(Robert I. Pfeffer, 1982, Revised 1984)

Purpose

This is a screening tool for assessing independence in daily activities designed for community studies of normal aging and mild senile dementia (1).

Conceptual Basis

The scale was intended to cover universal skills among older adults. Pfeffer followed the intuitively appealing concept of a hierarchy of skills proposed by Lawton and Brody and concentrated on higher level skills such as managing one's financial affairs and reading, which they had termed "social functions" (1).

Description

The Functional Activities Questionnaire (FAQ) is not self-administered but is completed by a lay informant such as the spouse, a relative, or a close friend. The original version described in the literature is shown in Exhibit 3.16; it has ten items concerned with performing daily tasks necessary for independent living. In 1984, the questionnaire was slightly expanded by adding four ADL items and an item on initiative; the first ten items are the same in both versions. For each activity, four levels ranging from dependence (scored 3) to independence (scored 0) are specified. For activities not normally undertaken by the person, the informant must specify whether the person would be unable to undertake the task if required (scored 1) or could do so if required (0). The total score is the sum of individual item scores; higher scores reflect greater dependency.

Reliability

The item-total correlations for all items exceeded 0.80 (1, Table 4).

Validity

In a study of 158 elderly people living in the community, ratings on the FAQ correlated 0.72 with Lawton and Brody's IADL scale (1, Table 3). Correlations with mental functioning tests were mostly in excess of 0.70; the lowest correlation (0.41) was with Raven's matrices. The highest correlation (0.83) was with a neurologist's global rating on a Scale of Functional Capacity

Exhibit 3.16 The Functional Activities Questionnaire

Activities questionnaire to be completed by spouse, child, close friend or relative of the participant.

Instructions: The following pages list ten common activities. *For each activity,* please read all choices, then choose the *one* statement which best describes the *current* ability of the participant. Answers should apply to *that person's* abilities, not your own. Please check off a choice for *each* activity; do not skip any.

1. Writing checks, paying bills, balancing checkbook, keeping financial records
   _____ A. Someone has recently taken over this activity completely or almost completely.
   _____ B. Requires frequent advice or assistance from others (e.g., relatives, friends, business associates, banker), which was *not previously necessary.*
   _____ C. Does without any advice or assistance, but more difficult than used to be or less good job.
   _____ D. Does without any difficulty or advice.
   _____ E. Never did and would find quite difficult to start now.
   _____ F. Didn't do regularly but can do normally now with a little practice if they have to.

2. Making out insurance or Social Security forms, handling business affairs or papers, assembling tax records
   _____ A. Someone has recently taken over this activity completely or almost completely, and that someone did not used to do any or as much.
   _____ B. Requires more frequent advice or more assistance from others than in the past.
   _____ C. Does without any more advice or assistance than used to, but finds more difficult or does less good job than in the past.
   _____ D. Does without any difficulty or advice.
   _____ E. Never did and would find quite difficult to start now, even with practice.
   _____ F. Didn't do routinely, but can do normally now should they have to.

3. Shopping alone for clothes, household necessities and groceries
   _____ A. Someone has recently taken over this activity completely or almost completely.
   _____ B. Requires frequent advice or assistance from others.
   _____ C. Does without advice or assistance, but finds more difficult than used to or does less good job.
   _____ D. Does without any difficulty or advice.
   _____ E. Never did and would find quite difficult to start now.
   _____ F. Didn't do routinely but can do normally now should they have to.

4. Playing a game of skill such as bridge, other card games or chess or working on a hobby such as painting, photography, woodwork, stamp collecting
   _____ A. Hardly ever does now or has great difficulty.
   _____ B. Requires advice, or others have to make allowances.
   _____ C. Does without advice, or assistance, but more difficult or less skillful than used to be.
   _____ D. Does without any difficulty or advice.
   _____ E. Never did and would find quite difficult to start now.
   _____ F. Didn't do regularly, but can do normally now should they have to.

5. Heat the water, make a cup of coffee or tea, and turn off the stove
   _____ A. Someone else has recently taken over this activity completely, or almost completely.
   _____ B. Requires advice or has frequent problems (for example, burns pots, forgets to turn off stove).
   _____ C. Does without advice or assistance but occasional problems.
   _____ D. Does without any difficulty or advice.
   _____ E. Never did and would find quite difficult to start now.
   _____ F. Didn't usually, but can do normally now, should they have to.

6. Prepare a balanced meal (e.g., meat, chicken or fish, vegetables, dessert)
   _____ A. Someone else has recently taken over this activity completely or almost completely.
   _____ B. Requires frequent advice or has frequent problems (for example, burns pots, forgets how to make a given dish).
   _____ C. Does without much advice or assistance, but more difficult (for example, switched to TV dinners most of the time because of difficulty).
   _____ D. Does without any difficulty or advice.
   _____ E. Never did and would find quite difficult to do now even after a little practice.
   _____ F. Didn't do regularly, but can do normally now should they have to.

Exhibit 3.16 *(Continued)*

93

Exhibit 3.16   *(Continued)*

7. Keep track of current events, either in the neighborhood or nationally
   _____ A. Pays no attention to, or doesn't remember outside happenings.
   _____ B. Some idea about *major* events (for example, comments on presidential election, major events in the news or major sporting events).
   _____ C. Somewhat less attention to, or knowledge of, current events than formerly.
   _____ D. As aware of current events as ever was.
   _____ E. Never paid much attention to current events, and would find quite difficult to start now.
   _____ F. Never paid much attention, but can do as well as anyone now when they try.

8. Pay attention to, understand, and discuss the plot or theme of a one-hour television program; get something out of a book or magazine
   _____ A. Doesn't remember, or seems confused by, what they have watched or read.
   _____ B. Aware of the *general idea,* characters, or nature while they watch or read, but may *not recall* later; may *not grasp theme* or have opinion about what they saw.
   _____ C. Less attention, or less memory than before, less likely to catch humor, points which are made quickly, or subtle points.
   _____ D. Grasps as quickly as ever.
   _____ E. Never paid much attention to or commented on T.V., never read much and would probably find very difficult to start now.
   _____ F. Never read or watched T.V. much, but read or watch as much as ever and get as much out of it as ever.

9. Remember appointments, plans, household tasks, car repairs, family occasions (such as birthdays or anniversaries), holidays, medications
   _____ A. Someone else has recently taken this over.
   _____ B. Has to be reminded some of the time (more than in the past or more than most people).
   _____ C. Manages without reminders but has to rely heavily on notes, calendars, schemes.
   _____ D. Remembers appointments, plans, occasions, etc. as well as they ever did.
   _____ E. Never had to keep track of appointments, medications or family occasions, and would probably find very difficult to start now.
   _____ F. Didn't have to keep track of these things in the past, but can do as well as anyone when they try.

10. Travel out of neighborhood; driving, walking, arranging to take or change buses and trains, planes
   _____ A. Someone else has taken this over completely or almost completely.
   _____ B. Can get around in own neighborhood but gets lost out of neighborhood.
   _____ C. Has more problems getting around than used to (for example, occasionally lost, loss of confidence, can't find car, etc.) but usually O.K.
   _____ D. Gets around as well as ever.
   _____ E. Rarely did much driving or had to get around alone and would find quite difficult to learn bus routes or make similar arrangements now.
   _____ F. Didn't have to get around alone much in past, but can do as well as ever when has to.

Reproduced from the Functional Activities Questionnaire provided by Dr. Robert I Pfeffer. With permission.

designed by Pfeffer (1, Table 3). The validity coefficients obtained for the FAQ were consistently higher than those obtained for the IADL. The FAQ and the IADL were used in multiple regression analyses as predictors of mental status and functional assessments and the FAQ consistently performed better.

Comparing the FAQ to diagnoses made by attending neurologists, the sensitivity was 85% at a specificity of 81% (1). The FAQ was found to correlate 0.76 with a Mental Function Index developed by Pfeffer (2). Scores on the FAQ in a longitudinal study reflected both clinical judgments of change and cognitive measures in 54 elderly patients (2, Table 8). The FAQ also showed significant contrasts between normal, depressed, and demented cases in a study of 195 respondents (3, Table 6).

Commentary

The Functional Activities Questionnaire is comparatively recent and the available validity results are promising. For the elderly population used in the validation study, the method seems clearly superior to Lawton and Brody's IADL on which it builds. The method differs somewhat from other IADL instruments in that the scale levels are defined primarily in terms of social function rather than physical capacities. This brings the scale close to some of the social health measurements described in Chapter 4.

REFERENCES

(1) Pfeffer RI, Kurosaki TT, Harrah CH, et al. Measurement of functional activities in older adults in the community. J Gerontol 1982;37:323–329.

(2) Pfeffer RI, Kurosaki TT, Chance JM, et al. Use of the Mental Function Index in older adults: reliability, validity, and measurement of change over time. Am J Epidemiol 1984;120:922–935.

(3) Pfeffer RI, Kurosaki TT, Harrah CH, et al. A survey diagnostic tool for senile dementia. Am J Epidemiol 1981;114:515–527.

THE LAMBETH DISABILITY SCREENING QUESTIONNAIRE
(Donald L. Patrick and Others, 1981)

Purpose

This postal questionnaire was designed to screen for physical disability in adults living in the community. It provides estimates of the prevalence of disability for use in planning health and social services.

Conceptual Basis

Based on the impairment, disability, and handicap triad, questions on disability concern mobility and self-care; they are phrased in terms of difficulty in performing various activities rather than in terms of reduced capacity. A section on impairments records the nature of the illnesses causing disability, and questions on handicap cover housework, employment, and social activities.

Description

This instrument was first used to screen for disability in the Lambeth Health Survey. The disabled persons and normal controls were interviewed using a British version of the Sickness Impact Profile called the Functional Limitations Profile (FLP). Data collected by the FLP were used in validating the screening instrument.

The original version of the Lambeth Questionnaire contained 31 questions drawn from the questionnaires of Bennett and Garrad, of Haber, and of Harris (1–3). Twenty-five of these questions were retained in the version used in the Lambeth survey (see Exhibit 3.17). Subsequently a third version was designed with 22 items, 13 of which were taken, unchanged, from the previous instrument; two were new, two were items reintroduced from the first version, and five were reworded from the second version (4). The third version is shown in Exhibit 3.18. All three versions record difficulties with body movement, ambulation and mobility, self-care, social activity, and sensory problems.

The second version (shown in Exhibit 3.17) is completed by one family member who reports for all members of a household. The respondent indicates the first name and age of each person who has any of the problems listed. As a screening instrument, it classifies people as disabled or not:

Respondents were classified as "disabled" if they reported difficulty with one or more of (a) the ambulation, mobility, body care, or movement items, except constipation or stress incontinence alone; (b) the sensory-motor items except giddiness when no associated illness condition was reported; and/or (c) the social activity items, except limitation in working at all or doing the job of choice where the respondent was over retirement age. (5, p66)

The third version (Exhibit 3.18) is interviewer-administered and collects data on the respondent only. It uses a yes/no response format and scoring weights are given (4, p304).

Exhibit 3.17   The Lambeth Disability Screening Questionnaire (Version 2)

The following questions apply to EVERYONE AGED 16 or over living in this household. Please answer every question as well as you can, as shown in the examples below.

EXAMPLE 1 *(for when someone has difficulty)*

WHO has difficulty with any of the following? ↓	The first names and ages of everyone having this difficulty are	No one
Getting around the house without help	*John (65)* .... *Mary (56)*	

EXAMPLE 2 *(for when no one has difficulty)*

↓ WHO has difficulty with any of the following?	The first names and ages of everyone having this difficulty are	No one
Getting around the house without help	....	✓

START HERE →

1. WHO has difficulty with any of the following?	The first names and ages of everyone having this difficulty are	No one
a. Walking without help	....	
b. Getting outside the house without help	....	
c. Crossing the road without help	....	
d. Travelling on a bus or train without help	....	

2. WHO has difficulty with any of the following?	The first names and ages of everyone having this difficulty are	No one
a. Getting in and out of bed or chair without help	....	
b. Dressing or undressing without help	....	

96

c. Kneeling or bending over without help	....	
d. Going up or down stairs without help	....	
e. Having a bath or all over wash without help	....	
f. Holding or gripping (for example a comb or a pen) without help	....	
g. Getting to and using the toilet without help	....	

3. WHO has any of the following problems?	The first names and ages of everyone having this difficulty are	No one
a. Difficulty with spells of giddiness or fits	....	
b. Frequent falls	....	
c. Weakness or paralysis of arms or legs	....	
d. A stroke	....	
e. Difficulty seeing newspaper print even with glasses	....	
f. Difficulty recognizing people across the road even with glasses	....	
g. Hearing difficulties	....	
h. Loss of whole or *significant part* of an arm, hand, leg or foot	....	
i. Controlling bowels or bladder	....	

Exhibit 3.17 *(Continued)*

Exhibit 3.17 *(Continued)*

4. WHO is limited in doing any of the following BECAUSE OF ILLNESS OR DISABILITY?	The first names and ages of everyone having this difficulty are	No one
a. Working at all	....	
b. Doing the job of their choice	....	
c. Doing housework	....	
d. Visiting family or friends	....	

5. *If you have written ANY names in Questions 1–4,* please tell us what their major illness or disability is?

First names and ages of anyone mentioned in Questions 1–4	Please describe their major illness or disability below

6. Does *anyone else* in your household have an illness or disability which affects their activities in any way?

First names and ages of anyone with illness or disability	What is the major illness or disability?	Please describe activity (e.g., playing sports, sewing, going to the pub)

All Information Confidential

Please complete below EVEN IF NO ONE IS ILL OR DISABLED. We need this information to plan services for EVERYONE in Lambeth.

List Below EVERYONE, INCLUDING YOURSELF, living in this household.
Give the full name together with details for EVERYONE

7.	NAME Write below Surname—Forename(s)	SEX Tick box Male Female (1) (2)		YEAR OF BIRTH Write Below	MARITAL STATUS Write below—Single, Married, Widowed, Divorced or Separated	CURRENTLY EMPLOYED? Tick box Yes (1) No (2)	
0							
1							
2							
3							
4							
5							
6							
7							
8							
9							

Since work can affect health, please complete for the head of your household only
(Person with responsibility for supporting household or for rent/accommodation).

First Name and Age of HEAD OF HOUSEHOLD	What job does he/she do? (If Head is retired, unemployed, or not present, what was the job he/she held for most of his/her working life?)

Exhibit 3.17 *(Continued)*

Exhibit 3.17 *(Continued)*

Is (or was) the Head of the Household. . . .	☐ a manager working for an employer?	☐ a foreman or supervisor working for an employer?	☐ working for an employer	☐ self-employed?
What qualifications, if any, were needed to obtain this job?	....			
What does the firm or organization do or make?	....			

We appreciate your co-operation, Thank you.   ....
Please check carefully that ALL questions on every page are answered.   Signature of person fillling in form

Reproduced from Patrick DL, ed. Health and care of the physically disabled in Lambeth. Phase I report of the Longitudinal Disability Interview Survey. London: St Thomas's Hospital Medical School, Department of Community Medicine, 1981. With permission.

Reliability

Sixty-eight people identified as disabled on the first version of the questionnaire were interviewed three to six months later. All were still classified as disabled in the follow-up interview, although there were discrepancies in replies to several individual items (1). No reliability information is available for versions two and three of the questionnaire.

Validity

Peach et al. reported low levels of agreement between self-ratings and assessments made by family physicians. The low agreement was attributed primarily to the doctors' ignorance of the patients' disabilities (1).

In the Lambeth Health Survey, the screening questionnaire was followed six to 12 months later by an interview survey of 892 respondents identified as disabled, and a comparison group of 346 nondisabled (6). Compared to the Functional Limitations Profile, the Lambeth questionnaire showed a sensitivity of 87.7% and a speci-

ficity of 72.2% (6, pp31–35). Because a change in health status may have occurred between the two assessments, these figures provide low estimates of the validity of the questionnaire.

Charlton et al. compared version three of the questionnaire to the FLP (4). The sample of 839 was randomly divided into two groups. Using 65% of the respondents, a regression equation was derived to predict the FLP scores; the equation was then applied to the replies of the second group. For the physical subscale of the FLP, the actual scores correlated 0.79 with those predicted from the screening instrument; for the psychosocial scales the correlation was 0.50 (4, p302).

Commentary

The second version of the Lambeth questionnaire (Exhibit 3.17) is one of very few validated postal screening instruments available. The instrument proved acceptable to respondents: a response rate of 86.6% was obtained in the Lambeth survey

Exhibit 3.18   The Lambeth Disability
Screening Questionnaire (Version 3)

Because of illness, accident or anything related to
your health, do you have difficulty with any of the
following? *Read out individually and code.*
   a. Walking without help
   b. Getting outside the house without help
   c. Crossing the road without help
   d. Travelling on a bus or train without help
   e. Getting in and out of bed or chair without
      help
   f. Dressing or undressing without help
   g. Kneeling or bending without help
   h. Going up or down stairs without help
   i. Having a bath or all over wash without help
   j. Holding or gripping (for example a comb or
      pen) without help
   k. Getting to and using the toilet without help
   l. Eating or drinking without help

Because of your health, do you have. . .
   m. Difficulty seeing newspaper print even with
      glasses
   n. Difficulty recognizing people across the road
      even with glasses
   o. Difficulty in hearing a conversation even with
      a hearing aid
   p. Difficulty speaking

Because of your health, do you have difficulty. . .
   q. Preparing or cooking a hot meal without help
   r. Doing housework without help
   s. Visiting family or friends without help
   t. Doing any of your hobbies or spare time
      activities
   u. Doing paid work of any kind (if under 65)
   v. Doing paid work of your choice (if under 65)

Reproduced from Charlton JRH, Patrick DL, Peach H. Use
of multivariate measures of disability in health surveys. J Epidemiol Community Health 1983;37:304. With permission.

of 11,659 households. Of the remainder,
8% could not be contacted, 0.2% provided
information too inadequate to analyze, and
only 5.2% refused (5). Locker et al. discussed methods for reducing the bias in-
curred in estimating prevalence due to nonresponse (3). The use of one person to
record details about other family members
was apparently successful.

The Lambeth Questionnaire is based on
an established conceptual approach to disability, although the wording of the questions may not indicate performance, as intended. Questions ask, "Do you have
difficulty with . . . ?" a wording that seems
to lie between performance and capacity:

it does not tell us whether the person does
or does not do the activity in question, or
whether he cannot. Indeed, question phrasing is crucial: Patrick et al. attributed lower
disability prevalence estimates obtained in
previous surveys to their use of capacity
question phrasing (5). This questionnaire
appears to be the best of the three survey
methods that we review, making it unfortunate that the data set from Lambeth has not
been fully analyzed to provide estimates
of internal consistency and validity for all
versions. We would like to see this instrument more fully tested before being recommended for widespread use.

REFERENCES

(1) Peach H, Green S, Locker D, et al. Evalua-
    tion of a postal screening questionnaire to
    identify the physically disabled. Int Rehabil
    Med 1980;2:189–193.
(2) Patrick DL. Screening for disability in
    Lambeth: a progress report on health and
    care of the physically handicapped. Lon-
    don: St. Thomas's Hospital Medical
    School, Department of Community Medi-
    cine, 1978.
(3) Locker D, Wiggins R, Sittampalam Y, et al.
    Estimating the prevalence of disability in
    the community: the influence of sample
    design and response bias. J Epidemiol Com-
    munity Health 1981;35:208–212.
(4) Charlton JRH, Patrick DL, Peach H. Use of
    multivariate measures of disability in health
    surveys. J Epidemiol Community Health
    1983;37:296–304.
(5) Patrick DL, Darby SC, Green S, et al.
    Screening for disability in the inner city. J
    Epidemiol Community Health 1981;
    35:65–70.
(6) Patrick DL, ed. Health and care of the phys-
    ically disabled in Lambeth. Phase I report
    of The Longitudinal Disability Interview
    Survey. London: St. Thomas's Hospital
    Medical School, Department of Commu-
    nity Medicine, 1981.

THE DISABILITY INTERVIEW
SCHEDULE
(A.E. Bennett and Jessie Garrad, 1970)

Purpose

This Disability Interview Schedule was designed to measure the prevalence and sever-

ity of disability in epidemiological surveys for planning health and welfare services.

Conceptual Basis

This interview schedule follows the standard distinction between disability and impairment. Disability was defined as limitation of performance in "essential" activities of daily living, severe enough to entail dependence upon another person. Impairment was defined as an anatomical, pathological, or psychological disorder that may cause or be associated with disability (1).

Description

Bennett and Garrad's 1966 survey of the prevalence of disability in London, England, used a brief screening questionnaire, followed by a 20-page interview schedule. Bennett also described 18-item and 15-item disability screening questionnaires that are not reviewed here (2).

The present review covers only the disability section from the detailed schedule which was applied to a sample of 571 respondents aged 35 to 74 years, drawn from those identified as disabled and/or impaired by the screening questionnaire. The schedule shown in Exhibit 3.19 is administered by interviewers trained to probe to identify actual levels of performance. The questions use performance rather than capacity wording, and the highest level of performance is recorded. If an answer falls between two defined levels, the less severe grade of limitation is recorded. Recognizing that there are reasons other than disability why people may not perform an activity, allowances are made in scoring the schedule—for example, men who do not perform domestic duties (1, 2). Details of the scoring system are not clear, although separate scores are provided for each topic, rather than a single score, which "masks different levels of performance in different areas, results in loss of information, and can be misleading." (1, p101)

Reliability

Complete agreement was obtained on test–retest ratings for 80% of 153 subjects after a 12-month delay (1, p103). For 28 of the 31 respondents exhibiting some change on the questionnaire, medical records corroborated that there had been a change in impairment or disability status.

Guttman analyses of the questions gave a coefficient of reproducibility of 0.95 and a coefficient of scalability of 0.69 for females and 0.71 for males (3, p73). There were slight differences in the ordering of items in scales derived for males and for females (4, Tables I–III).

Validity

Data from medical and social work records of 52 outpatients were compared with information obtained with the interview schedule. The clinical records listed disability in a total of 118 areas, of which 108 (91.5%) were reflected in the interview schedule (1, p102).

Commentary

This instrument is one of relatively few disability measurements designed for survey use; the clear format of the questionnaire is a notable feature. The instrument is, however, old and lacks extensive validity testing; potential users should consider the OECD instrument (next review) as an alternative. The Disability Interview Schedule serves as an example for those designing new survey measurements of disability.

REFERENCES

(1) Garrad J, Bennett AE. A validated interview schedule for use in population surveys of chronic disease and disability. Br J Prev Soc Med 1971;25:97–104.

(2) Bennett AE, Garrad J, Halil T. Chronic disease and disability in the community: a prevalence study. Br Med J 1970;3:762–764.

(3) Williams RGA, Johnston M, Willis LA, et al. Disability: a model and measurement technique. Br J Prev Soc Med 1976;30:71–78.

(4) St. Thomas's health survey in Lambeth: disability survey. London: St. Thomas's Hospital Medical School, Department of Clinical Epidemiology and Social Medicine, 1971.

Exhibit 3.19 The Disability Interview Schedule

Note: Cross in any box marked with an asterisk indicates presence of disability.

MOBILITY

Walking
Do you walk outdoors in the street (with crutch or stick if used)?

If 'Yes': one mile or more ☐	If 'No':	and:
¼ mile ☐	Between rooms [*]	Unaccompanied ☐
100 yds. [*]	Within room [*]	Accompanied [*]
10 yds. [*]	Unable to walk [*]	Acc. & support [*]

Stairs

Do you walk up stairs?

To 1st floor or above ☐	Unacc. ☐
5–8 steps or stairs [*]	Acc. [*]
2–4 steps or stairs [*]	Acc. & Supp. [*]
1 step [*]	No need to mount stairs ☐
mount stairs other than by walking [*]	
unable to mount stairs [*]	

Do you walk down stairs?

From 1 floor to another ☐	Unacc. ☐
5–8 steps or stairs [*]	Acc. [*]
2–4 steps or stairs [*]	Acc. & Supp. [*]
1 step [*]	No need to descend stairs ☐
goes down stairs other than by walking [*]	
unable to descend stairs [*]	

Transfer

	Yes	No		Yes	No
Do you need help to get into bed?.............................	[*]	☐	Do you need help to sit down in a chair?................................	[*]	☐
Do you need help to get out of bed?.............................	[*]	☐	Do you need help to stand up from a chair?................................	[*]	☐
Bedfast	[*]		Not applicable.....................................		☐

Travel

Do you drive yourself in a car?

| Normal (unadapt.) ☐ |
| Adapted ☐ |
| Invacar [*] |
| Self-propelled vehicle (outdoors) [*] |
| Does not drive ☐ |

Do you travel by bus or train?

If 'Yes':		If 'No':	
Whenever necessary ☐		Unable to use bus and train [*]	
Only out of rush hour [*]		Unable to use bus, train and car [*]	
and:			
Unaccompanied ☐		Does not travel by choice ☐	
Accompanied [*]		Uses private transport by choice ☐	

SELF CARE

Are you able to feed yourself:	Are you able to dress yourself completely:	Are you able to undress yourself completely:	Are you able to use the lavatory:	Are you able to wash yourself:
Without any help ☐	Without any help ☐	Without any help ☐	Without any help ☐	Without any help ☐
With specially prepared food or containers [*]	With help with fastenings [*]	With help with fastenings [*]	Receptacles without assistance [*]	With assistance for shaving, combing hair, etc. [*]
With assistance [*]	With help other than fastenings [*]	With help other than fastenings [*]	Lavatory with assistance [*]	With help for bodily washing [*]
Not at all, must be fed [*]	Does not dress [*]	Not applicable [*]	Receptacles with assistance [*]	Not at all [*]

Exhibit 3.19 *(Continued)*

103

Exhibit 3.19   *(Continued)*

DOMESTIC DUTIES

Do you do your own:

	all	part	none	preference	unable
Shopping	☐	☐	☐	☐	☐*
Cooking	☐	☐	☐	☐	☐*
Cleaning	☐	☐	☐	☐	☐*
Clothes washing	☐	☐	☐	☐	☐*
Men with no household duties	☐				

OCCUPATION

Do you have a paid job at present?

If 'Yes':   and: If 'No':

If 'Yes':		and:		If 'No':			
Full-time	☐	Normal working	☐	Males 65 and over	{	Age retired	☐
Part-time	☐	Modified working	☐*	Females 60 and over		Prem. retired	☐*
		Sheltered employment	☐*			Non-employed	☐
				Males 64 and under	{	Unemployed	☐
				Females 59 and under		Unfit	☐*
						Non-employed	☐

Reproduced from an original obtained from Dr. AE Bennett. With permission.

THE OECD LONG-TERM DISABILITY QUESTIONNAIRE
(Organization for Economic Cooperation and Development [OECD], 1981)

Purpose

The OECD questionnaire is a survey instrument that summarizes the impact of ill health on essential daily activities. It was intended to permit international comparisons of disability and, through national surveys, to monitor changes in disability over time (1).

Conceptual Basis

In 1976, the OECD sponsored an international effort to develop various social and health indicators.[1] The health survey questionnaire measured disability in terms of limitations in activities essential to daily living: mobility, self-care, and communication. The disruption of normal social activity was seen as the central theme (1).

[1]Participating countries included Canada, Finland, France, West Germany, The Netherlands, Switzerland, the United Kingdom, and the United States.

Two aspects of disability were considered: temporary alterations in functional levels and long-term restrictions such as those arising from congenital anomalies. A person's current functional performance reflects the presence of any long-term disability, overlaid by short-term fluctuations. Indicators of short-term disability already exist in the form of restricted activity or disability days. The OECD group considered these adequate and therefore devoted the questionnaire to measuring long-term disability among adults (2).

Description

Of the 16 questions, ten can be used as an abbreviated instrument and represent a core set of items for international comparisons. They are shown in Exhibit 3.20. No time specification is attached to these questions to signify long-term disability. Rather, the respondent is asked what he can usually do on a normal day, excluding any temporary difficulties. Four response categories were proposed: (1) yes, without difficulty; (2) yes, with minor difficulty; (3) yes, with major difficulty; (4) no, not able

Exhibit 3.20 The OECD Long-Term
Disability Questionnaire

Note: The ten questions with an asterisk are included in the abbreviated version.

---

* 1. Is your eyesight good enough to read ordinary newspaper print? (with glasses if usually worn).

2. Is your eyesight good enough to see the face of someone from 4 metres? (with glasses if usually worn).

3. Can you hear what is said in a normal conversation with 3 or 4 other persons? (with hearing aid if you usually wear one).

* 4. Can you hear what is said in a normal conversation with one other person? (with hearing aid if you usually wear one).

* 5. Can you speak without difficulty?

* 6. Can you carry an object of 5 kilos for 10 metres?

7. Could you run 100 metres?

* 8. Can you walk 400 metres without resting?

* 9. Can you walk up and down one flight of stairs without resting?

* 10. Can you move between rooms?

* 11. Can you get in and out of bed?

* 12. Can you dress and undress?

13. Can you cut your toenails?

14. Can you (when standing), bend down and pick up a shoe from the floor?

* 15. Can you cut your own food? (such as meat, fruit, etc.).

16. Can you both bite and chew on hard foods? (for example, a firm apple or celery).

Reproduced from McWhinnie JR. Disability assessment in population surveys: results of the OECD common development effort. Rev Epidémiol Santé Publique 1981;29:417, Masson SA, Paris. With permission.

to. These were not strictly adhered to in the field trials and sometimes categories 2 and 3 were merged into "yes, with difficulty." A detailed presentation of the rationale for question selection and administration is given in the OECD report (2).

Reliability

Wilson and McNeil used 11 of the questions, slightly modified, in interviews that were repeated after a two-week delay (N = 223) (3). It was not always possible to reinterview the original respondent, and in about half of the cases a proxy report was used. The agreement between first and second interviews was low, ranging from about 30% to 70% for the 11 items. Considering the scale as a whole, less than two-thirds of those who reported disabilities on either interview reported them on both interviews. Analyses showed that the inconsistencies were not due to using proxy respondents (3).

A Dutch survey compared the responses to a self-administered version of the questionnaire (N = 940) with an interview version (N = 500). Although the two groups were very similar in age and sex, there was a systematic bias toward more disability being reported in the self-administered version: on average, 3.1% more people declared some level of disability in the written version (4, p466).

Validity

Twelve of the OECD questions were included in a Finnish national survey (N = 2,000). With the exception of people over 65 years of age, the great majority expressed no difficulty with any of the activities covered (5, Table 1). Similar findings were obtained in the United States and in the Netherlands (3, 4). The questions were applied to 1,600 Swiss respondents aged 65 and over, and Raymond et al. reported sensitivity results (6). For different medical conditions, sensitivity ranged from 61% to 85%, being highest for those with eyesight, hearing and speech problems. Specificity was 76% (6, p455).

In Canada, the questions were tested in interviews with 104 rehabilitation outpatients. Correlations between the questions concerned with physical movements and a physicians's rating of mobility ranged between 0.21 and 0.61 (7, Table II). Item-total correlations ranged from 0.14 to 0.54.

Commentary

The OECD questionnaire represents an early attempt to develop an internationally applicable set of disability items; the Euro-Qol project described in Chapter 9 offers a more recent example. As well as the studies cited here, the method has been used in France (8), Japan, and West Germany. The questions continue to be used in Canadian national surveys in self-administered and interview formats (9, 10). Many of the questions are similar to those in the Rand Corporation scales and in the American Social Security Administration disability surveys.

Although the idea of an internationally standardized scale is commendable, it was not fully achieved. Most studies exhibit slight variations in the questions or answer categories. There are also certain illogicalities in the scale: although it is intended to measure the behavioral consequences of disability, the questions use a capacity rather than a performance wording. The method is designed as a survey instrument, but the questions cover relatively severe levels of disability so that few people in the general adult population answer affirmatively; the questions are most relevant to people over 65. The low test–retest reliability reported in the United States is cause for concern; the authors suggested that the distinction between short- and long-term disability may not have been adequately explained to the respondents, who may have reported minor and transient difficulties rather than long-term problems (3). The distinction between acute and chronic disability is hard to draw, especially where a respondent has problems of both types that may interact. Linked to this, the instructions to the respondents lack clarity. Unfortunately, none of the original contributing authors is still directly involved with this instrument, so it may not see further improvement.

Although it has been widely used, there are problems with this scale. Reliability and validity results are poor. The instrument is narrow in scope compared, for example, to the Lambeth questionnaire, which covers employment and social activities as well as the ADL and IADL themes included in the OECD instrument.

REFERENCES

(1) McWhinnie JR. Disability assessment in population surveys: results of the OECD common development effort. Rev Epidémiol Santé Publique 1981;29:413–419.
(2) McWhinnie JR. Disability indicators for measuring well-being. Paris: OECD Social Indicators Programme, 1981.
(3) Wilson RW, McNeil JM. Preliminary analysis of OECD disability on the pretest of the post census disability survey. Rev Epidémiol Santé Publique 1981;29:469–475.
(4) Van Sonsbeek JLA. Applications aux Pays-Bas des questions de l'OCDE relatives à l'incapacité. Rev Epidémiol Santé Publique 1981;29:461–468.
(5) Klaukka T. Application of the OECD disability questions in Finland. Rev Epidémiol Santé Publique 1981;29:431–439.
(6) Raymond L, Christe E, Clemence A. Vers l'établissement d'un score global d'incapacité fonctionnelle sur la base des questions de l'OCDE, d'après une enquête en Suisse. Rev Epidémiol Santé Publique 1981; 29:451–459.
(7) McDowell I. Screening for disability. An examination of the OECD survey questions in a Canadian study. Rev Epidémiol Santé Publique 1981;29:421–429.
(8) Mizrahi A, Mizrahi A. Evaluation de l'état de santé de personnes âgées en France, à l'aide de plusieurs indicateurs, dont les questions de l'OCDE. Rev Epidémiol Santé Publique 1981;29:441–450.
(9) McDowell I, Praught E. Report of the Canadian health and disability survey, 1983–1984. Ottawa, Canada: Minister of Supply and Services, 1986. (Catalogue No. 82–55E).
(10) Furrie AD. A national database on disabled persons: making disability data available to users. Ottawa, Canada: Statistics Canada, 1987.

THE HEALTH ASSESSMENT QUESTIONNAIRE
(James F. Fries, 1980)

Purpose

The Stanford Health Assessment Questionnaire (HAQ) measures difficulty in performing activities of daily living. It was originally designed for the clinical assessment of adult arthritics but has been used in a wide range of research settings to evaluate care.

Conceptual Basis

The HAQ is based on a hierarchical model that considers the effects of a disease in terms of death, disability, discomfort, the side effects of treatment, and medical costs (1–4). Except for death, these dimensions are divided into subdimensions, such as upper- and lower-limb problems for the disability dimension and physical and psychological problems for the discomfort dimension. The subdimensions are then divided into components, which are further divided into individual question topics (1, Figure 1; 2, Figure 1). Fries followed a parsimonious approach in selecting questions, noting that there may be no need to measure apparently distinct aspects of disability that are correlated. This allows an instrument to represent a content area without addressing every possible question (4). The hierarchic model expresses results at various levels of generality: question scores may be combined to form component (e.g., eating or dressing) and dimension (e.g., disability) scores (5). However, Fries argued against combining dimension scores to give an overall score, as this would involve value judgments of the relative importance of dimensions that may not hold across patients. Empirically, correlations across dimensions are lower than within dimensions, so Fries argued that "Disability, discomfort, psychologic outcomes, cost, and death have been identified as separable outcomes. The full number of dimensions seems likely to be between 5 and 8" (5, p701).

The HAQ model also considers the economic costs of disease and the possible side effects of treatment. A separate dimension considers medical and surgical complications such as gastrointestinal problems or infection. These are recorded from an audit of hospital records and death certificates; weights have so far been developed for rating several possible side effects (1,

p120). The economic impact of disease is assessed through direct (cost of drugs and doctor visits) and indirect effects such as work loss. Costs can be rated using standard computations based on average costs for various types of disease (1, p121).

Development of the HAQ has concentrated on the disability and discomfort dimensions; these are the most commonly used and are described in detail in this review. Considerable further development will be required to complete the scale and realize the overall conceptual framework Fries presented.

Description

The disability dimension of the HAQ includes 20 questions on daily functioning during the past week. These cover eight component areas: dressing and grooming, arising, eating, walking, hygiene, reach, grip, and outdoor activities. Earlier versions also included sexual activity. Each component includes two or three questions drawn from previous measures (2, p138); a description of the development of the HAQ is given by Fries et al. (4). The scale may be self-administered, or it may be applied in a telephone or personal interview (3, p30). It can be completed in five to eight minutes and scored in less than one (4). Where patients had previously completed the HAQ, Wolfe et al. found that 88% of patients completed it in less than three minutes; it took 15 to 22 seconds to score (6, p1485). The questions are shown in Exhibit 3.21.

Each response is scored on a four-point scale of ability patterned after the American Rheumatism Association functional classification (3, p31). The response scales range from "without any difficulty" to "unable to do" and a check list records any aids used or assistance received. The highest score in each of the eight components is added to form a total (range 0–24); this is divided by 8 to provide a 0–3 continuous score, termed the Functional Disability Index (6, p1481). Scoring in-

Exhibit 3.21 The Health Assessment Questionnaire

> In this section we are interested in learning how your illness affects your ability to function in daily life. Please feel free to add any comments on the back of this page.

- **Please check the one response which best describes your usual abilities OVER THE PAST WEEK:**

	Without ANY Difficulty	With SOME Difficulty	With MUCH Difficulty	UNABLE To Do
DRESSING & GROOMING Are you able to:				
—Dress yourself, including tying shoelaces and doing buttons?	_____	_____	_____	_____
—Shampoo your hair?	_____	_____	_____	_____
ARISING Are you able to:				
—Stand up from an armless straight chair?	_____	_____	_____	_____
—Get in and out of bed?	_____	_____	_____	_____
EATING Are you able to:				
—Cut your meat?	_____	_____	_____	_____
—Lift a full cup or glass to your mouth?	_____	_____	_____	_____
—Open a new milk carton?	_____	_____	_____	_____
WALKING Are you able to:				
—Walk outdoors on flat ground?	_____	_____	_____	_____
—Climb up five steps?	_____	_____	_____	_____

- **Please check any AIDS OR DEVICES that you usually use for any of these activities:**

_____	Cane	_____	Devices Used for Dressing (button hook, zipper pull, long-handled shoe horn, etc.)
_____	Walker	_____	Built Up or Special Utensils
_____	Crutches	_____	Special or Built Up Chair
_____	Wheelchair	_____	Other (Specify: _____)

- **Please check any categories for which you usually need HELP FROM ANOTHER PERSON:**

_____	Dressing & Grooming	_____	Eating
_____	Arising	_____	Walking

- **Please check the one response which best describes your usual abilities OVER THE PAST WEEK:**

	Without ANY Difficulty	With SOME Difficulty	With MUCH Difficulty	UNABLE To Do
HYGIENE Are you able to:				
—Wash and dry your entire body?	_____	_____	_____	_____

	Without ANY Difficulty	With SOME Difficulty	With MUCH Difficulty	UNABLE To Do
—Take a tub bath?	_____	_____	_____	_____
—Get on and off the toilet?	_____	_____	_____	_____

REACH

Are you able to:

—Reach and get down a 5 pound object (such as a bag of sugar) from just above your head?	_____	_____	_____	_____
—Bend down to pick up clothing from the floor?	_____	_____	_____	_____

GRIP

Are you able to:

—Open car doors?	_____	_____	_____	_____
—Open jars which have been previously opened?	_____	_____	_____	_____
—Turn faucets on and off?	_____	_____	_____	_____

ACTIVITIES

Are you able to:

—Run errands and shop?	_____	_____	_____	_____
—Get in and out of a car?	_____	_____	_____	_____
—Do chores such as vacuuming or yardwork?	_____	_____	_____	_____

- **Please check any AIDS OR DEVICES that you usually use for any of these activities:**

_____	Raised Toilet Seat	_____	Bathtub Bar
_____	Bathtub Seat	_____	Long-Handled Appliances for Reach
_____	Jar Opener (for jars previously opened)	_____	Long-Handled Appliances in Bathroom
			Other (Specify: _____)

- **Please check any categories for which you usually need HELP FROM ANOTHER PERSON:**

_____	Hygiene	_____	Gripping and Opening Things
_____	Reach	_____	Errands and Chores

We are also interested in learning whether or not you are affected by pain because of your illness.

- **How much pain have you had because of your illness IN THE PAST WEEK?**

NO PAIN   *PLACE A MARK ON THE LINE TO INDICATE THE SEVERITY OF THE PAIN*   VERY SEVERE PAIN

|——|

0   100

---

structions are given in Exhibit 3.22. Siegert et al. suggested the following interpretations of overall scores: "0.0–0.5: the patient is completely self-sufficient . . . 0.5–1.25: the patient is reasonably self-sufficient and experiences some minor and even major difficulties in performing ADL; 1.25–2.0: the patient is still self-sufficient, but has many major problems with ADL; 2.0–3.0: the patient may be called severely handicapped" (7, p309).

The discomfort dimension of the HAQ includes a single question on physical pain in the past week. It uses a 15-cm visual analogue pain scale, with the end points labeled "no pain" and "very severe pain." Scores are measured in centimeters from the left and are multiplied by 0.2 to give a range from 0 to 3; scores are rounded to two decimal places. Fries noted: "Attempts to elaborate pain activity by part of the body involved, times during the day which

Exhibit 3.22   Instructions for Scoring the Health Assessment Questionnaire

---

DAILY FUNCTION (Disability Index)

This section is composed of eight components (Dressing and Grooming, Arising, Eating, etc), each of which has at least two questions. These components each contribute a score from 0 to 3 which are then collapsed into a 0 to 3 Disability Index.

Possible responses for the questions are:

Without ANY difficulty   =   0
With SOME difficulty   =   1
With MUCH difficulty   =   2
UNABLE to do   =   3

The highest score for any question determines the score for that component. If a question is left blank or the response is too ambiguous to assign a score, then the score for that component is determined by the remaining completed question(s).

If either devices and/or help from another person is checked for a component, the score = 2. This may determine the score unless the score on any other component question = 3. For example, the response to "Dress yourself . . ." is with SOME difficulty (score 1). The patient has checked the use of a device for dressing, thereby increasing the score to 2. The response to "Shampoo your hair" is UNABLE to do (score = 3). Therefore, the score for the DRESSING category is 3.

Devices associated with each component:

DRESSING & GROOMING   —   Devices used for dressing (button hook, zipper pull, long handled shoe horn, etc.)
ARISING   —   built up or special chair
EATING   —   built up or special utensils
WALKING   —   cane, walker, crutches
HYGIENE   —   raised toilet seat
                           bathtub seat
                           bathtub bar
                           long handled appliances in bathroom
REACH   —   long handled appliances for reach
GRIP   —   jar opener (for jars previously opened)

Devices written in the "Other" sections are considered only if they would be used for any of the stated components.

Disability Index Calculation:

The index is calculated by adding the scores for each of the components and dividing by the number of components answered. This gives a score in the 0 to 3 range.

PAIN AND DISCOMFORT

Pain is measured on a visual analog scale, 15 cm. long, with "no pain" or 0 at one end and "very severe pain" or 100 at the other. A score from 0 to 3 is determined, based on the location of the respondent's mark. Using a metric rule, measure the distance from the left hand side of the line to the mark (0 to 15 cm.) and multiply by 0.2 to obtain a value from 0 to 3.

Adapted from Stanford Arthritis Center Disability and Discomfort Scales, 1981. With permission.

were painful, and severity of pain in different body parts failed to yield indexes that outperformed a simple analog scale" (3, p31).

The HAQ has been very widely used, and considerable evidence for reliability and validity have accumulated. A review by Ramey et al. summarizes evidence from more than 100 articles on the HAQ (1).

Reliability

Fries compared interview and self-administered versions of the disability scale (N = 20). The Spearman correlation for the disability index was 0.85, while correlations for individual sections ranged from 0.56 (IADL activities and hygiene) to 0.85 (eating) (2, Table 1).

During the development of the HAQ, Fries abbreviated the questionnaire and removed questions that correlated highly with others in the scale. Not surprisingly, therefore, item-total correlations are modest, ranging from 0.51 to 0.81 (2, Table 3). Pincus et al. reported somewhat higher alpha coefficients for the questions in each category, ranging from 0.71 (reaching) to 0.89 (eating) (8, Table 2). Milligan et al. found an alpha coefficient of 0.94 for the complete instrument, with maximum inter-item correlations of 0.75 (9).

Two-week test–retest reliability of the disability section was investigated with 37 rheumatoid arthritics, showing no significant difference by t-test and a Spearman correlation of 0.87 (3, p31). Goeppinger et al. reported a one-week test–retest reliability of 0.95 (N = 30 rheumatoid arthritis patients) and 0.93 (N = 30 osteoarthritis patients) (10). Fries et al. administered the HAQ on successive occasions and obtained a retest correlation of 0.98 after six months (4, p791).

Validity

Fries compared self-administered HAQ responses to observations of performance made during a home visit (N = 25). The Spearman correlation for the overall score was 0.88, while correlations for component

scores ranged from 0.47 (arising) to 0.88 (walking) (2, Table 2). Fitzpatrick et al. compared the HAQ to indicators of disease activity in 105 arthritics. Correlations of the overall score were highest with grip strength (-0.73) and with the Ritchie articular index (0.69). The correlation was 0.38 with erythrocyte sedimentation rate (ESR) and 0.41 with a rating of morning stiffness (11, Table II). Wolfe et al. also showed significant associations between the HAQ disability score and joint count, grip strength, anxiety and depression, and ESR (6). They demonstrated the validity of the HAQ in predicting health services utilization, clinical progression, and mortality. For predicting mortality, the relative risk associated with a one-point increase in baseline disability score was 1.77 (6, p1484). Ramey et al. listed several dozen studies that have compared the HAQ with clinical and laboratory variables; they also cited several studies that have used it as an outcome measure in randomized trials (1, Tables 6 and 8).

Principal component analyses have broadly confirmed the dimensions originally postulated by Fries: one main factor underlay 15 of the disability questions (2, Table 4). The eight disability subscales are substantially correlated with each other: a median correlation of 0.44 among them has been reported (12, p948). Brown et al. tested the factorial structure of the HAQ, showing a two-factor solution with the eight disability components loading on the first factor and the pain scale on the second in a small study of 48 patients with rheumatoid arthritis (13). Milligan et al. obtained one factor relating to movements involving the large limbs (rising, walking) and a second for fine movements such as grasping and eating (9).

Brown et al. compared the HAQ with the Arthritis Impact Measurement Scale (AIMS). The correlations were 0.91 for the disability dimension and 0.64 for the pain questions (14, p160). The two scales correlated 0.89 in another study (15). Liang et al. compared responses of 50 arthritics on the HAQ, the Sickness Impact Profile (SIP), the Functional Status Index (FSI), the AIMS, and the Quality of Well-Being Scale (QWB). The overall score on the HAQ correlated 0.84 with the AIMS, 0.78 with the SIP, 0.75 with the FSI, and 0.60 with the QWB (16, Table 4). For the mobility scale, correlations of the HAQ and the other instruments were lower than the correlations among the other four scales.

Liang et al. compared the relative efficiency of five measures, indicating their ability to identify change within subjects before and after hip or knee surgery. The rank order of five measures in terms of this statistic placed the HAQ in fourth place (16, Table 5). They subsequently replicated broadly similar findings: the overall and mobility scores on the HAQ would require larger sample sizes to demonstrate a significant effect of treatment than would equivalent scores from the AIMS or the SIP (17, Table 3). However, the HAQ may be more sensitive to change than physical measures such as ESR, grip strength, or morning stiffness. Hawley and Wolfe showed the HAQ more responsive than physical measures or depression following methotrexate treatment for rheumatoid arthritis; the HAQ pain score was especially responsive (18, p133). The HAQ also reflected the progressive nature of the condition better than did physical indicators: at five- and ten-year follow-up assessments, the HAQ showed large declines in function (effect sizes of -1.6 and -2.4). Fitzpatrick et al. found sensitivity to improvement in disease state over 15 months to be modest, at 65% (specificity 61%), while sensitivity to deterioration was 60% (specificity 73%) (11, Table IV). Hawley and Wolfe's findings may suggest, however, that the problem lies not with the HAQ so much as with the lack of sensitivity of the traditional "gold standard" measures.

Alternative Forms

Pincus et al. abbreviated the HAQ by retaining only one question in each of the eight disability components; they also added questions on satisfaction and change in activities. This has been called the "Modified HAQ" or MHAQ. The test–retest reliability at one month was higher for the revised version (0.91) than for the original HAQ (0.78) (8, p1350). A further test of the eight-item HAQ showed correlations of -0.53 with grip strength, 0.44 with walking time, and 0.60 with the ARA functional class (19, Table 1). Callahan and Pincus also evaluated the ratio of the pain score to the eight-item disability score as an approach to discriminating between early rheumatoid arthritis and diffuse musculoskeletal pain (20).

Pincus et al. also proposed "transition questions" such as "Compared with three months ago, how difficult is it now (this week) to . . . [Dress yourself, Get in and out of bed . . .]" (8, p1347). Subsequent testing showed these questions to be more sensitive to detecting change in rheumatoid status than the overall HAQ scores (21).

A modified version of the HAQ has been proposed for patients with spondylitis. This adds five questions covering handicaps arising from back problems (12). A children's version of the HAQ has also been proposed (1, p122).

The "AIDS-HAQ" includes 14 items from the Medical Outcomes Study instruments and 16 items from the HAQ. The items cover physical function, mental health, cognitive function, energy levels, and general health (22; 23, p94).

The HAQ has been adapted for use in many countries (1, Table 3); these include Britain (24), Sweden (25), Spanish-speaking countries (26–29) and Holland (7, 30, 31). French translations are available from France (32, 33) and Canada (34). The one-week test–retest reliability of the Swedish version was 0.91, and results correlated 0.76 with observational ratings of the patients carrying out the activities included in the scale (25, p267). Test–retest reliability of the Italian version ranged from 0.81 to 0.99 in several centers (35).

Commentary

The HAQ has become the most widely used instrument in a field that pays close attention to rigorous measurement. It has been included in the American Rheumatism Association Medical Information System, and the National Health and Nutrition Survey in the U.S. (3, p30). The design of the HAQ offers a scale that is broad in scope yet brief enough to be completed by patients while waiting to see their physician. Compared to the Functional Limitations Profile, the HAQ showed similar agreement with clinical indicators and similar sensitivity to change over time (11). And yet, the FLP takes about four times longer to complete than the HAQ. The available evidence shows the HAQ to have strong reliability and validity. The correlation of 0.91 between the AIMS and HAQ physical scales is remarkably high (13). A further strength lies in the continued involvement of the originator of the scale in coordinating its development; this has helped to control the proliferation of different versions that typifies other scales. The reader of Ramey's review, for example, gains the impression of a well-planned development effort (1).

In terms of improvements to the HAQ, it would be valuable to see a fuller exploitation of the large studies in which the method has been used—for example, to provide population reference standards for people with a range of disabilities; we also have little information on its adequacy in non-arthritics.

The criticisms of the HAQ have focused on its scoring, which was designed for simplicity and may have been achieved at the cost of precision. By counting only the highest score in each section, the HAQ summarizes the patient's major difficulty but does not use all the information collected. In comparing scores over time, therefore, improvements in less severely affected areas of functioning may be missed, which may account for the high test–retest reliability of the HAQ, combined with its comparative insensitivity to measuring change (36). Liang et al. concluded that "the HAQ and Index of Well-Being (IWB) are judged to be poor candidates for use when mobility change is a major functional outcome" (16, p547). Certainly, it seems curious to ask questions that are not incorporated into the scoring system; to include all questions would increase sensitivity. The study by Ziebland et al. raised the possibility that asking patients to rate their own progress may form a valuable adjunct to repeated administration of the basic HAQ (21). We conclude that the scale is a good descriptive instrument, but may be less appropriate as a tool for measuring clinical change in outcome studies.

REFERENCES

(1) Ramey DR, Raynauld J-P, Fries JF. The Health Assessment Questionnaire 1992: status and review. Arthritis Care Res 1992;5:119–129.

(2) Fries JF, Spitz P, Kraines RG, et al. Measurement of patient outcome in arthritis. Arthritis Rheum 1980;23:137–145.

(3) Fries JF, Spitz PW. The hierarchy of patient outcomes. In: Spilker B, ed. Quality of life assessments in clinical trials. New York: Raven Press, 1990:25–35.

(4) Fries JF, Spitz PW, Young DY. The dimensions of health outcomes: the Health Assessment Questionnaire, disability and pain scales. J Rheumatol 1982;9:789–793.

(5) Fries JF. Toward an understanding of patient outcome measurement. Arthritis Rheum 1983;26:697–704.

(6) Wolfe F, Kleinheksel SM, Cathey MA, et al. The clinical value of the Stanford Health Assessment Questionnaire functional disability index in patients with rheumatoid arthritis. J Rheumatol 1988;15:1480–1488.

(7) Siegert CEH, Vleming L-J, Van Den Broucke JP, et al. Measurement of disability in Dutch rheumatoid arthritis patients. Clin Rheumatol 1984;3:305–309.

(8) Pincus T, Summey JA, Soraci SA Jr, et al. Assessment of patient satisfaction in activities of daily living using a modified Stanford Health Assessment Questionnaire. Arthritis Rheum 1983;26:1346–1353.

(9) Milligan SE, Hom DL, Ballou SP, et al.

An assessment of the Health Assessment Questionnaire functional ability index among women with systemic lupus erythematosus. J Rheumatol 1993;20:972–976.

(10) Goeppinger J, Doyle M, Murdock B. Self-administered function measures: the impossible dream? Arthritis Rheum 1985; 28(suppl):145.

(11) Fitzpatrick R, Newman S, Lamb R, Shipley M. A comparison of measures of health status in rheumatoid arthritis. Br J Rheumatol 1989;28:201–206.

(12) Daltroy LH, Larson MG, Roberts WN, Liang MH. A modification of the Health Assessment Questionnaire for the spondyloarthropathies. J Rheumatol 1990; 17:946–950.

(13) Brown JH, Kazis LE, Spitz PW, et al. The dimensions of health outcomes: a cross-validated examination of health status measurement. Am J Public Health 1984; 74:159–161.

(14) Cavanaugh SA. Depression in the hospitalized inpatient with various medical illnesses. Psychother Psychosom 1986; 45:97–104.

(15) Hakala M, Nieminen P, Manelius J. Joint impairment is strongly correlated with disability measured by self-report questionnaires. Functional status assessment of individuals with rheumatoid arthritis in a population based series. J Rheumatol 1994;21:64–69.

(16) Liang MH, Larson MG, Cullen KE, et al. Comparative measurement efficiency and sensitivity of five health status instruments for arthritis research. Arthritis Rheum 1985;28:542–547.

(17) Liang MH, Fossel AH, Larson MG. Comparisons of five health status instruments for orthopedic evaluation. Med Care 1990;28:632–642.

(18) Hawley DJ, Wolfe F. Sensitivity to change of the Health Assessment Questionnaire (HAQ) and other clinical and health status measures in rheumatoid arthritis: results of short-term clinical trials and observational studies versus long-term observational studies. Arthritis Care Res 1992;5:130–136.

(19) Pincus T, Callahan LF, Brooks RH, et al. Self-report questionnaire scores in rheumatoid arthritis compared with traditional physical, radiographic, and laboratory measures. Ann Intern Med 1989; 110:259–266.

(20) Callahan LF, Pincus T. A clue from a self-report questionnaire to distinguish rheumatoid arthritis from noninflammatory diffuse musculoskeletal pain. Arthritis Rheum 1990;33:1317–1322.

(21) Ziebland S, Fitzpatrick R, Jenkinson C, et al. Comparison of two approaches to measuring change in health status in rheumatoid arthritis: the Health Assessment Questionnaire (HAQ) and modified HAQ. Ann Rheum Dis 1992;51:1202–1205.

(22) Lubeck DP, Fries JF. Changes in quality of life among persons with HIV infection. Qual Life Res 1992;1:359–366.

(23) Hays RD, Shapiro MF. An overview of generic health-related quality of life measures for HIV research. Qual Life Res 1992;1:91–97.

(24) Kirwan JR, Reeback JS. Stanford Health Assessment Questionnaire modified to assess disability in British patients with rheumatoid arthritis. Br J Rheumatol 1986; 25:206–209.

(25) Ekdahl C, Eberhardt K, Andersson SI, et al. Assessing disability in patients with rheumatoid arthritis. Scand J Rheumatol 1988;17:263–271.

(26) Bosi-Ferraz M, Oliveira LM, Araujo PMP, et al. Cross-cultural reliability of the physical ability dimension of the Health Assessment Questionnaire. J Rheumatol 1990; 17:813–817.

(27) Cardiel MH, Abello-Banfi M, Ruiz-Mercado R, et al. Quality of life in rheumatoid arthritis: validation of a Spanish version of the disability index of the Health Assessment Questionnaire. Arthritis Rheum 1991;34(suppl 9):S183.

(28) Perez ER, MacKenzie CR, Ryan C. Development of a Spanish version of the Modified Health Assessment Questionnaire. Arthritis Rheum 1990;33(suppl 9):S100.

(29) Esteve-Vives J, Batelle-Gualda E, Reig A. Spanish version of the Health Assessment Questionnaire: reliability, validity and transcultural equivalency. J Rheumatol 1993;20:2116–2122.

(30) van der Heidje DMFM, Van Riel PLCM, Van de Putte LBA. Sensitivity of a Dutch Health Assessment Questionnaire in a trial comparing hydroxychloroquine vs sulphasalazine. Scand J Rheumatol 1990; 19:407–412.

(31) van der Heide A, Jacobs JW, van Albada-Kuipers GA, et al. Self report functional disability scores and the use of devices: two distinct aspects of physical function in rheumatoid arthritis. Ann Rheum Dis 1993;52:497–502.

(32) Guillemin F, Briançon S, Pourel J. Measurement of the functional capacity in rheumatoid polyarthritis: a French adaptation of the Health Assessment Questionnaire

(HAQ). Rev Rhum Mal Osteoartic 1991;58:459–465.

(33) Guillemin F, Briançon S, Pourel J. Validity and discriminant ability of a French version of the Health Assessment Questionnaire in early RA. Disabil Rehabil 1992;14:71–77.

(34) Raynauld J-P, Singh G, Shiroky JB, et al. A French-Canadian version of the Health Assessment Questionnaire. Arthritis Rheum 1992;35(suppl 9):S125.

(35) Ranza R, Marchesoni A, Calori G, et al. The Italian version of the Functional Disability Index of the Health Assessment Questionnaire. A reliable instrument for multicenter studies on rheumatoid arthritis. Clin Exp Rheumatol 1993;11:123–128.

(36) Gardiner PV, Sykes HR, Hassey GA, et al. An evaluation of the Health Assessment Questionnaire in long-term longitudinal follow-up of disability in rheumatoid arthritis. Br J Rheumatol 1993;32:724–728.

THE FUNCTIONAL INDEPENDENCE MEASURE

(Carl V. Granger and Byron B. Hamilton, 1987)

Purpose

The Functional Independence Measure (FIM) assesses physical and cognitive disability in terms of burden of care. It is used to monitor patient progress and to assess outcomes of rehabilitation. It is a rating scale applicable to patients of all ages and diagnoses, by clinicians or by non-clinicians, and has been widely adopted by rehabilitation facilities in the United States and elsewhere (1).

Conceptual Basis

To simplify medical payments in the United States, a standard remuneration system bases payment for acute care on diagnosis rather than on the care actually provided. However, as the amount of care required for rehabilitation is based on level of disability rather than on diagnosis, an alternative assessment system was needed to form the basis for estimating payments in rehabilitation medicine. In 1983, a national task force designed a Uniform Data System for Medical Rehabilitation (UDS) to achieve uniform definitions and measurements of disability; the FIM is the central measurement of this scheme (2, 3). In addition, the UDS includes further items covering demographic characteristics, diagnoses, impairment groups, length of hospital stay, and hospital charges.

The UDS distinguishes between alterations in structure or function ("impairment," in WHO terms), activity (disability) and role (handicap). The FIM covers the activity and role levels, termed life functions (1, p138). Life functions are reduced by a disabling condition and rehabilitation seeks to restore them. The FIM is not seen as comprehensive, but as a basic indicator, collecting the minimum information required for assessing disability (4). The FIM focuses on burden of care: the level of a patient's disability indicates the burden of caring for them and items are scored on the basis of how much assistance is required for the individual to carry out activities of daily living (4). As human or physical resources have to be used to substitute for the individual's reduced function, disability entails an opportunity cost to society, as the resources cannot be applied to other uses. "The helper cost is measured in hours or energy consumed (e.g., heavy lifting), stress of concern or responsibility for the individual's safety (e.g., falling), and the frustration of being on call constantly" (1, p142).

Several stages of rehabilitation are identified and efficiency of care may be estimated by dividing the increase in life function (e.g., measured by improvement in FIM scores) by the cost of the rehabilitation services.

Description

The FIM includes 18 items covering independence in self-care, sphincter control, mobility, locomotion, communication, and social cognition (5). The physical items were based on the Barthel Index and cover self-care, sphincter control, mobility, and locomotion. Three cognition items cover social interaction, problem solving, and memory (see Exhibit 3.23). A pocket-sized

SELF-CARE

Eating. Includes use of suitable utensils to bring food to mouth, chewing and swallowing, once meal is appropriately prepared.
Grooming. Includes oral care, hair grooming, washing hands and face, and either shaving or applying makeup.
Bathing. Includes bathing the body from the neck down (excluding the back), either tub, shower or sponge/bed bath. Performs safely.
Dressing—Upper Body. Includes dressing above the waist as well as donning and removing prosthesis or orthosis when applicable.
Dressing—Lower Body. Includes dressing from the waist down as well as donning or removing prosthesis or orthosis when applicable.
Toileting. Includes maintaining perineal hygiene and adjusting clothing before and after toilet or bed pan use. Performs safely.

SPHINCTER CONTROL

Bladder Management. Includes complete intentional control of urinary bladder and use of equipment or agents necessary for bladder control.
Bowel Management. Includes complete intentional control of bowel movement and use of equipment or agents necessary for bowel control.

MOBILITY

Transfers: Bed, Chair, Wheelchair. Includes all aspects of transferring to and from bed, chair, and wheelchair, and coming to a standing position, if walking is the typical mode of locomotion.
Transfer: Toilet. Includes getting on and off a toilet.
Transfers: Tub or Shower. Includes getting into and out of a tub or shower stall.

LOCOMOTION

Walking or Using Wheelchair. Includes walking, once in a standing position, or using a wheelchair, once in a seated position, on a level surface.
  Check most frequent mode of locomotion. If both are about equal, check W *and* C. If initiating a rehabilitation program, check the mode for which training is intended.
( )W = Walking ( )C = Wheelchair
Stairs. Goes up and down 12 to 14 stairs (one flight) indoors.

COMMUNICATION

Comprehension. Includes understanding of either auditory or visual communication (e.g. writing, sign language, gestures).
  Check and evaluate the most usual mode of comprehension. If both are about equally used, check A *and* V.
( )A = Auditory ( )V = Visual
Expression. Includes clear vocal or non-vocal expression of language. This item includes both intelligible speech or clear expression of language using writing or a communication device.
  Check and evaluate the most usual mode of expression. If both are about equally used, check V *and* N.
( )V = Vocal ( )N = Nonvocal

SOCIAL COGNITION

Social Interaction. Includes skills related to getting along and participating with others in therapeutic and social situations. It represents how one deals with one's own needs *together* with the needs of others.
Problem Solving. Includes skills related to solving problems of daily living. This means making reasonable, safe, and timely decisions regarding financial, social and personal affairs and initiating, sequencing and self-correcting tasks and activities to solve the problems.
Memory. Includes skills related to recognizing and remembering while performing daily activities in an institutional or community setting. It includes ability to store and retrieve information, particularly verbal and visual. A deficit in memory impairs learning as well as performance of tasks.

DESCRIPTION OF THE LEVELS OF FUNCTION AND THEIR SCORES

INDEPENDENT—Another person is not required for the activity (NO HELPER).
7 COMPLETE INDEPENDENCE—All of the tasks described as making up the activity are typically performed safely, without modification, assistive devices, or aids, and within a reasonable time.
6 MODIFIED INDEPENDENCE—Activity requires any one or more than one of the following: an assistive device, more than reasonable time, or there are safety (risk) considerations.
  DEPENDENT—Another person is required for either supervision or physical assistance in order for the activity to be performed, or it is not performed (REQUIRES HELPER).
  MODIFIED DEPENDENCE—The subject expends half (50%) or more of the effort. The levels of assistance required are:
5 Supervision or setup—Subject requires no more help than standby, cuing or coaxing, without physical contact. Or, helper sets up needed items or applies orthoses.
4 Minimal contact assistance—With physical contact the subject requires no more help than touching, and subject expends 75% or more of the effort.

3 Moderate assistance—Subject requires more help than touching, or expends half (50%) or more (up to 75%) of the effort.

COMPLETE DEPENDENCE—The subject expends *less* than half (*less* than 50%) of the effort. Maximal or total assistance is required, or the activity is not performed. The levels of assistance required are:

2 Maximal assistance—Subject expends less than 50% of the effort, but at least 25%.

1 Total assistance—Subject expends less than 25% of the effort.

Adapted from Guide for the use of the Uniform Data Set for Medical Rehabilitation. Version 3.0. Buffalo, New York: Uniform Data System for Medical Rehabilitation, The Buffalo General Hospital, 1990.

chart summarizing the items and scoring system is shown in Exhibit 3.24. Ratings consider performance rather than capacity and may be based on observation, a patient interview, or medical records. A decision tree is available from the UDS that indicates the questions to ask to rate each item in a telephone interview. Evaluators are usually physicians, nurses, or therapists, but they may be laypersons. It takes about one hour to train raters to use the FIM and about 30 minutes to administer and score the scale for each patient (1, p145). Training workshops can be arranged through the UDS group at Buffalo, NY.

The seven-point ratings represent gradations of independence and reflect the amount of assistance a patient requires. For each item, two levels of independent functioning distinguish complete independence from modified independence—when the activity is performed with some delay, safety risk, or with an assistive device. Two dependent levels refer to the provision of assistance: modified dependence is when the assistant provides less than half the effort required to complete the task, and complete dependence is when the assistant provides more than half the effort. Within each level are finer gradations of assistance. Fuller details and illustrations are contained in the guide (6), while details of how to rate unusual cases are contained in the periodic "UDS Update" publication available from the UDS group (address follows). A total score sums the individual ratings; higher scores indicate more independent function. Scores range from a low of 18 to a maximum of 126. Granger et al. outline a Rasch analysis based on over 27,000 patients that translates this ordinal score into an interval scale; they provide charts that show the conversion and the rank order of severity of each item (7, Figures 2, 5, 6; 8, Figure 4). As an alternative scoring approach, Linacre and Heinemann argue that the 13 physical items should be scored separately from the five cognitive items in the communication and social cognition groups (8, 9).

Reliability

Inter-rater tests were carried out on patients from 25 facilities by physicians, nurses, and therapists. The intraclass correlation (for the four-point rating version) was 0.86 for 303 pairs of clinical assessments at admission and 0.88 for 184 pairs at discharge (1, p145; 2, p871). Kappa indices of agreement for the 18 items averaged 0.54. Turning to the seven-point rating version, intraclass correlations for pairs of clinicians rating 263 patients ranged from 0.93 (locomotion subscale) to 0.96 (self-care and mobility). The mean kappa index of agreement between ratings for each item was 0.71 (10).

Alpha coefficients of 0.93 (admission) and 0.95 (discharge) were found in a study of 11,102 rehabilitation patients. The internal consistency of the locomotion subscale was lower, at 0.68 (11, p533).

Validity

During the early development of the FIM, content validity was tested by asking clinicians to judge its scope and ease of administration. This led to the addition of two new items (social adjustment and cognition) and the expansion of the answer categories to include modified dependence and complete dependence (12, p12). A Rasch analysis

Exhibit 3.24   Functional Independence Measure (FIM)

L E V E L S	7 Complete Independence (Timely, Safely) 6 Modified Independence (Device)	NO HELPER
	Modified Dependence 　5 Supervision 　4 Minimal Assist (Subject = 75%+) 　3 Moderate Assist (Subject = 50%+) Complete Dependence 　2 Maximal Assist (Subject = 25%+) 　1 Total Assist (Subject = 0%+)	HELPER

	ADMIT	DISCHG	FOL-UP
Self-Care			
A. Eating			
B. Grooming			
C. Bathing			
D. Dressing - Upper Body			
E. Dressing - Lower Body			
F. Toileting			
Sphincter Control			
G. Bladder Management			
H. Bowel Management			
Transfers			
I. Bed, Chair, Wheelchair			
J. Toilet			
K. Tub, Shower			
Locomotion			
L. Walk/wheelchair	Walk / Wheelchair / Both	Walk / Wheelchair / Both	Walk / Wheelchair / Both
M. Stairs			
Motor Subtotal Score			
Communication			
N. Comprehension	Auditory / Visual / Both	Auditory / Visual / Both	Auditory / Visual / Both
O. Expression	Vocal / Non-vocal / Both	Vocal / Non-vocal / Both	Vocal / Non-vocal / Both
Social Cognition			
P. Social Interaction			
Q. Problem Solving			
R. Memory			
Cognitive Subtotal Score			
Total FIM			

Note: Leave no blanks; enter 1 if patient not testable due to risk supported the division into motor and cognitive components; contrasting patterns of responses of different patient groups reflected the types of disability to be expected from their diagnoses (7, pp86, 88).

Granger et al. recorded the time required to provide help for personal-care tasks for 24 multiple sclerosis patients over a seven-day period. The FIM items predicted this rating ($R^2 = 0.77$); correlations for several items exceeded 0.80; a change of one point on the FIM total score represented 3.8 minutes of care per day (2, Tables 2, 3). The R^2 improved to 0.99 when five cases with visual impairments were omitted from the analyses: the FIM does not reflect the amount of time required to care for someone because of vision problems. Similar analyses for 21 stroke patients yielded an R^2 of 0.65. A change of one point in the FIM score was related to an average of 2.2 minutes of help per day (13, pp136–137). Disler et al. found FIM scores to correlate −0.39 with an estimate of the hours of care required for 75 neurological patients; after removing three patients with cognitive or visual impairments, the Pearson correlation rose to −0.76 (14, p141). Each point of the FIM total score reflected 4.1 minutes of care per day (14, p142).

Dodds et al. in a large study of 11,102 patients found that FIM scores improved between admission and discharge and reflected the patient's destination. Scores also reflected the presence of coexisting conditions and the severity of impairments (11, pp533–534).

An attempt to evaluate the FIM cognitive items by comparison with a neuropsychological test battery failed because almost all of the 41 spinal cord injury patients achieved maximum scores on the FIM items (15). Davidoff et al. commented: "These findings underscore the potentially misleading nature of a 'normal' score of 6 or 7 on the Social Cognition and Communication subscale items of the FIM. The false negative rate for detection of cognitive deficit using the FIM varied from 0% to 63% for each neuropsychologic test" (15, p328).

Correlations with other measures include 0.84 with the Barthel Index, 0.68 with Katz's Index of ADL, and 0.45 with Spitzer's Quality of Life Index (16, Table 2).

The FIM designed for adults has also been used with children as young as 7 years; overall and component scores showed significant associations with clinical prediction of duration of disability (17).

Alternative Forms

The FIM has been translated into French, German, Japanese, and Swedish. A prototype FIM for children aged 6 months to 7 years (the "WeeFIM") is under development. It is a direct adaptation of the adult measure, with 18 items covering six domains (18).

Reference Standards

Granger and Hamilton have produced annual reports from the UDS that show mean scores and subscores at admission and discharge for various categories of rehabilitation patients. These are based on large numbers of patients: 44,997 in the 1991 report (5).

Transition norms, describing the progress measured in FIM scores made by patients during rehabilitation, are also beginning to appear (19, 20). These results might also be used in computing the transition probabilities for prognostic indices such as the Quality of Well-Being Scale.

Commentary

The Functional Independence Measure was based on the Barthel Index, a widely used scale with proven reliability and validity; the FIM was developed with the consensus of a national advisory committee which continues to oversee its refinement. It was carefully designed, with comprehensive item definitions, standard administration procedures, and reliability. Documentation on the FIM is outstanding. The manual is thorough, and regular "UDS Update" newsletters are written in an upbeat style that conveys the sense of participating in a large family of users. The newsletters provide information on training workshops and on validity results, explain the scoring of unusual cases, and answer readers' questions. Training videos are available. A data management service oversees the collation of data from user groups, and these data form the basis for many validity and reliability studies. It is evident that considerable resources are being channelled into developing and standardizing this instrument.

A major strength of the FIM lies in the size of the UDS enterprise. As of 1990, 140 rehabilitation facilities were participating in the Data Management Service, and an estimated 100 additional facilities use the Uniform Data System in the United States, Canada, Australia, France, Japan, Sweden, and West Germany. Several of the validation studies report data from 10,000 or more cases, unique in the field of functional measurement. The physical components of the FIM appear comparable to the best among the other ADL instruments. The cognitive and social communication dimensions may have low sensitivity (15); refinement may be desirable. Overall, the FIM is a sound instrument which benefits from outstanding support services. Viewed as a brief disability measure rather than a general health instrument, it deserves close consideration as a patient assessment tool and also as an evaluative instrument.

Address

Information and guidelines are available from the UDS Data Management Service, 82 Farber Hall, SUNY, South Campus, Buffalo, NY, USA 14214

REFERENCES

(1) Hamilton BB, Granger CV, Sherwin FS, et al. A uniform national data system for medical rehabilitation. In: Fuhrer MJ, ed. Rehabilitation outcomes: analysis and measurement. Baltimore, Maryland: Paul H. Brookes, 1987:137–147.

(2) Granger CV, Cotter AC, Hamilton BB, et al. Functional assessment scales: a study of persons with multiple sclerosis. Arch Phys Med Rehabil 1990;71:870–875.

(3) Granger CV, Hamilton BB, Keith RA, et al. Advances in functional assessment for medical rehabilitation. Top Geriatr Rehabil 1986;1:59–74.

(4) UDS Data Management Service. Uniform Data Set for Medical Rehabilitation: update. Buffalo, NY: UDS Data Management Service, SUNY, 1990.

(5) Granger CV, Hamilton BB. The Uniform Data System for Medical Rehabilitation report of first admissions for 1991. Am J Phys Med Rehabil 1993;72:33–38.

(6) UDS Data Management Service. Guide for use of the Uniform Data Set for Medical Rehabilitation including the Functional Independence Measure. Version 3.0. Buffalo, NY: Uniform Data System for Medical Rehabilitation, The Buffalo General Hospital, 1990.

(7) Granger CV, Hamilton BB, Linacre JM, et al. Performance profiles of the Functional Independence Measure. Am J Phys Med Rehabil 1993;72:84–89.

(8) Linacre JM, Heinemann AW, Wright BD, et al. The structure and stability of the Functional Independence Measure. Arch Phys Med Rehabil 1994;75:127–132.

(9) Heinemann AW, Linacre JM, Wright BD, et al. Relationships between impairment and physical disability as measured by the Functional Independence Measure. Arch Phys Med Rehabil 1993;74:566–573.

(10) Hamilton BB, Laughlin JA, Granger CV, et al. Interrater agreement of the seven level Functional Independence Measure (FIM). Arch Phys Med Rehabil 1991;72:790.

(11) Dodds TA, Martin DP, Stolov WC, et al. A validation of the Functional Independence Measurement and its performance among rehabilitation inpatients. Arch Phys Med Rehabil 1993;74:531–536.

(12) Keith RA, Granger CV, Hamilton BB, et al. The Functional Independence Measure: a new tool for rehabilitation. In: Eisenberg MG, Grzesiak RC, eds. Advances in clinical rehabilitation. Vol. 1. New York: Springer, 1987:6–18.

(13) Granger CV, Cotter AC, Hamilton BB, et al. Functional assessment scales: a study of persons after stroke. Arch Phys Med Rehabil 1993;74:133–138.

(14) Disler PB, Roy CW, Smith BP. Predicting hours of care needed. Arch Phys Med Rehabil 1993;74:139–143.

(15) Davidoff GN, Roth EJ, Haughton JS, et al. Cognitive dysfunction in spinal cord

injury patients: sensitivity of the Functional Independence Measure subscales vs neuropsychologic assessment. Arch Phys Med Rehabil 1990;71:326–329.

(16) Rockwood K, Stolee P, Fox RA. Use of goal attainment scaling in measuring clinically important change in the frail elderly. J Clin Epidemiol 1993;46:1113–1118.

(17) Di Scala C, Grant CC, Brooke MM, et al. Functional outcome in children with traumatic brain injury: agreement between clinical judgment and the Functional Independence Measure. Am J Phys Med Rehabil 1992;71:145–148.

(18) McCabe MA, Granger CV. Content validity of a pediatric Functional Independence Measure. Appl Nurs Res 1990;3:120–122.

(19) Long WB, Sacco WJ, Coombes SS, et al. Determining normative standards for Functional Independence Measure transitions in rehabilitation. Arch Phys Med Rehabil 1994;75:144–148.

(20) Hamilton BB, Granger CV. Disability outcomes following inpatient rehabilitation for stroke. Phys Ther 1994;74:494–503.

CONCLUSION: IADL SCALES

The IADL scales reviewed in this section represent a bridge between the traditional, physical measurements represented by ADL scales and other indices such as social functioning scales. The broader approach of the IADL instruments is increasingly supplanting the older ADL methods, and it is clear that they have been more thoroughly tested and are more sensitive to minor variations in a patient's condition.

We criticized the ADL scales on several grounds: most were developed in relative isolation from other methods, and few were founded on a clear conceptual basis or critique of earlier work. The IADL scales show some signs of overcoming these weaknesses, although little work has yet been done to establish the formal correspondence among the various measurements, with the exception of the work of Jette. We regard research that compares different scales as a crucial stage in consolidating the discipline of measurement; this has been achieved in some fields such as that of psychological well-being (Chapter 5), but not yet in the field of functional disability measurement.

Several themes emerge from our review of the IADL scales. The content of the scales stresses the patient's functioning within her particular environment, more closely reflecting handicap than impairment or disability. This theme is picked up and expanded in the indicators of social health, many of which define social health in terms of the ability to perform one's normal social roles. Perhaps because these topics require greater reliance on subjective data collected by self-report than do the more traditional indicators of physical functioning, more attention has been paid to establishing the validity and reliability of IADL scales than is the case with the older ADL methods. Because they are sensitive to lower levels of disablement, the IADL scales are more suited to use as survey methods for general population studies. It is also plausible that the IADL approach will come to rival, and perhaps replace, the traditional ADL scales in clinical studies. In their turn, however, the IADL scales may come to be replaced by the broader-ranging general measurement methods described in Chapter 9. There is no essential distinction between the IADL scales described here and the IADL component of several of the general health measurements covered in Chapter 9.

4

Social Health

The theme of social health is less familiar to us and is less frequently discussed, measured, and researched than the topics of physical and psychological health. Being less familiar, several potential misconceptions about social health must be addressed at the outset. As the word "social" does not refer to a characteristic of individuals, it may not be immediately clear how a person can be rated in terms of social health. And, indeed, there is an important tradition of regarding social health as a characteristic of society rather than of individuals: "A society is healthy when there is equal opportunity for all and access by all to the goods and services essential to full functioning as a citizen" (1, p75). Indicators of social health in this sense might include the distribution of economic wealth, the public accessibility of the decision-making process, and the accountability of public officials. In keeping with our approach in this book, however, we will not discuss indicators of the health of a society; we will consider only measurements of the rather less intuitively obvious concept of the social health of individuals. A representative definition of this theme would describe social health as "that dimension of an individual's well-being that

concerns how he gets along with other people, how other people react to him, and how he interacts with social institutions and societal mores" (1, p75). The definition is broad; it incorporates elements of personality and social skills and it also in part reflects the norms of the society in which the individual finds himself. In fact, most measurements of the social health of individuals do not employ the word "healthy" but speak instead of "well-being," "adjustment," "performance," or "social functioning." Why, then, should we regard this sphere of human interaction as a part of health at all?

Since the creation of the WHO definition of health, the emphasis on treating patients as social beings who live in a complex social context has permeated many branches of medicine. Those who are well integrated into their communities tend to live longer and may have an increased capacity to recover from disease; conversely, social isolation is a risk factor for disease. People with serious disease or disability generally need social support to remain in the community, and the social view of medicine holds that the ultimate aim of care should be to reintegrate people into productive lives in society rather than merely to treat their medical symptoms. All these arguments created a demand for new measurement scales to assess need for care and to evaluate outcomes. But aside from the philosophical appeal of considering social adjustment as a component of health, there are practical reasons for measuring an individual's social well-being and adjustment. The expense of institutional care and the resulting emphasis on discharging patients as early as possible implies a need to assess their readiness to live independently in the community. The movement away from institutional care in the mental health field, which has been responsible for partially emptying and sometimes closing large mental hospitals, has fostered studies of the quality of adjustment to community living or social functioning, especially among older patients (2). Studies of this type are equally relevant in the area of physical rehabilitation, and indices of social functioning can be used to evaluate the outcomes of rehabilitation in terms of social restoration: has the individual returned to a productive and stable position in society (3)? A further reason to measure social health, albeit in a slightly different sense, is to examine the influence of social support and social ties on a person's physical and psychological well-being. This treats the social adjustment not as a dependent, but as an independent, variable. Reviews of this field are given by Antonovsky (4), Berkman and Breslow (5), and Murawski et al. (6).

These contrasting ways of defining social health—in terms of adjustment, social support or the ability to perform normal roles in society—and the measurements that have been developed for each are further examined in the following sections.

SOCIAL ADJUSTMENT AND SOCIAL ROLES

The approach to social health that views it in terms of social or community adjustment derived primarily from the work of sociologists and, in the health field, of psychia-

trists. Psychiatric interest in social health arose because problems in personal or social relationships and communication represent the most common reason for seeking care for nonpsychotic mental disorders. The adequacy of a person's social adjustment and interaction may therefore indicate need for care; they may also form indicators of its outcome, especially that of psychotherapy. The development of adjustment scales also coincided with a gradual shift in psychiatry away from medical concepts of mental illness that emphasized disease or deviance, toward a concern with mental distress viewed in terms of inadequate social integration and adjustment: can the individual function adequately in personal relationships? This is most commonly expressed as social adjustment, broadly definable in terms of the interplay between the individual and his social environment and his success in chosen social roles (7). Linn has viewed adjustment in a dynamic sense, covering the person's equilibrium or success in reducing tensions and in satisfying needs (2). Interest in social adjustment is, of course, not peculiar to psychiatry: school curricula stress the importance of learning to function as a social being.

Social adjustment may be measured either by considering a person's satisfaction with his relationships or by studying his performance of various social roles. The subjective approach to measuring social adjustment records affective responses such as discontent, unhappiness (as measured, for example, by Linn's Social Dysfunction Rating Scale), and anxiety. This area of measurement is diffuse, and there are no clear boundaries between measurements of social health in this sense and measurements of life satisfaction, happiness, or quality of life. These scales are therefore often subsumed under the general heading of "subjective well-being," but we have attempted to form a finer classification. Measurements of happiness and general affective well-being that are not specifically related to social relationships, such as the

Bradburn scale, are included in Chapter 5, which addresses psychological well-being. Measurements of related themes such as life satisfaction and adjustment are also included in Chapter 5. Measurements of affective responses that focus on social relationships are included in the present chapter (e.g., Linn's scale). Quality of life scales are described in Chapter 9.

One of the major problems with measurements of social adjustment is selecting an appropriate standard against which to evaluate adjustment. Norms vary greatly from one culture to another, ranging from an emphasis on "oneness with nature" and rejection of worldly values in Asian cultures to an emphasis on material possessions in some sectors of contemporary Western society (3). Expectations also vary among social classes within a culture, making it difficult to compare adjustment between times, places, and groups. The most common way to avoid these problems is to focus the measurement on specific social roles for which there is some agreement about appropriate behavior.

The social role approach to assessing adjustment is based loosely on sociological role theory and implies a valuation: how adequately is the person performing compared to normal social expectations? A person who cannot function in a way that meets the normal demands of his situation may be considered socially disabled (8). Although this does not eliminate the problem of defining what is normal, there are, at least, recognized norms for many roles. These may be formally couched in law or in less formal regulations, traditions, or agreements among individuals. Although approaches based on norms seem to offer promise, they are not sufficiently refined to indicate what should be included in a social health questionnaire. Ultimately the selection of topics appears to be a more-or-less arbitrary process. Most operational definitions of social roles consider housework, occupation, community involvement, marital and parental roles, and leisure activities.

Most of these topics are also covered in the IADL scales (see Chapter 3), so the role approach to measuring social health brings it conceptually very close to indices of functional handicap. A social role approach is used in the measurement methods of Weissman and of Gurland, reviewed in this chapter.

There are several conceptual problems with using role theory as an approach to measuring social health. Assumptions have to be made regarding how to evaluate performance: should it be compared to some ideal, to the person's own aspirations, or to other peoples' expectations of her performance? The first tends to be insufficient: while there are recognized norms for much behavior, there is little consensus over what constitutes a socially "correct" definition of the marital role, for example. Norms vary between social strata, and there is little agreement over the relative importance of different roles. Alternative approaches also suffer problems: comparing a person's performance to the aspirations of her spouse, for example, makes it hard to evaluate pathology, as the partner may have unrealistically high or low expectations. The role approach has been criticized as being rigid and conservative; it may be impractical to evaluate the legitimacy of individual reasons for not behaving in a "normal" way. Platt argued that the role approach implies viewing the "ideal individual as an object which passively shapes itself to the culture and the external environment. He should be satisfied with his situation and if he is not, then he is not fully adjusted" (9, p103). Pursuing this criterion further, one might argue that the world of the socially healthy is "characterized by harmony, happiness and consensus, and is inhabited by men and women who are consistently interested, active, friendly, adequate, guilt-free, nondistressed and so on. If they show anything less than interest in their work they are maladjusted" (9, p106). Functioning in social roles may evidently be influenced by many factors other than health status.

While respondents may be asked to identify only problems that are due to their health, this is often a very complex judgment to make as problems rarely have a single cause. Nor are changes in role function specific to any one type of health problem: social and role limitations can be caused by depression or physical disability. Hence it can be difficult to know how to classify indicators of social or role functioning: as indicators of physical, mental, or social health?

Recognizing these potential problems, several scales, such as that of Remington and Tyrer, avoid imposing fixed definitions of what constitutes normal or adequate performance. The Katz Adjustment Scales use another approach that combines the objective assessments of the role approach with subjective evaluations of satisfaction made by the respondent: to evaluate how important it is that the individual does or does not fulfill her social role requires information as to how she views that role. This is close to the concept of the *person–environment fit;* rather than stressing adherence to somewhat arbitrary principles of behavior, the socially healthy person would be one who has found a comfortable niche in which to operate to the best of her capacities, and to the satisfaction of those around her.

SOCIAL SUPPORT

Many studies in the field of social epidemiology have highlighted the importance of social support in attenuating the effects of stressful events and thereby reducing the incidence of disease (10–12). In addition, social support contributes to positive adjustment in the child and adult and encourages personal growth. Because of the importance of social integration and social support, we review some social support scales in this chapter.

"Social support" is generally defined in terms of the availability of people whom the individual trusts, on whom he can rely, and who make him feel cared for and valued as a person. Social support may be distinguished from the related concept of social networks, which refers to the roles and ties that link individuals along definable paths of kinship, friendship, or acquaintance. Social networks may be seen as the structure through which support is provided (13), while most indices of social support take a functional approach.

An early scale that covered aspects of social support was the Berle Index, published in 1952 (14). For 30 years there were few other formal measurements of social support, and many studies relied on indirect, structural indicators such as marital status or other sociodemographic variables (13). The field has, however, become an important area of growth in sociomedical indices, and many scales have been proposed. Important stimuli for the development of more formal measurement indices came from conceptual discussions of support, including Bowlby's theories of attachment (15) and Weiss's functional analysis (16). Weiss saw social support as performing both instrumental and expressive functions for the individual: it provides for social integration, nurturance, alliance and guidance, and also fosters feelings of worth and intimacy. Support is of various types and Sherbourne and Stewart distinguished five categories: (a) providing emotional support, love, and empathy, (b) providing instrumental or tangible support, (c) providing information, guidance, or feedback on behavior, (d) offering appraisal support which helps the person to evaluate themselves, and (e) giving companionship in leisure and recreational activities (17, p705). Measures of structural support cover the existence and quantity of social relationships (numbers of relatives or friends) and the interconnectedness of the person's network (how closely the person's friends know each other). Issues in the measurement of social support include whether it is the number of social contacts a person has or their quality that is important and how to compare the value of formal affiliations and informal friendships. In general, the emphasis now lies with assessing the functional and qualitative aspects of relationships rather than their number or type. A research agenda might include evaluating how these different dimensions of social support relate to outcomes.

SCOPE OF THE CHAPTER

We present measures of social support and social adjustment. The theme of social support is represented here by McFarlane's Social Relationship Scale, by Sarason's Social Support Questionnaire, by two Duke scales, and by two scales from the Rand/ MOS group: the Rand Social Health Battery, which measures social interaction, conceptually close to social support, and the social support scale of Sherbourne and Stewart. References to other scales that are still in the process of development are given at the end of the chapter. There are also relevant scales in other chapters in the book, such as the Functional Assessment Inventory of Crewe and Athelstan in Chapter 9, which review the resources that may assist a patient in coping with physical handicaps.

The topic of social adjustment is treated in a sequence running from scales suited for general application, toward instruments designed for use with psychiatric and other patient groups. We begin with the Katz Adjustment Scales, followed by the Social Functioning Schedule, which covers problems in social functioning, the Interview Schedule for Social Interaction of Henderson et al., and Weissman's Social Adjustment Scale. We then review the Social Maladjustment Schedule of Clare, Linn's Social Dysfunction Rating Scale, and finally Gurland's Structured and Scaled Interview to Assess Maladjustment. Table 4.1 provides a quick reference comparison of the format and quality of these scales. The conclusion to the chapter mentions other scales that we considered for inclusion and which may be of value to researchers unable to find what they require in the main review section.

REFERENCES

(1) Russell RD. Social health: an attempt to clarify this dimension of well-being. Int J Health Educ 1973;16:74–82.
(2) Linn MW. Assessing community adjustment in the elderly. In: Raskin A, Jervik LF, eds. Assessment of psychiatric symptoms and cognitive loss in the elderly. Washington, DC: Hemisphere Press, 1979:187–204.
(3) Berger DG, Rice CE, Sewall LG, et al. Posthospital evaluation of psychiatric patients: the Social Adjustment Inventory Method. Psychiatr Studies Projects 1964; 2:2–30.
(4) Antonovsky A. Health, stress, and coping. San Francisco: Jossey-Bass, 1980.
(5) Berkman LF, Breslow L. Health and ways of living: the Alameda County Study. New York: Oxford University Press, 1983.
(6) Murawski BJ, Penman D, Schmitt M. Social support in health and illness: the concept and its measurement. Cancer Nurs 1978;1:365–371.
(7) Weissman MM, Sholomskas D, John K. The assessment of social adjustment: an update. Arch Gen Psychiatry 1981; 38:1250–1258.
(8) Ruesch J, Brodsky CM. The concept of social disability. Arch Gen Psychiatry 1968;19:394–403.
(9) Platt S. Social adjustment as a criterion of treatment success: just what are we measuring? Psychiatry 1981;44:95–112.
(10) Broadhead WE, Kaplan BH, James SA, et al. The epidemiologic evidence for a relationship between social support and health. Am J Epidemiol 1983;117:521–537.
(11) Mitchell RE, Billings AG, Moos RH. Social support and well-being: implications for prevention programs. J Primary Prev 1982;3:77–98.
(12) Bruhn JG, Philips BU. Measuring social support: a synthesis of current approaches. J Behav Med 1984;7:151–169.
(13) Lin N, Dean A, Ensel WM. Social support scales: a methodological note. Schizophr Bull 1981;7:73–89.
(14) Berle BB, Pinsky RH, Wolf S, et al. A clinical guide to prognosis in stress diseases. JAMA 1952;149:1624–1628.
(15) Bowlby J. Attachment and loss. Vol. I, Attachment. London: Hogarth, 1969.
(16) Weiss RS. The provisions of social rela-

Table 4.1 Comparison of the Quality of Social Health Measurements*

Measurement	Scale	Number of items	Application	Administered by (time)	Studies using method	Reliability Thoroughness	Reliability Results	Validity Thoroughness	Validity Results
Social Relationship Scale (McFarlane, 1981)	ordinal	6	research	self, interviewer assisted	few	+	++	+	0
Social Support Questionnaire (Sarason, 1983)	ordinal	27	research	self	several	++	++	++	++
Rand Social Health Battery (Rand, 1978)	ordinal	11	survey	self	few	++	+	++	+
Medical Outcomes Study Social Support Survey (Sherbourne, 1991)	ordinal	20	survey	self	few	++	++	++	++
Duke–UNC Functional Social Support Questionnaire (Broadhead, 1988)	ordinal	8	clinical	self	few	+	+	++	+
Duke Social Support and Stress Scale (Parkerson, 1989)	ordinal	24	research	self	few	++	+	++	+
Katz Adjustment Scales (Katz, 1963)	ordinal	205†	clinical	self (45–60 min)	many	++	++	++	++
Social Functioning Schedule (Tyrer, 1979)	ordinal	121	clinical	expert (10–20 min)	few	+	+	++	++
Interview Schedule for Social Interaction (Henderson, 1980)	ordinal	52	research, clinical	interviewer (45 min)	several	++	++	+++	++
Social Adjustment Scale—Self–Report (Weissman, 1971)	ordinal	42	clinical	self (15–20 min) interviewer (45–60 min)	many	+++	++	++	++
Social Maladjustment Schedule (Clare, 1978)	ordinal	42	clinical, survey	interviewer (45 min)	few	+	+	++	+
Social Dysfunction Rating Scale (Linn, 1969)	ordinal	21	research	staff (30 mins)	several	+	++	+	++
Structured & Scaled Interview to Assess Maladjustment (SSIAM) (Gurland, 1972)	ordinal	60	clinical, research	interviewer (30 min)	several	+	++	++	++

*For an explanation of the categories used, see Chapter 1, pages 6–7.

†There are 205 items in the five sections of this instrument. The questions can be answered twice, once by the patient and once by a relative.

tionships. In: Rubin Z, ed. Doing unto others. Englewood Cliffs, New Jersey: Prentice-Hall, 1974:17–26.

(17) Sherbourne CD, Stewart AL. The MOS Social Support Survey. Soc Sci Med 1991;32:705–714.

THE SOCIAL RELATIONSHIP SCALE
(Allan H. McFarlane, 1981)

Purpose

The Social Relationship Scale (SRS) was developed to measure the extent of an individual's network of social relationships and its perceived helpfulness in cushioning the effects of life stresses on health (1). This social support scale was intended primarily as a research instrument for use in studies of life events in general population samples.

Conceptual Basis

The notion that social support is a buffer against disease formed the stimulus for the development of this scale: social bonds are considered necessary for the individual to cope with adverse events. The scale was designed to summarize the qualitative and quantitative aspects of a person's network of relationships that help him to deal with stresses (1).

Description

The SRS is a self-administered scale that is introduced by a trained interviewer who orients the respondent and who prompts the respondent at the end to review possible relationships that may have been forgotten. The scale originally formed one section in a larger questionnaire concerned with the impact of life changes on emotional well-being in which the respondent was asked to identify the people who supported him in each of six areas in which he had experienced life changes (2). The SRS can also be used as a social support indicator on its own.

The scale covers six areas of life change and the question stem and response scale are standard for each. The six areas of life change include work-related events, monetary and financial events, home and family events, personal health events, personal and social events, and society in general. The format of the scale is shown in Exhibit 4.1. The scale shown in the exhibit is applied six times, referring to each of the six topics just listed here. Respondents are asked to give the initials of the person they talked to; these indicate the type of relationship (spouse, close family, distant family, friend, fellow worker, professional) and rate the helpfulness of the discussion on a seven-point scale. They also rate whether that person would come to them to discuss similar problems, as an indication of reciprocity in the relationship (2).

Three scores may be calculated. The quality of the network is estimated from the average of the seven-point helpfulness ratings, while the extent of the network is estimated from a count of the total number of different individuals the respondent mentions (3). A score reflecting the degree of reciprocity is established by counting the number of people named who the respondent thinks would come to him to discuss similar problems. McFarlane et al. designated a relationship as multiplex if a support person was named in three separate problem areas (2).

Reliability

Test–retest reliability was assessed on 73 students after a one-week interval. Correlations for the numbers of individuals in the person's network ranged from 0.62 to 0.99, with a median of 0.91 (1, p92). Correlations for the helpfulness score were lower, ranging from 0.54 to 0.94, giving a median of 0.78 (1, p93).

Validity

Content validity was ensured via a review by four psychiatrists who made recommendations for improvements that were subsequently incorporated in the scale. Discriminal validity was assessed by comparing 15 couples with known marital or family

Exhibit 4.1   Format of the Social Relationship Scale

Example 1: Home and family

Please list the people with whom you generally discuss home and family, using the first name or initials only. After each name or set of initials fill in a one- or two-word description of the relation each person has to you. Then go on to check the circle which indicates the degree of helpfulness or unhelpfulness of your discussions with each person, and lastly, check off yes or no if you feel this person would come to you to discuss home and family. Don't feel you have to fill up all the spaces provided. If you find you need more spaces, please inform the interviewer.

I discuss home and family with:

Name or initials	Relation	Helpfulness of discussion *(Check one circle)*				Would this person come to you to discuss home and family?	
		makes things a lot worse	makes things a bit worse	helps things a bit	helps things a lot	Yes	No
_____	_____	○ ○	○ ○	○ ○	○	( )1	( )2
_____	_____	makes things a lot worse ○	makes things a bit worse ○	helps things a bit ○	helps things a lot ○	( )1	( )2
_____	_____	makes things a lot worse ○	makes things a bit worse ○	helps things a bit ○	helps things a lot ○	( )1	( )2
_____	_____	makes things a lot worse ○	makes things a bit worse ○	helps things a bit ○	helps things a lot ○	( )1	( )2
_____	_____	makes things a lot worse ○	makes things a bit worse ○	helps things a bit ○	helps things a lot ○	( )1	( )2
_____	_____	makes things a lot worse ○	makes things a bit worse ○	helps things a bit ○	helps things a lot ○	( )1	( )2
_____	_____	makes things a lot worse ○	makes things a bit worse ○	helps things a bit ○	helps things a lot ○	( )1	( )2
_____	_____	makes things a lot worse ○	makes things a bit worse ○	helps things a bit ○	helps things a lot ○	( )1	( )2

Reproduced from McFarlane AH, Neale KA, Norman GR, Roy RJ, Streiner DL. Methodological issues in developing a scale to measure social support. Schizophr Bull 1981;7:91. With permission.

problems with 18 couples judged to communicate effectively with each other. The scale showed significant differences in its ratings of the marital relationship between these groups. Response bias was also examined, to ascertain whether respondents tended to give socially desirable replies. This was tested on 19 postgraduate students by altering the question stem so as to deliberately encourage a biased response and then assessing how far this differed from the responses given with the standard question stem. The results suggested that the standard wording showed significantly less bias toward a socially desirable response in all areas (1).

Reference Standards

McFarlane et al. provided descriptive statistics by sex and marital status for the SRS scores, derived from a sample of 518 general population respondents (1, Table 5).

Commentary

This brief rating scale provides more information than most social support measures. It covers both the quantity of social contacts and their supportive quality and covers giving as well as receiving support. It also covers negative aspects of relationships and satisfaction. The structure of the questionnaire is similar to that used in Part I of the Personal Resource Questionnaire developed by Brandt and Weinert (4). McFarlane et al. have used the SRS in a study of reactions to life events and have drawn several conclusions concerning the role of social support. For example, the quality of social supports, that is, the helpfulness of relationships, had greater impact than quantity (2); Henderson made the same point in discussing the Interview Schedule for Social Interaction. Those who felt least helped by their social networks had larger networks, made more contact with them, and reported more stressful events in their current, as well as their past, life (2). The early results appear promising, but before we can fully recommend the SRS, further

reliability and validity tests on larger samples and in other centers are necessary.

REFERENCES

(1) McFarlane AH, Neale KA, Norman GR, et al. Methodological issues in developing a scale to measure social support. Schizophr Bull 1981;7:90–100.
(2) McFarlane AH, Norman GR, Streiner DL, et al. Characteristics and correlates of effective and ineffective social supports. J Psychosom Res 1984;28:501–510.
(3) McFarlane AH, Norman GR, Streiner DL, et al. The process of social stress: stable, reciprocal, and mediating relationships. J Health Soc Behav 1983;24:160–173.
(4) Brandt PA, Weinert C. The PRQ—a social support measure. Nurs Res 1981;30:277–280.

THE SOCIAL SUPPORT QUESTIONNAIRE
(Irwin G. Sarason, 1983)

Purpose

The Social Support Questionnaire (SSQ) is intended to quantify the availability of, and satisfaction with, social support (1). It was designed primarily as a research instrument and can be used with any type of respondent.

Conceptual Basis

As with McFarlane's scale, the development of this instrument was stimulated by the numerous studies that link social support with health. Sarason et al. noted that social support contributes to positive adjustment and personal development and provides a buffer against the effects of stress (1). After reviewing alternative conceptual approaches to social support, Sarason et al. focused on two central elements in the concept: the perception that there are sufficient people available to help in times of need and the degree of satisfaction with the support available (1, 2).

Description

The SSQ is a 27-item self-administered scale; the items were drawn from a larger pool by discarding those with low intercor-relations (1). Each question requires a two-part answer: respondents are asked to list the people to whom they could turn and on whom they could rely in specified sets of circumstances (availability), and to rate how satisfied they are with the available support (satisfaction). A maximum of nine persons can be listed as supports for each topic, their identity being indicated by their initials and relationship to the respondent. The satisfaction rating is the same for each item and uses a six-point scale running from "very satisfied" to "very dissatisfied." The instructions and questions are shown in Exhibit 4.2.

A support score for each item is the number of support persons listed (the "number score"). The mean of these scores across the 27 items gives an overall support score (SSQN). An overall satisfaction score (SSQS) is based on the mean of the 27 satisfaction scores.

Reliability

For the number scores, inter-item correla-tions ranged from 0.35 to 0.71, with a mean of 0.54. The correlations of each item with the total score (after omitting that item from the total score) ranged from 0.51 to 0.79; the alpha coefficient of internal reliability was 0.97. For the satisfaction scores, the inter-item correlations ranged from 0.21 to 0.74, with a coefficient alpha of 0.94 (N = 602) (1, p130).

Test–retest correlations of 0.90 for the overall number score and 0.83 for the sat-isfaction score were obtained from 105 students after a four-week interval (1, p130).

Validity

Separate factor analyses were performed for the two types of score. In both cases a strong first factor was identified, account-ing for 82% of the variance in the numbers score and 72% in the satisfaction score (1). Sarason concluded that the two scores represent different dimensions of social support. The correlation between the num-ber and satisfaction scores has been studied in several samples and ranged from 0.21 to 0.34 (1, pp130–131).

Criterion validity was studied in samples of psychology students. Significant negative correlations were obtained between the SSQ and a depression scale (correlations ranged from −0.22 to −0.43) (1, Table 2). For females only, both scales of the SSQ correlated negatively with hostility and lack of protection scales; for both sexes there was a slight, but not significant, cor-relation between the satisfaction score and a social desirability scale (coefficients ranged from 0.16 to 0.24) (1, Table 2). A correlation of 0.57 was obtained between the satisfaction score and an optimism scale, while the number score correlated 0.34 (1, p132).

With 295 students, a significant associa-tion was found between the numbers of positive life events and the number score, with more positive events reported among those with higher SSQ scores (1). Those with more social support also felt more able to control the occurrence of life events (1, Table 3). In a study of 163 men in military training, respondents who had many negative life events and less support showed a higher frequency of chronic ill-ness than other groups (2). From this study, Sarason et al. showed significant agreement between an experimenter's rating of the social competence of the respondent and the number score; those in high and low support groups differed significantly in their scores on a loneliness questionnaire and a social competence questionnaire (3).

Alternative Forms

In 1987, Sarason et al. described a six-item abbreviation of the SSQ (4). The six items were selected through factor analyses in two samples and were all items that loaded highly on the SSQN and SSQS scales; they are items 9, 17, 19, 20, 23, and 25 in our exhibit. Internal consistency of the SSQ-6 was $\alpha = 0.90$ and $\alpha = 0.93$ in two sam-ples; correlations with the full SSQ were 0.95 for SSQN and 0.96 for SSQS (after

Exhibit 4.2   The Social Support Questionnaire

Note: The answer categories and the satisfaction rating are the same for all questions and are therefore shown only for the first question in the exhibit.

The following questions ask about people in your environment who provide you with help or support. Each question has two parts. For the first part, list all the people you know, excluding yourself, whom you can count on for help or support in the manner described. Give the person's initials and their relationship to you (see example). Do not list more than one person next to each of the letters beneath the question.

For the second part, circle how satisfied you are with the overall support you have.

If you have no support for a question, check the words "No one," but still rate your level of satisfaction. Do not list more than nine persons per question.

Please answer all questions as best you can. All your responses will be kept confidential.

EXAMPLE

Who do you know whom you can trust with information that could get you in trouble?

No one   1) T.N. (brother)   4) T.N. (father)   7)
                    2) L.M. (friend)   5) L.N. (employer)   8)
                    3) R.S. (friend)   6)   9)

How satisfied?

6—very satisfied	5—fairly satisfied	4—a little satisfied	3—a little dissatisfied	2—fairly dissatisfied	1—very dissatisfied

1. Whom can you really count on to listen to you when you need to talk?

No one   1)   4)   7)
                    2)   5)   8)
                    3)   6)   9)

How satisfied?

6—very satisfied	5—fairly satisfied	4—a little satisfied	3—a little dissatisfied	2—fairly dissatisfied	1—very dissatisfied

2. Whom could you really count on to help you if a person whom you thought was a good friend insulted you and told you that he/she didn't want to see you again?

3. Whose lives do you feel that you are an important part of?

4. Whom do you feel would help you if you were married and had just separated from your spouse?

5. Whom could you really count on to help you out in a crisis situation, even though they would have to go out of their way to do so?

6. Whom can you talk with frankly, without having to watch what you say?

7. Who helps you feel that you truly have something positive to contribute to others?

8. Whom can you really count on to distract you from your worries when you feel under stress?

9. Whom can you really count on to be dependable when you need help?

10. Whom could you really count on to help you out if you had just been fired from your job or expelled from school?

11. With whom can you totally be yourself?

12. Whom do you feel really appreciates you as a person?

13. Whom can you really count on to give you useful suggestions that help you to avoid making mistakes?

14. Whom can you count on to listen openly and uncritically to your innermost feelings?

15. Who will comfort you when you need it by holding you in their arms?

16. Whom do you feel would help if a good friend of yours had been in a car accident and was hospitalized in serious condition?

17. Whom can you really count on to help you feel more relaxed when you are under pressure or tense?
18. Whom do you feel would help if a family member very close to you died?
19. Who accepts you totally, including both your worst and your best points?
20. Whom can you really count on to care about you, regardless of what is happening to you?
21. Whom can you really count on to listen to you when you are very angry at someone else?
22. Whom can you really count on to tell you, in a thoughtful manner, when you need to improve in some way?
23. Whom can you really count on to help you feel better when you are feeling generally down-in-the-dumps?
24. Whom do you feel truly loves you deeply?
25. Whom can you count on to console you when you are very upset?
26. Whom can you really count on to support you in major decisions you make?
27. Whom can you really count on to help you feel better when you are very irritable, ready to get angry at almost anything?

Reproduced from the Social Support Questionnaire obtained from Dr. Irwin G Sarason. With permission.

deleting the six common items). Correlations with the Beck Depression Inventory and with other social support measures were high and similar to those of the full SSQ. The abbreviated version appears appropriate for use when time constraints do not permit use of the complete scale.

Commentary

The SSQ seems to be a valid and reliable scale, although the evidence is not extensive. Considerable reliance was placed on psychology students in testing the instrument, and it will be important to assess how the scale performs with other samples and how it correlates with other social support scales.

The response categories used in assessing social support vary from scale to scale. The Medical Outcomes Study (MOS) Social Support Scale asks how much of the time each form of support is available, McFarlane's scale counts the helpfulness of each supportive person, while Sarason counts the number of people available to help and the perceived adequacy of this support. This diversity reflects the difficulty of selecting appropriate answer categories; it is not certain that counting numbers of people available (number score) is the most relevant indicator. Perhaps the link between numbers of contacts and perceived support is not linear, in that having too

few people and also reporting large numbers under every category would both indicate problems. The number score also does not reflect the extent of overlap between people identified in different questions and hence does not indicate the overall size of the network or McFarlane's theme of multiplexity. While asking about who provides support and about satisfaction for each question lengthens the instrument, it is likely that having the respondent think about all the people who provide support improves the accuracy of reports of satisfaction.

The SSQ appears to offer a sound, but longer, alternative to the MOS instrument described later in this chapter.

REFERENCES

(1) Sarason IG, Levine HM, Basham RB, et al. Assessing social support: the Social Support Questionnaire. J Pers Soc Psychol 1983;44:127–139.
(2) Sarason IG, Sarason BR, Potter EH, et al. Life events, social support, and illness. Psychosom Med 1985;47:156–163.
(3) Sarason BR, Sarason IG, Hacker TA, et al. Concomitants of social support: social skills, physical attractiveness, and gender. J Pers Soc Psychol 1985;49:469–480.
(4) Sarason IG, Sarason BR, Shearin EN, et al. A brief measure of social support: practical and theoretical implications. J Soc Personal Relations 1987;4:497–510.

THE RAND SOCIAL HEALTH BATTERY
(Rand Corporation, 1978)

Purpose

The Rand Social Health Battery records social interaction and resources for social support; it does not rate the subjective experience of support. It is intended for use in general population surveys.

Conceptual Basis

Originally, Donald and Ware used the concepts of social well-being and support interchangeably (1, 2), but later, distinctions were drawn between social functioning, role functioning, and social support; a series of measures was developed to tap each of these constructs. The instrument reviewed here forms an overall measure of social functioning, defined as "the ability to develop, maintain, and nurture major social relationships" (3, p173). This may be measured in terms of relatively objective behavioral indicators such as the numbers of social resources a person has and the frequency of contact with friends and relatives (1, 2). Social support is somewhat independent of social functioning, for a person may have good social functioning but derive little support, while conversely a chronically ill person who is unable to function socially may receive strong support from family or relatives (3). Likewise, social functioning in personal relationships was distinguished from role functioning; a separate measure of role functioning was developed (4). Finally, a separate four-item scale focused on restrictions to social functioning produced by illness (3).

Description

This self-administered scale was developed along with the Rand physical and psychological scales as an outcome measurement for the Health Insurance Experiment. The 11 items include predominantly objective indicators covering social resources (e.g., number of friends) and contacts (e.g., the frequency of seeing friends or involvement in group activities). The scale covers home and family, friendships, and social and community life; it specifically excludes work-related performance and items that need not involve interaction, such as attending sports events (2). Nor does the scale cover satisfaction with relationships. The development of the questionnaire is described by Donald and Ware (2), and it is shown in Exhibit 4.3.

Forced choice and open-ended responses are used. A scoring format developed by Donald and Ware is used to recode the printed response options: this is shown in Exhibit 4.4. High scores indicate more favorable social contacts, although the authors give no guidance about critical scores that might differentiate good from poor adjustment. On the basis of factor analyses, the items may be grouped to form two subscales and an overall score (1). The first subscale, social contacts, includes items 3, 4 and 5 from Exhibit 4.3; a group participation scale includes items 10 and 11. An overall score uses all the items except for 7 (writing letters) and 8 (getting along with others), although the authors recommend using scores for individual items and subscales rather than the overall score, pending additional validity studies (1). They also recommend standardizing items to a mean of 0 and a standard deviation of 1 before forming subscores (2). Item 7 (writing letters) was dropped from analyses of scale results because few people answered affirmatively and it did not correlate with the total score. It could be deleted (C. D. Sherbourne, personal communication).

Reliability

The inter-item correlations are low, with only five of 45 correlations exceeding 0.40 (1, Table 8). Internal consistency coefficients for the three subscores were 0.72 for social contacts, 0.84 for group participation, and 0.68 for the overall index (1, Table 11). The corresponding one-year test–retest coefficients were 0.55, 0.68, and 0.68 while coefficients for individual items ranged from 0.23 to 0.80.

Exhibit 4.3 The Rand Social Health Battery

1. About how many families in your neighborhood are you well enough acquainted with, that you visit each other in your homes?
   _____ families

2. About how many *close* friends do you have—people you feel at ease with and can talk with about what is on your mind? (You may include relatives.) (Enter number on line)
   _____ close friends

3. Over a year's time, about how often do you get together with friends or relatives, like going out together or visiting in each other's homes? (Circle one)

Every day	1
Several days a week	2
About once a week	3
2 or 3 times a month	4
About once a month	5
5 to 10 times a year	6
Less than 5 times a year	7

4. During the *past month*, about how often have you had friends over to your home? (Do *not* count relatives.) (Circle one)

Every day	1
Several days a week	2
About once a week	3
2 or 3 times in past month	4
Once in past month	5
Not at all in past month	6

5. About how often have you visited with friends at *their* homes during the *past month?* (Do not count relatives.) (Circle one)

Every day	1
Several days a week	2
About once a week	3
2 or 3 times in past month	4
Once in past month	5
Not at all in past month	6

6. About how often were you on the telephone with close friends or relatives during the *past month?* (Circle one)

Every day	1
Several times a week	2
About once a week	3
2 or 3 times	4
Once	5
Not at all	6

7. About how often did you write a letter to a friend or relative during the *past month?* (Circle one)

Every day	1
Several times a week	2
About once a week	3
2 or 3 times in past month	4
Once in past month	5
Not at all in past month	6

8. In general, how well are you getting along with other people these days—would you say better than usual, about the same, or not as well as usual? (Circle one)

Better than usual	1
About the same	2
Not as well as usual	3

9. How often have you attended a religious service during the *past month?* (Circle one)

Every day	1
More than once a week	2

Exhibit 4.3 *(Continued)*

135

Exhibit 4.3   *(Continued)*

Once a week	3
2 or 3 times in past month	4
Once in past month	5
Not at all in past month	6

10. About how many voluntary groups or organizations do you belong to—like church groups, clubs or lodges, parent groups, etc. ("Voluntary" means because you want to.)
    _____ groups or organizations   (Write in number. If none, enter "0.")

11. How active are you in the affairs of these groups or clubs you belong to? (If you belong to a great many, just count those you feel closest to. If you don't belong to any, circle 4.)   (Circle one)

Very active, attend most meetings	1
Fairly active, attend fairly often	2
Not active, belong but hardly ever go	3
Do not belong to any groups or clubs	4

Validity

Preliminary validation results were drawn from 4,603 interviews in the Health Insurance Experiment. Correlations were calculated between each item and three criterion scores: a nine-item self-rating of health in general, a three-item measure of emotional ties, and a nine-item psychological well-being scale. The correlations were low, with only three of 33 Pearson correlations equal to or above 0.20 (1, Table 4). Correlations for the three aggregated indices were somewhat higher; the overall index correlated 0.32 with the psychological well-being scale and 0.20 with emotional ties (1, Table 13). The overall score was found to predict variations in mental health, as measured by the Rand Mental Health Inventory, explaining 12% of the variance (5). The question on writing letters was found not to correlate with two of the criterion scores and was not used in calculating overall scores or in further analyses of the scale.

For a sample of 256 patients with multiple sclerosis, the social index scores showed

Exhibit 4.4   Scoring Method for the Rand Social Health Battery

Abbreviated item content	Recoding rule
Neighborhood family acquaintances	(0 = 0) (1 = 1) (2 = 2) (3 = 3) (4 = 4) (5 thru 10 = 5) (11 or higher = 6)
Close friends and relatives	(0 = 0) (1 = 1) (2 = 2) (3 = 3) (4 = 4) (5 thru 9 = 5) (10 thru 20 = 6) (21 thru 25 = 7) (26 thru 35 = 8) (36 or higher = 9)
Visits with friends/relatives	(1 thru 3 = 4) (4 = 3) (5,6 = 2) (7 = 1)
Home visits by friends	(1 thru 4 = 3) (5 = 2) (6 = 1)
Visits to homes of friends	(1 thru 3 = 3) (4,5 = 2) (6 = 1)
Telephone contacts	(1 = 5) (2 = 4) (3,4 = 3) (5 = 2) (6 = 1)
Getting along	(1 = 3) (2 = 2) (3 = 1)
Attendance at religious services	(1,2 = 5) (3 = 4) (4 = 3) (5 = 2) (6 = 1)
Voluntary group membership	(0 = 0) (1 = 1) (2 = 2) (3 = 3) (4 = 4) (5 or higher = 5)
Level of group activity	(1 = 4) (2 = 3) (3 = 2) (4 = 1)

moderate deterioration as disease severity increased (Spearman $\rho = -0.31$) (6, p307).

Reference Standards

Table 7 in Donald and Ware's report shows the response patterns for ten items for 4,603 respondents from the Rand study (1).

Commentary

This scale was based on an extensive review of social health measurements and was designed to reflect areas identified as important by current literature (7). It is one of the few scales we review that was not designed for use with patients, and the authors made some interesting observations on the point beyond which an increase in social contacts does not bring additional benefits to a person's well-being.

The preliminary testing of the method had the advantage of a large, representative sample, but the design of the scale complicated the validation process. That is, items were deliberately chosen to represent a concept of social health independent of physical and psychological well-being, so the low intercorrelations obtained in the validation studies may be expected. This is a dilemma of discriminant validity: showing that a scale does not correlate with something it is supposed to differ from does not prove that it would correlate with another scale closer in meaning. The results so far published do not suggest high levels of validity or reliability, and further studies are required to indicate how the instrument compares with alternative social health measurements and how well it agrees with assessments made by independent observers. Given the currently slender evidence for validity and reliability, we recommend that potential users of the scale first check for additional evidence on its quality. Readers may also consider the MOS Social Support Survey that we review next. It was developed by the same team and examines the functional and structural aspects of support.

REFERENCES

(1) Donald CA, Ware JE Jr. The measurement of social support. Res Community Ment Health 1984;4:325–370.
(2) Donald CA, Ware JE Jr. The quantification of social contacts and resources. Santa Monica, California: Rand Corporation, 1982. (R-2937–HHS).
(3) Sherbourne CD. Social functioning: social activity limitations measure. In: Stewart AL, Ware JE Jr, eds. Measuring functioning and well-being: the Medical Outcomes Study approach. Durham, North Carolina: Duke University Press, 1992:173–181.
(4) Sherbourne CD, Stewart AL, Wells KB. Role functioning measures. In: Stewart AL, Ware JE Jr, eds. Measuring functioning and well-being: the Medical Outcomes Study approach. Durham, North Carolina: Duke University Press, 1992:205–219.
(5) Williams AW, Ware JE Jr, Donald CA. A model of mental health, life events, and social supports applicable to general populations. J Health Soc Behav 1981;22:324–336.
(6) Harper AC, Harper DA, Chambers LW, et al. An epidemiological description of physical, social and psychological problems in multiple sclerosis. J Chronic Dis 1986;39:305–310.
(7) Donald CA, Ware JE Jr, Brook RH, et al. Conceptualization and measurement of health for adults in the Health Insurance Study. Vol. IV, Social health. Santa Monica, California: Rand Corporation, 1978.

THE MEDICAL OUTCOMES STUDY SOCIAL SUPPORT SURVEY
(Cathy Sherbourne and Anita Stewart, 1991)

Purpose

The Social Support Survey offers a brief, self-administered indicator of the availability of four categories of social support. It is intended for use in survey research and can be used with general population samples (1).

Conceptual Basis

The Rand and Medical Outcomes Study (MOS) teams have developed several measures of social health, including the social functioning measure described in this chapter, a measure of social role functioning (2), and the present measure of social support. Social functioning refers to the ability to develop and maintain major social relationships; a person may derive social support from these, but the connection is not strong as social relationships may not always be supportive (3). Support includes tangible and emotional support, and empirical evidence shows that these help people in coping with stress or illness, although the mechanisms involved are not fully clear.

Existing measures of social support generally cover the structural (size of social network, how closely the friends know each other) or the functional (perception of support) aspects. Functional support appears the most important and can be of various types: *(i)* providing emotional support, love, and empathy, *(ii)* providing instrumental or tangible support, *(iii)* providing information, guidance, or feedback, *(iv)* providing appraisal support, which helps the person evaluate herself, and *(v)* providing companionship in leisure and recreational activities (1, p705). The focus on perceived support is justified because "the fact that a person does not receive support during a given time period does not mean that the person is unsupported. Received support is confounded with need and may not accurately reflect the amount of support that is available to a person." (1, p706)

Description

An initial pool of 50 items was reduced to 19 functional support items that were hypothesized to cover five dimensions: emotional support, informational support, tangible support, positive social interaction, and affection. To reduce respondent burden, the scale does not ask about who provides the support; each question asks about how often each form of support is available to them. One structural support item asks about the respondent's number of close friends or relatives.

The instrument is self-administered and uses five-point answer scales (Exhibit 4.5).

Empirical analyses indicated that the emotional and informational support items should be scored together, so four subscales are derived: tangible support (items 2, 5, 12, 15), affectionate (items 6, 10, 20), positive social interaction (items 7, 11, 14, 18), and emotional or informational support (items 3, 4, 8, 9, 13, 16, 17, 19). Subscale scores sum the responses checked for the relevant items; these scores are rescaled to a 0-to-100 range for each subscale with high scores indicating more support. A total score is calculated from the mean of the subscale scores, although Sherbourne and Stewart recommend using the subscale scores rather than the total score (1, p712). The structural item is not included in the subscores.

Reliability

Internal consistency for the overall scale was high ($\alpha = 0.97$) and values for the subscales ranged from $\alpha = 0.91$ to 0.96. Item-scale correlations all exceeded 0.72 (1, pp709–710). One-year test–retest reliability was also high at 0.78 (0.72 to 0.76 for each subscale) (1, Table 3).

Validity

Criterion validity was tested using variables included in the Medical Outcomes Study. The Social Support Survey showed significant convergent correlations with loneliness ($r = -0.53$ to -0.69), marital and family functioning (0.38 to 0.57), and mental health (0.36 to 0.45) (1, Table 4). Discriminant correlations ranged from -0.14 to -0.30 with physical symptoms and role limitations and -0.14 to -0.21 with pain severity. Correlations with indicators of social activity were intermediate, in the range 0.24 to 0.33 (1, Table 4).

Factor analyses confirmed that the 19 items could reasonably be fit into an overall index, and also that the four subscales were internally consistent and distinct from each other. Correlations between the four subscales ranged from 0.69 to 0.82 (1, p710). Item 1, the single item measure of structural support, showed low correlations

Exhibit 4.5   The Medical Outcomes Study Social Support Survey

Next are some questions about the support that is available to you.
1. About how many close friends and close relatives do you have (people you feel at ease with and can talk to about what is on your mind)?

Write in number of close friends and close relatives: ☐☐

People sometimes look to others for companionship, assistance, or other types of support. How often is each of the following kinds of support available to you if you need it?

	None of the Time	A Little of the Time	Some of the Time	Most of the Time	All of the Time
2. Someone to help you if you were confined to bed	1	2	3	4	5
3. Someone you can count on to listen to you when you need to talk	1	2	3	4	5
4. Someone to give you good advice about a crisis	1	2	3	4	5
5. Someone to take you to the doctor if you needed it	1	2	3	4	5
6. Someone who shows you love and affection	1	2	3	4	5
7. Someone to have a good time with	1	2	3	4	5
8. Someone to give you information to help you understand a situation	1	2	3	4	5
9. Someone to confide in or talk to about yourself or your problems	1	2	3	4	5
10. Someone who hugs you	1	2	3	4	5
11. Someone to get together with for relaxation	1	2	3	4	5
12. Someone to prepare your meals if you were unable to do it yourself	1	2	3	4	5
13. Someone whose advice you really want	1	2	3	4	5
14. Someone to do things with to help you get your mind off things	1	2	3	4	5
15. Someone to help with daily chores if you were sick	1	2	3	4	5
16. Someone to share your most private worries and fears with	1	2	3	4	5
17. Someone to turn to for suggestions about how to deal with a personal problem	1	2	3	4	5
18. Someone to do something enjoyable with	1	2	3	4	5
19. Someone who understands your problems	1	2	3	4	5
20. Someone to love and make you feel wanted	1	2	3	4	5

Sherbourne CD, Stewart AL. The MOS Social Support Survey. Soc Sci Med 1991;32:713–714. With permission.

with the four subscale scores (range 0.18 to 0.24) (1, p709).

Reference Standards

Sherbourne and Stewart reported mean scores and standard deviations for each item taken from 2,987 participants in the MOS; these represent an ambulatory sick population each of whom had screened positive for one of four medical conditions (1, Table 2).

Commentary

The MOS questionnaire was carefully developed from previous instruments and was based on a sound theoretical formulation.

Sherbourne and Stewart criticized existing support scales as weak in design, narrow in content, and unimpressive in psychometric properties. There is still a need for multidimensional instruments that are psychometrically sound, yet relatively short. The preliminary evidence for reliability and validity is impressive. The criterion validity coefficients are logical, and higher than those for other scales. Although the scale was designed for use in a study of chronically ill patients, items are universally applicable. We do not yet have information on the validity of the scale in a general population sample, but it should be carefully considered for use in surveys and epidemiological studies of chronic disease etiology. This instrument demonstrates that functional social support is distinct from the structural aspects of support, a distinction like that between availability and adequacy of support.

REFERENCES

(1) Sherbourne CD, Stewart AL. The MOS Social Support Survey. Soc Sci Med 1991;32:705–714.
(2) Sherbourne CD, Stewart AL, Wells KB. Role functioning measures. In: Stewart AL, Ware JE Jr, eds. Measuring functioning and well-being: the Medical Outcomes Study approach. Durham, North Carolina: Duke University Press, 1992:205–219.
(3) Sherbourne CD. Social functioning: social activity limitations measure. In: Stewart AL, Ware JE Jr, eds. Measuring functioning and well-being: the Medical Outcomes Study approach. Durham, North Carolina: Duke University Press, 1992:173–181.

THE DUKE–UNC FUNCTIONAL SOCIAL SUPPORT QUESTIONNAIRE (W.E. Broadhead, 1988)

Purpose

The Duke–UNC Functional Social Support Questionnaire (DUFSS) measures a person's satisfaction with the functional and affective aspects of their social support. It was intended for clinical use in family practice settings to identify people at risk of isolation and in research applications to examine the interactions between social support and other determinants of health.

Conceptual Basis

Social support has direct and buffering effects on health, and most research has demonstrated that the quality of social relationships predicts health and well-being better than the number of friends or frequency of contact. Previous work had shown that quantity and quality of support "are minimally intercorrelated and that it may be inappropriate to combine them into summary measures" (1, p710). The Duke Functional Support Questionnaire covers the qualitative, or functional, aspects of support. It was originally designed to cover four content areas: confidant relationship, affective support, quantity of support, and instrumental assistance. Fourteen items were tested but those covering instrumental assistance and quantity of support were found unreliable and were deleted, leaving eight items in the final instrument.

Description

Of the eight items in the DUFSS, numbers 1, 2, and 8 cover affective support (an emotional form of caring) and the remaining five cover confidant support (reflecting a relationship in which important life concerns can be discussed). The five-point answer scales range from "as much as I would like" to "much less than I would like" (see Exhibit 4.6). A summary score is formed by adding item scores, and subscores can also be formed.

Reliability

Two-week test–retest reliability for the items ranged from 0.50 to 0.77. The average item-total correlations were 0.62 for confidant support and 0.64 for affective support (1, pp714–715).

Validity

Discriminant validity correlations for each item were derived from a sample of 401

Exhibit 4.6   The Duke–UNC Functional Social Support Questionnaire

Here is a list of some things that other people do for us or give us that may be helpful or supportive. Please read each statement carefully and place a check (✔) in the blank that is *closest* to your situation.

	As much as I would like			Much less than I would like
Here is an example: I get...				
enough vacation time	.	.　✔　.	.	.

If you put a check where we have, it means that you get *almost* as much vacation time as you would like, but not quite as much as you would like.

Answer each item as best you can. There are *no* right or wrong answers.

	As much as I would like			Much less than I would like
I get...				
1. people who care what happens to me	.	. .	.	.
2. love and affection	.	. .	.	.
3. chances to talk to someone about problems at work or with my housework	.	. .	.	.
4. chances to talk to someone I trust about my personal and family problems	.	. .	.	.
5. chances to talk about money matters	.	. .	.	.
6. invitations to go out and do things with other people	.	. .	.	.
7. useful advice about important things in life	.	. .	.	.
8. help when I'm sick in bed	.	. .	.	.

Adapted from Broadhead WE, Gehlbach SH, de Gruy FV, Kaplan BH. The Duke–UNC Functional Social Support Questionnaire: measurement of social support in family medicine patients. Med Care 1988;26:722–723.

family-practice patients. Divergent correlations between confidant and affective support and physical function ranged from 0.08 to 0.17, correlations with symptom status ranged from 0.18 to 0.30, and correlations with emotional function ranged from 0.34 to 0.41 (1, Table 4). However, correlations with a social function scale derived from the Duke Health Profile were low, 0.15 for the affective scale and 0.17 for the confidant support scale (1, Table 6). Correlations with social functioning measures drawn from the Rand studies were also low, although some showed an appropriate pattern. For example, the correlation of the confidant scale with a measure of social contacts ($r = 0.35$) was higher than that of the affective support score (0.17); the equivalent correlations with a question on socializing with other people were 0.29 and 0.22 (1, Table 6). The overall impression is of very low associations: correlations with group participation for both scales were 0.08, lower than the correlations with physical or mental health measures.

Factor analyses confirmed the presence of two factors, with loadings ranging from 0.52 to 0.72 (1, Table 3).

Construct validity was assessed in a number of ways. Level of support was found to be linked to number of office visits to general practitioners, such that those with low support made more visits (2, Table 3). In particular, those with low confidant support made more longer-than-average office visits (2, Table 4). The association was stronger than that between utilization and structural measures of support (e.g., numbers of friends). The DUFSS scores showed no correlation with demographic variables (race, age, employment) but were correlated with whether or not the respondent lived alone (1, Table 5).

Commentary

This Duke questionnaire is the briefest of the social support measures we review; its practicality in a clinical setting is a strong asset. Its focus on the quality rather than the amount of support reflects the trend of previous research; the items are very similar to those in the MOS Social Support Survey. The preliminary reliability results are adequate: item-total correlations of 0.62 will translate into an alpha of about 0.80–0.85; the retest correlations are appropriate. The divergent validity correlations with symptoms are very similar to those reported for the MOS Social Support Survey.

The convergent validity findings, however, cause concern: associations with other social support indicators were low, even if statistically significant owing to the large sample. Broadhead et al. did not address this issue but presented the correlations as statistically significant and as indicating that "the new scales are measuring constructs similar, but not identical, to the existing scales" (1, p718). Perhaps the criterion measures against which the DUFSS was tested are not ideal, but nonetheless the shared variance between the new and existing scales ranged from only 0.5% to a high of 12%, which seems to underscore the "not identical" more than the "similar." Broadhead et al. noted that two items ("help when sick in bed" and "invitations to go out") were not predicted to load on the factors on which empirical analyses placed them. The extent to which the two factors were distinct was not reported, and future analyses may show less separation between them. Some of the items are grammatically awkward (e.g., "I get people who care what happens to me . . . As much as I would like").

Before this instrument can be recommended for general use, further examination of its agreement with other measures of social support should be undertaken. Readers are referred to other scales developed by this team. A review of the Duke Social Support and Stress Scale follows, and their general health measurement is reviewed in Chapter 9.

REFERENCES

(1) Broadhead WE, Gehlbach SH, de Gruy FV, et al. The Duke–UNC Functional Social Support Questionnaire: measurement of social support in family medicine patients. Med Care 1988;26:709–723.
(2) Broadhead WE, Gehlbach SH, de Gruy FV, et al. Functional versus structural social support, and health care utilization in a family medicine outpatient practice. Med Care 1989;27:221–233.

THE DUKE SOCIAL SUPPORT AND STRESS SCALE
(George R. Parkerson, 1989)

Purpose

The Duke Social Support and Stress Scale (DUSOCS) rates family and non-family relationships in terms of the amount of support they provide and the amount of stress they cause. It is a family practice research instrument to be used in studying the family environment as a determinant of health (1).

Conceptual Basis

The links between stress, social support, and health have been extensively studied, and Parkerson et al. addressed the role that family members play in this process with an emphasis on the person's perceptions of the supportiveness or stressfulness of their relationships (1, p218).

Description

The DUSOCS is self-administered; 12 items covering perceived support and 12 covering stress are rated on three-point scales for six categories of family members and four categories of nonfamily members. In addition, the most supportive and most stressful relationships are identified (Exhibit 4.7).

Four scores are created: family support and stress and non-family support and stress. Total support and stress scores can be created by adding family and non-family scores. Responses are coded as follows: "none" = 0, "some" = 1, "a lot" = 2, "yes" = 2, "no" = 0, and "there is no such person" = 0. Blank responses are considered as 0 unless all items in the entire section (A, B, or C) are left blank, in which case no score can be generated for that section. The family support score is calculated by summing the responses in section A; if the reply to section C identified a family member, 2 is added to the support score. The resulting total is divided by 14 to give a 0-to-1 score. The same approach is used in scoring family stress and for the two nonfamily scores, except that the total nonfamily score is divided by 10 to provide a 0-to-1 score. The total stress and support scores are calculated by summing the raw scores in sections A, B, and C and dividing this by 22. Scores can also be reported on a 0-to-100 scale, from lowest to highest stress or support for the four scales.

Reliability

Two-week test–retest correlations were 0.76 for family support, 0.67 for nonfamily support, 0.68 for nonfamily stress, but only 0.40 for family stress (1, p222). The sample was, however, selected as experiencing low family stress. Test–retest correlations were reported from a sample of 314 ambulatory patients: 0.58 for family stress and 0.27 for nonfamily stress, 0.73 for family support and 0.50 for nonfamily support. Alpha coefficients ranged from 0.53 to 0.70 (2, Table 1).

Validity

Initial validity findings were based on a sample of 249 adults who attended a family medicine center. A Spearman correlation of $\rho = 0.43$ was obtained between the DUSOCS family support score and Olson's Family Strength measure; a correlation of $\rho = 0.45$ was found between the family stress score and an independent measure of intrafamily and marital strains (1, p222). Equivalent figures from a subsequent study were 0.51 and 0.33 (3, p690). The family stress measure correlated −0.32 with symptom status from the Duke–UNC Health Profile (DUHP); the correlation with emotional function was −0.44. Correlations for the family support measures fell in the opposite direction and were somewhat weaker, at 0.20 and 0.37, respectively. The equivalent correlations for the Olson Family Strength measure, however, were higher, at 0.29 and 0.59 (1, Table 3). In a separate study, the Olson instrument again correlated more strongly ($\rho = 0.17$ to 0.53) with scales from the DUKE measure than did the DUSOCS family support measure ($\rho = 0.07$ to 0.33) (4, Table 1). Again, the DUSOCS stress measure showed stronger (but reversed) correlations than the support scores: ρ ranging from 0.07 to 0.43 (4, Table 1).

The comparison between family and nonfamily measures showed inconsistent trends: in some instances the nonfamily scores showed stronger associations with criterion measures, while in others the family measures were more strongly associated (1, Table 4; 4, Table 2). In the study of 314 ambulatory patients, DUSOCS family stress scores were significantly associated with all subscores of the DUKE Health Profile (5, Table 1). Family stress scores

Exhibit 4.7   The Duke Social Support and Stress Scale

I. People Who Give Personal **Support**

(A *supportive* person is one who is helpful, will listen to you or who will back you up when you are in trouble.)

Instructions: Please look at the following list and decide how much each person (or group of persons) is supportive for you at this time in your life. Check your answer.

A. Family Members

	This person is supportive now:			There is No Such Person
	None	Some	A Lot	
1. Your wife, husband, or significant other person				
2. Your children or grandchildren				
3. Your parents or grandparents				
4. Your brothers or sisters				
5. Your other blood relatives				
6. Your relatives by marriage (for example: in-laws, ex-wife, ex-husband)				

B. Non-Family Members

	None	Some	A Lot	There is No Such Person
7. Your neighbors				
8. Your co-workers				
9. Your church members				
10. Your other friends				

C. Special Supportive Person

	Yes	No
11. Do you have one particular person whom you trust and to whom you can go with personal difficulties?		

12. If you answered "yes", which of the above types of person is he or she? (for example: child, parent, neighbor) _____

II. People Who Cause Personal **Stress**

(A person who *stresses* you is one who causes problems for you or makes your life more difficult.)

Instructions: Please look at the following list and decide how much each person (or group of persons) is a stress for you at this time in your life. Check your answer.

A. Family Members

	I feel stressed by this person now:			There is No Such Person
	None	Some	A Lot	
1. Your wife, husband, or significant other person				
2. Your children or grandchildren				
3. Your parents or grandparents				
4. Your brothers or sisters				

144

5. Your other blood relatives .....

6. Your relatives by marriage
(for example: in-laws, ex-
wife, ex-husband) ....

B. Non-Family Members

7. Your neighbors ....

8. Your co-workers ....

9. Your church members ....

10. Your other friends ....

C. Most Stressful Person

                                                       Yes   No

11. Is there one particular person who is causing you the most
personal stress now? ....

12. If you answered "yes", which of the above types of person is
he or she? (for example: child, parent, neighbor) _____

also predicted subsequent health care utilization over an 18-month period (5, Tables 2–5).

Commentary

The developers at Duke consider simplicity and general applicability to be the main advantages of the DUSOCS. Some concerns arise from the results of the preliminary validity testing. The retest reliability coefficients are low, apparently because the constructs change over time. The comparatively low reliability may account for the low validity coefficients: correlations of only 0.07 with the DUHP social function score or of 0.31 with the DUKE social health score (see Chapter 9) are not strong indicators of convergent validity. The correlations for the criterion measures and the Olson scale exceeded those for the DUSOCS, suggesting that the Olson scale may be superior. The stress component of the DUSOCS may be more adequate than the support component.

The DUSOCS is innovative and somewhat provocative in combining support and stress in the same measure, but this potential does not seem to have been fully exploited. Parkerson does not, for example,

discuss the possibility of forming balance scores in which the stress scores are subtracted from the support scores, along the lines used by Bradburn's Affect Balance Scale, to provide an indicator of the net effects of family and acquaintances. The resulting scores might correlate more strongly with health outcomes than either component alone. Correlations between support and stress scores were not reported, so we do not know if these are the obverse of each other, or whether respondents can report feeling both supported and also stressed in their relationships.

Further testing, including comparisons with other social support scales, is required before the DUSOCS can be recommended as a rival to some of the other scales we review. The reader should also consider the other brief social support instrument developed by the same team (see previous review) and their multidimensional measurement included in Chapter 9.

REFERENCES

(1) Parkerson GR Jr, Michener JL, Wu LR, et al. Associations among family support, family stress, and personal functional

health status. J Clin Epidemiol 1989;42: 217–229.

(2) Parkerson GR Jr, Broadhead WE, Tse C-KJ. Quality of life and functional health of primary care patients. J Clin Epidemiol 1992; 45:1303–1313.

(3) Parkerson GR Jr, Michener JL, Wu LR, et al. The effect of a telephone family assessment intervention on the functional health of patients with elevated family stress. Med Care 1989;27:680–693.

(4) Parkerson Gr Jr, Broadhead WE, Tse C-KJ. Validation of the Duke Social Support and Stress Scale. Fam Med 1991;23:357–360.

(5) Parkerson GR Jr, Broadhead WE, Tse C-KJ. Perceived family stress as a predictor of health-related outcomes. Arch Fam Med 1995;4:253–260.

THE KATZ ADJUSTMENT SCALES
(Martin M. Katz, 1963)

Purpose

Katz developed this set of scales to measure the social adjustment of psychiatric patients following treatment; the scales incorporate judgments made by the patient and by a relative. The assessments cover psychiatric symptoms, social behavior, and home and leisure activities. The scales have also been used in population surveys.

Conceptual Basis

Katz and Lyerly viewed the aims of psychiatric treatment in terms of enhancing the patient's adjustment to living in the community. Adjustment was defined as a balance between the individual and his environment; it is a positive concept, implying more than the absence of negative behaviors. It includes freedom from symptoms of psychopathology and absence of personal distress, but also suitable patterns of social interaction and adequate performance in social roles (1). This conceptual approach brings the adjustment scales close to indices of positive mental well-being. In addition to the individual's own feelings of well-being and satisfaction, the assessment of social adjustment must reflect the view of others in his milieu: "the extent to which

persons in the patient's social environment are satisfied with his type and level of functioning" (1, p509). This led to the approach of basing the measurement on judgments made by the individual and by those close to him.

Description

Two sets of scales are used, one completed by the patient (S scales) and the other by a relative (R scales). There are five scales in each set. The scales are introduced by an interviewer but are completed by the patient or relative; the questions use nontechnical language. The patient reports on his or her somatic symptoms, mood, level of activities, and personal satisfaction. A relative who has been in close contact with the patient reports on the patient's behavior and indicates the extent to which other people are satisfied with his functioning. Full administration takes 45 to 60 minutes but the scales need not be administered as a set.

On form R1 (127 items) the relative rates the patient's psychiatric symptoms (e.g., "looks worn out," "laughs or cries for no reason"). Form R1 also covers social behavior (e.g., "dependable" or "gets into fights with people"). Four-point scales indicate the frequency of each symptom and these may be summed into 12 or more scales and an overall score. Form R2 contains 16 items on the individual's performance of socially expected activities: social responsibilities, self-care, community activities. Three-point frequency response scales are used. The items and response scales on form R3 are identical to those on R2, save that the relative now indicates his expectation of the patient's level of performance in these activities. A score indicating the relative's satisfaction with the patient's performance may be derived from the discrepancy between expectations (form R3) and actual performance (form R2) (1). In a similar manner, a pair of 23–item forms (R4 and R5) covers the relative's ratings of the patient's level of free-time activities and the relative's expectations for this. Items cover hobbies and social, community, and self-improvement activities.

The patient also completes five forms. Form S1 contains 55 items derived from the Hopkins Symptom Checklist on somatic symptoms and mood from which a total score may be calculated. The other four forms are equivalent to the relative's rating forms R2 to R5 and include the same items with minor changes in wording. Because the wording of the fourth set of forms is identical, Katz refers to these as RS4.

The forms are too long to reproduce here; a summary of the items is given in Katz and Lyerly's article (1, Tables 1–3). Since the questions in form R2 cover social health, we include a summary of them in Exhibit 4.8.

Reliability

Kuder–Richardson internal consistency coefficients for 11 subscores on form R1 were calculated on two samples of patients. Coefficients ranged from 0.41 to 0.87, with a median coefficient of 0.72 (N = 315) (1, Table 7). Six of the scales did not reach the level of 0.70 normally used as indicative of an acceptable internal consistency. Alpha internal consistency values for 13 scores derived from scale R1 were only moder-

ately high, ranging from 0.61 to 0.87 in a U.S. study; similar figures were reported from Japanese and West African studies (2, Table 3). A recent study reported alpha coefficients for 12 R1 scores ranging from 0.57 to 0.89; seven scales failed to meet the criterion of 0.70 (3, Table 1).

Inter-rater agreement has been reported for the R forms. Agreement between fathers and mothers in rating adult schizophrenics showed median correlations of 0.71 for the R1 rating; figures for role performance and recreation were 0.85 and 0.47, respectively (4, p213). Katz et al. reported an indirect measure of inter-rater agreement, showing that there was no difference between ratings made by different types of rater (father, mother, or spouse) for most ratings; significant differences were found on only four out of 26 comparisons (2, pp340–341).

Vickrey et al. altered the scoring procedure for scale R1 by increasing the number of items that are used in the eventual score. This significantly improved its reliability (3).

Validity

The relative's forms discriminated significantly between patients judged on clinical

---

Exhibit 4.8   The Katz Adjustment Scale Form R2 (Level of Performance of Socially Expected Activities) and Form R3 (Level of Expectations for Performance of Social Activities)

Note: The two forms are used to derive separate measures and in combination, to provide a "level of satisfaction" measure.

1. Helps with household chores	9. Goes to parties and other social activities
2. Visits his friends	10. Gets along with neighbors
3. Visits his relatives	11. Helps with family shopping
4. Entertains friends at home	12. Helps in the care and training of children
5. Dresses and takes care of himself	13. Goes to church
6. Helps with the family budgeting	14. Takes up hobbies
7. Remembers to do important things on time	15. Works
8. Gets along with family members	16. Supports the family

The response scales for form R2 include three categories: "is not doing," "is doing some," and "is doing regularly." For form R3, the response are: "did not expect him to be doing," "expected him to be doing some" and "expected him to be doing regularly."

Reproduced with permission from Katz, M.M., and Lyerly, S.B. Methods for measuring adjustment and social behavior in the community: I. Rationale, description, discriminative validity and scale development. *Psychological Reports*, 1963, 13, 503–535, Table 2.

grounds to be well adjusted and those who were poorly adjusted. Hogarty quotes multiple correlations ranging from 0.70 to 0.83 between the scale scores and global ratings made by a psychologist and social worker (4, p214). The data published by Hogarty and Katz indicate consistent contrasts in responses between psychiatric patients and a general population sample (5). Scores for the 127 items in form R1 were factor analyzed and found to fall on 13 factors (2, Table 2). A profile analysis of variance was used to compare responses to the 13 scales between subtypes of schizophrenia; the contrast was highly significant for a sample in India but not in Nigeria (2, p343). The R1 Adjustment Scale showed significant differences between the Indian and Nigerian samples which broadly corresponded to differences in presenting symptoms observed with the Present State Examination (2, p347).

Correlations with the Sickness Impact Profile were 0.45 for the overall score, 0.57 for the withdrawal subscale, and 0.36 for the psychoticism scale (6, Table 5).

Alternative Forms

The Katz Adjustment Scales have been translated and used in a variety of languages and settings, including most of Europe, Japan, India, Hong Kong, Turkey, and West Africa. References to these studies are given by Katz et al. (2).

The R1 form includes 127 items, of which Katz and Lyerly originally included only 76 in forming 12 subscales. Vickrey et al. evaluated a modified scoring procedure that increased the number of items scored to 126 items, forming 14 subscales. The alpha reliability of these ranged from 0.66 to 0.88, considerably higher than the figures obtained using the original scoring approach (3, Table 2). The revised scale scores discriminated between different grades of epilepsy (3, p68).

Reference Standards

Hogarty and Katz reported reference standards for the 13 factor scores on form R1, derived from a sample of 450 community respondents aged 15 years and over. The standards are presented by age, sex, social class, and marital status (5, Table 1).

Commentary

For some time the Katz Adjustment Scales were taken as the standard approach to measuring social adjustment, and they benefit from a clear theoretical foundation. While the conceptual formulation mentions positive adjustment, it is primarily the negative aspects of adjustment that are scored (7, p616). The scales also permit comparison of actual and expected levels of performance, and of the relative's and the patient's assessments. The use of the relative's forms permits assessment of patients with cognitive problems.

Given the widespread use of the scales, it is surprising how little evidence has been published on their validity. Many studies have used the scales, but virtually none presents data from which conclusions may be drawn concerning reliability and validity of the measurements; many of the results reviewed in one article come from unpublished studies (4). We cannot, therefore, agree with the conclusion of Chen and Bryant, who claimed that "extensive efforts were made to establish the different forms of reliabilities and validities, all of which were found satisfactory" (8). Nonetheless, the Katz scales have had a considerable impact on the design of subsequent methods. For example, the approach of combining ratings by a patient and a relative was followed in subsequent scales, such as that of Clare. Considering the age of the Katz scales and the scant evidence for their reliability and validity, we recommend their use only if none of the other scales we describe applies.

REFERENCES

(1) Katz MM, Lyerly SB. Methods for measuring adjustment and social behavior in the community. I. Rationale, description, discriminative validity and scale development. Psychol Rep 1963;13:503–535.

(2) Katz MM, Marsella A, Dube KC, et al. On the expression of psychosis in different cultures: schizophrenia in an Indian and in a Nigerian community. Cult Med Psychiatry 1988;12:331–355.

(3) Vickrey BG, Hays RD, Brook RH, et al. Reliability and validity of the Katz Adjustment Scales in an epilepsy sample. Qual Life Res 1992;1:63–72.

(4) Hogarty GE. Informant ratings of community adjustment. In: Waskow IE, Parloff MB, eds. Psychotherapy change measures. Rockville, Maryland: National Institute of Mental Health, 1975:202–221. (DHEW Publication No. ADM 74–120).

(5) Hogarty GE, Katz MM. Norms of adjustment and social behavior. Arch Gen Psychiatry 1971;25:470–480.

(6) Temkin NR, Dikmen S, Machamer J, et al. General versus disease-specific measures: further work on the Sickness Impact Profile for head injury. Med Care 1989; 27(suppl):S44–S53.

(7) Linn MW. A critical review of scales used to evaluate social and interpersonal adjustment in the community. Psychopharmacol Bull 1988;24:615–621.

(8) Chen MK, Bryant BE. The measurement of health—a critical and selective overview. Int J Epidemiol 1975;4:257–264.

THE SOCIAL FUNCTIONING SCHEDULE
(Marina Remington and P.J. Tyrer, 1979)

Purpose

The Social Functioning Schedule (SFS) is a semistructured interview designed to assess the problems a person experiences in 12 areas of social functioning. The scale was designed for evaluating treatment of neurotic outpatients.

Conceptual Basis

The SFS uses a role performance approach to assess functioning but does not impose external standards to define adequate performance. Instead, the patient is asked to record difficulties experienced, in effect comparing behavior with his own expectations. The questions are phrased in terms of difficulties; they do not specify what form the difficulties may take (1).

Description

The SFS includes 12 sections: employment, household chores, contribution to household, money, self-care, marital relationship, care of children, patient–child relationships, patient–parent and household relationships, social contacts, hobbies, and spare-time activities. The first two, the fourth, and the last sections are subdivided into problems in managing activities in that area and the feelings of distress that result. Sections that are irrelevant for a particular respondent may be omitted.

The SFS is intended for use by a psychologist or physician in clinical practice settings. It is a rating scale based on "a number of suggested questions designed to encompass the range of difficulty encountered with neurotic out-patients. The examiner is free to adapt and add questions where this is necessary to gain sufficient information" (2, p1). The schedule includes a total of 121 questions, not all of which would be relevant to every respondent. After asking the questions in each section, the interviewer rates the level of problems in that area on a visual analogue scale running from "none" to "severe difficulties." The ratings cover only difficulties reported by the patient; the rater avoids making normative judgments. Ratings refer to the past four weeks with the exception of six months for the employment questions, and the interview takes 10 to 20 minutes. Numerical scores are derived from the analogue scales by measurement, and an overall score is calculated as the average of the relevant subsections; lower scores represent better adjustment.

The SFS is too long to reproduce here; as an illustration, the section on work problems is shown in Exhibit 4.9. Note that the version shown is a slight revision of that originally described by Remington and Tyrer (1). Copies of the complete instrument may be obtained from Dr. Tyrer.

Reliability

Intraclass inter-rater reliability figures ranged from 0.45 to 0.81 for different sec-

Exhibit 4.9 Example of a Section from the Social Functioning Schedule

1. Work problems—behavior

   1a Performance: As far as you know, how has S [the Subject] been coping with work? Does S have any difficulties? (Rate performance at work tasks.)

	0	1	2
Not known *Not applicable*	no problems	reduced output/given easier job	unable to perform his job/others have taken over

   1b Time keeping: Does S usually get to work on time?

	0	1	2
Not known *Not applicable*	usually arrives at a reasonable time	has occasionally missed $1/2$–1 hour, or been more than 1 hour late	has been more than 1 hour late on more than two occasions in last 4 weeks

   1c Overactivity: Does S take on too much? (Is he rushed? Does he miss breaks or work late a lot?)

	0	1	2
Not known *Not applicable*	does a day's work but no more—work does not intrude on personal time	rushes to complete jobs, on a tight schedule and/or occasionally works late or brings work home	work frequently occupies evenings and weekends

   Other problems (specify) _____

   _____

1. Rate work problems—behaviour

none   severe difficulties

   ├———┤

2. Work problems—stress

Does S talk about work? Has S complained about work recently? Has S seemed upset about work or under strain because of work?

   2a Interest and satisfaction: Does S say that he likes his work? Has S complained that he is bored or fed up with work?

	0	1	2
Not known *Not applicable*	S seems reasonably satisfied with work situation	S reports that he is disinterested or somewhat dissatisfied with work	S indicates that he is utterly bored or dissatisfied with work

   2b Distress: Does S seem to take work in his stride, or does work get him down? Does he appear troubled when he gets home from work? Does S complain that he has lost confidence? (Exclude boredom and dissatisfaction; include worry, strain, anxiety and anger).

	0	1	2
Not known *Not applicable*	no noticeable discomfort due to work	some degree of distress occasionally reported or observed	S reports extreme distress or informant observes this most of the time

   2c Work relationships—friction: Has S talked about other people at work? In general how does he get on with them? Has S mentioned any quarrels or friction recently? (Include overt interpersonal difficulty with both clients and colleagues regardless of degree of associated distress).

	0	1	2
Not known *Not applicable*	generally, smooth easy relationships	some friction or quarrelling during each week	friction or quarrelling is a constant feature of work situation

2d Work relationships—exploitation: Has S complained that he is treated unfairly at work? Has he complained that he feels put upon or dominated?

	0	1	2
Not known *Not applicable*	S reports no exploitation	S reports occasional injustices or exploitation	S complains of extreme exploitation

Other problems (specify) _____

_____

1. Rate work problems—stress

none   severe difficulties

|—————————————————————————————————|

tions (average, 0.62) (1, p153). Ratings made by patients were compared with those made by spouses; correlations ranged from 0.45 to 0.80 (1, Table 1).

Validity

Virtually all of the evidence comes from studies of discriminant validity. Discriminant ability was originally tested by comparing ratings of patients with personality disorders, other psychiatric outpatients (mainly psychotic patients on maintenance therapy), and the spouses of patients. The SFS distinguished between the personality-disordered patients and the other groups, but not between normals and other psychiatric cases. In a study of 171 general practice patients referred for psychiatric consultation, the SFS showed significant differences between patients rated with various levels of certainty as psychiatric cases by a psychiatrist (3). The scale was not, however, able to differentiate among clinically defined categories of personality disorder. In another study, the SFS score correlated strongly ($r = 0.69$) with the total score of the Present State Examination (PSE) (3, p7). A correlation of 0.65 was obtained with a five-point indicator of level of alcohol consumption used as the outcome of an alcohol detoxification program for 27 patients (4, Table 1). The SFS showed significant differences between patients with phobia, anxiety, and depression before treatment (5, p60). Finally, Casey

and Tyrer compared SFS scores in randomly drawn rural and urban community samples. Social functioning was significantly worse in urban than rural settings, worse among people defined as psychiatric cases using the PSE, and significantly worse among people with depression than those with anxiety (6, p367). The PSE score correlated 0.75 with the SFS scores (6, Table 4).

Commentary

The Social Functioning Schedule covers problems in social interaction and role performance and the patient's satisfaction with this, in a manner similar to that of Weissman's and Gurland's scales. It does not indicate the level of social support available to the patient, nor does it cover positive levels of functioning: the highest rating in each section is expressed in terms of the absence of identifiable problems. This is comparable to the approach used in several of the scales we review, as is the semi-structured interview format. The scale is being used in current research and preliminary validity and reliability analyses are available.

Potential criticisms of the SFS include the possibility of interviewer bias in translating responses into the visual analogue ratings. This may have caused the relatively low inter-rater reliability results, although the intraclass correlations used here give a coefficient as much as 0.20 lower than a

Pearson correlation computed on the same data. More reliability testing is desirable, particularly as the rating system depends on the judgment of the interviewer. Because the scale is broad in scope, it naturally sacrifices detail in most areas when compared with alternative scales. Nonetheless, where an expert rater is available to make the ratings and where summary ratings of a patient's problems (rather than assets) are required, this scale should be considered for use. Because of its semistructured design, the method may be better suited for formulating rather than testing hypotheses.

Address

P.J. Tyrer, MD, FRCP, FRCPsych, Consultant Psychiatrist, St. Charles Hospital, Exmoor Street, London, England W10 6DZ

REFERENCES

(1) Remington M, Tyrer P. The Social Functioning Schedule—a brief semi-structured interview. Soc Psychiatry 1979;14:151–157.
(2) Tyrer PJ. Social Functioning Schedule—short version. (Manuscript, nd).
(3) Casey PR, Tyrer PJ, Platt S. The relationship between social functioning and psychiatric symptomatology in primary care. Soc Psychiatry 1985;20:5–9.
(4) Griggs SMLB, Tyrer PJ. Personality disorder, social adjustment and treatment outcome in alcoholics. J Stud Alcohol 1981;42:802–805.
(5) Tyrer P, Remington M, Alexander J. The outcome of neurotic disorders after outpatient and day hospital care. Br J Psychiatry 1987;151:57–62.
(6) Casey PR, Tyrer PJ. Personality, functioning and symptomatology. J Psychiatr Res 1986;20:363–374.

THE INTERVIEW SCHEDULE FOR SOCIAL INTERACTION
(Scott Henderson, 1980)

Purpose

The Interview Schedule for Social Interaction (ISSI) is a research instrument that assesses the availability and supportive quality of social relationships. The interview was designed as a survey method to measure social factors associated with the development of neurotic illness; it may also be used to evaluate the outcomes of care for psychiatric patients (1).

Conceptual Basis

Henderson's approach to measuring social relationships was guided by his research goal of identifying how social bonding and support protect against neurotic disorders in the presence of adversity (2). For this, he required a measure of the independent variable: the supportive quality of relationships (3). Following the conceptual work of Robert Weiss, Henderson identified six benefits that are offered by lasting social relationships: a sense of attachment and security, social integration, the opportunity to care for others, the provision of reassurance as to one's personal worth, a sense of reliable alliance, and the availability of help and guidance when needed (1). The first of these themes, attachment, was considered especially important, and refers to "that attribute of relationships which is characterized by affection and which gives the recipient a subjective sense of closeness. It is also pleasant and highly valued, commonly above all else." (4, p725)

Social ties may be evaluated in terms of their objective availability, or in terms of the person's subjective assessment of their adequacy. The ISSI "seeks to establish the availability of most of the six provisions proposed by Weiss by ascertaining the availability of persons in specified roles. Questions about adequacy follow each of the availability items." (1, p34)

Description

The ISSI is a 45-minute interview that records details of a person's network of social attachments, covering both quantity and quality of social support in the last 12 months. The questions cover close, intimate relationships such as those with family, parents, and very close friends and also more diffuse ties, such as those with neighbors, acquaintances, or work associates. Four principal indices are formed: *(i)* the availability of close and emotionally intimate relationships and *(ii)* their adequacy, *(iii)* the availability of more diffuse relationships and friendships that provide social integration and *(iv)* the adequacy of these relationships. The interviewer mentions a particular type of social relationship and asks the respondent if she has such a relationship; the interviewer then asks if the amount of this type of relationship is adequate. Adequacy covers friendship, attachment, nurturance, reassurance of worth, and reliable alliances (5). In addition, the respondent is asked to name the main person who provides each of several different facets of attachment relationships. This information is summarized on an attachment table that records the degree of closeness of the respondent to each of the people she cites as emotionally close to her. Details of the identity of these individuals are recorded, as is an indication of their accessibility to the respondent. The table is also used to indicate the extent to which social provisions are concentrated on few or many people.

The instrument is too long to reproduce here; it is available, along with guide notes, in the appendices of the book by Henderson et al. (1, pp203–230). As an illustration, Exhibit 4.10 shows one question from the ISSI.

Initial analyses indicated that the results obtained from the questionnaire did not fully reflect the complexity of the conceptual formulation, so a simplified scoring system was proposed. Four scores summarize the extent and adequacy of social support:

availability of attachment (AVAT, 8 items)
adequacy of attachment (ADAT, 12 items)
availability of social integration (AVSI, 16 items)
adequacy of social integration (ADSI, 17 items)

Detailed discussions of scoring procedures are available (1, pp37–39; 5). The scores

Exhibit 4.10   Example of an Item from the Interview Schedule for Social Interaction

33. At present, do you have someone you can share your most private feelings with (confide in) or not?	
No one (Go to Q. 33D)	0
Yes	1

A. Who is this mainly? (Fill in only one on Attachment Table)

B. Do you wish you could share more with _____ or is it about right?

About right	1
Depends on the situation	2
More	3
Not applicable	9

C. Would you like to have someone else like this as well, would you prefer not to use a confidant, or is it just about right for you the way it is?

Prefers no confidant	1
About right	2
Depends on the situation	3
Like someone else as well	4
Not applicable	9

(Go to Q. 34)

(If no one)

D. Would you like to have someone like this or would you prefer to keep your feelings to yourself?

Keep things to self	1
Like someone	2
Not applicable	9

Reprinted from *Neurosis and the social environment* by S Henderson with DG Byrne and P Duncan-Jones, Academic Press, Sydney, 1981, 214. With permission.

are complex in that they reflect the idea that scores should not necessarily increase or decrease monotonically: both too much and too little support may constitute less-than-ideal replies. An alternative, simpler scoring system, and the questions that are included in forming the four scores shown here, are given in Appendix III of the book by Henderson et al.

Reliability

The alpha internal consistency of four scores ranged from 0.67 to 0.79 (N = 756), and 18-day test–retest correlations ranged from 0.71 to 0.76 (N = 51) (1, p47). For 221 respondents, stability correlations were calculated using a structural modeling approach that corrects for the imperfect internal consistency of the scores. The stability results at four, eight, and 12 months ranged from 0.66 to 0.88 (1, 4).

Validity

Preliminary comparisons were made between the structure of the scale and the conceptual definition of its content. A detailed presentation is given by Duncan-Jones (6). Henderson et al. concluded that the dimensions of availability and adequacy of "reliable alliance" and "reassurance of worth" could be distinguished but could not be very well separated from friendship. The attempt to measure Weiss's concept of "opportunity for nurturing" was not successful and, finally, the results showed that a more general dimension of "social integration" could be formed by combining acquaintance, friendship, reassurance of worth, and reliable alliance (1, p38).

The ISSI was shown to discriminate significantly between groups that would be expected to differ in social adjustment: recent arrivals in a city compared with residents, and separated or divorced people compared with those who were married (1). Similar analyses compared scores by living arrangements, marital status, and the presence of an extended family; there were clear and logical associations with the ISSI scores (7, pp383–384).

Correlations between the four scores and trait neuroticism measured by the Eysenck Personality Inventory ranged from 0.18 to 0.31 for 225 respondents (1). Henderson described the pattern of associations as "coherent." Correlations between the respondent's scores and an informant's score reflecting his perception of the respondent's social world ranged from 0.26 to 0.59 (N = 114) (4, p731). To estimate the effect of response sets, the scale was correlated with two lie scales, and a maximum of 10.6% of variance in the ISSI scores could be explained by socially desirable response styles (4). Other validity data include a comparison with the Health Locus of Control Scale: $\rho = 0.40$ with the availability of social integration score, showing greater social integration with greater internality (8).

In a study of predictive validity over four months, Henderson showed that 30% of the variance in the General Health Questionnaire (GHQ) was shared by the ISSI in a population experiencing many life changes (9). Concurrent correlations between the GHQ-30 and the four ISSI scores ranged from −0.16 to −0.38 (9, Table 1). A significant association between the GHQ-12 and the ISSI AVAT score was found, in which those with lower support tended to be more disturbed (10, Table 3).

Changes in health may not be reflected in changes in ISSI scores: in a 12-month study of anxious patients, reductions in the level of anxiety were not mirrored by changes in ISSI scores (11).

Alternative Forms

Henderson et al. made minor changes to item wording to suit elderly respondents (7, p381).

Reference Standards

Henderson et al. reported mean scores and standard deviations for population samples in Canberra, Australia, by age and marital status (1, Tables 3.1–3.3; 7, Table 1).

Commentary

The ISSI has already offered stimulating insights into the relationships between support, life change, coping, and morbidity (3). Thus, for example, Henderson was able to show that the quality, rather than the quantity, of support provided the best predictor of resistance to psychological disorder. The ISSI is one of the few scales that measures social support rather than social roles. Like Linn's Social Dysfunction Rating Scale and Brandt and Weinert's Personal Resource Questionnaire (12), the ISSI assesses both availability and adequacy of relationships. Evidence for reliability and validity are quite good and hopefully will continue to accumulate.

Henderson reviews some criticisms of the ISSI and provides an interesting comparison with the measurement approach used by George Brown in London (3). The ISSI covers feelings of attachment more than the actual provision of support, and Henderson notes that the two may not completely correspond. Brown's Social Evaluation and Social Support Schedule, by contrast, collects more detailed information on the nature of support provided by each person (3, p75).

It is noticeable that, as was the case with Weissman's scale, empirical analyses of the structure of the scale do not match the conceptual framework that it was designed to reflect. This seems to be a problem in this field, as with quality of life measurements. In comparison with the validity and reliability results of the other scales that we review, the ISSI is sufficiently successful that we recommend its use in studies of neurotic and other psychiatric patients where a 45-minute interview is practical. Where a shorter rating of social support is required, we recommend McFarlane's or Sarason's scales, reviewed in this chapter, or one of the scales developed by Brandt or Norbeck.

REFERENCES

(1) Henderson S, Byrne DG, Duncan-Jones P. Neurosis and the social environment. Sydney, Australia: Academic Press, 1981.

(2) Henderson S. A development of social psychiatry: the systematic study of social bonds. J Nerv Ment Dis 1980;168:63–69.

(3) Henderson AS, Brown GW. Social support: the hypothesis and the evidence. In: Henderson AS, Burrows GD, eds. Handbook of social psychiatry. Amsterdam: Elsevier, 1988:73–85.

(4) Henderson S, Duncan-Jones P, Byrne DG, et al. Measuring social relationships: the Interview Schedule for Social Interaction. Psychol Med 1980;10:723–734.

(5) Duncan-Jones P. The structure of social relationships: analysis of a survey instrument, part 1. Soc Psychiatry 1981;16:55–61.

(6) Duncan-Jones P. The structure of social relationships: analysis of a survey instrument, part 2. Soc Psychiatry 1981; 16:143–149.

(7) Henderson AS, Grayson DA, Scott R, et al. Social support, dementia and depression among the elderly living in the Hobart community. Psychol Med 1986;16:379–390.

(8) Thomas PD, Hooper EM. Healthy elderly: social bonds and locus of control. Res Nurs Health 1983;6:11–16.

(9) Henderson S. Social relationships, adversity and neurosis: an analysis of prospective observations. Br J Psychiatry 1981; 138:391–398.

(10) Singh B, Lewin T, Raphael B, et al. Minor psychiatric morbidity in a casualty population: identification, attempted intervention and six-month follow-up. Aust NZ J Psychiatry 1987;21:231–240.

(11) Parker G, Barnett B. A test of the social support hypothesis. Br J Psychiatry 1987; 150:72–77.

(12) Brandt PA, Weinert C. The PRQ—a social support measure. Nurs Res 1981;30:277–280.

THE SOCIAL ADJUSTMENT SCALE
(Myrna M. Weissman, 1971)

Purpose

The Social Adjustment Scale (SAS) was designed as an outcome measurement to evaluate drug treatment and psychotherapy for depressed patients. It has since been used in studying a broader range of patients and healthy respondents.

Conceptual Basis

The development of this self-report scale reflected a growing interest in measuring successful adjustment to community living, as distinct from problems in role performance. This approach is particularly relevant to patients receiving psychotherapy who do not, for the most part, present with clinical symptoms (1). The conceptual approach and item content were derived from Gurland's Structured and Scaled Interview to Assess Maladjustment (SSIAM—discussed later in this chapter) and from prior empirical studies by Paykel and Weissman. The scale assesses interpersonal relationships in various roles, covering feelings, satisfaction, friction, and performance. The structure reflects two separate dimensions: six role areas (such as work, family) and five aspects of adjustment that are applied, depending on the appropriateness, to each role area (2).

Description

There are two versions of the SAS—an interview schedule that is available, with a manual and scoring guide, from Dr. Weissman, and the self-report version, the SAS-SR, shown in Exhibit 4.11. The latter was developed from the interview, and its advantages are that it is inexpensive to administer and free from interviewer bias (1). It is generally completed by the respondent but can also be completed by a relative.

Both the interview and self-report versions contain 42 questions covering role performance in six areas of role functioning: work (as employee, housewife, or student) (questions 1–18); social and/or leisure activities (questions 19–29); relationships with extended family (questions 30–37); and roles as spouse (questions 38–46), parent (questions 47–50), and member of the family unit (questions 51–54). The method provides alternative questions on

work relations for students, housewives, and the employed, so the scale includes a total of 54 questions of which respondents answer 42. In each role area, questions cover the patient's performance over the past two weeks, the amount of friction he experiences with others, finer aspects of interpersonal relationships (e.g., level of independence), inner feelings (e.g., shyness, boredom), and satisfaction. Five- and six-point response scales are used; higher scores represent increasing impairment. Two scoring methods are used: a mean score for each section (e.g., work, leisure), or an overall score obtained by summing the item scores and dividing by the number of items checked.

The self-report version takes 15 to 20 minutes to complete, while the interview version takes about 45 to 60 minutes and includes an additional six global judgments (1). The SAS-SR is usually completed in the presence of a research assistant, who can explain the format, answer questions, and check on the completeness of replies.

Reliability

For 15 depressed patients the correlation between the patient's replies on the self-report instrument and a rating made by the spouse or other informant was 0.74; the correlation between patient and interviewer assessments was 0.70 (1, Table 5). Patients rated themselves as more impaired than the interviewer rated them. Scores on the self-report and interview versions of the SAS correlated 0.72 for 76 depressed patients; agreement for the various sections ranged from 0.40 to 0.76 (1, Table 3). Item-total correlations for the various role areas ranged between 0.09 and 0.83 for the interviewer-administered SAS (2, Table 2). An alpha internal consistency coefficient of 0.74 and a mean test–retest coefficient of 0.80 were reported (3, p324). Agreement between raters was assessed for the interview version for 31 patients. The raters agreed completely on 68% of all items, with a further 27% of ratings falling within

Exhibit 4.11   The Social Adjustment Scale—Self-Report

Social Adjustment Self-Report Questionnaire

We are interested in finding out how you have been doing in the last *two weeks*. We would like you to answer some questions about your work, spare time and your family life. There are no right or wrong answers to these questions. Check the answers that best describe how you have been in the last *two weeks*.

WORK OUTSIDE THE HOME

Please check the situation that best describes you.

I am 1 ☐ a worker for pay   4 ☐ retired
2 ☐ a housewife   5 ☐ unemployed
3 ☐ a student

Do you usually work for pay more than 15 hours per week?

1 ☐ YES   2 ☐ NO

Did you work any hours for pay in the last two weeks?

1 ☐ YES   2 ☐ NO

Check the answer that best describes how you have been in the last two weeks.

1. How many days did you miss from work in the last two weeks?
   1 ☐ No days missed.
   2 ☐ One day.
   3 ☐ I missed about half the time.
   4 ☐ Missed more than half the time but did make at least one day.
   5 ☐ I did not work any days.
   8 ☐ On vacation all of the last two weeks.

If you have not worked any days in the last two weeks, go on to Question 7.

2. Have you been able to do your work in the last 2 weeks?
   1 ☐ I did my work very well.
   2 ☐ I did my work well but had some minor problems.
   3 ☐ I needed help with work and did not do well about half the time.
   4 ☐ I did my work poorly most of the time.
   5 ☐ I did my work poorly all the time.

3. Have you been ashamed of how you do your work in the last 2 weeks?
   1 ☐ I never felt ashamed.
   2 ☐ Once or twice I felt a little ashamed.
   3 ☐ About half the time I felt ashamed.
   4 ☐ I felt ashamed most of the time.
   5 ☐ I felt ashamed all the time.

4. Have you had any arguments with people at work in the last 2 weeks?
   1 ☐ I had no arguments and got along very well.
   2 ☐ I usually got along well but had minor arguments.
   3 ☐ I had more than one argument.
   4 ☐ I had many arguments.
   5 ☐ I was constantly in arguments.

5. Have you felt upset, worried, or uncomfortable while doing your work during the last 2 weeks?
   1 ☐ I never felt upset.
   2 ☐ Once or twice I felt upset.
   3 ☐ Half the time I felt upset.
   4 ☐ I felt upset most of the time.
   5 ☐ I felt upset all of the time.

6. Have you found your work interesting these last two weeks?
   1 ☐ My work was almost always interesting.
   2 ☐ Once or twice my work was not interesting.
   3 ☐ Half the time my work was uninteresting.
   4 ☐ Most of the time my work was uninteresting.
   5 ☐ My work was always uninteresting.

WORK AT HOME—HOUSEWIVES ANSWER QUESTIONS 7–12. OTHERWISE, GO ON TO QUESTION 13.

7. How many days did you do some housework during the last 2 weeks?
   1 ☐ Every day.
   2 ☐ I did the housework almost every day.
   3 ☐ I did the housework about half the time.
   4 ☐ I usually did not do the housework.
   5 ☐ I was completely unable to do housework.
   8 ☐ I was away from home all of the last two weeks.

8. During the last two weeks, have you kept up with your housework? This includes cooking, cleaning, laundry, grocery shopping, and errands.
   1 ☐ I did my work very well.

Exhibit 4.11   *(Continued)*

Exhibit 4.11   *(Continued)*

2 ☐ I did my work well but had some minor problems.

3 ☐ I needed help with my work and did not do it well about half the time.

4 ☐ I did my work poorly most of the time.

5 ☐ I did my work poorly all of the time.

9. Have you been ashamed of how you did your housework during the last 2 weeks?

1 ☐ I never felt ashamed.

2 ☐ Once or twice I felt a little ashamed.

3 ☐ About half the time I felt ashamed.

4 ☐ I felt ashamed most of the time.

5 ☐ I felt ashamed all the time.

10. Have you had any arguments with salespeople, tradesmen or neighbors in the last 2 weeks?

1 ☐ I had no arguments and got along very well.

2 ☐ I usually got along well, but had minor arguments.

3 ☐ I had more than one argument.

4 ☐ I had many arguments.

5 ☐ I was constantly in arguments.

11. Have you felt upset while doing your housework during the last 2 weeks?

1 ☐ I never felt upset.

2 ☐ Once or twice I felt upset.

3 ☐ Half the time I felt upset.

4 ☐ I felt upset most of the time.

5 ☐ I felt upset all of the time.

12. Have you found your housework interesting these last 2 weeks?

1 ☐ My work was almost always interesting.

2 ☐ Once or twice my work was not interesting.

3 ☐ Half the time my work was uninteresting.

4 ☐ Most of the time my work was uninteresting.

5 ☐ My work was always uninteresting.

FOR STUDENTS

Answer Questions 13–18 if you go to school half time or more. Otherwise, go on to Question 19.

What best describes your school program? (Choose one)

1 ☐ Full Time

2 ☐ 3/4 Time

3 ☐ Half Time

Check the answer that best describes how you have been the last 2 weeks.

13. How many days of classes did you miss in the last 2 weeks?

1 ☐ No days missed.

2 ☐ A few days missed.

3 ☐ I missed about half the time.

4 ☐ Missed more than half time but did make at least one day.

5 ☐ I did not go to classes at all.

8 ☐ I was on vacation all of the last two weeks.

14. Have you been able to keep up with your class work in the last 2 weeks?

1 ☐ I did my work very well.

2 ☐ I did my work well but had minor problems.

3 ☐ I needed help with my work and did not do well about half the time.

4 ☐ I did my work poorly most of the time.

5 ☐ I did my work poorly all the time.

15. During the last 2 weeks, have you been ashamed of how you do your school work?

1 ☐ I never felt ashamed.

2 ☐ Once or twice I felt ashamed.

3 ☐ About half the time I felt ashamed.

4 ☐ I felt ashamed most of the time.

5 ☐ I felt ashamed all of the time.

16. Have you had any arguments with people at school in the last 2 weeks?

1 ☐ I had no arguments and got along very well.

2 ☐ I usually got along well but had minor arguments.

3 ☐ I had more than one argument.

4 ☐ I had many arguments.

5 ☐ I was constantly in arguments.

8 ☐ Not applicable; I did not attend school.

17. Have you felt upset at school during the last 2 weeks?

1 ☐ I never felt upset.

2 ☐ Once or twice I felt upset.

3 ☐ Half the time I felt upset.

4 ☐ I felt upset most of the time.

5 ☐ I felt upset all of the time.

8 ☐ Not applicable; I did not attend school.

18. Have you found your school work interesting these last 2 weeks?

    1 ☐ My work was almost always interesting.

    2 ☐ Once or twice my work was not interesting.

    3 ☐ Half the time my work was uninteresting.

    4 ☐ Most of the time my work was uninteresting.

    5 ☐ My work was always uninteresting.

SPARE TIME—EVERYONE ANSWER QUESTIONS 19–27.

Check the answer that best describes how you have been in the last 2 weeks.

19. How many friends have you seen or spoken to on the telephone in the last weeks?

    1 ☐ Nine or more friends.

    2 ☐ Five to eight friends.

    3 ☐ Two to four friends.

    4 ☐ One friend.

    5 ☐ No friends.

20. Have you been able to talk about your feelings and problems with at least one friend during the last 2 weeks?

    1 ☐ I can always talk about my innermost feelings.

    2 ☐ I usually can talk about my feelings.

    3 ☐ About half the time I felt able to talk about my feelings.

    4 ☐ I usually was not able to talk about my feelings.

    5 ☐ I was never able to talk about my feelings.

    8 ☐ Not applicable; I have no friends.

21. How many times in the last two weeks have you gone out socially with other people? For example, visited friends, gone to movies, bowling, church, restaurants, invited friends to your home?

    1 ☐ More than 3 times.

    2 ☐ Three times.

    3 ☐ Twice.

    4 ☐ Once.

    5 ☐ None.

22. How much time have you spent on hobbies or spare time interests during the last 2 weeks? For example, bowling, sewing, gardening, sports, reading?

    1 ☐ I spent most of my spare time on hobbies almost every day.

    2 ☐ I spent some spare time on hobbies some of the days.

    3 ☐ I spent a little spare time on hobbies.

    4 ☐ I usually did not spend any time on hobbies but did watch TV.

    5 ☐ I did not spend any spare time on hobbies or watch TV.

23. Have you had open arguments with your friends in the last 2 weeks?

    1 ☐ I had no arguments and got along very well.

    2 ☐ I usually got along well but had minor arguments.

    3 ☐ I had more than one argument.

    4 ☐ I had many arguments.

    5 ☐ I was constantly in arguments.

    8 ☐ Not applicable; I have no friends.

24. If your feelings were hurt or offended by a friend during the last two weeks, how badly did you take it?

    1 ☐ It did not affect me or it did not happen.

    2 ☐ I got over it in a few hours.

    3 ☐ I got over it in a few days.

    4 ☐ I got over it in a week.

    5 ☐ It will take me months to recover.

    8 ☐ Not applicable; I have no friends.

25. Have you felt shy or uncomfortable with people in the last 2 weeks?

    1 ☐ I always felt comfortable.

    2 ☐ Sometimes I felt uncomfortable but could relax after a while.

    3 ☐ About half the time I felt uncomfortable.

    4 ☐ I usually felt uncomfortable.

    5 ☐ I always felt uncomfortable.

    8 ☐ Not applicable; I was never with people.

26. Have you felt lonely and wished for more friends during the last 2 weeks?

    1 ☐ I have not felt lonely.

    2 ☐ I have felt lonely a few times.

    3 ☐ About half the time I felt lonely.

    4 ☐ I usually felt lonely.

    5 ☐ I always felt lonely and wished for more friends.

27. Have you felt bored in your spare time during the last 2 weeks?

    1 ☐ I never felt bored.

    2 ☐ I usually did not feel bored.

    3 ☐ About half the time I felt bored.

Exhibit 4.11 *(Continued)*

Exhibit 4.11 *(Continued)*

4 ☐ Most of the time I felt bored.

5 ☐ I was constantly bored.

Are you a Single, Separated, or Divorced Person not living with a person of opposite sex; please answer below:

1 ☐ YES, Answer questions 28 & 29.

2 ☐ NO, go to question 30.

28. How many times have you been with a date these last 2 weeks?

1 ☐ More than 3 times.

2 ☐ Three times.

3 ☐ Twice.

4 ☐ Once.

5 ☐ Never.

29. Have you been interested in dating during the last 2 weeks? If you have not dated, would you have liked to?

1 ☐ I was always interested in dating.

2 ☐ Most of the time I was interested.

3 ☐ About half of the time I was interested.

4 ☐ Most of the time I was not interested.

5 ☐ I was completely uninterested.

FAMILY

Answer Questions 30–37 about your parents, brothers, sisters, in laws, and children not living at home. Have you been in contact with any of them in the last two weeks?

1 ☐ YES, Answer questions 30–37.

2 ☐ NO, Go to question 36.

30. Have you had open arguments with your relatives in the last 2 weeks?

1 ☐ We always got along very well.

2 ☐ We usually got along very well but had some minor arguments.

3 ☐ I had more than one argument with at least one relative.

4 ☐ I had many arguments.

5 ☐ I was constantly in arguments.

31. Have you been able to talk about your feelings and problems with at least one of your relatives in the last 2 weeks?

1 ☐ I can always talk about my feelings with at least one relative.

2 ☐ I usually can talk about my feelings.

3 ☐ About half the time I felt able to talk about my feelings.

4 ☐ I usually was not able to talk about my feelings.

5 ☐ I was never able to talk about my feelings.

32. Have you avoided contacts with your relatives these last two weeks?

1 ☐ I have contacted relatives regularly.

2 ☐ I have contacted a relative at least once.

3 ☐ I have waited for my relatives to contact me.

4 ☐ I avoided my relatives, but they contacted me.

5 ☐ I have no contacts with any relatives.

33. Did you depend on your relatives for help, advice, money or friendship during the last 2 weeks?

1 ☐ I never need to depend on them.

2 ☐ I usually did not need to depend on them.

3 ☐ About half the time I needed to depend on them.

4 ☐ Most of the time I depend on them.

5 ☐ I depend completely on them.

34. Have you wanted to do the opposite of what your relatives wanted in order to make them angry during the last 2 weeks?

1 ☐ I never wanted to oppose them.

2 ☐ Once or twice I wanted to oppose them.

3 ☐ About half the time I wanted to oppose them.

4 ☐ Most of the time I wanted to oppose them.

5 ☐ I always opposed them.

35. Have you been worried about things happening to your relatives without good reason in the last 2 weeks?

1 ☐ I have not worried without reason.

2 ☐ Once or twice I worried.

3 ☐ About half the time I worried.

4 ☐ Most of the time I worried.

5 ☐ I have worried the entire time.

8 ☐ Not applicable; my relatives are no longer living.

EVERYONE answer Questions 36 and 37, even if your relatives are not living.

36. During the last two weeks, have you been thinking that you have let any of your relatives down or have been unfair to them at any time?

1 ☐ I did not feel that I let them down at all.

2 ☐ I usually did not feel that I let them down.

160

3 ☐ About half the time I felt that I let them down.

4 ☐ Most of the time I have felt that I let them down.

5 ☐ I always felt that I let them down.

37. During the last two weeks, have you been thinking that any of your relatives have let you down or have been unfair to you at any time?

1 ☐ I never felt that they let me down.

2 ☐ I felt that they usually did not let me down.

3. ☐ About half the time I felt they let me down.

4 ☐ I usually have felt that they let me down.

5 ☐ I am very bitter that they let me down.

Are you living with your spouse or have been living with a person of the opposite sex in a permanent relationship?

1 ☐ YES, Please answer questions 38–46.

2 ☐ NO, Go to question 47.

38. Have you had open arguments with your partner in the last 2 weeks?

1 ☐ We had no arguments and we got along well.

2 ☐ We usually got along well but had minor arguments.

3 ☐ We had more than one argument.

4 ☐ We had many arguments.

5 ☐ We were constantly in arguments.

39. Have you been able to talk about your feelings and problems with your partner during the last 2 weeks?

1 ☐ I could always talk freely about my feelings.

2 ☐ I usually could talk about my feelings.

3 ☐ About half the time I felt able to talk about my feelings.

4 ☐ I usually was not able to talk about my feelings.

5 ☐ I was never able to talk about my feelings.

40. Have you been demanding to have your own way at home during the last 2 weeks?

1 ☐ I have not insisted on always having my own way.

2 ☐ I usually have not insisted on having my own way.

3 ☐ About half the time I insisted on having my own way.

4 ☐ I usually insisted on having my own way.

5 ☐ I always insisted on having my own way.

41. Have you been bossed around by your partner these last 2 weeks?

1 ☐ Almost never.

2 ☐ Once in a while.

3 ☐ About half the time.

4 ☐ Most of the time.

5 ☐ Always.

42. How much have you felt dependent on your partner these last 2 weeks?

1 ☐ I was independent.

2 ☐ I was usually independent.

3 ☐ I was somewhat dependent.

4 ☐ I was usually dependent.

5 ☐ I depended on my partner for everything.

43. How have you felt about your partner during the last 2 weeks?

1 ☐ I always felt affection.

2 ☐ I usually felt affection.

3 ☐ About half the time I felt dislike and half the time affection.

4 ☐ I usually felt dislike.

5 ☐ I always felt dislike.

44. How many times have you and your partner had intercourse?

1 ☐ More than twice a week.

2 ☐ Once or twice a week.

3 ☐ Once every two weeks.

4 ☐ Less than once every two weeks but at least once in the last month.

5 ☐ Not at all in a month or longer.

45. Have you had any problems during intercourse, such as pain these last two weeks?

1 ☐ None.

2 ☐ Once or twice.

3 ☐ About half the time.

4 ☐ Most of the time.

5 ☐ Always.

8 ☐ Not applicable; no intercourse in the last two weeks.

46. How have you felt about intercourse during the last 2 weeks?

1 ☐ I always enjoyed it.

2 ☐ I usually enjoyed it.

3 ☐ About half the time I did and half the time I did not enjoy it.

4 ☐ I usually did not enjoy it.

5 ☐ I never enjoyed it.

Exhibit 4.11 *(Continued)*

161

Exhibit 4.11 *(Continued)*

CHILDREN

Have you had unmarried children, stepchildren, or foster children living at home during the last two weeks?

1 ☐ YES, Answer questions 47–50.

2 ☐ NO, Go to question 51.

47. Have you been interested in what your children are doing—school, play or hobbies during the last 2 weeks?

   1 ☐ I was always interested and actively involved.

   2 ☐ I usually was interested and involved.

   3 ☐ About half the time interested and half the time not interested.

   4 ☐ I usually was disinterested.

   5 ☐ I was always disinterested.

48. Have you been able to talk and listen to your children during the last 2 weeks? Include only children over the age of 2.

   1 ☐ I always was able to communicate with them.

   2 ☐ I usually was able to communicate with them.

   3 ☐ About half the time I could communicate.

   4 ☐ I usually was not able to communicate.

   5 ☐ I was completely unable to communicate.

   8 ☐ Not applicable; no children over the age of 2.

49. How have you been getting along with the children during the last 2 weeks?

   1 ☐ I had no arguments and got along very well.

   2 ☐ I usually got along well but had minor arguments.

   3 ☐ I had more than one argument.

   4 ☐ I had many arguments.

   5 ☐ I was constantly in arguments.

50. How have you felt toward your children these last 2 weeks?

   1 ☐ I always felt affection.

   2 ☐ I mostly felt affection.

   3 ☐ About half the time I felt affection.

   4 ☐ Most of the time I did not feel affection.

   5 ☐ I never felt affection toward them.

FAMILY UNIT

Have you ever been married, ever lived with a person of the opposite sex, or ever had children? Please check

1 ☐ YES, Please answer questions 51–53.

2 ☐ NO, Go to question 54.

51. Have your worried about your partner or any of your children without any reason during the last 2 weeks, even if you are not living together now?

   1 ☐ I never worried.

   2 ☐ Once or twice I worried.

   3 ☐ About half the time I worried.

   4 ☐ Most of the time I worried.

   5 ☐ I always worried.

   8 ☐ Not applicable; partner and children not living.

52. During the last 2 weeks have you been thinking that you have let down your partner or any of your children at any time?

   1 ☐ I did not feel I let them down at all.

   2 ☐ I usually did not feel that I let them down.

   3 ☐ About half the time I felt I let them down.

   4 ☐ Most of the time I have felt that I let them down.

   5 ☐ I let them down completely.

53. During the last 2 weeks, have you been thinking that your partner or any of your children have let you down at any time?

   1 ☐ I never felt that they let me down.

   2 ☐ I felt they usually did not let me down.

   3 ☐ About half the time I felt they let me down.

   4 ☐ I usually felt they let me down.

   5 ☐ I feel bitter that they have let me down.

FINANCIAL—*EVERYONE PLEASE ANSWER QUESTION 54.*

54. Have you had enough money to take care of your own and your family's financial needs during the last 2 weeks?

   1 ☐ I had enough money for needs.

   2 ☐ I usually had enough money with minor problems.

   3 ☐ About half the time I did not have enough money but did not have to borrow money.

   4 ☐ I usually did not have enough money and had to borrow from others.

   5 ☐ I had great financial difficulty.

Reproduced from Social Adjustment Scale obtained from Dr. Myrna M Weissman. With permission.

one point of each other (4). Pearson correlations between the raters across all items averaged 0.83 (4, Table 3).

Validity

The SAS scores did not correlate significantly with age, social class, sex, or history of previous depression (N = 76), suggesting that scores are unaffected by sociodemographic status (1). A factor analysis applied to the interview version produced six factors: work performance, interpersonal friction, inhibited communication, submissive dependency, family attachment, and anxiety (2). These factors cut across the two-dimensional conceptual framework on which the method was constructed.

For 76 depressed patients, the self-report method was administered before and after four weeks of treatment. Significant improvements were recorded in all of the six areas covered in the questionnaire (1). Applied to samples of community residents, depressives, alcoholics, and schizophrenics, the SAS demonstrated consistent, although not strong, contrasts in responses (3). In an earlier study, significant differences had been shown between depressed patients and nonpatients for 40 out of the 48 items (5).

Weissman et al. presented correlations with independent ratings for various subsamples. Table 4.2 shows the resulting correlations with four independent assessments: the Hamilton Rating Scale for Depression and the Raskin Depression Scale, both applied by a clinician, and two self-administered scales: the Center for Epi-

demiologic Studies Depression Scale and the Symptom Checklist-90. A correlation of 0.42 was obtained with the Brief Psychiatric Rating Scale and one of 0.53 was found with a clinical rating of irritability (6, Table 2). Further details of the validation results are given in a review by Weissman et al. (4).

Reference Standards

Weissman et al. reported mean scores from a sample of 482 community respondents and 191 depressives (3). Richman reported scores by employment and marital status (7, Tables 2, 3).

Alternative Forms

An enlarged version (SAS-II), a semi-structured interview containing 56 items in eight role areas, has been developed for schizophrenic patients. The scale takes about one hour to complete and information may be obtained either from the patient or from a significant other. Agreement between self-report and ratings by significant others was studied for 56 schizophrenics, giving intraclass correlations from 0.27 to 0.81 (8, Table 2). The multiple correlation of the SAS-II with the section scores from the Brief Psychiatric Rating Scale was 0.58 for 98 schizophrenic patients (9, Table 1). Data on the inter-rater reliability of this version are given by Glazer et al. (8).

A British version of the SAS-SR modified item wording and standardized the rating scale for each question (10). Agreement between self-administered and interviewer versions was close: Pearson correlations of 0.63 for women who screened negative on

---

Table 4.2 Correlation of the SAS and Independent Rating Scales

Sample	Correlation with				
	Hamilton	Raskin	CES-D	SCL-90	(N)
Community sample	. . .	0.44	0.57	0.59	(482)
Acute depressives	0.36	0.18	0.49	0.66	(191)
Alcoholics	0.67	0.65	0.74	0.76	(54)
Schizophrenics	0.72	0.75	0.85	0.84	(47)

Adapted from Weissman MM, Prusoff BA, Thompson WD, Harding PS, Myers JK. Social adjustment by self-report in a community sample and in psychiatric outpatients. J Nerv Ment Dis 1978;166:324, Table 5.

the General Health Questionnaire (GHQ) and 0.80 for women who screened positive. Interestingly, the women's husbands appeared to be less familiar with their spouse's social adjustment: the equivalent correlations were lower, at 0.45 and 0.70, respectively (10, Table I). Correlations with the Present State Examination scores ranged from 0.33 to 0.64 among cases and from 0.17 to 0.53 among the non-cases; correlations with the Profile of Mood States ranged from 0.35 to 0.74 for both groups (10, p72).

Commentary

The Social Adjustment Scale was based on a clearly defined conceptual approach to the topic and drew items from another well-established scale, the SSIAM. Its emphasis on successful adjustment places it in contrast with the maladjustment measures of Linn, Gurland, and Remington. The SAS has been extensively used in psychiatric research, and Weissman provided a lengthy discussion of the dimensions of social health and of the components that may be modifiable through therapy for depression. The scale is one of the few designed to measure the outcomes of psychotherapy, which may seek less to alleviate clinical symptoms than to improve interpersonal skills and relationships. Information on administering, scoring, and interpreting the SAS is available from Dr. Weissman along with a bibliography of studies that have used the instrument.

Weissman has reviewed some of the limitations of the scale, including the difficulty of scoring patients who are too sick to undertake some of the roles (such as work). As originally proposed, sections that are not applicable to an individual are omitted, but this means that a patient who subsequently assumes a role (such as starting to work, perhaps at a low level) may receive a low score, thereby appearing to have deteriorated (4). A more adequate scoring approach is required for such instances. Factor analyses suggested a grouping that cut across the two-dimensional conceptual schema on which the instrument was constructed. It is therefore not clear that providing scores for each role area as Weissman did subsequently (1, 4) is the optimal way to score the SAS; further examination of this issue would seem to be indicated if the SAS is to reach its potential as an outcome measurement.

Address

Myrna M. Weissman, PhD, College of Physicians and Surgeons of Columbia University, 722 West 168th Street, Box 14, New York, New York, USA 10032

REFERENCES

(1) Weissman MM, Bothwell S. Assessment of social adjustment by patient self-report. Arch Gen Psychiatry 1976;33:1111–1115.

(2) Paykel ES, Weissman M, Prusoff BA, et al. Dimensions of social adjustment in depressed women. J Nerv Ment Dis 1971;152:158–172.

(3) Weissman MM, Prusoff BA, Thompson WD, et al. Social adjustment by self-report in a community sample and in psychiatric outpatients. J Nerv Ment Dis 1978; 166:317–326.

(4) Weissman MM, Paykel ES, Prusoff BA. Social Adjustment Scale handbook: rationale, reliability, validity, scoring, and training guide. (Manuscript, nd).

(5) Weissman MM, Paykel ES, Siegel R, et al. The social role performance of depressed women: comparisons with a normal group. Am J Orthopsychiatry 1971;41:390–405.

(6) Weissman MM, Klerman GL, Paykel ES. Clinical evaluation of hostility in depression. Am J Psychiatry 1971;128:261–266.

(7) Richman J. Sex differences in social adjustment: effects of sex role socialization and role stress. J Nerv Ment Dis 1984; 172:539–545.

(8) Glazer WM, Aaronson HS, Prusoff BA, et al. Assessment of social adjustment in chronic ambulatory schizophrenics. J Nerv Ment Dis 1980;168:493–497.

(9) Glazer W, Prusoff B, John K, et al. Depression and social adjustment among chronic schizophrenic outpatients. J Nerv Ment Dis 1981;169:712–717

(10) Cooper P, Osborn M, Gath D, et al. Evaluation of a modified self-report measure of social adjustment. Br J Psychiatry 1982;141:68–75.

THE SOCIAL MALADJUSTMENT SCHEDULE
(Anthony W. Clare, 1978)

Purpose

This rating form was designed to measure social maladjustment among adults with chronic neurotic disorders. Intended originally for use in psychiatric research, it has also been used in studies in family practice and with general population samples.

Conceptual Basis

Clare and Cairns argued that scales measuring social adjustment in terms of conformity to social roles and norms will not permit comparisons across social groups in which norms and social expectations differ. They designed their scale to combine an interviewer's objective assessment of the patient's material circumstances and performance with the patient's own ratings of satisfaction. The topics covered in the scale were derived from a review of previous measurements.

Description

The Social Maladjustment Schedule is a 26-page interview that covers six domains: housing, occupation and social role, economic situation, leisure and social activities, family relationships, and marriage. Questions in each domain cover three themes that were described by Clare and Cairns as follows:

... the social schedule examines each individual's life from 3 main standpoints: first, it attempts to assess what the individual *has*, in terms of his living conditions, money, social opportunities in a number of areas; secondly, it measures what he *does* with his life, what use he makes of his opportunities, how well he copes; finally, it measures what he *feels* about it, that is to say how satisfied he is with various aspects of his social situation. (1, p592)

A trained interviewer administers the semistructured interview in the respondent's home; the interviewer may also incorporate information collected from the spouse. The interview requires about 45 minutes; the schedule and a training manual are available, at cost, from Dr. Clare. The content of the schedule is summarized in Exhibit 4.12.

From the individual's responses the interviewer makes a total of 42 ratings on four-point scales that describe the extent of maladjustment in each of the three areas. Ten ratings cover material conditions, 14 refer to management of social opportunities and activities, and 18 cover satisfaction (2). The ratings concentrate on levels of maladjustment; no gradation is made of satisfactory functioning. An overall score may also be used, with higher scores indicating poorer adjustment.

Reliability

Inter-rater reliability was assessed using analyses of variance; agreement was close with the exception of three of the 25 items tested, for which significant differences were obtained (1, Table 3). Weighted kappas ranged from 0.55 to 0.94 with most coefficients falling above 0.70 (1, Table 4).

Validity

Factor analyses were applied to various samples, but the results did not clearly replicate the dimensions around which the schedule was constructed, and from this Clare and Cairns inferred the need to calculate an overall score. This overall maladjustment score was associated (at $p < 0.05$) with a rating made using Goldberg's standardized psychiatric interview. From Clare's data, a sensitivity of 30% and a specificity of 80% may be calculated, compared with the Goldberg rating (1, Table 7).

Alternative Forms

A 41-item self-report Social Problem Questionnaire has been derived from the Social Maladjustment Schedule (3).

Commentary

Clare and Cairns offer a thorough conceptual discussion of the development of indices of social health, reviewing the problems

Exhibit 4.12 Structure and Content of the Social Maladjustment Schedule

Subject Area	Material Conditions	Social Management	Satisfaction
		Rating category with each item rated shown below the appropriate category	
Housing	Housing conditions	Household care	Satisfaction with housing
	Residential stability	Management of housekeeping	
Occupation/social role	Occupational stability	Quality of personal interaction with workmates	Satisfaction with occupation/social role (includes housewives, unemployed, disabled, retired)
	Opportunities for interaction with workmates*		Satisfaction with personal interaction with workmates
Economic situation	Family income	Management of income	Satisfaction with income
Leisure/social activities	Opportunities for leisure and social activities*	Extent of leisure and social activities	Satisfaction with leisure and social activities
	Opportunities for interaction with neighbors	Quality of interaction with neighbors	Satisfaction with interaction with neighbors
			Satisfaction with heterosexual role
Family and domestic relationships	Opportunities for interaction with relatives*	Quality of interaction with relatives	Satisfaction with interaction with relatives
		Quality of solitary living	Satisfaction with solitary living
	Opportunities for domestic interaction (i.e., with unrelated others or adult offspring in household)	Quality of domestic interaction (i.e., with unrelated others or adult offspring in household)	Satisfaction with domestic interaction
	Situational handicaps to child management*	Child management	Satisfaction with parental role
Marital		Fertility and family planning	
		Sharing of responsibilities and decision-making	Satisfaction with marital harmony
		Sharing of interests and activities	Satisfaction with sexual compatibility

*This group of items rates objective restrictions which might be expected to impair functioning in the appropriate area. "Situational handicaps to child management" assesses difficulties likely to exacerbate normal problems of child-rearing, e.g., inadequate living space, an absent parent. Objective restrictions on leisure activities include extreme age, physical disabilities, heavy domestic or work commitments, isolated situation of the home, etc.

Reproduced with permission from Clare AW, Cairns VE, Design, development and use of a standardized interview to assess social maladjustment and dysfunction in community studies. Psychol Med 1978;8:592, Table 1. Copyright Cambridge University Press. Reprinted with the permission of Cambridge University Press.

of comparing social behavior across cultural groups and discussing the balance to be set between recording objective life circumstances and personal satisfaction. Although their scale was explicitly designed to reflect this distinction, empirical data from factor analyses did not confirm the intended conceptual structure.

The scale seems well designed, but it has not seen widespread use other than by its original authors (3–5), and beyond the initial development work little further evidence for the reliability and validity of the scale has been published. The scale covers only the negative aspects of social adjustment; for assessing social support or the positive indications of integration a different scale, such as that of Henderson or McFarlane, would be needed. The Social Maladjustment Schedule may find a role in studies that require detailed information on social maladjustment and that have the resources to carry out home interviews, but the decision to use the instrument should be taken in the light of future evidence on its validity and reliability.

Address

Anthony W. Clare, MD, Department of Psychological Medicine, St. Bartholomew's Hospital Medical School, West Smithfield, London, England EC1A 7BE

REFERENCES

(1) Clare AW, Cairns VE. Design, development and use of a standardized interview to assess social maladjustment and dysfunction in community studies. Psychol Med 1978;8:589–604.
(2) A manual for use in conjunction with the General Practice Research Unit's standardized social interview schedule. London: Institute of Psychiatry, 1979.
(3) Corney RH, Clare AW, Fry J. The development of a self-report questionnaire to identify social problems: a pilot study. Psychol Med 1982;12:903–909.
(4) Clare AW. Psychiatric and social aspects of pre-menstrual complaint. Psychol Med 1983;13(suppl 4):1–58.
(5) Corney RH. Social work effectiveness in the management of depressed women: a clinical trial. Psychol Med 1981;11:417–423.

THE SOCIAL DYSFUNCTION RATING SCALE
(Margaret W. Linn, 1969)

Purpose

The Social Dysfunction Rating Scale (SDRS) assesses the negative aspects of a person's social adjustment. This rating scale is applied by a clinician and is intended as a research instrument, mainly for use with the elderly.

Conceptual Basis

Effective social functioning, in Linn's conceptual formulation,

would suggest equilibrium within the person and in his interaction with his environment. ... Dysfunction, on the other hand, implies discontent and unhappiness, accompanied by negative self-regarding attitudes. It furthermore suggests handicapping anxiety and other pathological interpersonal functions that reduce flexibility in coping with stressful situations or achieving self-actualization in what is to that person a significant role.... From this standpoint, dysfunction is seen as coping with either personal, interpersonal, or geographic environment in a maladaptive manner. In this respect, the SDRS seeks to quantify the objective observations of man's dysfunctional interaction with his environment. (1, p299)

Linn viewed adjustment as a process of coping, problem solving, and achieving personal goals (2, p617). As a dysfunction scale, however, the SDRS concentrates on symptoms of low morale and reduced social participation; it does not assess positive adjustment. The assessments do not emphasize roles, which makes the instrument suitable for elderly people. "The SDRS is applicable to older patients, particularly with respect to assessing the meaningfulness of their life, their goals, and their satisfactions. It does not provide descriptive assessments of different kinds of activities. Work is rated on the basis of productive activities ... and whether these generate feelings of usefulness." (2, p617)

Description

The Social Dysfunction Rating Scale is applied by an interviewer, generally a social worker or other therapist familiar with the patient. The scale, shown in Exhibit 4.13, includes 21 symptoms of social and emotional problems, each judged on a six-point severity scale. The ratings are grouped into three classes: four items refer to the respondent's self-image, six refer to interpersonal relationships, and 11 concern lack of success and dissatisfaction in social situations. The questions are semi-structured and combine the interviewer's evaluations with the respondent's own self-evaluation (1, p301). For instance, the interviewer rates the availability of friends and social contacts, after which the respondent is asked if he feels a need for more friends. Hence, the person who has few friends and is discontent about this will receive a lower

Exhibit 4.13   The Social Dysfunction Rating Scale

Directions: Score each of the items as follows:

1. Not Present   3. Mild   5. Severe
2. Very Mild   4. Moderate   6. Very severe

Self system

1. _____ Low self concept (feelings of inadequacy, not measuring up to self ideal)
2. _____ Goallessness (lack of inner motivation and sense of future orientation)
3. _____ Lack of a satisfying philosophy or meaning of life (a conceptual framework for integrating past and present experiences)
4. _____ Self-health concern (preoccupation with physical health, somatic concerns)

Interpersonal system

5. _____ Emotional withdrawal (degree of deficiency in relating to others)
6. _____ Hostility (degree of aggression toward others)
7. _____ Manipulation (exploiting of environment, controlling at other's expense)
8. _____ Over-dependency (degree of parasitic attachment to others)
9. _____ Anxiety (degree of feeling of uneasiness, impending doom)
10. _____ Suspiciousness (degree of distrust or paranoid ideation)

Performance system

11. _____ Lack of satisfying relationships with significant persons (spouse, children, kin, significant persons serving in a family role)
12. _____ Lack of friends, social contacts
13. _____ Expressed need for more friends, social contacts
14. _____ Lack of work (remunerative or non-remunerative, productive work activities which normally give a sense of usefulness, status, confidence)
15. _____ Lack of satisfaction from work
16. _____ Lack of leisure time activities
17. _____ Expressed need for more leisure, self-enhancing and satisfying activities
18. _____ Lack of participation in community activities
19. _____ Lack of interest in community affairs and activities which influence others
20. _____ Financial insecurity
21. _____ Adaptive rigidity (lack of complex coping patterns to stress)

---

rating than the person with few friends but who is not concerned by this. The interview lasts about 30 minutes (2, p617).

Linn et al. provide definitions of the items and instructions for completing the scale. As an example, comments on item 4 read as follows:

4. *Self-health concern.* The frequency and severity of complaints of body illness are rated. Evaluation is based on degree to which the person believes that physical symptoms are an important factor in his total well-being. No consideration is given for actual organic basis of illness. Only the frequency and severity of complaints are rated. (1, p301)

Higher scores on the scale reflect greater dysfunction. Items are not weighted differentially, although Linn et al. considered using discriminant function coefficients as item weights (1, p305).

Reliability

The agreement between two raters in scoring 40 subjects was measured; intraclass correlations for the 21 items ranged from 0.54 to 0.86 (1, Table 1). The agreement between seven raters, who independently rated ten schizophrenics in group interviews, yielded a Kendall index of concordance of 0.91 (1, p303).

Validity

The scale was applied to schizophrenic outpatients and nonpsychiatric respondents. Using discriminant function analysis, it correctly classified 92% of the 80 respondents (1, Table 2). In the same study, a correlation of 0.89 was obtained between the total scale scores and a global judgment of adjustment made by a social worker who interviewed the respondents (1, p305). The data were factor analyzed, producing five factors: apathetic-detachment, dissatisfaction, hostility, health-finance concern, and manipulative-dependency (1).

Alternative Forms

A self-report version has been used by Linn, although she argued that "the original version of the scale provides a better assessment of adjustment when there are no serious limitations on staff and patient time." (2, p617)

Commentary

The SDRS was based on considerable conceptual work on the theme of social adjustment among the elderly (1–4). It is a broad-ranging instrument, overlapping in content with the morale and well-being scales described in Chapter 5. The inter-rater reliability can be high for overall scores, although agreement for individual scales shows a wide variation. There is little evidence on validity. Although it was first described in 1969 and has been used in several studies (5–8), the only validity results come from a single study of 80 subjects. The question of how best to score the scale also requires further investigation, especially as the empirical factor analysis results do not match the three subdivisions built into the scale (self-perceptions, interpersonal relations, and social performance). It is not clear whether a total score or subscores offer the best way to summarize the results. The Social Dysfunction Rating Scale offers a brief and rather narrower alternative to Clare's Social Maladjustment Schedule.

REFERENCES

(1) Linn MW, Sculthorpe WB, Evje M, et al. A Social Dysfunction Rating Scale. J Psychiatr Res 1969;6:299–306.
(2) Linn MW. A critical review of scales used to evaluate social and interpersonal adjustment in the community. Psychopharmacol Bull 1988;24:615–621.
(3) Linn MW. Studies in rating the physical, mental, and social dysfunction of the chronically ill aged. Med Care 1976; 14(suppl 5):119–125.
(4) Linn MW. Assessing community adjustment in the elderly. In: Raskin A, Jervik LF, eds. Assessment of psychiatric symptoms and cognitive loss in the elderly. Washington, DC: Hemisphere Press, 1979:187–204.
(5) Linn MW, Caffey EM Jr. Foster placement

for the older psychiatric patient. J Gerontol 1977;32:340–345.

(6) Linn MW, Caffey EM Jr, Klett CJ, et al. Hospital vs community (foster) care for psychiatric patients. Arch Gen Psychiatry 1977;34:78–83.

(7) Linn MW, Klett CJ, Caffey EM Jr. Foster home characteristics and psychiatric patient outcome: the wisdom of Gheel confirmed. Arch Gen Psychiatry 1980;37:129–132.

(8) Linn MW, Caffey EM, Klett CJ, et al. Day treatment and psychotropic drugs in the aftercare of schizophrenic patients. Arch Gen Psychiatry 1979;36:1055–1066.

THE STRUCTURED AND SCALED INTERVIEW TO ASSESS MALADJUSTMENT
(Barry J. Gurland, 1972)

Purpose

The Structured and Scaled Interview to Assess Maladjustment (SSIAM) provides a detailed clinical assessment of social role performance as an outcome indicator for psychotherapy. It has been used in both clinical and research applications (1).

Conceptual Basis

Gurland held that the relevance of measuring social maladjustment derives from the fact that much psychiatric treatment seeks to assist people in becoming more socially effective and in reducing distress, deviant behavior, and friction with others (2). The questions in the SSIAM "cover those aspects of social adjustment which are of interest to a clinician" (2). The scale was derived from Parloff's 1954 Social Ineffectiveness Scale. Gurland et al. distinguished between objective and subjective facets of maladjustment. Objectively, maladjustment is viewed as ineffective performance of social roles; subjectively, it refers to a failure to obtain satisfaction from one's social activities (2). The SSIAM covers both facets of maladjustment, indicating levels of distress, deviant behavior and friction. Assessments of maladjustment must also consider the patient's environment, because

an unfavorable environment may in part explain distress or disturbed behavior. To cover this, the SSIAM includes a rating by the interviewer in each section asking to what degree the ratings are due to a currently unfavorable environment.

Description

The instrument contains 60 items, 45 of which are grouped into five "fields": work, social relations, family, marriage, and sex. The remaining 15 items are used to record the interviewer's judgments on the level of stress in the patient's environment; on the patient's prognosis and willingness to change; and on aspects of positive mental health such as personality strengths.

Within each of the five fields the assessments follow a standard order: five deal with the patient's deviant behavior, one deals with friction between the patient and others, and three deal with the patient's distress (2). Questions refer to behavior over the past four months (1). Gurland et al. describe the structure of the questions as follows:

Each item has a caption indicating the disturbance covered, a question which the rater asks the patient, and a continuous scale with five anchoring definitions. The highest anchoring definition describes the maximum disturbance likely to be found in an outpatient psychoneurotic population. The lowest describes reasonable adjustment. The remaining three definitions represent successive levels of disturbance between the extremes. (2, pp261–262)

The questions are asked open-ended and the interviewer matches the reply to the answers printed on the interview schedule. If there is doubt about which rating best matches the reply, the interviewer reads the two most applicable categories (in a preset order), effectively implementing a forced-choice response (1). The scale positions of the defining phrases were determined by four psychotherapists in a scaling task (2). The response categories are unique to each item, thereby reducing the likelihood that an interviewer will use a particular response category across several questions. The questionnaire is too long to reproduce here, but an indication of the scope of the instrument is given in Exhibit 4.14. The interview takes about 30 minutes. Definitions of terms are given on the rating form as part of the item: an illustration is given in Exhibit 4.15. An instruction manual is included in the 30-page interview booklet (1).

Raw scores from 0 to 10 for each scale may be summed across each of the five fields, or each field may be scored in terms of deviant behavior, friction between the patient and others, and the patient's distress. Alternatively, factor scores may be used (see Validity section).

Reliability

Fifteen patients were each interviewed by one of three psychiatrists; all three then rated the patient, either during the interview or from a tape recording of it. Intraclass correlations among raters were calculated for six factor scores; the lowest coefficient was 0.78, the highest 0.97 (3, p265). Analyses of variance showed no significant differences among the raters, but small differences among them were obtained for the scores on social isolation and friction in relationships with people other than family members (3).

Validity

Using a sample of 164 adults "considered suitable for outpatient psychotherapy" (70% of whom were students), 33 of the 45 subjective items were factor analyzed. Nine items on marriage and three on sex were omitted from the 45 questions because nearly two-thirds of the sample had never been married. Twelve items were found not to load on factors and were discarded; the remaining 21 items loaded on six factors: social isolation, work inadequacy, friction with family, dependence on family, sexual dissatisfaction, and friction outside the family (3). For 89 patients, a relative or close friend of the patient was interviewed to provide independent ratings of the six topics identified in the factor analysis. There was significant agreement between the SSIAM and the informants' ratings for all factors except sexual dissatisfaction (3).

Serban has reported on the performance of the SSIAM with 100 schizophrenic patients (4, 5). The correlations between the SSIAM scores and the total score derived from a psychiatrist's evaluation using the Psychiatric Assessment Interview ranged from 0.21 and 0.41 (4, Table 1). The SSIAM correlated 0.45 with the Social Stress and Functioning Inventory for Psychotic Disorders (4, p950). Serban showed that the SSIAM discriminated significantly between different types of schizophrenic patients (5). The SSIAM has also been shown capable of identifying significant changes before and after psychotherapy (6).

Commentary

The descriptions of the SSIAM given by Gurland et al. are extremely clear. Great care was evidently taken in the design of the questionnaire and the interviewer instructions are exemplary. The conceptual basis for this scale, contrasting objective and subjective indices of adjustment, corresponds well to other available approaches, and the approach used in the SSIAM has influenced the design of subsequent measurements such as the OARS Multidimensional Functional Assessment Questionnaire and Weissman's Social Adjustment Scale. The SSIAM is one of the more widely used of the social health indices, having been applied in studies of depression (7) and as an outcome indicator for psychotherapy (6).

The expectation that three manifestations of maladjustment (behavior, friction, and distress) would appear across all five fields of maladjustment received little empirical support from the factor analytic study, so careful consideration must be given to how the instrument is scored. We would also like to see considerably more evidence for the reliability and validity of

Exhibit 4.14   Scope of the SSIAM Showing Arrangement of Items within Each Section

Fields of maladjustment	Type of item	Caption of items
WORK	Behavior	Unstable, inefficient, unsuccessful, over-working, over-submissive
	Friction	Friction
	Distress	Disinterested, distressed, feeling inadequate
	Inferential	Rater's assessment of environmental stress
SOCIAL	Behavior	Isolated, constrained, unadaptable, apathetic in leisure, unconforming
	Friction	Friction
	Distress	Distressed by company, lonely, bored by leisure
	Inferential	Rater's assessment of environmental stress
FAMILY	Behavior	Reticent, over-compliant, rebellious, family-bound, withdrawn
	Friction	Friction
	Distress	Guilt-ridden, resentful, fearful
	Inferential	Rater's assessment of environmental stress
MARRIAGE	Behavior	Constrained, submissive, domineering, neglectful, over-dependent
	Friction	Friction
	Distress	Distressed, feeling deprived, feeling inadequate
	Inferential	Rater's assessment of environmental stress
SEX	Behavior	Undesirous, inadequate, inactive, cold, promiscuous
	Friction	Rejected by partner
	Distress	Tension, feeling deprived, unwanted urges
	Inferential	Rater's assessment of environmental stress
OVERALL	Global	Extent of patient's distress, exaggerating, minimizing
	Prognostic	Duration, contrast with previous state, willingness to change, pressure from others to change
	Positive mental health	Strengths and assets, resourcefulness, constructive effort

the instrument, including correlations with other social health measurement scales. With these reservations, we recommend the SSIAM where time permits a thorough assessment of a broad range of types and levels of disorder.

REFERENCES

(1) Gurland BJ, Yorkston NJ, Stone AR, et al. Structured and Scaled Interview to Assess Maladjustment (SSIAM). New York: Springer, 1974.

(2) Gurland BJ, Yorkston NJ, Stone AR, et al. The Structured and Scaled Interview to Assess Maladjustment (SSIAM): I. Description, rationale, and development. Arch Gen Psychiatry 1972;27:259–264.

(3) Gurland BJ, Yorkston NJ, Goldberg K, et al. The Structured and Scaled Interview to Assess Maladjustment (SSIAM): II. Factor analysis, reliability, and validity. Arch Gen Psychiatry 1972;27:264–267.

(4) Serban G. Mental status, functioning, and stress in chronic schizophrenic patients in

Exhibit 4.15   An Example of Two Items Drawn from the SSIAM: Social and Leisure Life Section

Friction	Distress
S6 FRICTION	*S7 DISTRESSED BY COMPANY
Q: How smoothly and well do you get along with your friends and close acquaintances?	Q: Are you ill at ease, tense, shy or upset when with friends?
1) Rate overt behavior between the patient and others. The patient's subjective responses are rated under #S7	1) Only rate distress occurring in friendly and informal company.
	2) Mild initial shyness or mild anticipatory anxiety should be rated as "reasonable."
	3) Include distress from any other source which interferes with the enjoyment of company.
Higher first	Lower first
Frequently has furious clashes or is studiously avoided by others.	Company is mainly a source of agonizing distress.
Often irritates others or is treated with reserve by them.	Company is mainly a source of marked distress.
Sometimes relationships with others somewhat uneasy and tense.	Company is sometimes a source of distress but often enjoyable.
Not provocative but can not handle delicate social situations.	Company is unnecessarily distressing only in special circumstances but usually enjoyable.
Reasonably diplomatic.	Company is enjoyed with reasonable ease.
— Not known	— Not known
— Not applicable	— Not applicable
scope	*scope*
The frequency and intensity of his aggressive actions towards others, and the seriousness of the reaction he provokes in others.	The frequency and intensity of distress when in company, and enjoyment of company.

Reproduced from Gurland BJ, Yorkston NJ, Stone AR, Frank JD. Structured and Scaled Interview to Assess Maladjustment (SSIAM). New York: Springer. 1974:10. With permission.

community care. Am J Psychiatry 1979;136:948–952.

(5) Serban G, Gidynski CB. Relationship between cognitive defect, affect response and community adjustment in chronic schizophrenics. Br J Psychiatry 1979;134:602–608.

(6) Cross DG, Sheehan PW, Khan JA. Short- and long-term follow-up of clients receiving insight-oriented therapy and behavior therapy. J Consult Clin Psychol 1982; 50:103–112.

(7) Paykel ES, Weissman M, Prusoff BA, et al. Dimensions of social adjustment in depressed women. J Nerv Ment Dis 1971;152:158–172.

CONCLUSION

In addition to the scales reviewed here, we considered a large number of others for inclusion in this chapter. Several are described in review articles by Linn (1), Donald et al. (2), and Weissman et al. (3, 4). An extensive and useful conceptual discussion of social disability was given by Ruesch in presenting his Rating of Social Disability (5, 6). The scale itself summarizes physical and emotional impairment and describes the resulting impact on social role functioning; it is completed by a psychiatrist, social worker, or psychologist. Ruesch's scale has seldom been reported in the literature and there is no published evidence for its validity.

Roen's Community Adaptation Schedule was developed to evaluate the success of aftercare programs for mental patients discharged to the community (7, 8). It is a 202-item interview that covers work, family relationships, social interaction, social activities, and activities of daily living. It employs an interesting manner of collecting information in that each question is asked in three modes. The first records factual information on circumstances or describes behavior, the second covers affective responses to these, and the third assesses the patient's cognitive responses: for example, the plans the patient has made or his understanding of how other people feel about him. The scale fell into disuse after a spate of validation studies in the early 1970s, most of which showed only modest agreement with other scales (results that did not deter the authors from inferring good construct validity for the method) (9, 10). The interpretation of the scale remains unclear and more evidence is required on its association with other social scales—such as those in the present chapter—before we can recommend its use. Further references to validation studies can be found in the article by Harris and Brown (10).

The Social Disability Questionnaire by Branch deserves mention as one of the few scales designed for use in general population surveys. It is a self-report instrument that estimates need for help in performing daily tasks among elderly people in the general population (11). An innovative feature is its provision of a high risk score that anticipates the possible development of future problems. Termed a social disability questionnaire, the scale resembles the IADL scales in Chapter 3, but it also considers social support and social interaction. The scale lacks evidence on reliability and validity and has seen only limited use.

The Community Adjustment Profile System was designed for use in the long-term monitoring of patients' adjustment. Using 60 questions, it covers ten aspects of adjustment and was designed for computer scoring. Test-retest reliability was quoted at 0.83 and internal consistency of the scales ranged from 0.70 to 0.92 (12, p533). A newer instrument, the Social Functioning Scale, was developed for use with psychiatric patients and assesses strengths and weaknesses in the patient's social functioning. Preliminary evidence for reliability and validity are promising (13).

An early scale occasionally mentioned in introductory discussions, but seldom used in published studies, is the 1968 Personality and Social Network Adjustment Scale by Clark (14). This was designed to evaluate social adjustment among severe psychiatric patients receiving treatment in a therapeutic community. There is relatively good evidence for the validity and reliability of this scale and an abbreviated version is shown in Clark's report; it is worth consideration where a brief and simple rating is required. Another scale often cited as one of the seminal efforts in the field was developed by Renne (15). We have not described this as it has virtually no published validation data and has seldom been actually used.

A promising social support scale has been developed by Norbeck (16). The Norbeck Social Support Questionnaire is based on an explicit conceptual discussion of support, and it showed test–retest reliability coefficients between 0.85 and 0.92 as well as high internal consistency (16, p267). Another instrument, the Personal Resource Questionnaire developed by Brandt and Weinert, is in two sections. The first provides descriptive information on the person's resources and satisfaction with these, and the second section includes questions that reflect Weiss's dimensions of social support (17). Alpha internal consistency for the second part is 0.89 and validity coefficients ranged from 0.30 to 0.44. Validity coefficients for the first part were somewhat lower, ranging from 0.21 to 0.23 (17, p279). Finally, the Duke Social Support Index (DSSI) is designed for use with chronically ill elderly people. It should not be confused with the other Duke social support measures reviewed in this chapter. (More distinctive titles for these scales would be helpful.) The 35-item DSSI covers social network, social interactions, subjective feelings of social support, and instrumental or practical support. Abbreviated versions (23 and 11 items) have been produced (18). We recommend that readers planning to measure social support obtain recent evidence on the further testing of these scales.

Two types of scale have been reviewed in this chapter: social adjustment scales and measurements of social support. Among the former, the Social Adjustment Scale of Weissman is the most carefully developed and shows the highest levels of validity and reliability. Henderson's social interaction scale also shows attention to conceptual and empirical development, and study results have made contributions to the literature on social aspects of disease. Among the social support scales, none is clearly superior, mainly because they are all comparatively new and few have been widely tested. Of those we review, Sarason's scale appears to be the most promising, but we advise readers to search for more recent validity reports on the scales.

REFERENCES

(1) Linn MW. Assessing community adjustment in the elderly. In: Raskin A, Jervik LF, eds. Assessment of psychiatric symptoms and cognitive loss in the elderly. Washington, DC: Hemisphere Press, 1979:187–204.

(2) Donald CA, Ware JE Jr, Brook RH, et al. Conceptualization and measurement of health for adults in the Health Insurance Study. Vol. IV, Social Health. Santa Monica, California: Rand Corporation, 1978.

(3) Weissman MM. The assessment of social adjustment: a review of techniques. Arch Gen Psychiatry 1975;32:357–365.

(4) Weissman MM, Sholomskas D, John K. The assessment of social adjustment: an update. Arch Gen Psychiatry 1981; 38:1250–1258.

(5) Reusch J, Brodsky CM. The concept of social disability. Arch Gen Psychiatry 1968;19:394–403.

(6) Ruesch J, Jospe S, Peterson HW Jr, et al. Measurement of social disability. Compr Psychiatry 1972;13:507–518.

(7) Roen SR, Ottenstein D, Cooper S, et al. Community adaptation as an evaluative concept in community mental health. Arch Gen Psychiatry 1966;15:36–44.

(8) Burnes AJ, Roen SR. Social roles and adaptation to the community. Community Ment Health J 1967;3:153–158.

(9) Cook PE, Looney MA, Pine L. The Community Adaptation Schedule and the Adjective Check List: a validational study with psychiatric inpatients and outpatients. Community Ment Health J 1973;9:11–17.

(10) Harris DE, Brown TR. Relationship of the Community Adaptation Schedule and the Personal Orientation Inventory: two measures of positive mental health. Community Ment Health J 1974;10:111–118.

(11) Branch LG, Jette AM. The Framingham Disability Study: 1. social disability among

the aging. Am J Public Health 1981;71:1202–1210.

(12) Evenson RC, Sletten IW, Hedlund JL, et al. CAPS: an automated evaluation system. Am J Psychiatry 1974;131:531–534.

(13) Birchwood M, Smith J, Cochrane R, et al. The Social Functioning Scale: the development and validation of a new scale of social adjustment for use in family intervention programmes with schizophrenic patients. Br J Psychiatry 1990;157:853–859.

(14) Clark AW. The Personality and Social Network Adjustment Scale: its use in the evaluation of treatment in a therapeutic community. Hum Rel 1968;21:85–96.

(15) Renne KS. Measurement of social health in a general population survey. Soc Sci Res 1974;3:25–44.

(16) Norbeck JS, Lindsey AM, Carrieri VL. The development of an instrument to measure social support. Nurs Res 1981;30:264–269.

(17) Brandt PA, Weinert C. The PRQ—a social support measure. Nurs Res 1981;30:277–280.

(18) Koenig HG, Westlund RE, George LK, et al. Abbreviating the Duke Social Support Index for use in chronically ill elderly individuals. Psychosomatics 1993;34:61–69.

5

Psychological Well-Being

Of all the chapters in this book, the scope of the present one on psychological measurements has proved the most difficult to delimit. Unlike several other fields of health measurement, the problem here is the embarrassment of riches: there are many well-tested measurements and it was not easy to set criteria for what should be included. It would be possible to fill an entire book with measurements of psychological morbidity: anxiety scales, depression inventories, and psychiatric ratings. Depression scales are covered in Chapter 6 and cognitive functioning in Chapter 7, but anxiety scales and psychiatric ratings are not covered in the present edition. Methods designed for assessing severe levels of mental or psychiatric disorder such as schizophrenia have also been omitted, as have scales that would only be used in clinical settings. Then there exist many instruments that measure psychological health, or "subjective well-being," a common theme in social surveys. Our review of such scales cannot be exhaustive. We found it convenient to base our selection, and the way we have grouped scales in the chapter, on a classification of measurement methods proposed by Campbell (1). This taxonomy noted that early measurements of psychological well-being viewed it largely as a cognitive process in which the individual compared her aspirations to her perception of her current situation: well-being was seen in terms of life satisfaction (1). Examples reviewed here include the Life Satisfaction Index and the Philadelphia Geriatric Center Morale Scale. A second category of well-being scales has recorded affective responses to experience—the feeling states inspired by daily experience. We include two examples of this approach in the present chapter, represented by Bradburn's scale and the single-item indicators of well-being popularized by Andrews. A third approach to measuring psychological well-being is via questions that screen for psychological distress. Distress has long been considered a primary indicator of mental health, but it is not synonymous with it. Distress and well-being are often influenced by social and environmental circumstances: mentally healthy people are not immune from anxiety or depression. However, because distress is often a stimulus to seek care, measures of distress represent a clinical orientation, although the scales we review stop short of making diagnostic classifications; instead they screen for signs of general psychological distress. Measures of distress are narrow in that the best state they can distinguish is the absence of distress; scales of well-being are required to extend the conceptual range of measures of distress. A major issue in the early development of such measures was the balance to be set between affective and somatic symptoms (see the criticisms of the Health Opinion Survey). A common resolution of this debate comes from the recognition that in distinguishing mental disorders, both somatic and affective components must be assessed, while in assessing general well-being the somatic symptoms are not necessary. The measurements reviewed in this chapter cover short-term psychological states rather than lasting traits and describe human psychological responses in adapting to the environment, in a manner analogous to Selye's concept of stress, which covers the physiological process of adaptation.

There have been many attempts to specify what is being measured—to distinguish, for example, between "distress" and "disorder" and between "psychological," "emotional," and "mental" well-being. The attempts have not always been successful, and the development of this field has been checkered by disputes over the intent and conceptual interpretation of the scales. Unfortunately, this was exacerbated by the tendency, in the earlier scales at least, for the author not to explain conceptually what he was attempting to measure. Many of the earlier scales were developed empirically by selecting questions that distinguished between well and emotionally distressed persons. This fostered considerable dispute over the correct way to interpret the measurement, as seen with Langner's 22-item scale. The same set of questions has been said to indicate "mental health," "emotional adjustment," "psychological disturbance or disorder," "psychiatric or psychological symptoms," and "mental illness," and has even been considered a "psychiatric case identification instrument." This disagreement indicates the disadvantage of the empirical approach, but it also reflects the difficulty of establishing firm conceptual definitions—a problem

that we have seen over the past ten years in the area of quality-of-life measurement. Dohrenwend et al. have commented critically on indicators of "non-specific psychological distress":

As might be expected given the actuarial procedures and undifferentiated patient criterion groups used to construct them, none of the screening scales reflects a clearly specified conceptual domain. Thus, there is no ready correspondence between the content of the scales and conceptions of major dimensions or types of psychopathology such as mania, depression, hallucinations, or antisocial behavior. (2, p1229)

Dohrenwend et al. suggested that these scales give general indications of distress, analogous to the measurement of body temperature: elevated scores tell you that something is wrong, but not what is wrong. In this chapter we refer to distress rather than disorder, and we use the broad term "psychological" to connote a general level of discussion, commonly referring to emotional, and at times to mental, problems.

Perhaps because of these complexities, considerable attention has been paid to testing the validity of these methods. In many cases this has resulted in scales of very high quality, but there are examples in which the critical interest in a scale has backfired. This most commonly occurs where a clear conceptual explanation of the purpose is lacking; this can have the unfortunate effect of encouraging critics to make piecemeal and uncoordinated modifications to scales. A clear example is Macmillan's Health Opinion Survey, for which Exhibit 5.2 compares seven different, but widely used, versions. To complete the confusion, the versions all bear the same name. This problem is most acute with the older scales; the more recent methods reviewed in this chapter have somewhat clearer explanations of their purpose.

DESIGN OF PSYCHOLOGICAL MEASURES

Two approaches have been used in constructing the measurements reviewed in this chapter: symptom check lists that include behavioral and somatic symptoms of distress, and questions that ask directly about positive and negative feelings of well-being. The common arguments in support of the symptom check list hold that it is more objective and more adequately conceals the intent of the measurement; this is deemed necessary as respondents are expected to be reticent about reporting their true feelings. Indeed, it has been estimated that underreporting of emotional problems in surveys may be as high as 60% (3). Thus, for example, Macmillan deliberately named his screening scale the "Health Opinion Survey" and designed it as a symptom check list to obscure its intent. Conversely, symptom check lists almost certainly classify some physical disorders as psychological; they can also only detect more severe forms of disorder and they cannot identify emotional distress unless it is manifested somatically or behaviorally. Against these criticisms one must set the results of many validation studies that show that the symptom check lists can achieve high sensitivity and specificity when compared with psychiatric ratings. More recently, the argument that people will not respond honestly to direct questions about their emotional well-being has, in some measure, passed from favor. Influenced by the criticisms of the symptom check list approach and by the growing awareness in the later 1950s of the potential accuracy of subjective reports, Gurin, and later Bradburn, led a movement toward surveying feelings of happiness and emotional well-being. This trend also reflected the theme of positive mental health, a concept that may be traced back, through Jahoda's work (5), to the WHO conception of health. The extensive recent work on social support, on coping, and on health promotion emphasizes the need for questions on well-being as well as on symptoms of distress.

Later work suggested that the reaction against the symptom check list approach may have been too strong, for the check lists do succeed in detecting mental disorders even though, as Dohrenwend noted,

they do not provide diagnostic information. Thus, the trend from symptom check lists toward direct questions on feelings has many of the characteristics of a dialectical process, and more recent methods represent a synthesis of the two approaches. Scales such as those developed by Dupuy and by Goldberg have combined the check list and questionnaire approaches to form a hybrid, a trend that marks the convergence of the screening methods of Langner and Macmillan with life satisfaction scales. Perhaps these scales will offer the best of both worlds, and the coming years may see more use of them in studies of the protective impact of "positive mental health" (e.g., in preventing cancer) and of the epidemiology of "wellness" in general. Questions on feelings are necessary to tap the positive end of the mental health spectrum, as they can be phrased to differentiate levels of health among asymptomatic individuals.

Several of the scales we review share questions; most of the symptom check lists originally drew items from the U.S. Army's neuropsychiatric screening instrument (4). This contained symptoms of adverse reactions to stressful situations, selected empirically as being capable of identifying recruits who subsequently performed poorly in military combat. Although these questions were originally designed for use with healthy, young adult males, they were adapted by Macmillan, and later by Langner, for more widespread use in community surveys, forming the first generation of psychological well-being scales. Despite widespread criticism of these scales, they still see occasional use: Langner's questions, for example, are quite frequently used in studies of the impact of life events, stress, and social support on emotional health. We have reviewed the Macmillan and Langner scales for this reason and to provide a historical introduction to the field. More recent scales also share items in common: the Rand Mental Health Inventory incorporates many of Dupuy's questions from the General Well-Being Schedule, and these bear a strong family resemblance to items in Goldberg's General Health Questionnaire.

SCOPE OF THE CHAPTER

The scales we review in this chapter fall into five categories; all are suited for use in population surveys. The first category comprises brief screening scales for psychological distress that use a symptom check list approach; we illustrate this type of instrument by describing the Health Opinion Survey and Langner's 22-Item Screening Scale. These do not cover positive well-being, which is a feature of the second category of scales, illustrated by Bradburn's Affect Balance Scale and the Single-Item Indicators of Well-Being. The third category of scales refers to life satisfaction (which refers to feeling about the past) and morale (which refers to optimism for the future). These are illustrated here by the Life Satisfaction Index and the Morale Scale from the Philadelphia Geriatric Center. Both are intended for elderly populations and cover some of the negative feelings that may occur with aging. The final category of measures represents the current trend in this domain of measurement and includes scales that combine elements of general well-being survey measures and clinical instruments. Their items are more clearly grouped into symptom areas: anxiety, depression, and so forth. The General Well-Being Schedule and the Mental Health Inventory cover both positive and negative feelings; this more clinical orientation is then pursued in Goldberg's General Health Questionnaire, the final scale in the chapter. This method is explicitly designed to detect acute, psychiatrically diagnosable disorders in population studies, and has seen widespread use in many parts of the world. A comparative summary of the quality of the measurements in this chapter is shown in Table 5.1.

REFERENCES

(1) Campbell A. Subjective measures of well-being. Am Psychol 1976;31:117–124.
(2) Dohrenwend BP, Shrout PE, Egri G, et al. Nonspecific psychological distress and other dimensions of psychopathology. Arch Gen Psychiatry 1980;37:1229–1236.
(3) United States Department of Health, Education and Welfare. Net differences in interview data on chronic conditions and information derived from medical records. Washington, DC: Government Printing Office, DHEW Publication No. (HSM)73–1331, 1973. (Vital and Health Statistics, Series 2, No. 57).
(4) Stouffer SA, Guttman L, Suchman EA, et al. Measurement and prediction. Studies in social psychology in World War II. Volume IV. Princeton, New Jersey: Princeton University Press, 1950.
(5) Jahoda M. Current concepts of positive mental health. New York: Basic Books, 1958.

THE HEALTH OPINION SURVEY
(Allister M. Macmillan; First Used in 1951, Published in 1957)

Purpose

Macmillan developed the Health Opinion Survey (HOS) as a "psychological screening test for adults in rural communities" (1). It was designed to identify "psychoneurotic and related types of disorder." Subsequently the HOS has been widely used in epidemiological studies, in estimating need for psychiatric services and in evaluating their impact.

Conceptual Basis

No information is available. Macmillan used the title "Health Opinion Survey" to disguise the purpose of the scale and to make respondents less reticent in reporting emotional problems (1, 2).

Description

The HOS comprises 20 items that were found to discriminate between 78 diagnosed neurotic cases and 559 community respondents in a pilot study in Nova Scotia, Canada (1, 3). The 20 items are shown in Exhibit 5.1 (1).

More than is the case with other instruments, the HOS has frequently been modified by those who have used it. Indeed, the

Table 5.1 Comparison of the Quality of Psychological Indices*

Measurement	Scale	Number of items	Application	Administered by (time)	Studies using method	Reliability Thoroughness	Reliability Results	Validity Thoroughness	Validity Results
Health Opinion Survey (Macmillan, 1957)	ordinal	20	survey	self	many	++	++	+++	++
22–Item Screening Score (Langner, 1962)	ordinal	22	survey	self (5 min)	many	++	++	++	++
Affect Balance Scale (Bradburn, 1965)	ordinal	10	survey	self (few min)	many	++	++	++	++
Four Single-Item Indicators of Well-Being (Andrews, 1976)	interval	1**	survey	self (<1 min)	several	++	++	+	++
Life Satisfaction Index A (Neugarten, 1961)	ordinal	20	survey	self	many	++	++	+++	++
Philadelphia Geriatric Center Morale Scale (Lawton, 1972)	ordinal	22	clinical, survey	self	few	++	++	++	++
General Well-Being Schedule (Dupuy, 1977)	ordinal	18	survey	self (10 min)	several	+++	+++	+++	++
Rand Mental Health Inventory (Ware, 1979)	ordinal	38	survey	self	few	++	++	++	++
Health Perceptions Questionnaire (Ware, 1976)	ordinal	33	survey	self	several	+++	++	++	++
General Health Questionnaire (Goldberg, 1972)	ordinal	60	survey	self (6–8 min)	many	+++	+++	+++	+++

* For an explanation of the categories used, see Chapter 1, pages 6–7

** Andrews describes several, single-item rating scales.

Exhibit 5.1   The Original Version of the Health Opinion Survey

Note: The questions are not presented in the order as asked in the interview, but in decreasing rank order of their derived weights.

---

1. Do you have loss of appetite?

2. How often are you bothered by having an upset stomach?

3. Has any ill health affected the amount of work you do?

4. Have you ever felt that you were going to have a nervous breakdown?

5. Are you ever troubled by your hands sweating so that they feel damp and clammy?

6. Do you feel that you are bothered by all sorts (different kinds) of ailments in different parts of your body?

7. Do you ever have any trouble in getting to sleep and staying asleep?

8. Do your hands ever tremble enough to bother you?

9. Do you have any particular physical or health trouble?

10. Do you ever take weak turns?

11. Are you ever bothered by having nightmares? (Dreams that frighten or upset you very much?)

12. Do you smoke a lot?

13. Have you ever had spells of dizziness?

14. Have you ever been bothered by your heart beating hard?

15. Do you tend to lose weight when you have important things bothering you?

16. Are you ever bothered by nervousness?

17. Have you ever been bothered by shortness of breath when you were not exercising or working hard?

18. Do you tend to feel tired in the mornings?

19. For the most part, do you feel healthy enough to carry out the things that you would like to do?

20. Have you ever been troubled by "cold sweats"? (NOT a hot-sweat—you feel a chill, but you are sweating at the same time.)

Reproduced from Macmillan, AM. The Health Opinion Survey: technique for estimating prevalence of psychoneurotic and related types of disorder in communities. *Psychological Reports*, 1957,3,325–329, Table 1.

original 20 items were altered during the course of the studies in which Macmillan participated. Seven questions were deleted and replaced by questions on other topics, and nine were reworded. Subsequent users have not adhered strictly to either version; we present a comparison of the main variants in Exhibit 5.2, which gives Macmillan's original question topics and shows the variations made to his wording. This means that extreme caution is needed in interpreting results obtained with the scale, as it is seldom clear which version was used. Unfortunately, neither the results of the validation studies reported here nor the cutting points selected to distinguish sick from well respondents will be strictly comparable among different studies.

The HOS may be self- or interviewer-administered. A three-point answer scale ("often," "sometimes," "hardly ever or never") was used originally; other versions have employed four- or five-point scales. Macmillan proposed a scoring system by which the questions may be weighted to maximally discriminate between neurotic and healthy respondents (1). Other users have reported high correlations between weighted and unweighted scores; the advantage of weighted scores seems slight (4). Macmillan suggested a cutting point of 60.0 for the weighted scoring system to distinguish between neurotic and non-neurotic populations; for the unweighted score, 29.5 was optimal (4, p244). A computer program has been developed to provide depression and anxiety scores from the HOS (5).

Reliability

Leighton et al. reported a test–retest correlation of 0.87 "after a few weeks or months" (3, p208). Tousignant et al. obtained a coefficient of 0.78 for 387 respondents after a ten-month delay (4, p243). Schwab et al. showed a high degree of stability between surveys in 1970 and 1973 for 517 respondents (6). There was no difference in the mean scores at the two times; 53.4% of the variance in 1973 scores was attributable to the 1970 score. When classified into normal and abnormal scores, 81.5% of respondents did not change their classification between the two surveys (6, p183).

Butler and Jones reported item-total correlations ranging from 0.20 to 0.62; the coefficient alpha for their 18-item version of the questionnaire was 0.84 (7, p557). Tousignant et al. reported item-total correlations ranging from 0.21 to 0.60 (4, p244).

Validity

There are many validation studies of the variants of the HOS and our review cannot be exhaustive. Macmillan reported a sensitivity of 92% (at a cutting point of 60.0 for the weighted scoring system), and specificity levels ranging from 75% to 88% according to the socioeconomic status of the presumed healthy population (1, p332). Leighton et al. reported correlations between clinical judgments of psychiatric status and the HOS ranging from 0.37 to 0.57 (3, pp208–210). The HOS discriminated adequately between the extremes of well and psychiatrically sick but less adequately at intermediate stages of psychological distress (3).

Tousignant et al. administered the HOS to 88 psychiatric patients and to 88

Exhibit 5.2 Main Variants of the Health Opinion Survey

Note: A blank indicates that the question was omitted, " = " indicates identical wording, "V" indicates minor variation in wording, "R" indicates the question was reworded.

Macmillan No. of items:	Leighton 20	Denis 18	Butler 18	Gunderson 20	Spiro 13	Gurin 20	Schwartz 20
1. Loss of appetite	R	=	R	R	R	=	=
2. Upset stomach	=	R	=	=	=	=	R
3. Ill health affected work		R	=	=	R	=	=
4. Nervous breakdown	V				=	=	=
5. Hands sweating	R	R	R	R	R	R	R
6. Bothered by ailments	V	=	R	R	R	R	R
7. Trouble sleeping	R	R	R	R	R	R	R
8. Hands tremble	=	R	=	=		=	=
9. Particular health trouble	R	R		R		R	R
10. Weak turns		R	R	R			
11. Nightmares	V	R	R	R		R	R
12. Smokes	R		R	R			
13. Spells of dizziness		R	R	R		=	=
14. Heart beating hard	=	=	=	=	R	=	=
15. Lose weight		R	R	R		V	V
16. Bothered by nervousness					R	R	R
17. Shortness of breath		R	R	R	R	=	=
18. Tired in mornings	=	=	=	V	R	R	R
19. Feel healthy enough		=	=	V	R	=	V
20. "Cold sweats"	V		V	V	R		

matched community controls (4). All HOS items discriminated at $p < 0.001$; the sensitivity was 80.7%. A cutting point of 29.5 identified as sick 90% of the neurotic patients in the study, all the alcoholics, 70% of the 13 schizophrenics, 71% of 45 psychotics, but only 30% of manic depressives (8, p391). Gunderson et al. evaluated the ability of the HOS to classify over 4,000 Navy personnel into the categories "fit" and "not fit for duty" (2). Thirteen items showed significant differences between the groups. Eleven HOS questions discriminated between people receiving outpatient psychotherapy and others who were not (9). Four questions were included in a discriminant function that provided a sensitivity of 63% and a specificity of 89% (9, p111). Whereas Macmillan's patients were hospitalized, none in Spiro's study was, and this may account for the lower sensitivity level.

Macmillan compared the HOS scores with the judgment of a psychiatrist; for 64 respondents he reported a 14% disagreement (1, p335). However, the disagreement may be much higher according to how the substantial number of cases rated "uncertain" by the psychiatrist are classified (4). The agreement between the computer scoring system and a psychiatrist's rating is reported by Murphy et al. (5). The sensitivity was 89% for depression and 96% for anxiety; the specificity was 79% for depression and 48% for anxiety (5, Table 4). Receiver operating characteristic (ROC) curves were reported for the HOS scores for 154 patients diagnosed by psychiatrists as having neurotic disorders and 787 people designated as psychiatrically well. Using a dichotomous scoring for each item, the area under the ROC curve was 0.90, which rose to 0.91 using scores that took account of the frequency responses. The area under the curve rose to 0.97 for the computer scoring method (10, Figures 3–5).

Tousignant et al. showed that replies to the HOS were associated with use of medications, psychological symptoms, reports of behavioral disturbances, and judgments of disorder made by interviewers (4, Table 3). Denis et al. showed highly significant variations in HOS scores by age, sex, occupation, marital status, education, income, language, and geographical location (8). Butler and Jones obtained significant correlations with estimates of role conflict, family strain, and frequency of illness (7). Schwartz et al. correlated the HOS with the New Haven Schizophrenia Index ($r = 0.39$) and with the Psychiatric Evaluation Form ($r = 0.55$) (11, p268). The HOS was found to cover neurotic traits only; it did not cover the range of psychotic symptoms exhibited by schizophrenics.

Three factor analyses have identified factors that were interpreted as representing physical and psychological problems (7, 9, 12). There was, however, no clear correspondence between the factor placement of those questions common to the three studies.

Alternative Forms

In addition to the variants noted, Murphy used a questionnaire that included certain of the HOS items in a study in Vietnam (13). A French version was used in the Stirling County studies (3) and in Quebec by Tousignant et al. (4, 8).

Commentary

The HOS was extensively used during the 1960s and 1970s, including cross-cultural studies in Africa and North America (14, 15). There have also been a wide variety of validation studies and there is considerable evidence that it succeeds in its purpose as a screening test for neurotic disorders. Nonetheless, few would now recommend that the scale be used and, for the purposes of our review, there are several lessons to be learned from the history of the HOS.

The first comment illustrates our theme that indices should have a clear conceptual basis. Although the HOS can distinguish between neurotic patients and people without psychiatric diagnoses, it is not clear what a high score actually indicates: mental disorder or normal reactions to stress? Dohrenwend and Dohrenwend suggested that the symptoms covered in measures such as the HOS may reflect normal processes of responding to temporary stressors, rather than neurotic disorders (16). Butler and Jones, indeed, commented that "continued use of the HOS and related mental health indices appears to offer greater potential if they are approached more as stress indicators than as general indices of mental health" (7). Alternatively, the HOS has been said to measure a general demoralization, rather than diagnosable mental disorders, an interpretation that Murphy denies (17). Empirically, the high test–retest reliability results obtained by Tousignant, by Schwab, and by Leighton suggest that the HOS is measuring a comparatively stable construct rather than a transient state.

Our second comment is that the empirical way in which the HOS was developed has further compounded the interpretation problem. The tactic of using physical symptoms to disguise the intent of the scale complicates interpretation and may not have worked anyway: Tousignant et al. reported correlations between the HOS and a "lie scale" that indicated a tendency to avoid admitting to socially undesirable attributes (4, 8).[1] The studies that showed separate physical and psychological factors suggest that the HOS may reflect purely physical complaints as well as psychosomatic problems. Wells and Strickland have studied this bias and have suggested an approach to remove it from the scale (18). The unfortunate history of the development of so many versions of the HOS illustrates the confusion that can arise when health indices are modified piecemeal and without clear conceptual guidelines to define their content. Other more recent scales seem to have avoided this pitfall.

Ultimately, history may condemn the HOS, not because it does not work, but for reasons that relate to the uncertainty of exactly why it works and of how it should be interpreted. The problems with the HOS highlight the need for measurement methods to be founded on a secure conceptual basis that explains what they measure and how they should be interpreted. We cannot recommend the HOS for these reasons and because other scales, such as those of Goldberg and Dupuy, offer better alternatives.

REFERENCES

(1) Macmillan AM. The Health Opinion Survey: technique for estimating prevalence of psychoneurotic and related types of disorder in communities. Psychol Rep 1957;3:325–339.

(2) Gunderson EKE, Arthur RJ, Wilkins WL. A mental health survey instrument: the Health Opinion Survey. Milit Med 1968;133:306–311.

(3) Leighton DC, Harding JS, Macklin DB, et al. The character of danger: psychiatric symptoms in selected communities. Vol. III. New York: Basic Books, 1963.

(4) Tousignant M, Denis G, Lachapelle R. Some considerations concerning the validity and use of the Health Opinion Survey. J Health Soc Behav 1974;15:241–252.

(5) Murphy JM, Neff RK, Sobol AM, et al. Computer diagnosis of depression and anxiety: the Stirling County Study. Psychol Med 1985;15:99–112.

(6) Schwab JJ, Bell RA, Warheit GJ, et al. Social order and mental health: the Florida Health Study. New York: Brunner/Mazel, 1979.

(7) Butler MC, Jones AP. The Health Opinion Survey reconsidered: dimensionality, reliability, and validity. J Clin Psychol 1979;35:554–559.

(8) Denis G, Tousignant M, Laforest L. Prévalence de cas d'intérêt psychiatrique dans une région du Québec. Can J Public Health 1973;64:387–397.

(9) Spiro HR, Siassi I, Crocetti GM. What gets surveyed in a psychiatric survey? A case study of the Macmillan index. J Nerv Ment Dis 1972;154:105–114.

(10) Murphy JM, Berwick DM, Weinstein MC, et al. Performance of screening and diagnostic tests. Arch Gen Psychiatr 1987;44:550–555.

(11) Schwartz CC, Myers JK, Astrachan BM.

---

1. On a humorous note, the principle of trying to obscure the intent of a question was carried to its logical conclusion in the No-Nonsense Personality Inventory (a spoof on the MMPI). Concealed among items such as "Sometimes I find it hard to conceal the fact that I am not angry," or "Weeping brings tears to my eyes" is question 69. Question 69 is entirely blank. In: Scherr GH, ed. The best of the Journal of Irreproducible Results. New York: Workman Publishing, 1983.

Comparing three measures of mental status: a note on the validity of estimates of psychological disorder in the community. J Health Soc Behav 1973;14:265–273.

(12) Gurin G, Veroff J, Feld S. Americans view their mental health: a nationwide interview survey. New York: Basic Books, 1960.

(13) Murphy JM. War stress and civilian Vietnamese: a study of psychological effects. Acta Psychiatr Scand 1977;56:92–108.

(14) Beiser M, Benfari RC, Collomb H, et al. Measuring psychoneurotic behavior in cross-cultural surveys. J Nerv Ment Dis 1976;163:10–23.

(15) Jegede RO. Psychometric characteristics of the Health Opinion Survey. Psychol Rep 1977;40:1160–1162.

(16) Dohrenwend BP, Dohrenwend BS. The problem of validity in field studies of psychological disorder. J Abnorm Psychol 1965;70:52–69.

(17) Murphy JM. Diagnosis, screening, and 'demoralization': epidemiologic implications. Psychiatr Dev 1986;2:101–133.

(18) Wells JA, Strickland DE. Physiogenic bias as invalidity in psychiatric symptom scales. J Health Soc Behav 1982;23:235–252.

THE TWENTY-TWO ITEM SCREENING SCORE OF PSYCHIATRIC SYMPTOMS
(Thomas S. Langner, 1962)

Purpose

The 22-item scale is a screening method to provide a "rough indication of where people lie on a continuum of impairment in life functioning due to very common types of psychiatric symptoms" (1, p269). The scale is intended to identify mental illness, but not to specify its type or degree; nor does it detect organic brain damage, mental retardation, or sociopathic traits (1).

Conceptual Basis

No information is available.

Description

The items were taken mainly from the U.S. Army's Neuropsychiatric Screening Adjunct and from the Minnesota Multiphasic Personality Inventory and were developed for the Midtown Manhattan Study of the social context of mental disorder (2). Of 120 items originally tested, 22 were found to discriminate most adequately between "known well" people (as classified by a psychiatrist) and a group of psychiatric patients.

The scale consists of 22 closed-ended questions that cover somatic symptoms of anxiety, depression, and other neurotic disturbances and that also record subjective judgments of emotional states (3). Fabrega and McBee (4) and Muller (5) concluded that the score assesses mild neurotic and psychosomatic symptoms. In Langner's original work the questionnaire was administered by an interviewer; self-completed (6, 7) and telephone versions (8, 9) have also been used. The self-administered version requires few instructions and takes less than five minutes to complete.

The items and response categories are shown in Exhibit 5.3. The score consists of the total number of responses that indicate sickness, termed pathognomonic responses, designated by asterisks in the exhibit. Differential weights were not used in the original. Haese and Meile proposed a scoring system that provided a different weight for each item based on the conditional probability of having a particular diagnosis with a certain symptom pattern (10). A comparison of this technique with the simpler, summative scoring system showed few differences between their abilities to correctly classify patients and healthy respondents. Logan recommended that four or more symptoms provided a "convenient cutting point" for distinguishing well and sick groups (1). Twenty-eight percent of nonpatients reported four or more symptoms, compared with 50% of ex-patients and 60% of outpatients. Other commentators have set scores of 7 or 10 as cutting points (7, 8, 10).

Reliability

From a survey of over 11,000 respondents, Johnson and Meile obtained alpha reliability coefficients of 0.77 and an omega coefficient of 0.80 (this estimates internal consistency where items fall on more than one factor) (9). They found very little variation

Exhibit 5.3 Langner's Twenty-Two Item Screening Score of Psychiatric Symptoms

Note: An asterisk indicates the scored or pathognomonic responses. DK indicates Don't Know. NA indicates No Answer.

Item	Response
1. I feel weak all over much of the time.	*1. Yes 2. No 3. DK 4. NA
2. I have had periods of days, weeks or months when I couldn't take care of things because I couldn't "get going."	*1. Yes 2. No 3. DK 4. NA
3. In general, would you say that most of the time you are in high (very good) spirits, good spirits, low spirits, or very low spirits?	1. High 2. Good *3. Low *4. Very Low 5. DK 6. NA
4. Every so often I suddenly feel hot all over.	*1. Yes 2. No 3. DK 4. NA
5. Have you ever been bothered by your heart beating hard? Would you say: often, sometimes, or never?	*1. Often 2. Sometimes 3. Never 4. DK 5. NA
6. Would you say your appetite is poor, fair, good or too good?	*1. Poor 2. Fair 3. Good 4. Too Good 5. DK 6. NA
7. I have periods of such great restlessness that I cannot sit long in a chair (cannot sit still very long).	*1. Yes 2. No 3. DK 4. NA
8. Are you the worrying type (a worrier)?	*1. Yes 2. No 3. DK 4. NA
9. Have you ever been bothered by shortness of breath when you were *not* exercising or working hard? Would you say: often, sometimes, or never?	*1. Often 2. Sometimes 3. Never 4. DK 5. NA
10. Are you ever bothered by nervousness (irritable, fidgety, tense)? Would you say: often, sometimes, or never?	*1. Often 2. Sometimes 3. Never 4. DK 5. NA
11. Have you ever had any fainting spells (lost consciousness)? Would you say: never, a few times, or more than a few times?	1. Never 2. A few times *3. More than a few times 4. DK 5. NA

Exhibit 5.3 *(Continued)*

Exhibit 5.3 *(Continued)*

12. Do you ever have any trouble in getting to sleep or staying asleep? Would you say: often, sometimes, or never?

    *1. Often
    2. Sometimes
    3. Never
    4. DK
    5. NA

13. I am bothered by acid (sour) stomach several times a week.

    *1. Yes
    2. No
    3. DK
    4. NA

14. My memory seems to be all right (good).

    1. Yes
    *2. No
    3. DK
    4. NA

15. Have you ever been bothered by "cold sweats"? Would you say: often, sometimes, or never?

    *1. Often
    2. Sometimes
    3. Never
    4. DK
    5. NA

16. Do your hands ever tremble enough to bother you? Would you say: often, sometimes, or never?

    *1. Often
    2. Sometimes
    3. Never
    4. DK
    5. NA

17. There seems to be a fullness (clogging) in my head or nose much of the time.

    *1. Yes
    2. No
    3. DK
    4. NA

18. I have personal worries that get me down physically (make me physically ill).

    *1. Yes
    2. No
    3. DK
    4. NA

19. Do you feel somewhat apart even among friends (apart, isolated, alone)?

    *1. Yes
    2. No
    3. DK
    4. NA

20. Nothing ever turns out for me the way I want it to (turns out, happens, comes about, i.e., my wishes aren't fulfilled).

    *1. Yes
    2. No
    3. DK
    4. NA

21. Are you ever troubled with headaches or pains in the head? Would you say: often, sometimes, or never?

    *1. Often
    2. Sometimes
    3. Never
    4. DK
    5. NA

22. You sometimes can't help wondering if anything is worthwhile anymore.

    *1. Yes
    2. No
    3. DK
    4. NA

Reproduced from Langer TS. A twenty-two item screening score of psychiatric symptoms indicating impairment. J Health Hum Behav 1962;3:271–273.

in these results across age, sex, and educational categories (9, Table 1). Cochrane reported relatively low item-total correlations ranging from 0.17 to 0.54 (11, Table 3). He also reported an alpha of 0.83 and a one-week test–retest reliability of 0.88 (11, Table 4).

Wheaton studied two samples (N = 613 and 250) over four years and reported path coefficients of 0.68 and 0.81 between the initial and subsequent scores for ten items that Crandell and Dohrenwend (12) recommended be taken to form a psychological subscale (13, p399).

Validity

Using information obtained from an interview that included the 22 items among 100 psychiatric symptoms, two psychiatrists independently rated 1,660 respondents on their degree of psychiatric impairment in the Midtown Manhattan Study (1). Each of the 22 questions was then compared with this rating; correlations ranged from 0.41 to 0.79, confirming that psychiatrists had relied heavily on these items in forming their overall judgment (1, p273).

The data of Manis et al. yielded a sensitivity of 67% and a specificity of 63% at a cutting point of 4. A cutting point of 10 gave a sensitivity of 20% and a specificity of 96% (7, p111). These values are low and suggest the instrument has limitations as a screening tool. The positive predictive value of the test in the Midtown study was also low: around 13% for the cutting point of 4, 21% for the cutting point of 7. All 22 items in the scale discriminated between patients newly admitted to a mental hospital and samples drawn from the community (7, Table 1). A score derived from the nine most discriminative questions performed almost as well as the full scale (7). Manis reported a correlation of 0.65 with a 45-item scale of behavioral symptoms of mental health. Shader et al. reported a correlation of 0.77 between the scale and Taylor's Manifest Anxiety Scale (N = 566), and of 0.72 with a Minnesota Multiphasic Personality Inventory depression score, and of

0.72 with Eysenck's Neuroticism Scale (6, Table 8). Fabrega and McBee obtained correlations of 0.50 with psychiatrists' ratings of depression and anxiety, and 0.30 with scores indicating neuroticism (4).

Several studies have reviewed the meaning of the items in the 22-item scale. Crandell and Dohrenwend asked a sample of psychiatrists and internists to judge the content of each item. Ten items were judged to reflect psychological symptoms, five were psychophysiological, three were physical, and four could not be classified. Responses to these four types of items reveal variations by age, sex, and socioeconomic status (14, 15). A similar analysis was carried out by Seiler and Summers (16). Empirical studies of the structure of the scale have used cluster analysis (14, 15, 17) and factor analysis (9). The cluster analyses identified between three and five clusters that cut across the grouping made by psychiatrists in Crandell and Dohrenwend's study. Johnson and Meile factor analyzed the scale using data from a large community study. Three factors were identified, reflecting physical symptoms, psychological stress, and psychophysiological responses (9, Table 2). Johnson and Meile, as well as De Marco, concluded that the physical component in the scale did not act independently of the psychological or psychophysiological components, but rather contributed to the overall impression.

Commentary

Langner's scale has been widely used but has also received considerable critical attention. These criticisms, although now old, will be reviewed to illustrate an important phase in the development of psychological indices.

As with the HOS, a debate arose over precisely what the 22-item scale measures; this again illustrates the need for a clear conceptual formulation of the aims of an index (see Chapter 2). The questions have been variously said to indicate "psychiatric or psychological symptoms," "psychological disturbance or disorder," "psychophys-iological symptoms," "emotional adjust-ment," "mental health," or "mental illness" (3). The method has even been termed a "psychiatric case identification instrument" (10, p335). The debate is un-likely to be resolved, although Seiler's con-clusion that the scale is partly an indicator of psychological stress and partly of physi-ological malaise (16) is supported by sev-eral commentators. Both the HOS and Langner scales may falsely interpret purely physical symptoms as reflecting psychologi-cal disorder (8, 9, 12, 14, 16). Somatic symptoms may also not provide a consis-tent indicator of psychological distress across different social groups: lower social class respondents may both suffer more physical illness and tend to express psycho-logical disorders in physical, rather than psychological, terms (3, 8, 12). However, Meile has dissented and argued on the basis of large studies that the physical items did not provide evidence that diverged from that offered by the other questions in the scale (8, 9).

Several studies have shown a higher symptom response rate among women than men (15, 16, 18); this may reflect a re-porting bias because women are less inhib-ited about reporting their symptoms (12). Clancy and Gove, however, showed that males and females did not differ in their bias toward acquiescing to the items and that the difference in responses seemed to reflect a true difference in symptoms expe-rienced (18).

Seiler offered an extensive summary of the limitations of using the validation pro-cedure of "known groups" and estimated that one-third of the known mentally sick are not detected by the scale (3). Manis et al. commented that the scale holds some validity as a community survey technique but cannot indicate the health of individu-als (7). The interpretation of a high score may also not be clear: does this suggest an increasing probability of disorder or does it imply a more severe disorder? Wheaton answers this in terms of increasing scores indicating a higher probability of impair-ment (19, p28). The scale contains no items covering positive mental health, so a low score will not distinguish between the ab-sence of sickness and more positive states of well-being (3). As the 22-item scale does not claim to cover a number of important psychiatric problems, the low-scoring group may contain healthy people, plus various types of the mentally ill not identi-fied by the items. These problems in inter-preting the Langner scale have led to its virtual replacement by newer scales whose interpretation is clearer.

Wheaton's review of the Langner scale provides a balanced summary; he con-cludes that the psychological items provide a good indicator of the likelihood that a person scoring highly has a psychiatric dis-order. The psychophysiological items (numbers 1, 4, 15, 18, and 21 in our ex-hibit) are more problematic; their interpre-tation varies from group to group, they are often closely associated with physical illness, and they are not strongly associated with the chances of receiving a psychiatric diagnosis (19, p50).

REFERENCES

(1) Langner TS. A twenty-two item screening score of psychiatric symptoms indicating impairment. J Health Hum Behav 1962;3:269–276.
(2) Srole L, Langner TS, Michael ST, et al. Mental health in the metropolis: the Mid-town Manhattan Study. New York: New York University Press, 1978.
(3) Seiler LH. The 22-item scale used in field studies of mental illness: a question of method, a question of substance, and a question of theory. J Health Soc Behav 1973;14:252–264.
(4) Fabrega H Jr, McBee G. Validity features of a mental health questionnaire. Soc Sci Med 1970;4:669–673.
(5) Muller DJ. Discussion of Langner's psychi-atric impairment scale. Am J Psychiatry 1971;128:601.
(6) Shader RI, Ebert MH, Harmatz JS. Lang-ner's psychiatric impairment scale: a short screening device. Am J Psychiatry 1971; 128:596–601.
(7) Manis JG, Brawer MJ, Hunt CL, Kercher LC. Validating a mental health scale. Am Sociol Rev 1963;28:108–116.

(8) Meile RL. The 22-item index of psycho-physiological disorder: psychological or organic symptoms? Soc Sci Med 1972; 6:125–135.

(9) Johnson DR, Meile RL. Does dimensionality bias in Langner's 22-item index affect the validity of social status comparisons? An empirical investigation. J Health Soc Behav 1981;22:415–433.

(10) Haese PN, Meile RL. The relative effectiveness of two models for scoring the midtown psychological disorder index. Community Ment Health J 1967;3:335–342.

(11) Cochrane R. A comparative evaluation of the Symptom Rating Test and the Langner 22-item index for use in epidemiological surveys. Psychol Med 1980;10:115–124.

(12) Crandell DL, Dohrenwend BP. Some relations among psychiatric symptoms, organic illness, and social class. Am J Psychiatry 1967;123:1527–1537.

(13) Wheaton B. The sociogenesis of psychological disorder: reexamining the causal issues with longitudinal data. Am Sociol Rev 1978;43:383–403.

(14) Roberts RE, Forthofer RN, Fabrega H Jr. Further evidence on dimensionality of the index of psychophysiological stress. Soc Sci Med 1976;10:483–490.

(15) Roberts RF, Forthofer RN, Fabrega H Jr. The Langner items and acquiescence. Soc Sci Med 1976;10:69–75.

(16) Seiler LH, Summers GF. Toward an interpretation of items used in field studies of mental illness. Soc Sci Med 1974;8:459–467.

(17) De Marco R. Relationships between physical and psychological symptomatology in the 22-item Langner's scale. Soc Sci Med 1984;19:59–65.

(18) Clancy K, Gove W. Sex differences in mental illness: an analysis of response bias in self-reports. Am J Sociol 1974;80:205–216.

(19) Wheaton B. Uses and abuses of the Langner Index: a reexamination of findings on psychological and psychophysiological distress. In: Mechanic D, ed. Symptoms, illness behavior and help-seeking. New York: Prodist, 1982:25–53.

THE AFFECT BALANCE SCALE
(Norman M. Bradburn, 1965, Revised 1969)

Purpose

The ten questions developed by Norman Bradburn were designed to indicate the psychological reactions (positive and negative) of people in the general population to events in their daily lives. Bradburn described his scale as an indicator of happiness or of general psychological well-being; these terms denote an individual's ability to cope with the stresses of everyday living. The scale is not concerned with detecting psychiatric or psychological *disorders*, which Bradburn viewed as reactions that persist after removal of the stressful conditions or that are out of proportion to the magnitude of the stress (1).

Conceptual Basis

From their early studies, Bradburn and Caplovitz suggested that subjective feelings of well-being could be indicated by a person's position on two independent dimensions, termed "positive" and "negative affect" (2). Overall well-being is expressed as the balance between these two compensatory forces: an "individual will be high in psychological well-being in the degree to which he has an excess of positive over negative affect and will be low in well-being in the degree to which negative affect predominates over positive" (1, p9). Positive factors (e.g., being complimented) can compensate for the negative feelings to keep the overall sense of well-being at a constant level. The "affect balance score" represents this theme.

Beyond simply compensating for each other, positive and negative feelings were found empirically to be relatively independent of one another; they were not simply the opposite ends of a single dimension of well-being. To indicate the independence of the dimensions, Bradburn cited the example of a man who has an argument with his wife, which may increase their negative feelings without changing their positive feelings. Different circumstances were found to contribute to the presence of positive and negative affects.

Description

Bradburn's research formed part of the National Opinion Research Center's investigations into mental health at about the same time that Macmillan, Leighton, Gurin, and Langner were working on similar themes. The original scale developed by Bradburn consisted of 12 questions, seven measuring positive and five measuring negative affect. Responses were coded on a frequency scale ("once," "sometimes," "often"). Four questions were deleted and two others were added to give the ten questions (five positive, five negative) that have been widely used. They are shown in Exhibit 5.4.

The wording of the questions has remained constant in most studies, but the wording of the question stem has varied. Bradburn specified a time referent (originally "the past week," subsequently, "the past few weeks"); some users have changed this to "the past few months" (3), while others have asked, "How often do you feel each of these ways?" (4, 5).

The scale is self-administered, and replies may use a dichotomous yes/no reply or a scale of three, four, or five points representing the frequency of experiencing the feelings; a three-point scale ("often," "sometimes," "never") has been most commonly used. Differential weights were tested but did not significantly alter the results and so are not used (6). The affect balance score is calculated as the positive score minus the negative. The resulting balance scale has occasionally been collapsed into one with fewer categories (4, 5).

Reliability

Bradburn reported test–retest reliability results over three days for 174 respondents. The resulting test–retest associations (Yule's Q) exceeded 0.90 for nine of the items, while the question "excited or interested" had a reliability of 0.86 (1).

Internal consistency results from a number of subsamples ranged from 0.55 to 0.73 for the positive scale and from 0.61 to 0.73 for the negative scale (7, p196). Warr obtained median item-total correlations for the positive scale of 0.47 and 0.48 for the negative scale (8, p114). Correlations among the items in the two scales were modest, in the range of 0.24 to 0.26 (8). Warr also summarized the response patterns to the questions from five studies; although the absolute rates of affirmative replies varied between studies, the rank ordering of the questions by response rates was remarkably consistent. Himmelfarb and Murrell obtained alpha coefficients of 0.65 (community sample) and 0.70 (clinical sample) (9, Table 1).

Validity

Bradburn provided extensive evidence of agreement between the questions and other indices of self-reported well-being. He gave evidence of discriminant validity by showing contrasts in response patterns between employed and unemployed, between rich and poor, and between different occupa-

Exhibit 5.4   The Affect Balance Scale

During the past few weeks, did you ever feel _____   (Yes/No)

  A. Particularly excited or interested in something?

  B. Did you ever feel so restless that you couldn't sit long in a chair?

  C. Proud because someone complimented you on something you had done?

  D. Very lonely or remote from other people?

  E. Pleased about having accomplished something?

  F. Bored?

  G. On top of the world?

  H. Depressed or very unhappy?

  I. That things were going your way?

  J. Upset because someone criticized you?

Reproduced from Bradburn NM. The structure of psychological well-being. Chicago: Aldine, 1969: 267. With permission.

tional levels (1). Positive affect was shown to be related to social participation, satisfaction with social life, and engaging in novel activities. Several of these findings have been confirmed in subsequent studies. The independence of positive and negative affect scores and their lack of association with age have been widely replicated (7, 8, 10–12). Similarly, correlations have frequently been reported with ratings of overall happiness (10, 11), employment status (8, 13), and social participation (3, 7, 11, 13). Kushman and Lane reported significant associations with minority status and the sex of the respondent (13).

Berkman used eight of the questions in the Alameda County survey and reported a correlation of 0.48 with a 20-item Index of Neurotic Traits (5). Warr reported significant correlations between the affect scales and an anxiety rating and a scale of feelings about one's present life among steelworkers who had been laid off (8). Beiser obtained a correlation of 0.42 between negative affect and a psychiatrist's rating of "psychiatric caseness" (11).

Cherlin and Reeder reported results of a factor analysis of the ten items; these formed two clearly distinct factorial groups, although the authors questioned whether these measured affect (see Commentary section). A detailed analysis of the items was gained by interviewing respondents about their responses (14). Three items, in particular, were identified as problematic: "on top of the world," "proud," and "restless." A significant number of respondents found the idiom of these items inappropriate, and it appeared that a negative answer to them implied discontent with the question rather than the absence of the affect in question (14, pS273).

Alternative Forms

A French translation was made in Canada (15); a German version has been published (16).

Reference Standards

Reference standards for the Canadian population are available from the 1978–1979

Canada Health Survey (sample size 23,000) (15, 17).

Commentary

There are several important strengths in Bradburn's scale. The questions have been widely and consistently used in many, large surveys, so findings can be compared across studies; reference standards are available. The fact that the question wording has remained virtually unchanged is a major advantage of this method. The clear conceptual description of the purpose of the scale seems to have prevented some of the misconceptions and disputes over interpretation that have characterized the HOS and Langner scales. Bradburn's scale was also innovative in its inclusion of both positive and negative questions. This has permitted empirical examination of the concept of positive mental health.

At the same time, detailed criticisms have been made of the method by Cherlin and Reeder (7), Beiser et al. (3, 11), and Brenner (12). The Bradburn scale is brief and broad in scope, so it inevitably suffers some resulting psychometric weaknesses: the internal consistency, for example, is low compared with that of the HOS and Langner scales. The interpretation of several questions has been challenged; Cherlin and Reeder argued that the theme covered by the questions is broader than that implied by Bradburn's term "affect": the positive dimension includes activation or participation (7). Beiser implied a similar criticism when he altered the term "positive affect" to "pleasurable involvement" to reflect the item content more adequately; he also discarded the item "on top of the world" (3, 11).

Behind criticisms of individual questions lies the general issue of the adequacy of Bradburn's two-component model of emotional well-being. Reality appears to be more complex (7), and the somewhat surprising finding of statistical independence between positive and negative affect may be an artifact of the question phrasing, a possibility that Bradburn had recognized (1). Five questions refer to specific events (e.g., "upset because someone criticized you") and these do, indeed, seem to be independent of one another (7). The positive and negative questions covering more general feelings tend, however, to show a comparatively strong inverse relationship (12). In commenting on the General Health Questionnaire, Goodchild and Duncan-Jones noted that positively worded items seem to tap more transient, and the negative items more stable, states (18). Because of these criticisms, Cherlin and Reeder questioned the affect balance score as the summary statistic because it may entail a loss of information compared with reporting positive and negative scores separately (7). Kammann et al. (19) commented on the continuing debate over the independence of positive and negative affect; the theme will be discussed further in our review of the Rand Mental Health Inventory.

The Bradburn scale was instrumental in stimulating research in the measurement of subjective well-being and happiness. It served to demonstrate that these qualities can be measured, a claim that was disputed when the scale was introduced.[2] Nonetheless, the scale is 30 years old, and despite its historic significance, users should seriously consider applying an alternative scale such as the General Well-Being Schedule or the Rand Mental Health Inventory.

REFERENCES

(1) Bradburn NM. The structure of psychological well-being. Chicago: Aldine, 1969.

(2) Bradburn NM, Caplovitz D. Reports on happiness: a pilot study of behavior related to mental health. Chicago: Aldine, 1965.

(3) Beiser M, Feldman JJ, Egelhoff CJ. Assets and affects: a study of positive mental health. Arch Gen Psychiatry 1972; 27:545–549.

(4) Berkman PL. Life stress and psychological well-being: a replication of Langner's analysis in the Midtown Manhattan Study. J Health Soc Behav 1971;12:35–45.

(5) Berkman PL. Measurement of mental health in a general population survey. Am J Epidemiol 1971;94:105–111.

(6) Bradburn NM, Miles C. Vague quantifiers. Public Opin Q 1979;43:92–101.

(7) Cherlin A, Reeder LG. The dimensions of psychological well-being: a critical review. Sociol Methods Res 1975;4:189–214.

(8) Warr P. A study of psychological well-being. Br J Psychol 1978;69:111–121.

(9) Himmelfarb S, Murrell SA. Reliability and validity of five mental health scales in older persons. J Gerontol 1983;38:333–339.

(10) Gaitz CM, Scott J. Age and the measurement of mental health. J Health Soc Behav 1972;13:55–67.

(11) Beiser M. Components and correlates of mental well-being. J Health Soc Behav 1974;15:320–327.

(12) Brenner B. Quality of affect and self-evaluated happiness. Soc Indicat Res 1975;2:315–331.

(13) Kushman J, Lane S. A multivariate analysis of factors affecting perceived life satisfaction and psychological well-being among the elderly. Soc Sci Q 1980;61:264–277.

(14) Perkinson MA, Albert SM, Luborsky M, et al. Exploring the validity of the Affect Balance Scale with a sample of family caregivers. J Gerontol 1994;49:S264–S275.

(15) Health and Welfare Canada. The health of Canadians: report of the Canada Health Survey. Ottawa, Canada: Ministry of Supply and Services, 1981. (Catalogue No. 82–538E).

(16) Noelle-Neumann E. Politik und Glück. In: Baier H, ed. Freiheit und Sachzwang Beiträge zu Ehren Helmut Schelskys. Opladen, Germany: West Deutscher Verlag, 1977:207–262.

(17) McDowell I, Praught E. On the measurement of happiness: an examination of the Bradburn scale in the Canada Health Survey. Am J Epidemiol 1982;116:949–958.

(18) Goodchild ME, Duncan-Jones P. Chronicity and the General Health Questionnaire. Br J Psychiatry 1985;146:55–61.

(19) Kammann R, Farry M, Herbison P. The analysis and measurement of happiness as a sense of well-being. Soc Indicat Res 1984;15:91–115.

2. Such research now appears very common. In one of Unger's Herman cartoons a Martian survey researcher, his flying saucer parked nearby, is inquiring whether the bemused simpleton Herman is " 'extremely happy,' 'happy,' 'average,' or 'bored stiff'?"

FOUR SINGLE-ITEM INDICATORS OF WELL-BEING
(F.M. Andrews, 1976)

Purpose

These scales may be used to assess satisfaction with life in general or with more specific topics such as health, economic status, or housing. They have most commonly been used in population surveys but can also be used in clinical settings.

Conceptual Basis

Andrews stressed the subjective, evaluative component of ratings of quality of life: "The quality of life is not just a matter of the conditions of one's physical, interpersonal and social setting but also of how these are judged and evaluated by oneself and others." (1, p12)

Description

Self-ratings of life satisfaction and quality of life are frequently made on single-item response scales that vary in design and format; their use is exemplified in the studies by Campbell et al. (2). Although no single author developed these methods, it is convenient to review them in a description of the work of Frank M. Andrews, who formally compared the validity of several single-item scales.

Of the scales tested by Andrews, we have selected the four shown to be most valid in his analyses. They may refer to life as a whole—"How happy are you these days?" or to reactions to particular life concerns such as health, income, or housing. In either case, the scales are used to assess the affective component of quality of life rather than the physical and social conditions in which a person lives. According to the question phrasing, the scales may refer to the present or to the past, or may be used to express the respondent's hopes for the future.

To measure change with these scales Andrews uses difference scores. If this approach is complicated by an attenuation of the range of improvement where the initial score is already high, scores can be expressed as a proportion of the possible change (F. Andrews, personal communication, 1984).

The four scales are:

1. The Delighted-Terrible Scale. This is a seven-point scale ranging from delighted to terrible (see Exhibit 5.5). Respondents are told, "We want to find out how you feel about various parts of your life, and life in this country as

Exhibit 5.5 The Delighted-Terrible Scale

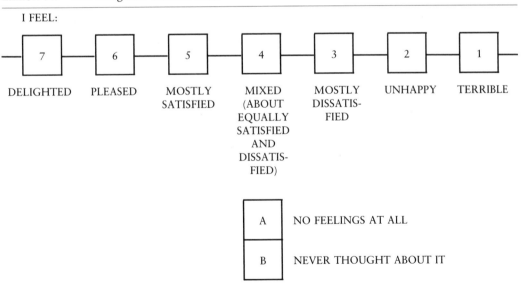

you see it. Please indicate the feelings you have now—taking into account what has happened in the last year and what you expect in the near future. . . . How do you feel about _____?" (3, p5).

2. The Faces Scale. This is a seven-point scale consisting of stylized faces (see Exhibit 5.6). Each face consists of a circle with eyes that do not change and a mouth that varies from a smile of almost a half-circle to a similar half-circle upside down, representing gloom. Respondents were told, "Here are some faces expressing various feelings. . . . Which face comes closest to expressing how you feel about your _____?" (3, p5).

3. Ladder Scale. This scale (shown in Exhibit 5.7) is drawn as a ladder with nine rungs, derived from the ladder scale of Hadley Cantril (4). It has been used frequently and the instructions show slight variations (5–7). The phrasing of Andrews and Withey is typical: the top rung is labeled "Best I could expect to have" and the bottom rung, "Worst I could expect to have." Respondents are told, "Here is a picture of a ladder. At the bottom of this ladder is the worst situation you might reasonably expect to have. At the top is the best you might expect to have. The other rungs are in between. . . . Where on the ladder is your _____? On which rung would you put it?" The scale is often termed self-anchoring because ratings are made relative to each person's conception of her own maximum and minimum life satisfaction.

4. The Circles Scale. Each of nine circles in this scale is divided into eight slices, each containing plus or minus signs. Circles are ordered so that they contain progressively more pluses and fewer minuses. The instruction reads, "Here are some circles that we can imagine represent the lives of different people. Circle 0 has all minuses in it, to represent a person who has all bad things in his or her life. Circle 8 has all pluses in it, to represent a person who has all good things in his or her life. Other circles are in between. Which circle comes closest to matching how you feel about _____?" (3). The Circles Scale is shown in Exhibit 5.8.

Reliability

Reliability estimates from various surveys using the scales were combined by Andrews, who estimated an average test–retest reliability for each scale (applied twice in the same interview) of about 0.70. He noted that 92% of respondents provided an answer on retest that was identical or immediately adjacent to their previous answer (1). Two-year test–retest reliability in a community sample was 0.40 for the Ladder Scale and 0.41 for an 11-point satisfaction rating scale. For respondents who reported no major changes in life circumstances, coefficients were 0.47 and 0.43, respectively (8). Agreement between self-ratings and judgments by acquaintances averaged 0.33 for 16 areas rated on the Delighted–Terrible Scale. Correlations between alternative forms of the question stem (both using the Delighted–Terrible Scale) averaged 0.71 over 16 areas (9, Fig-

Exhibit 5.6   The Faces Scale

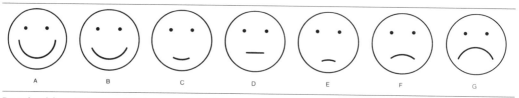

Exhibit 5.7 The Ladder Scale

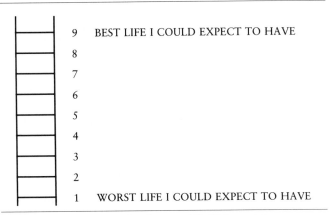

9   BEST LIFE I COULD EXPECT TO HAVE

8

7

6

5

4

3

2

1   WORST LIFE I COULD EXPECT TO HAVE

Reproduced from Andrews and Withey, page 370. With permission.

ure 1). Lehman et al. reported internal consistency reliabilities for the Delighted–Terrible Scales between 0.74 and 0.87 on a sample of chronic mental patients (10, p1272).

Validity

Validity analyses (N = 222) took the form of a multimethod-multitrait investigation in which six aspects of well-being were each assessed by the four methods, using the LISREL method of partitioning variance (3). The results show median validity coefficients of 0.82 for the Delighted–Terrible Scale, 0.82 for the Faces Scale, 0.70 for the Ladder Scale, and of 0.80 for the Circles Scale. Full results are presented by Andrews and Crandall (3, Table 1). The validity coefficients remained consistent when different aspects of life quality were assessed by the same method (3). Several other single-item scales tested by Andrews showed much lower validity.

The Ladder Scale has been frequently used, although rarely validated. Using the Ladder Scale, Palmore and Kivett showed considerable stability in life satisfaction in a longitudinal study of 378 community residents aged 46 to 70 (5). Self-rated health levels formed the strongest predictors of overall life satisfaction, accounting for two thirds of the explained variance (5, 6). Atkinson showed significant associations between the Ladder Scale results and life events (8).

Lehman et al. showed the Delighted–Terrible Scale capable of indicating consistent contrasts between mental patients liv-

Exhibit 5.8 The Circles Scale

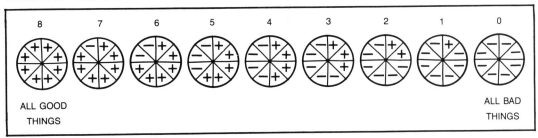

ALL GOOD THINGS

ALL BAD THINGS

Reproduced from Andrews and Withey, page 370. With permission.

ing in the community and population reference values derived from Andrews's data (10). They also presented correlations between the subjective ratings and objective life circumstances, with coefficients falling in the range 0.07 to 0.57 (10, Table 3).

Commentary

These methods are equivalent to the numerical and visual analogue pain rating scales discussed in Chapter 8. The scales are simple to apply, and there are advantages to the nonverbal format. A scale such as the Faces Scale may provide a more direct representation of the feelings involved in quality of life than would a verbal translation of the response in a conventional question. The nonverbal scales may be used with children and others who would have difficulty completing a questionnaire. A Faces Scale has, for example, been used in measuring pain in children ages 3 to 15 years (11). We presume that they provide measurements on an interval scale.

Because of their simplicity, these scales are likely to be widely used in survey research. However, it is strongly desirable that more evidence be collected on their reliability and validity. The Ladder Scale was originally used by Cantril without formal validation. Brown et al. used the Ladder Scale to examine life satisfaction among 84 people with various chronic conditions, and their work represents an example of this type of study in the medical field (7). There is some data on the agreement between single-item scales and Neugarten's Life Satisfaction Index (see Table 5.2 in the review that follows.) Correlations ranged from 0.40 to 0.47: only about one-quarter of the variance is shared by the two approaches, suggesting that although both may have some strengths, they do not agree closely as indicators of life satisfaction.

REFERENCES

(1) Andrews FM, Withey SB. Social indicators of well-being: Americans' perceptions of life quality. New York: Plenum, 1976.

(2) Campbell A, Converse PE, Rodgers WL. The quality of American life: perceptions, evaluations, and satisfactions. New York: Russell Sage, 1976.

(3) Andrews FM, Crandall R. The validity of measures of self-reported well-being. Soc Indicat Res 1976;3:1–19.

(4) Cantril H. The pattern of human concerns. New Brunswick, New Jersey: Rutgers University Press, 1965.

(5) Palmore E, Kivett V. Change in life satisfaction: a longitudinal study of persons aged 46–70. J Gerontol 1977;32:311–316.

(6) Palmore E, Luikart C. Health and social factors related to life satisfaction. J Health Soc Behav 1972;13:68–80.

(7) Brown JS, Rawlinson ME, Hilles NC. Life satisfaction and chronic disease: exploration of a theoretical model. Med Care 1981;19:1136–1146.

(8) Atkinson T. The stability and validity of quality of life measures. Soc Indicat Res 1982;10:113–132.

(9) Crandall R. Validation of self-report measures using ratings by others. Soc Methods Res 1976;4:380–400.

(10) Lehman AF, Ward NC, Linn LS. Chronic mental patients: the quality of life issue. Am J Psychiatry 1982;139:1271–1276.

(11) McGrath PA, de Veber LL, Hearn MT. Multidimensional pain assessment in children. In: Fields HL, Dubner R, Cervero F, eds. Advances in pain research and therapy. Vol. 9. New York: Raven Press, 1985:387–393.

THE LIFE SATISFACTION INDEX
(Bernice L. Neugarten and Robert J. Havighurst, 1961)

Purpose

The Life Satisfaction Index (LSI) covers general feelings of well-being among older people to identify "successful" aging (1).

Conceptual Basis

As used by Neugarten, Havighurst, and Tobin, the concept of life satisfaction is closely related to morale, adjustment, and psychological well-being. Discussing these terms, they noted:

The term "adjustment" is unsuitable because it carries the implication that conformity is the most desirable pattern of behavior. "Psychological well-being" is, if nothing else, an awkward phrase. "Morale," in many ways, cavptures best the qualities here being described, but there was the practical problem that there are already in use in gerontological research two different scales entitled Morale. The term Life Satisfaction was finally adopted on the grounds that, although it is not altogether adequate, it comes close to representing the five components (1, p137).

Neugarten et al. criticized earlier, single-dimensional approaches to measuring morale or well-being; from a review of previous measurement instruments they identified five components of life satisfaction which the LSI was intended to measure. These include zest (as opposed to apathy), resolution and fortitude, congruence between desired and achieved goals, positive self-concept, and mood tone (1). Positive well-being is indicated by the individual taking pleasure to his daily activities, finding life meaningful, reporting a feeling of success in achieving major goals, a positive self-image, and optimism (1).

Description

There exist several versions of the LSI. The original, the Life Satisfaction Index A (LSIA), comprises 20 items, of which 12 are positive and eight are negative. An agree/disagree response format is used. A second and little-used version, the LSIB, contains 12 questions using three-point answer scales (1). A third version, the LSIZ, was proposed by Wood et al. as a refinement of the LSIA and contains 13 of the 20 items (2, 3). Finally, Adams recommended deleting items 11 and 14 from the LSIA, forming an 18-item version which he also called the LSIA. This was later used by Harris in two large national surveys, although he confusingly named it the LSIZ (4). Exhibit 5.9 shows the original 20-item LSIA.

The LSIA was developed empirically by administering a draft questionnaire to two groups of people known to differ in their level of life satisfaction on the basis of the Life Satisfaction Rating Scale, also developed by Neugarten et al. The Rating Scale is scored by an expert and also reflects the five components of life satisfaction hypothesized by the authors (1). Questions that differentiated successfully between high and low scorers on the Rating Scale were selected for the LSIA, which is self-administered.

There are two ways to score the LSI. In the original method, a two-point agree/disagree score rated items 0 for a response indicating dissatisfaction and 1 for satisfaction. Problems with coding "undecided" responses then prompted the use of a three-point scale, rating a satisfied response as 2, an uncertain response as 1, and a dissatisfied response as 0 (3). This approach was used by Harris in his national surveys and is shown in Exhibit 5.9. Ray, however, showed little advantage of this approach over the two-point method (5).

Reliability

Adams calculated item-total correlations for his 18-item LSIA, but only reported results for a few of the items (2). The alpha internal consistency of Wood's 13-item LSIZ was 0.79 (3, p467). Stock and Okun obtained an alpha of 0.80 with 325 older persons (6, p626). In a study of 1,288 older men, Dobson et al. used the 13-item LSIZ and reported alphas of 0.70 for two-point responses, and 0.76 for five-point answer scales (7, p571). Internal consistency appears to improve for the subset of ten items identified by Adams as loading on a factor analysis: Edwards and Klemmack obtained an alpha of 0.90 (8, p498). Himmelfarb reported an alpha of 0.74 for 264 community subjects, and 0.84 for 101 patients (9, Table 1).

Test–retest reliability for the LSIZ ranged from 0.80 to 0.90 in three samples of patients with chronic disease (10, p352).

Validity

Life satisfaction and quality of life have been defined either in terms of objective indicators such as wealth or via subjective feelings. The LSI is a subjective indicator

Exhibit 5.9　The Life Satisfaction Index A

Here are some statements about life in general that people feel differently about. Would you read each statement in the list, and if you agree with it, put a check mark in the space under "AGREE." If you do not agree with a statement, put a check mark in the space under "DISAGREE." If you are not sure one way or the other, put a check mark in the space under "?"
Please be sure to answer every question on the list.

	Agree	Disagree	?
1. As I grow older, things seem better than I thought they would be.	2	0	1
2. I have gotten more of the breaks in life than most of the people I know.	2	0	1
3. This is the dreariest time of my life.	0	2	1
4. I am just as happy as when I was younger.	2	0	1
5. My life could be happier than it is now.	0	2	1
6. These are the best years of my life.	2	0	1
7. Most of the things I do are boring or monotonous.	0	2	1
8. I expect some interesting and pleasant things to happen to me in the future.	2	0	1
9. The things I do are as interesting to me as they ever were.	2	0	1
10. I feel old and somewhat tired.	0	2	1
11. I feel my age, but it does not bother me.	2	0	1
12. As I look back on my life, I am fairly well satisfied.	2	0	1
13. I would not change my past life even if I could.	2	0	1
14. Compared to other people my age, I've made a lot of foolish decisions in my life.	0	2	1
15. Compared to other people my age, I make a good appearance.	2	0	1
16. I have made plans for things I'll be doing a month or a year from now.	2	0	1
17. When I think back over my life, I didn't get most of the important things I wanted.	0	2	1
18. Compared to other people, I get down in the dumps too often.	0	2	1
19. I've gotten pretty much what I expected out of life.	2	0	1
20. In spite of what people say, the lot of the average man is getting worse, not better.	0	2	1

Reproduced from Neugarten BL, Havighurst RJ, Tobin SS. The measurement of life satisfaction. J Gerontol 1961;16:141. With permission. Scoring system based on Wood V, Wylie ML, Sheafor B. An analysis of a short self-report measure of life satisfaction correlation with rater judgments. J Gerontol 1969;24:467.

and it is of interest to study whether or not it also reflects objective circumstances. Neugarten and Havighurst showed that replies to the LSIA did not correlate with sex, socioeconomic status, age, or geographical location, concluding that the scale is not merely an indicator of objective environmental circumstances (1, 11). Other studies have not replicated this finding, however: Cutler obtained significant correlations with socioeconomic status (12). Harris found positive correlations with income, employment, and education (4). Using multiple regression analysis, Edwards showed that socioeconomic status, perceived health status, and social participation together explained 24% of the variance in LSIA scores (8). By contrast, Markides and Martin found that a self-rating health score, income, and education explained 50% of the variance on the LSIA scores for males and 40% for females (13).

Convergent validity has been studied extensively. Neugarten et al. reported a correlation of 0.55 between the LSIA and the fuller Life Satisfaction Rating Scale for 92 respondents aged 50 to 90 years and of 0.39 with a psychologist's clinical assessment of 51 respondents (1, p142). A separate study again compared the LSIA and the Rating Scale, reporting a virtually identical correlation of 0.56 (3, p467). Lohmann compared the LSIA with other indicators of life satisfaction administered to 259 elderly people (14). The scales included the LSIB, the LSIZ, the Philadelphia Geriatric Center Morale Scale, the Kutner Morale Scale, and a global life satisfaction rating: "How satisfied are you with your life?" The results of the analyses are shown in Table 5.2. The Kutner Morale Scale shares four items with the LSIB, which may account for their high correlation. The LSIZ correlated 0.74 with the Philadelphia Geriatric Center Morale Scale in a nursing-home sample (15, pS163). Stock and Okun reported correlations of 0.33 with the positive affect score on the Bradburn scale and of −0.39 with the negative affect score (6, Table 1). The LSIZ correlated −0.31 with the psychological dimension scores on the Sickness Impact Profile (15, pS163).

Because the LSI is based on a specified conceptual definition of life satisfaction, several studies have examined its factor structure empirically. Adams identified three interpretable factors from a sample of 508 community respondents. The results showed an important general factor (34% of the variance) reflecting mood tone. The second factor corresponded to the original concept of zest for life; the third reflected congruence between desired and achieved goals. The interpretation of a fourth factor was unclear, and two items did not fall on any factor (2). Liang concluded that three first-order factors (mood tone, zest, and congruence between hopes and reality) and one second-order factor (representing general subjective well-being) described the structure of the LSIA (16). The congruence factor was found to vary across age groups, while the other factors remained stable (17). Extensive exploratory and confirmatory factor analyses were carried out by Hoyt and Creech (N = 2,651) (18). The best model they identified was a three-factor solution that resembled Adams's results: congruence, mood tone, and optimism. Using multiple regression analyses, Knapp showed that different demographic and health variables predicted each factor score, thus confirming the multidimensional nature of the scale (19). Although the LSI does cover several dimensions, Adams, like Hoyt and Creech, stressed that

Table 5.2 Correlations of the LSIA with Other Scales

	LSIA	LSIB	LSIZ	Kutner	PGC	Global rating
LSIA	1.00					
LSIB	0.63	1.00				
LSIZ	0.94	0.64	1.00			
Kutner	0.65	0.88	0.67	1.00		
PGC	0.76	0.74	0.79	0.74	1.00	
Global rating	0.41	0.40	0.40	0.40	0.47	1.00

Adapted from Lohmann N. Correlations of life satisfaction, morale and adjustment measures. J Gerontol 1977;32:74, Table 1.

the empirical findings did not closely replicate the original conceptual formulation given by Neugarten and Havighurst (18, p115). The factor structure also seems to vary from sample to sample (20, 21).

Alternative Forms

An eight-item Life Satisfaction Index—Well-Being (LSIW) was derived from the LSIA and has been used in Britain. The eight items load on two factors with alpha coefficients of 0.65 and 0.41 (22, p649).

Reference Standards

Neugarten et al. obtained a mean LSIA score of 12.4 (SD, 4.4) (1, p142). Very similar results have been obtained by other users for the 20-item scale and two-point responses: 11.6, (3, p466), 12.5, (2, p470), and 12.1 (SD, 3.9) (11, p76). For the 18-item scale, using three-point responses, Harris reported mean scores of 26.7 for those 18 to 64 years (N = 1,457) and 24.4 for those over 65 years (N = 2,797) (4, p159).

Commentary

The Life Satisfaction Index has been extensively used and has several strengths, including reliability, strong correlations with other scales, and availability of reference standards. The consistency of the validity findings and, in particular, of the factor structure, is striking: many other scales reviewed in this book show much less consistency between replications of factorial studies.

Despite these strengths, there have been a number of critical reviews of the LSI from which several points emerge. The question of precisely what the scale does measure is open to debate. It is agreed that the scale does not fully reflect the subtleties implied in the five-component conceptual model of life satisfaction proposed by Neugarten and Havighurst. Hoyt and Creech were critical: their results "raise serious questions about the structure and interpretation of the measures in the LSIA" (18). Indeed, measurement techniques (such as the LSI) have not managed to reflect the conceptual distinctions that have been drawn between concepts such as quality of life, anomie, happiness, and morale (7, 23). Klemmack et al. noted, "Although the distinction between life satisfaction and social isolation may have some justification on theoretic grounds, there is no reason to anticipate, on the basis of our data, that the subtleties between the two concepts are reflected on an empirical level" (23, p270). The failure of the measurement methods to reflect the distinctions among these concepts is shown by Lohmann's findings of strong associations between the LSI and the morale scales, although both were only weakly associated with a global life satisfaction rating scale of the type used by Andrews. This is probably due to the multidimensional nature of scales like the LSI, which introduces another criticism of the scale. Neugarten and Havighurst proposed a single score, which appears to obscure the multidimensional nature of the scale. A more adequate scoring system should be developed. Finally, Connidis has criticized the wording of some of the items in the LSI, suggesting that the values implicit in the wording may lead some respondents to disagree with the item even though they were not dissatisfied (24).

Some commentators have attempted to modify Neugarten and Havighurst's conceptual formulation to bring it more into line with empirical evidence. Lieberman noted, "Life satisfaction, rather than being merely a reflection of a person's current level of goal achievement, is more like a set or orientation to one's environment which is acquired fairly early and remains moderately stable throughout life" (11, p75). Despite the conceptual uncertainties over the LSI and despite its age, we do not recommend discarding it in favor of other life satisfaction scales, most of which have been less thoroughly evaluated. Its psychometric properties rival those of the best among comparable indices; the task is to identify clearly what, in conceptual terms, the scale measures.

REFERENCES

(1) Neugarten BL, Havighurst RJ, Tobin SS. The measurement of life satisfaction. J Gerontol 1961;16:134–143.

(2) Adams DL. Analysis of a Life Satisfaction Index. J Gerontol 1969;24:470–474.

(3) Wood V, Wylie ML, Sheafor B. An analysis of a short self-report measure of life satisfaction: correlation with rater judgments. J Gerontol 1969;24:465–469.

(4) Harris L. The myth and reality of aging in America. Washington, DC: National Council on the Aging, 1975.

(5) Ray RO. The Life Satisfaction Index-Form A as applied to older adults: technical note on scoring patterns. J Am Geriatr Soc 1979;27:418–420.

(6) Stock WA, Okun MA. The construct validity of life satisfaction among the elderly. J Gerontol 1982;37:625–627.

(7) Dobson C, Powers EA, Keith PM, et al. Anomie, self-esteem, and life satisfaction: interrelationships among three scales of well-being. J Gerontol 1979;34:569–572.

(8) Edwards JN, Klemmack DL. Correlates of life satisfaction: a re-examination. J Gerontol 1973;28:479–502.

(9) Himmelfarb S, Murrell SA. Reliability and validity of five mental health scales in older persons. J Gerontol 1983;38:333–339.

(10) Burckhardt CS, Woods SL, Schultz AA, et al. Quality of life of adults with chronic illness: a psychometric study. Res Nurs Health 1989;12:347–354.

(11) Lieberman LR. Life satisfaction in the young and the old. Psychol Rep 1970;27:75–79.

(12) Cutler SJ. Voluntary association participation and life satisfaction: a cautionary research note. J Gerontol 1973;28:96–100.

(13) Markides L, Martin HW. A causal model of life satisfaction among the elderly. J Gerontol 1979;34:86–93.

(14) Lohmann N. Correlations of life satisfaction, morale and adjustment measures. J Gerontol 1977;32:73–75.

(15) Rothman ML, Hedrick S, Inui T. The Sickness Impact Profile as a measure of the health status of noncognitively impaired nursing home residents. Med Care 1989;27(suppl):S157–S167.

(16) Liang J. Dimensions of the Life Satisfaction Index A: a structural formulation. J Gerontol 1984;39:613–622.

(17) Liang J, Tran TV, Markides KS. Differences in the structure of Life Satisfaction Index in three generations of Mexican Americans. J Gerontol 1988;43:S1–S8.

(18) Hoyt DR, Creech JC. The Life Satisfaction Index: a methodological and theoretical critique. J Gerontol 1983;38:111–116.

(19) Knapp MRJ. Predicting the dimensions of life satisfaction. J Gerontol 1976;31:595–604.

(20) Wilson GA, Elias JW, Brownlee LJ Jr. Factor invariance and the Life Satisfaction Index. J Gerontol 1985;40:344–346.

(21) Cutler NE. Age variations in the dimensionality of life satisfaction. J Gerontol 1979;34:573–578.

(22) James O, Davies ADM, Ananthakopan S. The Life Satisfaction Index-Well-Being: its internal reliability and factorial composition. Br J Psychiatry 1986;149:647–650.

(23) Klemmack DL, Carlson JR, Edwards JN. Measures of well-being: an empirical and critical assessment. J Health Soc Behav 1974;15:267–270.

(24) Connidis I. The construct validity of the Life Satisfaction Index A and Affect Balance Scales: a serendipitous analysis. Soc Indicat Res 1984;15:117–129.

THE PHILADELPHIA GERIATRIC CENTER MORALE SCALE
(M. Powell Lawton, 1972)

Purpose

The Philadelphia Geriatric Center Morale Scale was designed to measure dimensions of emotional adjustment in persons aged 70 to 90. It is applicable both to community residents and to people in institutions.

Conceptual Basis

Lawton viewed morale as "a generalized feeling of well-being with diverse specific indicators" (1). The indicators of morale include "freedom from distressing symptoms, satisfaction with self, feeling of syntony between self and environment, and ability to strive appropriately while still accepting the inevitable" (1). The interrelationship among these components may or may not be close: a pessimistic ideology "may or may not accompany an ability to accept the status quo." Morale is viewed as a feeling that is not necessarily related to behavior; the relationship resembles that between attitudes and behavior (1).

The person of high morale has a feeling of having attained something in his life, of being useful now, and thinks of himself as an adequate person. . . . High morale also means a feeling that there is a place in the environment for oneself . . . a certain acceptance of what cannot be changed. (1, p148)

Description

The Morale Scale is one of a series of geriatric assessment scales developed by the Philadelphia Geriatric Center. Their Multi-level Assessment Instrument is described in Chapter 9. Others include the Mental Status Questionnaire, the Instrumental Role Maintenance Scale, and the Minimal Social Behavior Scale (2).

A preliminary version of the Morale Scale with 41 items was tested on 300 healthy people with an average age of 78 years. Twenty-two items that were significantly associated with an independent ranking of the respondents according to morale, and that also loaded on a factor analysis, were retained for the main version of the scale, shown in Exhibit 5.10. Lawton subsequently recommended a further abbreviation of the scale to 17 items, as indicated by asterisks in the exhibit (3). Most of the items have a dichotomous response; the method can be self- or interviewer-administered. Liang and Bollen suggested that scores be calculated to form three subscales (agitation, dissatisfaction, and atti-

Exhibit 5.10   The Philadelphia Geriatric Center Morale Scale

Note: Asterisks indicate the 17 items retained for the shortened version. Responses indicating satisfaction are shown on the right.

Item	Positive response
* 1. Things keep getting worse as I get older	no
* 2. I have as much pep as I did last year	yes
* 3. How much do you feel lonely? (not much, a lot)	not much
* 4. Little things bother me more this year	no
* 5. I see enough of my friends and relatives	yes
* 6. As you get older you are less useful	no
7. If you could live where you wanted, where would you live?	here
* 8. I sometimes worry so much that I can't sleep	no
* 9. As I get older, things are (better, worse, same) than/as I thought they would be	better
*10. I sometimes feel that life isn't worth living	no
*11. I am as happy now as I was when I was younger	yes
12. Most days I have plenty to do	no
*13. I have a lot to be sad about	no
14. People had it better in the old days	no
*15. I am afraid of a lot of things	no
16. My health is (good, not so good)	good
*17. I get mad more than I used to	no
*18. Life is hard for me most of the time	no
*19. How satisfied are you with your life today? (satisfied, not satisfied)	satisfied
*20. I take things hard	no
21. A person has to live for today and not worry about tomorrow	yes
*22. I get upset easily	no

Derived from Lawton MP. The dimensions of morale. In: Kent DP, Kastenbaum R, Sherwood S, eds. Research planning and action for the elderly: the power and potential of social science. New York: Behavioral Publications, 1972:152–153. Also from Lawton MP. The Philadelphia Geriatric Center Morale Scale: a revision. J Gerontol 1975;30:78, Table 1.

tudes toward one's own aging) and this has been widely followed; an overall score reflecting global life satisfaction can also be formed (4).

Reliability

Lawton studied reliability for several groups of respondents following varying delays. Test–retest correlations ranged from 0.91 after five weeks to 0.75 after three months (1, p150).

For 300 respondents a split-half reliability of 0.79 was obtained with the 22-item scale (1). The Kuder-Richardson internal consistency was 0.81. Internal consistency reliability for the three subscales ranged from 0.57 to 0.61 (5, p80).

Differences were found between Black and White respondents in the reliability of only two items: "I am afraid of a lot of things" and "Life is hard for me" (6, p427).

Validity

For 199 elderly subjects, the 22-item scale correlated 0.47 with an independent ranking of their morale. Because of the low reliability of the independent ranking, this result probably represents an underestimate of the validity of the scale. A correlation of 0.57 was obtained with the Life Satisfaction Index (LSI), applied by a psychologist (1, p151). The Morale Scale correlated 0.74 with the LSIZ in a mixed community and hospital sample (7, Table 1); a correlation of 0.74 was also obtained in a nursing-home sample; the correlation with the psychological dimension of the Sickness Impact Profile was −0.40 (8, pS163).

Much attention has been paid to the factor structure of the Morale Scale. From the replies of 300 subjects in Lawton's original study, six factors were extracted: surgency—a feeling of optimism and willingness to be involved; attitudes toward own aging; satisfaction with the status quo; anxiety; depression versus optimism; and loneliness and dissatisfaction (1). Test–retest reliability on the factor scores ranged

from 0.75 to 0.80. Morris and Sherwood examined the factorial structure in two samples of elderly and moderately handicapped patients (5). They obtained similar results from the two samples, but their findings differed from those of Lawton: satisfaction with the status quo and surgency were not replicated. Three factors (attitudes toward aging, agitation, and loneliness) were, however, present in all samples.

Morris and Sherwood factor analyzed an abbreviated version of the scale. Three factors were obtained with internal consistencies ranging from 0.62 to 0.76 (5, p81). Lawton replicated this analysis on 828 elderly community residents (3). Seventeen items formed three factors which were comparable to those obtained by Morris and Sherwood: agitation (six items), attitude toward one's own aging (five items), and lonely dissatisfaction (six items). They obtained alpha internal consistency coefficients of 0.85, 0.81, and 0.85, respectively (3, p87). Lawton recommended that these 17 items (indicated by asterisks in Exhibit 5.10) be referred to as the "Revised PGC Morale Scale," a conclusion supported by Morris and Sherwood (3).

Liang and Bollen analyzed the factor structure of the scale for a sample of 3,996 community elderly respondents. Using a structural equation modeling approach, they identified three first-order factors (agitation, dissatisfaction, and attitudes toward one's own aging) and one second-order factor (global life satisfaction), which linked the three first-order factors (4). They subsequently reported that this structure applied well to both males and females (9). The same three-factor structure was further replicated by McCulloch using a confirmatory factor analysis. The model did not hold constant over time, however (10, pP256). For a sample of 4,000 people aged 65 and older, Schooler factored a pool of morale-related items that included 21 of the original 22 items of the morale scale. The results "closely reproduced the three factors" obtained by Lawton (3). Liang et al. further showed that the three-factor solution applied in a Japanese study (11).

Commentary

The Philadelphia Geriatric Center Morale Scale appears a reliable and internally consistent scale that correlates strongly with the most comparable alternative, the Life Satisfaction Index. More data are, however, needed on the validity of the scale in terms of its prediction and correlation with other quality of life scales. Nevertheless, the consistency of results across several studies suggests that Lawton's scale offers a reliable measurement of a relatively stable concept.

As Lawton noted, the Morale Scale might benefit from the addition of more positive affect items (3). There is some divergence of opinion over the number of items to include: Morris and Sherwood and Liang and Bollen found that two questions (numbers 3 and 5 in Exhibit 5.10) were conceptually different from the rest of the scale and should be omitted, but Lawton recommends retaining them. Liang and Bollen reviewed the scale in some detail and provide a thoughtful discussion of the alternative ways of scoring and interpreting the instrument (4).

REFERENCES

(1) Lawton MP. The dimensions of morale. In: Kent DP, Kastenbaum R, Sherwood S, eds. Research planning and action for the elderly: the power and potential of social science. New York: Behavioral Publications, 1972:144–165.

(2) Lawton MP. Assessing the competence of older people. In: Kent DP, Kastenbaum R, Sherwood S, eds. Research planning and action for the elderly: the power and potential of social science. New York: Behavioral Publications, 1972:122–143.

(3) Lawton MP. The Philadelphia Geriatric Center Morale Scale: a revision. J Gerontol 1975;30:85–89.

(4) Liang J, Bollen KA. The structure of the Philadelphia Geriatric Center Morale Scale: a reinterpretation. J Gerontol 1983;38:181–189.

(5) Morris JN, Sherwood S. A retesting and modification of the Philadelphia Geriatric Center Morale Scale. J Gerontol 1975; 30:77–84.

(6) Liang J, Lawrence RH, Bollen KA. Race differences in factorial structures of two measures of subjective well-being. J Gerontol 1987;42:426–428.

(7) Kozma A, Stones MJ. Social desirability in measures of subjective well-being: a systematic evaluation. J Gerontol 1987;42:56–59.

(8) Rothman ML, Hedrick S, Inui T. The Sickness Impact Profile as a measure of health status of noncognitively impaired nursing home residents. Med Care 1989;27 (suppl):S157–S167.

(9) Liang J, Bollen KA. Sex differences in the structure of the Philadelphia Geriatric Center Morale Scale. J Gerontol 1985; 40:468–477.

(10) McCulloch BJ. A longitudinal investigation of the factor structure of subjective well-being: the case of the Philadelphia Geriatric Center Morale Scale. J Gerontol 1991;46:P251–P258.

(11) Liang J, Asano H, Bollen KA, et al. Cross-cultural comparability of the Philadelphia Geriatric Center Morale Scale: an American-Japanese comparison. J Gerontol 1987;42:37–43.

THE GENERAL WELL-BEING SCHEDULE
(Harold J. Dupuy, 1977)

Purpose

The General Well-Being Schedule (GWB) offers a brief but broad-ranging indicator of subjective feelings of psychological well-being and distress for use in community surveys.

Conceptual Basis

The only conceptual description of the content of the GWB is contained in an unpublished paper by Dupuy (1). Reflecting the theories of Kurt Lewin, the scale assesses how the individual feels about his "inner personal state," rather than about external conditions such as income, work environment, or neighborhood (1). The scale reflects both positive and negative feelings: six dimensions cover anxiety, depression, general health, positive well-being, self-control, and vitality.

Description

The GWB is a self-administered questionnaire that was developed for the U.S. Health and Nutrition Examination Survey (HANES I) (2). A draft instrument contained 68 items, 18 of which were used in the HANES study and form the usual set of questions referred to as the GWB. They are shown in Exhibit 5.11.

The GWB includes both positive and negative questions. Each item has the time frame "during the last month" and the first 14 questions use six-point response scales representing intensity or frequency. The ordinal qualities of these response options were checked empirically (1). The remaining four questions use 0-to-10 rating scales defined by adjectives at each end. In coding replies, the polarity of certain questions is reversed, so a low score represents more severe distress. Dupuy used a total score running from 0 to 110 and for this 14 is subtracted from the score derived from the codes shown in Exhibit 5.11. Dupuy proposed cutting points to represent three levels of disorder: scores of 0 to 60 reflect "severe distress," 61 to 72 "moderate distress," while 73 to 110 represent "positive well-being" (1). Six subscores may be formed as we show in Exhibit 5.12. Using the labels proposed by Brook et al. (3), the subscores measure anxiety, depression, positive well-being, self-control, vitality, and general health.

Reliability

Using the HANES data, Monk reported test–retest reliability coefficients (after three months) of 0.68 and 0.85 for "two different groups" (2, p183). Fazio reported a retest coefficient of 0.85 after three months for 195 college students (4, p10). Edwards et al. obtained a retest coefficient of 0.68 for 98 college graduates (5, Table 3).

The internal consistency of the GWB is very high: in Fazio's study the coefficients were 0.91 for 79 males and 0.95 for 116 females (4, p11). Himmelfarb and Murrell reported alpha coefficients of 0.88 in a community sample, and 0.92 in a clinical sample (6, Table 1). Ware et al. reviewed three other studies that reported internal consistency; all provided coefficients over 0.90 (7). The HANES data provided an internal consistency of 0.93 (N = 6,913) (1, p7). Fazio reported correlations among the subscores ranging from 0.16 to 0.72 (4, Table 6). Edwards et al. reported an alpha of 0.95 (5, Table 2).

Validity

There is considerable evidence for the correlational validity of the GWB. In Fazio's validation study, the GWB total score correlated 0.47 with an interviewer's rating of depression, 0.66 with Zung's Self-rating Depression Scale, and 0.78 with the Personal Feelings Inventory—Depression (4, Table B). The average correlation of the GWB and six independent depression scales was 0.69; the average correlation was 0.64 with three anxiety scales (4, p10). Simpkins and Burke obtained correlations of 0.70 with a ten-item depression score, 0.58 with the Lubin Depression Adjective Checklist, and 0.80 with Zung's Self-rating Depression Scale (7, Table 9; 8). Brook et al. reported correlations between the GWB subscales and reports of stress at home and at work ranging from 0.17 to 0.59 (3, Table 12).

Correlations between individual GWB subscales and criterion ratings were reported by Fazio (4) and by Ware et al. (7). In the main, such correlations were high, frequently falling between 0.65 and 0.90. Using an interviewer's rating as the criterion, Fazio noted that three short subscales of the GWB correlated with the criterion about as well or better than many longer scales (4, p8 and Table A). Correlations with use of services were summarized by Ware et al. and fell in the range of 0.09–0.48 (7, pp48–49). The draft version of the GWB contained a validation question: "Have you had severe enough personal, emotional, behavior or mental problems that you felt you needed help DURING

Exhibit 5.11 The General Well-Being Schedule

READ—This section of the examination contains questions about how you feel and how things have been going with you. For each question, mark (X) beside the answer which best applies to you.

1. How have you been feeling in general?
   (DURING THE PAST MONTH)

   1 ☐ In excellent spirits
   2 ☐ In very good spirits
   3 ☐ In good spirits mostly
   4 ☐ I have been up and down in spirits a lot
   5 ☐ In low spirits mostly
   6 ☐ In very low spirits

2. Have you been bothered by nervousness or your "nerves"? (DURING THE PAST MONTH)

   1 ☐ Extremely so—to the point where I could not work or take care of things
   2 ☐ Very much so
   3 ☐ Quite a bit
   4 ☐ Some—enough to bother me
   5 ☐ A little
   6 ☐ Not at all

3. Have you been in firm control of your behavior, thoughts, emotions, OR feelings? (DURING THE PAST MONTH)

   1 ☐ Yes, definitely so
   2 ☐ Yes, for the most part
   3 ☐ Generally so
   4 ☐ Not too well
   5 ☐ No, and I am somewhat disturbed
   6 ☐ No, and I am very disturbed

4. Have you felt so sad, discouraged, hopeless, or had so many problems that you wondered if anything was worthwhile? (DURING THE PAST MONTH)

   1 ☐ Extremely so—to the point that I have just about given up
   2 ☐ Very much so
   3 ☐ Quite a bit
   4 ☐ Some—enough to bother me
   5 ☐ A little bit
   6 ☐ Not at all

5. Have you been under or felt you were under any strain, stress, or pressure? (DURING THE PAST MONTH)

   1 ☐ Yes—almost more than I could bear or stand
   2 ☐ Yes—quite a bit of pressure
   3 ☐ Yes—some, more than usual
   4 ☐ Yes—some, but about usual
   5 ☐ Yes—a little
   6 ☐ Not at all

6. How happy, satisfied, or pleased have you been with your personal life? (DURING THE PAST MONTH)

   1 ☐ Extremely happy—could not have been more satisfied or pleased
   2 ☐ Very happy
   3 ☐ Fairly happy
   4 ☐ Satisfied—pleased
   5 ☐ Somewhat dissatisfied
   6 ☐ Very dissatisfied

7. Have you had any reason to wonder if you were losing your mind, or losing control over the way you act, talk, think, feel, or of your memory? (DURING THE PAST MONTH)

   1 ☐ Not at all
   2 ☐ Only a little
   3 ☐ Some—but not enough to be concerned or worried about
   4 ☐ Some and I have been a little concerned
   5 ☐ Some and I am quite concerned
   6 ☐ Yes, very much so and I am very concerned

8. Have you been anxious, worried, or upset? (DURING THE PAST MONTH)	1 ☐	Extremely so—to the point of being sick or almost sick
	2 ☐	Very much so
	3 ☐	Quite a bit
	4 ☐	Some—enough to bother me
	5 ☐	A little bit
	6 ☐	Not at all
9. Have you been waking up fresh and rested? (DURING THE PAST MONTH)	1 ☐	Every day
	2 ☐	Most every day
	3 ☐	Fairly often
	4 ☐	Less than half the time
	5 ☐	Rarely
	6 ☐	None of the time
10. Have you been bothered by any illness, bodily disorder, pains, or fears about your health? (DURING THE PAST MONTH)	1 ☐	All the time
	2 ☐	Most of the time
	3 ☐	A good bit of the time
	4 ☐	Some of the time
	5 ☐	A little of the time
	6 ☐	None of the time
11. Has your daily life been full of things that were interesting to you? (DURING THE PAST MONTH)	1 ☐	All the time
	2 ☐	Most of the time
	3 ☐	A good bit of the time
	4 ☐	Some of the time
	5 ☐	A little of the time
	6 ☐	None of the time
12. Have you felt down-hearted and blue? (DURING THE PAST MONTH)	1 ☐	All the time
	2 ☐	Most of the time
	3 ☐	A good bit of the time
	4 ☐	Some of the time
	5 ☐	A little of the time
	6 ☐	None of the time
13. Have you been feeling emotionally stable and sure of yourself? (DURING THE PAST MONTH)	1 ☐	All the time
	2 ☐	Most of the time
	3 ☐	A good bit of the time
	4 ☐	Some of the time
	5 ☐	A little of the time
	6 ☐	None of the time
14. Have you felt tired, worn out, used-up, or exhausted? (DURING THE PAST MONTH)	1 ☐	All the time
	2 ☐	Most of the time
	3 ☐	A good bit of the time
	4 ☐	Some of the time
	5 ☐	A little of the time
	6 ☐	None of the time

Exhibit 5.11   *(Continued)*

Exhibit 5.11   *(Continued)*

	For each of the four scales below, note that the words at each end of the 0 to 10 scale describe opposite feelings. Circle any number along the bar which seems closest to how you have generally felt DURING THE PAST MONTH
15. How concerned or worried about your HEALTH have you been? (DURING THE PAST MONTH)	0 1 2 3 4 5 6 7 8 9 10 Not concerned at all Very concerned
16. How RELAXED or TENSE have you been? (DURING THE PAST MONTH)	0 1 2 3 4 5 6 7 8 9 10 Very relaxed Very tense
17. How much ENERGY, PEP, VITALITY have you felt? (DURING THE PAST MONTH)	0 1 2 3 4 5 6 7 8 9 10 No energy AT ALL, listless Very ENERGETIC, dynamic
18. How DEPRESSED or CHEERFUL have you been? (DURING THE PAST MONTH)	0 1 2 3 4 5 6 7 8 9 10 Very depressed Very cheerful

Reproduced from Fazio AF. A concurrent validational study of the NCHS General Well-Being Schedule. Hyattsville, Maryland: U.S. Department of Health, Education and Welfare, National Center for Health Statistics, 1977:34–36. With permission.

THE PAST YEAR?" Dupuy showed a correlation of 0.53 between the GWB total score and this question (N = 2,007 from the HANES survey); Simpkins and Burke reported a correlation of 0.67 (8, Table 9).

Using the HANES data, Dupuy constructed a sociodemographic index (reflecting social class and size of household), a somatic index (which covered use of medications, self-report of symptoms of anxiety and a self-rating of general health), and a psychological problem index. The multiple correlation between the GWB overall score and the last two of these indices was 0.73 (1, p9). The GWB was only weakly related to sociodemographic status (r = 0.25), and this association disappeared when the so-

matic and the psychological problem indices were controlled (1). Fifty-five questions covering clinical symptoms and self-perceptions of health in the HANES study explained 31% of the variance in GWB scores (9).

Edwards et al. showed a significant contrast between psychiatric day patients and non-patient volunteers (5, Table 1). They also showed the GWB to be capable of detecting progress made by 21 psychiatric day patients following two weeks of treatment. Simpkins and Burke's comparison of community and psychiatric patient samples yielded a point biserial correlation of 0.56 with the GWB scores (8, p38).

From the HANES data, Wan and Livie-

Exhibit 5.12   The General Well-Being Schedule: Subscore
Labels and Question Topics

Subscore labels	Question topics
Anxiety	2. nervousness
	5. strain, stress, or pressure
	8. anxious, worried, upset
	16. relaxed, tense
Depression	4. sad, discouraged, hopeless
	12. down-hearted, blue
	18. depressed
Positive well-being	1. feeling in general
	6. happy, satisfied with life
	11. interesting daily life
Self-control	3. firm control of behavior, emotions
	7. afraid losing mind, or losing control
	13. emotionally stable, sure of self
Vitality	9. waking fresh, rested
	14. feeling tired, worn out
	17. energy level
General health	10. bothered by illness
	15. concerned, worried about health

ratos reported factor analyses of the GWB items, providing three factors that explained 51% of the variance (9, Table 2). The first factor included items suggesting anxiety, tension, and depression, and accounted for 18% of total variance. The second contained items on health and energy and the third comprised positive well-being or life satisfaction items.

In an interesting study, Stephens analyzed U.S. and Canadian survey data to show a significant association between mental well-being measured by the GWB and the level of physical activity, controlling for education, age, and physical health status (10).

Alternative Forms

The GWB items shown in Exhibit 5.11 were incorporated with modifications in the draft version of the Rand Mental Health Inventory and extensive scaling, reliability, and validity tests were carried out. The considerable overlap between the GWB and the draft Rand instrument (which they termed the HIS-GWB) has led us to include some of the Rand findings

here as suggestive of the quality of the GWB questions. The same 22 items were later termed the Psychological General Well-Being (PGWB) Index by Dupuy (11).

The validity of Dupuy's hypothesized grouping of items into six subscales was evaluated empirically on 1,209 respondents using multitrait and factor analyses (7). A six-factor solution provided results that agreed closely with the structure hypothesized by Dupuy, providing scores indicating anxiety, depression, self-control, positive well-being, general health, and vitality. Internal consistency coefficients for the six subscales ranged from 0.72 to 0.88 (7, Table 20; 11, Table II). One-week test–retest reliability estimates were made for the anxiety and positive well-being scales, and were 0.70 and 0.74, respectively (N = 437) (7, Table 20). Test–retest reliability declined to 0.50 when the interval exceeded one month (7, p77). Validity was examined by correlating GWB subscales and overall scores with 24 validating variables covering stress, recognition of mental problems, life satisfaction, and use of mental health care. Of 192 correlations, 158 were statistically significant at $p \leq 0.01$ in the hypothesized direction. The nonsignificant associations pertained to stressful life events, which occurred rarely in the sample under study (7, Table 22). Dupuy reported correlations between the PGWB and the Center for Epidemiologic Studies Depression Scale (−0.72), the Beck Depression Inventory (−0.68), the Zung index (−0.75), the Langner 22-item score (−0.77), and the Health Opinion Survey (−0.59) (11, Table III). Alpha reliability for the PGWB Index ranged from 0.90 to 0.94 in seven samples (11, Table VI). Fifteen of the GWB items were retained for use in the final version of the Rand Mental Health Inventory, which we describe in a separate review (7, p94; 12).

A ten-item version of the GWB has been developed, called the Psychological Mental Health Index (13). Four subscales are included: positive well-being (items 1 and 6 from Exhibit 5.11), depressed mood (items 4, 12), behavioral–emotional control (items 3, 7, and 13), and tension–anxiety (items 2, 5, and 8). Administered to chronic psychotic patients, a retest coefficient of 0.27 was obtained; internal consistency alpha scores ranged from 0.69 to 0.85. The item-total correlations were low, ranging from 0.38 to 0.64 (13, p233). The ten-item scale correlated 0.45 with a therapist-rated symptom score. In the light of these low coefficients, Ulin concluded that further research is needed to test this abbreviation of the GWB before it can be recommended for general use.

Reference Standards

Dupuy derived U.S. national reference standards from the HANES data (11, Table II). Seventy-one percent of the adult population fell into the "positive well-being" category (scores 73 to 110); 15.5% showed moderate distress (scores 61 to 72); and 13.5% were classified as experiencing "severe distress" (scores 0 to 60) (1, p10). About 60% of the population were both free of severe problems over the past year and in a state of positive well-being during the past month. Other reference figures are presented by Fazio (4, Table 1).

Commentary

The General Well-Being Schedule improves upon the older methods reviewed in this chapter in several respects. Like the Bradburn scale, it includes positive well-being but, reflecting a criticism of the Bradburn scale, it divides the positive questions into separate dimensions. It avoids reference to physical symptoms of emotional distress and so avoids the interpretation problems seen with the HOS and Langner scales. The available reliability and validity tests show extremely good results—the internal consistency is higher than for other scales and there is wide evidence of agreement with other, purpose-built depression and anxiety scales. A possible weakness in the performance of the scale was noted by Edwards et al., who showed that, while the internal consistency of the scale was excellent, the test–retest reliability was low (5). A measurement that contains fluctuations over time may be of little use in assessing individuals, although it may be adequate for groups.

Given the quality of the General Well-Being Schedule, it is unfortunate that so many of the validation studies remain unpublished. Analyses of the psychometric properties of the scale could be produced from the HANES data, for example. The most useful document summarizing the unpublished material is the Rand review by Ware et al. (7). Fazio's study indicated that the GWB performed as well as several other leading scales in assessing emotional distress in a student sample. He concluded: "the GWB emerged as the single most useful instrument in measuring depression" (4). Although Dupuy's description of the conceptual structure of the GWB is vague, the results of a large factor analytic study provided data that support the dimensions originally built into the scale. This consistency is rare indeed.

Some debate has arisen over the most useful way to score the GWB. The internal consistency of the 18 items is very high, so forming subscores may be redundant. Wan and Livieratos argued that the three factors obtained from the HANES data did not offer a suitable approach to scoring; inclusion of all 18 items in a single score may be the most appropriate method. Having very few items, subscales would inevitably provide only crude measurements; Fazio's results did, indeed, show lower internal consistency for the subscales than for the instrument as a whole.

Because of its outstanding reliability and validity results, we recommend that the General Well-Being Schedule be seriously considered for use where a general population indicator of subjective well-being is required. We know less about its adequacy as a case-detection instrument, for which the General Health Questionnaire is recommended.

REFERENCES

(1) Dupuy HJ. Self-representations of general psychological well-being of American adults. Paper presented at American Public Health Association Meeting, Los Angeles, October, 1978.

(2) Monk M. Blood pressure awareness and psychological well-being in the Health and Nutrition Examination Survey. Clin Invest Med 1981;4:183–189.

(3) Brook RH, Ware JE Jr, Davies-Avery A, et al. Overview of adult health status measures fielded in Rand's Health Insurance Study. Med Care 1979;17(suppl):1–131.

(4) Fazio AF. A concurrent validational study of the NCHS General Well-Being Schedule. Hyattsville, MD: U.S. Department of Health, Education and Welfare, National Center for Health Statistics, 1977. (Vital and Health Statistics Series 2, No. 73. DHEW Publication No. (HRA) 78–1347).

(5) Edwards DW, Yarvis RM, Mueller DP, et al. Test-taking and the stability of adjustment scales: can we assess patient deterioration? Evaluation Q 1978;2:275–291.

(6) Himmelfarb S, Murrell SA. Reliability and validity of five mental health scales in older persons. J Gerontol 1983;38:333–339.

(7) Ware JE Jr, Johnston SA, Davies-Avery A, et al. Conceptualization and measurement of health for adults in the Health Insurance Study. Vol. III. Mental health. Santa Mon-

ica, California: Rand Corporation, 1979. (Publication No. R-1987/3-HEW).

(8) Simpkins C, Burke FF. Comparative analyses of the NCHS General Well-Being Schedule: response distributions, community vs. patient status discriminations, and content relationships. Nashville, Tennessee: Center for Community Studies, George Peabody College, 1974. (Contract No. HRA 106–74–13).

(9) Wan TTH, Livieratos B. A validation of the General Well-Being Index: a two-stage multivariate approach. Paper presented at American Public Health Association Meeting, Washington, DC, November 1977.

(10) Stephens T. Physical activity and mental health in the United States and Canada: evidence from four population surveys. Prev Med 1988;17:35–47.

(11) Dupuy HJ. The Psychological General Well-Being (PGWB) Index. In: Wenger NK, Mattson ME, Furberg CD, Elinson J, eds. Assessment of quality of life in clinical trials of cardiovascular therapies. New York: LeJacq, 1984:170–183.

(12) Veit CT, Ware JE Jr. The structure of psychological distress and well-being in general populations. J Consult Clin Psychol 1983;51:730–742.

(13) Ulin PR. Measuring adjustment in chronically ill clients in community mental health care: an assessment of the Psychological Mental Health Index. Nurs Res 1981;30:229–235.

THE RAND MENTAL HEALTH INVENTORY
(Rand Corporation and John E. Ware, 1979)

Purpose

The Rand Mental Health Inventory (MHI) measures mental health in terms of psychological distress and well-being, focusing on affective states (1, p105). It was developed for use in population surveys.

Conceptual Basis

Veit and Ware discussed the limitations of early screening tests such as the HOS and the Langner scale. Because of their physical orientation, such methods may not be able to distinguish changes in mental health from changes in physical health, and many of the symptoms they include are rarely encountered in the general population (2). Veit and Ware noted:

a substantial proportion of people in a general population rarely or never report occurrences of even the most prevalent psychological distress symptoms. To increase measurement precision, it may be necessary to extend the definition of mental health ... to include characteristics of psychological well-being (e.g., feeling cheerful, interest in and enjoyment of life). Psychological well-being items have the potential to improve the precision of mental health measurement by distinguishing among persons who receive perfect scores on measures of psychological distress. (2, p730)

As well as being developed as a screening instrument, the MHI was also used to examine the structure of mental health: are distress and positive well-being separate dimensions (as argued by Bradburn), and are these concepts themselves multidimensional, implying that they should be further subdivided (2)? To develop an instrument that could reflect the multidimensional nature of psychological well-being, Ware et al. incorporated four factors hypothesized by Dupuy—anxiety, depression, loss of behavioral/emotional control, and general positive affect—and added a fifth factor, emotional ties, to form the basis for the MHI (2). The behavioral control dimension covers emotional stability and control of behavior or thoughts and feelings, including fear of losing one's mind. A fuller discussion of the relationships among these constructs is given by Stewart et al. (1, pp106–107).

Description

The MHI formed the primary mental health measurement in the Rand Health Insurance Experiment. It focuses on mood and symptoms of anxiety and of loss of control over feelings, thoughts, and behavior (3). The MHI used 15 items from Dupuy's General Well-Being Schedule: the GWB items covering general health and vitality were discarded because they failed discriminant tests of validity (2). Twenty items were drawn from other scales to cover anxiety, depression, general positive

affect, and loss of behavioral or emotional control; three items were written to cover the fifth hypothesized factor, emotional ties. To these 38 items, another eight may be added to assess a socially desirable response set (3). Details of the development of the MHI and the origin of the questions are given in several sources (1–3). The questions and response scales are shown in Exhibit 5.13 along with the factor placement of each item. The MHI is self-administered and items refer to the past month. Most of the response scales have six options. To ensure comparability, the response options were kept close to those used in the questionnaires from which the items were originally drawn.

As well as an overall score known as the Mental Health Index, subscores are available for psychological distress and psychological well-being (see the final column of Exhibit 5.13). Three distress scores include anxiety, depression, and loss of behavioral or emotional control; two well-being scores represent general positive affect and emotional ties (1, p105). The subscales can be scored and interpreted separately or scores can be aggregated into the overall Mental Health Index (2). When combining all the scores it is necessary to reverse the scoring of the positive section. This may be done by subtracting the raw score from 67.

Reliability

The MHI was tested on a representative population sample of 5,089 respondents in the Rand Health Insurance Experiment. One-year test–retest results were based on 3,525 respondents, and coefficients ranged from 0.56 (for the depression scale) to 0.63 (for anxiety). Test–retest reliability of the overall score was 0.64 (2). Internal consistency coefficients ranged from 0.83 to 0.92 for the five scales; the coefficient was 0.96 for the overall score (2, Table 6).

Validity

Veit and Ware presented an extensive discussion of the factorial structure of the MHI, from which they derived a hierarchi-

Exhibit 5.13 The Rand Mental Health Inventory, Showing Response Scales and Factor Placement of Each Item

Note: The answer scales vary from question to question and are shown at the foot of the table. Letters to the right of each question indicate the response scale that is applicable: T refers to the answer scale indicating time or frequency, AN indicates the scale running from always to never, and U indicates a unique answer category. The factor placement of each item is shown in the right-hand column: Anx = anxiety, Dep = depression, Behave = behavioral/emotional control, Pos = general positive affect and Emotion = emotional ties.

Question	Response scale	Factor
How happy, satisfied, or pleased have you been with your personal life during the past month?	U1	Pos
How much of the time have you felt lonely during the past month?	T	Emotion
How often did you become nervous or jumpy when faced with excitement or unexpected situations during the past month?	AN	Anx
During the past month, how much of the time have you felt that the future looks hopeful and promising?	T	Pos
How much of the time, during the past month, has your daily life been full of things that were interesting to you?	T	Pos
How much of the time, during the past month, did you feel relaxed and free of tension?	T	Pos
During the past month, how much of the time have you generally enjoyed the things you do?	T	Pos
During the past month, have you had any reason to wonder if you were losing your mind, or losing control over the way you act, talk, think, feel, or of your memory?	U2	Behav
Did you feel depressed during the past month?	U3	Dep
During the past month, how much of the time have you felt loved and wanted?	T	Emotion
How much of the time, during the past month, have you been a very nervous person?	T	Anx
When you got up in the morning, this past month, about how often did you expect to have an interesting day?	AN	Pos
During the past month, how much of the time have you felt tense or "high-strung"?	T	Anx
During the past month, have you been in firm control of your behavior, thoughts, emotions, feelings?	U4	Behav
During the past month, how often did your hands shake when you tried to do something?	AN	Anx
During the past month, how often did you feel that you had nothing to look forward to?	AN	Behav
How much of the time, during the past month, have you felt calm and peaceful?	T	Pos
How much of the time, during the past month, have you felt emotionally stable?	T	Behav
How much of the time, during the past month, have you felt downhearted and blue?	T	Dep
How often have you felt like crying, during the past month?	AN	Behav
During the past month, how often did you feel that others would be better off if you were dead?	AN	Behav
How much of the time, during the past month, were you able to relax without difficulty?	T	Anx
During the past month, how much of the time did you feel that your love relationships, loving and being loved, were full and complete?	T	Emotion
How often, during the past month, did you feel that nothing turned out for you the way you wanted it to?	AN	Behav

Exhibit 5.13 *(Continued)*

215

Exhibit 5.13 *(Continued)*

Question	Response scale	Factor
How much have you been bothered by nervousness, or your "nerves," during the past month?	U5	Anx
During the past month, how much of the time has living been a wonderful adventure for you?	T	Pos
How often, during the past month, have you felt so down in the dumps that nothing could cheer you up?	AN	Behav
During the past month, did you ever think about taking your own life?	U6	Behav
During the past month, how much of the time have you felt restless, fidgety, or impatient?	T	Anx
During the past month, how much of the time have you been moody or brooded about things?	T	Dep
How much of the time, during the past month, have you felt cheerful, lighthearted?	T	Pos
During the past month, how often did you get rattled, upset, or flustered?	AN	Anx
During the past month, have you been anxious or worried?	U7	Anx
During the past month, how much of the time were you a happy person?	T	Pos
How often during the past month did you find yourself having difficulty trying to calm down?	AN	Anx
During the past month, how much of the time have you been in a low or very low spirits?	T	Dep
How often, during the past month, have you been waking up feeling fresh and rested?	U8	Pos
During the past month, have you been under or felt you were under any strain, stress, or pressure?	U9	Dep

Response scales and scores:

T

(1)	All of the time	(4)	Some of the time
(2)	Most of the time	(5)	A little of the time
(3)	A good bit of the time	(6)	None of the time

AN

(1)	Always	(4)	Sometimes
(2)	Very often	(5)	Almost never
(3)	Fairly often	(6)	Never

U1

(1) Extremely happy, could not have been more satisfied or pleased
(2) Very happy most of the time
(3) Generally satisfied, pleased
(4) Sometimes fairly satisfied, sometimes fairly unhappy
(5) Generally dissatisfied, unhappy
(6) Very dissatisfied, unhappy most of the time

U2

(1) No, not at all
(2) Maybe a little
(3) Yes, but not enough to be concerned or worried about it
(4) Yes, and I have been a little concerned
(5) Yes, and I am quite concerned
(6) Yes, and I am very much concerned about it

U3

(1) Yes, to the point that I did not care about anything for days at a time
(2) Yes, very depressed almost every day

U4

(3) Yes, quite depressed several times
(4) Yes, a little depressed now and then
(5) No, never felt depressed at all

U4

(1) Yes, very definitely
(2) Yes, for the most part
(3) Yes, I guess so
(4) No, not too well
(5) No, and I am somewhat disturbed
(6) No, and I am very disturbed

U5

(1) Extremely so, to the point where I could not take care of things
(2) Very much bothered
(3) Bothered quite a bit by nerves
(4) Bothered some, enough to notice
(5) Bothered just a little by nerves
(6) Not bothered at all by this

U6

(1) Yes, very often
(2) Yes, fairly often
(3) Yes, a couple of times
(4) Yes, at one time
(5) No, never

U7

(1) Yes, extremely so, to the point of being sick or almost sick
(2) Yes, very much so
(3) Yes, quite a bit
(4) Yes, some, enough to bother me
(5) Yes, a little bit
(6) No, not at all

U8

(1) Always, every day
(2) Almost every day
(3) Most days
(4) Some days, but usually not
(5) Hardly ever
(6) Never wake up feeling rested

U9

(1) Yes, almost more than I could stand or bear
(2) Yes, quite a bit of pressure
(3) Yes, some, more than usual
(4) Yes, some, about normal
(5) Yes, a little bit
(6) No, not at all

Adapted from Veit CT, Ware JE Jr.. The structure of psychological distress and well-being in general populations. J Consult clin Psychol 1983;51:733,Table 1. Also from Ware JE Jr. Johnston SA, Davies-Avery A, Brook RH. Conceptualization and measurement of health for adults in the Health Insurance Study: Vol. III, Mental Health. Santa Monica, California: Rand Corporation, 1979, Table 27 and Appendix E.

cal model of the structure of the scores it provides. The items were found to fall into the five factors indicated in Exhibit 5.13. Correlations among the factors ranged from −0.39 to 0.77 and the five factors were, in turn, grouped into two higher-order factors termed psychological distress (incorporating the negative items) and psychological well-being. These factors correlated −0.75 and may be regarded as forming a bipolar distress versus well-being measurement of general mental health. This result supported the multidimensional model of emotional well-being that was hypothesized, although a strong general factor underlies the instrument (2).

Ware et al. showed a strong association between MHI scores and the use of ambulatory mental health services in a prospective study (2, 4). The results lent added support to the inclusion of items covering positive psychological well-being. Correlations between the MHI and criterion measurements are shown by Ware et al. (5). The correlations between the various sections of the MHI and a life events scale ranged from 0.12 to 0.26; correlations with life satisfaction ran from 0.40 to 0.51, and correlations with an indicator of severe emotional problems ranged from 0.48 to 0.58 (5, Table 4).

Alternative Forms

As with all of the Rand measurements, several abbreviated forms of the MHI have been developed. We list a select few of these, reassuring readers that there are yet others; fuller details are given by Stewart et al. (1, Table 7-2).

A five-item version (the MHI5) is quite widely used (6, 7). The items are introduced by the question, "How much of the time, during the last month, have you . . ."

1. ". . . been a very nervous person?"
2. ". . . felt calm and peaceful?"
3. ". . . felt downhearted and blue?"
4. ". . . been a happy person?"
5. ". . . felt so down in the dumps that nothing could cheer you up?"

The first four items use the "T" response scale shown at the foot of Exhibit 5.13 while the fifth uses scale "AN." The MHI5 was subsequently incorporated into the Short-Form-20 and -36 instruments described in Chapter 9. Item-total correlations ranged from 0.54 to 0.81; alpha was 0.90 in one study and 0.86 in another (1, pp128, 134).

An 18-item version of the MHI was developed for telephone administration. It contained at least four items from the anxiety, depression, behavioral control, and positive affect subscales of the MHI, including the five items listed above (1,

p110). Berwick et al. compared the MHI5 and the MHI18, the 30-item General Health Questionnaire (GHQ), and a 28-item Somatic Symptom Inventory (SSI) against a criterion diagnosis using the Diagnostic Interview Schedule (DIS) (6, 7). The MHI5 performed almost as well as the 18-item MHI in detecting any DIS disorder, with areas under the ROC curve of 0.79 and 0.80, respectively (6, Table 1). The GHQ performed slightly less well (0.77), and the SSI was the least accurate (0.71) (6, Figure 1). In detecting depressive symptoms, the two versions of the MHI performed as well as the GHQ, while the SSI was again less successful. The item on feeling downhearted and blue detected nearly three-quarters of the DIS disorders, with only a 5% false-positive rate, forming "a powerful nonspecific detector for all of the five diagnostic clusters" (6, p173). In a separate analysis, the MHI performed better than the GHQ, showing an AUC of 0.76 for the MHI and 0.68 for the GHQ (7, Table 3).

Some subsequent versions of the MHI18 omit the question on ability to relax without difficulty, making a 17-item version (1, Table 7-2). This has an internal consistency between 0.94 and 0.96 in different samples (1, Table 7-13).

A new, revised version of the MHI was created for use in the Medical Outcomes Study. This contained 33 items, of which 24 are identical to items in the 38-item MHI described here and six others contain slight variations in wording or response categories (1, Table 7-2). This was tested, along with the MHI5 and MHI17, in various parts of the Medical Outcomes Study. Item-total correlations ranged from 0.50 to 0.87 (1, p128).

A validation of a Chinese version of the MHI has been reported (8).

Reference Standards

Veit and Ware presented mean scores for each section of the MHI, although these figures are based on slightly different numbers of items from those shown in Exhibit 5.13 (2, Table 6).

Commentary

The MHI and its derivatives have been used in several large studies and to predict service use (2). The inventory incorporates the most adequate questions from some of the leading mental health scales; it has been carefully constructed and appears to have been used without alterations to the wording of the questions. The MHI deliberately focused on affective indicators of well-being and therefore avoided the problems that beset the earlier scales such as the HOS and the Langner scale.

Stewart et al. provide an insightful discussion of the relative merits of the various abbreviations of the MHI and of the concepts the scales assess (1, p139–141). They also mention the possible problem of response bias whereby some people underreport distress and others overreport. It did not prove feasible to create a balanced set of positively and negatively worded items for the MHI (1, p141).

The MHI should be seriously considered as an alternative to the General Well-Being Schedule in general population surveys because more published material is available and because it has extended the scope of Dupuy's scale. A direct comparison of the sensitivity and specificity of the two methods would be beneficial. The abbreviated forms of the scale perform well, at least when presented as overall scores. The stability of the subscores from the abbreviated instruments may be limited, however. The success of the single question on feeling downhearted and blue is remarkable and commends it as an option when a single-item screen for mental distress is required. As Berwick et al. noted, the "downhearted and blue" question identified nearly three quarters of those with any disorder in a primary care population, with a false-positive rate of only 5% (6, p175). The strength of single screening items supports the approach of the Dartmouth COOP Charts described in Chapter 9; these non-specific items seem to act as flags for a wide range of psychological distress in primary care populations.

REFERENCES

(1) Stewart AL, Ware JE Jr, Sherbourne CD, et al. Psychological distress/well-being and cognitive functioning measures. In: Stewart AL, Ware JE Jr, eds. Measuring functioning and well-being: the Medical Outcomes Study approach. Durham, North Carolina: Duke University Press, 1992:102–142.

(2) Veit CT, Ware JE Jr. The structure of psychological distress and well-being in general populations. J Consult Clin Psychol 1983;51:730–742.

(3) Ware JE Jr, Johnston SA, Davies-Avery A, et al. Conceptualization and measurement of health for adults in the Health Insurance Study. Vol. III. Mental health. Santa Monica, California: Rand Corporation, 1979. (Publication No. R-1987/3-HEW).

(4) Ware JE Jr, Manning WG Jr, Duan N, et al. Health status and the use of ambulatory mental health services. Am Psychol 1984;39:1090–1100.

(5) Ware JE Jr, Davies-Avery A, Brook RH. Conceptualization and measurement of health for adults in the Health Insurance Study: Vol. VI. Analysis of relationships among health status measures. Santa Monica, California: Rand Corporation, 1980. (Publication No. R-1987/6-HEW).

(6) Berwick DM, Murphy JM, Goldman PA, et al. Performance of a five-item mental health screening test. Med Care 1991;29:169–176.

(7) Weinstein MC, Berwick DM, Goldman PA, et al. A comparison of three psychiatric screening tests using receiver operating characteristic (ROC) analysis. Med Care 1989;27:593–607.

(8) Liang J, Wu SC, Krause NM, et al. The structure of the Mental Health Inventory among Chinese in Taiwan. Med Care 1992;30:659–676.

THE HEALTH PERCEPTIONS QUESTIONNAIRE
(John E. Ware, 1976)

Purpose

The Health Perceptions Questionnaire (HPQ) is a self-report instrument that records perceptions of past, present, and future health, resistance to illness, and attitudes toward sickness (1). It is a survey instrument that has been used as an outcome measurement in the Rand Health Insurance Experiment (HIE) and as a predictor of use of care (2).

Conceptual Basis

"Health perceptions are personal beliefs and evaluations of general health status" and refer to whether people see themselves as well or unwell (3, p143). This is a subjective concept and perceptions may reflect a person's feelings and beliefs more than her actual physical health. Ware et al. wrote:

measures of general health perceptions differ from other health status measures in that they do not specify one or more components of health (physical, mental, or social). Rather, respondents are asked only for an assessment of their "health." In theory, this difference in measurement strategy makes it possible to achieve two important goals. First, general health ratings may constitute one kind of overall health status index if respondents consider all health components when they make their ratings. Second, general health ratings may reflect the objective information people have about their health status as well as their evaluation of that information and may, thereby, help solve the problem of aggregating the two kinds of health status data. (4, page v)

This is relevant because subjective perceptions of health, rather than objective measures of health status, predict utilization of care; health perceptions fit within the conceptual framework of the Health Belief Model which seeks to explain health behavior (3, p144). Whereas previous measurements of health perceptions had generally used single items, the Rand group developed a multi-item scale to test hypothesized dimensions of the overall concept (5).

Description

The HPQ contains the 33 items shown in Exhibit 5.14. The questions were originally tested for the Rand Health Insurance Experiment; further items did not satisfy scaling criteria and were discarded (6, Table 1). The items form six subscales: current health (nine items), prior health (three items), health outlook (four items), resistance to illness (four items), health worry/

concern (five items), and sickness orientation (two items). The items comprising each are indicated in the right-hand column of Exhibit 5.14. The 22 items used in forming an overall General Health Rating Index (GHRI) are also identified. Six items are not used in the subscales; these cover rejection of the sick role and attitudes toward going to the doctor (7). Where an indication of general health is required but space does not permit fielding the 22-item GHRI, either the nine items forming the current health subscale can be used or a four-item version can be used which includes items I, Q, V, and Z (7, p103). The questions use five-point, Likert-type responses and the full instrument is self-administered in seven to 11 minutes (8).

Scores are calculated for each of the six subscales and an overall score is derived for the General Health Rating Index. It is first necessary to reverse the scores on several items. For each scale a higher score represents more of the quality implied in the title of the scale; two subscales (health worry and sickness orientation) are negative in theme. Scores for the following items are therefore reversed by subtracting the response from 6: items C, E, F, I, K, L, R, T, Z, CC, and DD. The score for question 6 is also reversed by subtracting it from 5. Ware et al. handled missing data for individual items by substituting the mean score on the remaining items of that scale, after the appropriate item scores have been reversed (7, p227). Subscores are then calculated by summing response codes for the items identified in the exhibit. Because item-total correlations are similar, differential weights are not used in computing these scores (9). Raw subscale scores and the GHRI may be transformed to a 0 to 100 scale. The formula is:

Transformed score = [(Actual raw score − Lowest possible raw score) / (Highest possible raw score − Lowest possible raw score)] × 100

Full details of scoring are given by Davies et al. (7).

Exhibit 5.14 The Health Perceptions Questionnaire, Showing the Items Included in Each Subscore

Note: In copy given to respondent, the two columns on the right are omitted.

Please read each of the following statements, and then circle one of the numbers on each line to indicate whether the statement is true or false for you.

There are no right or wrong answers.
    If a statement is definitely true for you, circle 5.
    If it is mostly true for you, circle 4.
    If you don't know whether it is true or false, circle 3.
    If it is mostly false for you, circle 2.
    If it is definitely false for you, circle 1.

Some of the statements may look or seem like others. But each statement is different, and should be rated by itself.

		Definitely true	Mostly true	Don't know	Mostly false	Definitely false	GHRI	Subscale*
A.	According to the doctors I've seen, my health is now excellent	5	4	3	2	1	•	CH
B.	I try to avoid letting illness interfere with my life	5	4	3	2	1		
C.	I seem to get sick a little easier than other people	5	4	3	2	1	•	RI
D.	I feel better now than I ever have before	5	4	3	2	1	•	CH
E.	I will probably be sick a lot in the future	5	4	3	2	1	•	HO
F.	I never worry about my health	5	4	3	2	1	•	HW
G.	Most people get sick a little easier than I do	5	4	3	2	1	•	RI
H.	I don't like to go to the doctor	5	4	3	2	1		
I.	I am somewhat ill	5	4	3	2	1	•	CH
J.	In the future, I expect to have better health than other people I know	5	4	3	2	1	•	HO
K.	I was so sick once I thought I might die	5	4	3	2	1	•	PH
L.	I'm not as healthy now as I used to be	5	4	3	2	1	•	CH
M.	I worry about my health more than other people worry about their health	5	4	3	2	1	•	HW

Exhibit 5.14 *(Continued)*

Exhibit 5.14 *(Continued)*

		Definitely true	Mostly true	Don't know	Mostly false	Definitely false	GHRI	Subscale*
N.	When I'm sick, I try to just keep going as usual	5	4	3	2	1		
O.	My body seems to resist illness very well	5	4	3	2	1	•	RI
P.	Getting sick once in a while is a part of my life	5	4	3	2	1		SO
Q.	I'm as healthy as anybody I know	5	4	3	2	1	•	CH
R.	I think my health will be worse in the future than it is now	5	4	3	2	1	•	HO
S.	I've never had an illness that lasted a long period of time	5	4	3	2	1	•	PH
T.	Others seem more concerned about their health than I am about mine	5	4	3	2	1		HW
U.	When I'm sick, I try to keep it to myself	5	4	3	2	1		
V.	My health is excellent	5	4	3	2	1	•	CH
W.	I expect to have a very healthy life	5	4	3	2	1	•	HO
X.	My health is a concern to my life	5	4	3	2	1		HW
Y.	I accept that sometimes I'm just going to be sick	5	4	3	2	1		SO
Z.	I have been feeling bad lately	5	4	3	2	1	•	CH
AA.	It doesn't bother me to go to a doctor	5	4	3	2	1		
BB.	I have never been seriously ill	5	4	3	2	1	•	PH
CC.	When there is something going around, I usually catch it	5	4	3	2	1	•	RI
DD.	Doctors say that I am now in poor health	5	4	3	2	1	•	CH
EE.	When I think I am getting sick, I fight it	5	4	3	2	1		
FF.	I feel about as good now as I ever have	5	4	3	2	1	•	CH

During the *past 3 months,* how much has your health worried or concerned you?

(circle one)   HW

A great deal 1
Somewhat 2
A little 3
Not at all 4

*Subscale labels: CH = Current Health; PH = Prior Health; HO = Health Outlook; RI = Resistance to Illness; HW = Health Worry/Concern; SO = Sickness Orientation

Derived from Davies AR, Sherbourne CD, Peterson JR, Ware JE Jr. Scoring manual: adult health status and patient satisfaction measures used in Rand's Health Insurance Experiment. Santa Monica, California: Rand Corporation, 1988: Figures 5.1 and 5.2.

Reliability

Reliability figures for the subscales are available from several sources. There are extensive data on internal consistency and test–retest reliability from several large population samples. Typical results are summarized in Table 5.3. The first column shows median alpha coefficients from four field tests (total N ≈ 2000) (4, p42; 6, Table 4). The second column gives alpha coefficients reported by Davies et al., using data from the main Health Insurance Experiment. The final column gives one-year test–retest figures, drawn from the Seattle center of the HIE (7, p107).

Reliability results were slightly lower in low socioeconomic status groups, among those with less education and among older people (4, p43; 7, p97), but remain adequate for group comparisons.

Test–retest reliability figures for the GHRI at intervals of one, two, and three years for adults in HIE were 0.66, 0.59, and 0.56 (1, p185).

Validity

The HPQ was designed to measure six postulated aspects of health perceptions. Factor analyses of data from the preliminary field tests confirmed the existence of six main factors and indicated that each scale contributed some unique information about health perceptions (6). Furthermore, the results were similar across different samples. The resistance to illness subscale showed the least clear separation, and a higher-order factor analysis which factor analyzed the scale scores rather than the individual items showed that it overlapped with several other factors (4, p49).

Ware and others have presented numerous correlations between the subscales and

Table 5.3 Reliability of Health Perceptions Questionnaire Scales

Scale	Alpha		One-year stability (N = 1,200)
	(N = 1,790)	(N = 4,700)	
Current health (9 items)	0.91	0.88	0.58
Current health (4 items)	(NA)	0.81	(NA)
Prior health	0.73	0.65	0.67
Health outlook	0.75	0.73	0.59
Resistance to illness	0.71	0.70	0.65
Health worry/concern	0.60	0.64	0.50
Sickness orientation	0.59	0.53	0.55
General Health Rating Index	(NA)	0.89	0.67

criterion variables such as disability days, number of chronic problems, pain level, and psychological well-being (4; 6, Tables 6–8; 9, pp49–60). The great majority of coefficients were as hypothesized; for example, current health and prior health showed significant positive relationships with variables defining favorable health states, and negative relationships with variables defining poor health. Coefficients typically fell in the range of 0.30 to 0.60 (4, p52). Correlations with health behavior variables (such as number of doctor visits, hospitalizations) were lower than those with health status variables. Associations between age and health perceptions are generally negative, while greater income and higher education are generally positively correlated with general health perceptions (5, p48). Connelly et al. controlled for differences in level of physical health and found significant associations between health perceptions scores and anxiety, depression, worry, and utilization behaviors such as numbers of physician visits and telephone calls to the physician (10). Indeed, 5% of office visits were attributed to poor health perceptions alone, in the absence of any medical indication for the visit (10, pS107).

The GHRI correlated 0.46 with the Quality of Well-Being Scale (QWB) and 0.52 with the Sickness Impact Profile (SIP) (8, Table 4). Convergent validity correlations suggest that the GHRI offers a general indicator of self-perceived health that shows relatively weak associations with more objective indicators. Scores on the GHRI correlated 0.71 with the question, "How would you rate your overall health: excellent, good, fair or poor?" The equivalent correlations for the QWB and the SIP were lower, at 0.43 and 0.51 (8, Table 4). Conversely, the QWB and SIP showed generally stronger correlations with other indicators, such as numbers of health problems recorded in the patient's chart, utilization of care, level of disability, a mental health indicator, and employment status, than did the GHRI (8, Table 5).

Alternative Forms

A modified version of the HPQ was developed for the Medical Outcomes Study and is described by Stewart et al. (3, Table 8-8). This contains 36 items that cover the same dimensions as the original scale, except that sickness orientation was replaced by a health distress scale, and a new energy/fatigue scale was developed.

A general health perceptions measurement for children has been described by Eisen et al. (11). Seven questions cover current health, resistance to illness, and prior health.

Reference Standards

Means, standard deviations, and complete frequency tables are available for each subscale and for the overall GHRI from Appendix A of the manual by Davies et al. (7, pp184–194).

Commentary

The HPQ is an important extension of the previously used, single-item measures with the format, "How would you rate your health today: good, fair, or poor?" It was carefully developed and has been widely tested in large, national studies. For example, Davies and Ware report on an experiment that studied the effect of altering the sequence of questions; this may seem unremarkable but the study involved three different testing sites and over 2,800 respondents (9, p41).

Evidence for reliability and validity is promising. The hypothesized subscores are largely supported by empirical evidence and, while all six scales are related positively, the correlations among them are low enough to suggest that they tap separate dimensions (5, p35). The high stability over time suggests that it may be more suitable as a trait indicator than as an outcome measure that is sensitive to changes. The correlation of 0.71 with an overall self-rating question both confirms the general nature of the GHRI and suggests that the single question may offer an effective alternative. Most of the concurrent validity correlations were drawn from survey measurements of disability or health care utilization; it would be valuable to see correlations between the HPQ subscales and other, established health indices.

REFERENCES

(1) Ware JE Jr. General health rating index. In: Wenger NK, Mattson ME, Furberg CD, Elinson J, eds. Assessment of quality of life in clinical trials for cardiovascular therapies. New York: LeJacq, 1984:184–188.
(2) Ware JE Jr, Manning WG Jr, Duan N, et al. Health status and the use of ambulatory mental health services. Am Psychol 1984;39:1090–1100.
(3) Stewart AL, Hays RD, Ware JE Jr. Health perceptions, energy/fatigue, and health distress measures. In: Stewart AL, Ware JE Jr, eds. Measuring functioning and well-being: the Medical Outcomes Study approach. Durham, North Carolina: Duke University Press, 1992:143–172.
(4) Ware JE Jr, Davies-Avery A, Donald CA. Conceptualization and measurement of health for adults in the Health Insurance Study: Vol. V. General health perceptions. Santa Monica, California: Rand Corporation, 1978. (Publication No. R-1987/5-HEW).
(5) Brook RH, Ware JE Jr, Davies-Avery A, et al. Overview of adult health status measures fielded in Rand's Health Insurance Study. Med Care 1979;17(suppl):1–131.
(6) Ware JE Jr. Scales for measuring general health perceptions. Health Serv Res 1976;11:396–415.
(7) Davies AR, Sherbourne CD, Peterson JR, et al. Scoring manual: adult health status and patient satisfaction measures used in Rand's Health Insurance Experiment. Santa Monica, California: Rand Corporation, 1988. (Publication No. N-2190-HHS).
(8) Read JL, Quinn RJ, Hoefer MA. Measuring overall health: an evaluation of three important approaches. J Chronic Dis 1987;40(suppl 1):S7–S21.
(9) Davies AR, Ware JE Jr. Measuring health perceptions in the Health Insurance Experiment. Santa Monica, California: Rand Corporation, 1981. (Publication No.R-2711-HHS).
(10) Connelly JE, Philbrick JT, Smith GR, et al. Health perceptions of primary care patients and the influence on health care utilization. Med Care 1989;27(suppl):S99–S109.
(11) Eisen M, Ware JE Jr, Donald CA, et al. Measuring components of children's health status. Med Care 1979;17:902–921.

THE GENERAL HEALTH QUESTIONNAIRE
(David Goldberg, 1972)

Purpose

The General Health Questionnaire (GHQ) is a self-administered screening instrument designed to detect current, diagnosable psychiatric disorders. The method may be used in surveys or clinical settings to identify potential cases, leaving the task of diagnosing actual disorder to a psychiatric interview (1).

Conceptual Basis

The GHQ is designed to identify two main classes of problem: "inability to carry out one's normal 'healthy' functions, and the appearance of new phenomena of a distressing nature" (2). It focuses on breaks in normal functioning rather than on life-long traits; therefore it only covers personality disorders or patterns of adjustment where these are associated with distress. The GHQ was not intended to detect severe illness such as schizophrenia or psychotic depression, although subsequent experience with the scale suggests that these conditions are detected (3).

The GHQ was designed to cover four identifiable elements of distress: depression, anxiety, social impairment, and hypochondriasis (chiefly indicated by organic symptoms) (1). Subsequent empirical analyses of the factor structure of the GHQ have largely confirmed this coverage (4). Goldberg suggests that his approach to psychiatric disorder is close to the lowest level of the hierarchy of mental illness outlined by Foulds and Bedford, which they term dysthymic states. "An individual falling into any of these states might be said to be *disturbed*, emotionally stirred up, altered in this respect from his normal self" (3). Such individuals will be prone to minor

somatic symptoms and may show out-
wardly observable changes in social behaviors.

Although the GHQ does cover separate
types of distress, it is not intended to distinguish among psychiatric disorders or to be
used in making diagnoses. No assumptions
were made concerning a hierarchy among
the symptoms included in the questionnaire: probable cases are identified on the
basis of checking any 12 or more of the 60
symptoms included, and the results express
the likelihood of psychiatric disorder.

Description

The GHQ was designed for use in general
population surveys, in primary medical
care settings, or among general medical
outpatients (3). It was meant to be a first-
stage screening instrument for psychiatric
illness that could then be verified and diagnosed. The questions ask whether the respondent has recently experienced a particular symptom (like abnormal feelings or
thoughts) or type of behavior. Emphasis is
on changes in condition, not on the absolute level of the problem, so items compare
the present state to the person's normal
situation with responses ranging from "less
than usual" to "much more than usual"
(3). The questionnaire begins with relatively neutral questions and leads to the
more overtly psychiatric items toward the
end. The questions were drawn from existing instruments or were created especially for this application, and those that
discriminated between severely ill and
mildly ill psychiatric patients and healthy
people were retained. Details of the item
selection procedure are given by Goldberg
(1, 3). The GHQ is normally completed by
the patient; Goldberg reports that more
than 95% of respondents could do this and
were remarkably frank in admitting
symptoms.

The main version of the GHQ, shown
in Exhibit 5.15, contains 60 items, and
Goldberg recommends using this version
where possible because of its superior validity. However, from the outset Goldberg

proposed alternative, shorter versions for
use where all 60 questions could not be
asked. These include 30-, 20-, and 12-item
abbreviations, and the GHQ-28 or "Scaled
GHQ" that contains four scales derived
from factor analyses (2). We show the
items included in the abbreviated versions
in Exhibit 5.16. Note that the exhibits give
the original wording of the items; some
may be rephrased using an American idiom
and these are shown under Alternative
Forms. The GHQ-28 provides four scores,
measuring somatic symptoms, anxiety and
insomnia, social dysfunction, and severe
depression, and is intended for studies in
which an investigator requires more information than is provided by a single severity
score (2). There is only a partial overlap
between the GHQ-28 and the GHQ-30,
which share just 14 items. The 30-, 20-,
and 12-item versions are balanced in terms
of "agreement sets"—that is, in each version half of the questions are worded to
indicate illness if answered "yes" and half
indicate illness if answered "no." The
shortened versions also discard 12 questions that were answered positively by
physically ill patients (1). It takes six to
eight minutes to complete the GHQ-60 and
three to four minutes for the GHQ-30 (3).

Items may be scored using conventional
0–1–2–3 Likert scores for the response
categories shown in Exhibit 5.15. Alternatively, a two-point score rates each problem
as present or absent, ignoring frequency
(3). In the latter approach, known as "the
GHQ score," replies are coded 0–0–1–1.
There appears little advantage to the Likert
approach; correlations between the two
scoring methods lie between 0.92 and 0.94
(5, Table 3), so Goldberg recommended
the simpler system (2). Weights for each
item held little advantage and so were discarded in the interests of simplicity, although a variant of this approach was re-
vived by Surtees and Miller (6). While
Goldberg originally rated only changes in
condition, Goodchild and Duncan-Jones
argued that ratings should cover changes
from what is normal in the population

Exhibit 5.15 The General Health Questionnaire (60-Item Version)

Please read this carefully:

We should like to know if you have had any medical complaints, and how your health has been in general, *over the past few weeks.* Please answer ALL the questions on the following pages simply by underlining the answer which you think most nearly applies to you. Remember that we want to know about present and recent complaints, not those that you had in the past.

It is important that you try to answer ALL the questions.

Thank you very much for your co-operation.

Have you recently:

1. been feeling perfectly well and in good health?	Better than usual	Same as usual	Worse than usual	Much worse than usual
2. been feeling in need of a good tonic?	Not at all	No more than usual	Rather more than usual	Much more than usual
3. been feeling run-down and out of sorts?	Not at all	No more than usual	Rather more than usual	Much more than usual
4. felt that you are ill?	Not at all	No more than usual	Rather more than usual	Much more than usual
5. been getting any pains in your head?	Not at all	No more than usual	Rather more than usual	Much more than usual
6. been getting a feeling of tightness or pressure in your head?	Not at all	No more than usual	Rather more than usual	Much more than usual
7. been able to concentrate on whatever you're doing?	Better than usual	Same as usual	Less than usual	Much less than usual
8. been afraid that you were going to collapse in a public place?	Not at all	No more than usual	Rather more than usual	Much more than usual
9. been having hot or cold spells?	Not at all	No more than usual	Rather more than usual	Much more than usual
10. been perspiring (sweating) a lot?	Not at all	No more than usual	Rather more than usual	Much more than usual
11. found yourself waking early and unable to get back to sleep?	Not at all	No more than usual	Rather more than usual	Much more than usual
12. been getting up feeling your sleep hasn't refreshed you?	Not at all	No more than usual	Rather more than usual	Much more than usual
13. been feeling too tired and exhausted even to eat?	Not at all	No more than usual	Rather more than usual	Much more than usual
14. lost much sleep over worry?	Not at all	No more than usual	Rather more than usual	Much more than usual
15. been feeling mentally alert and wide awake?	Better than usual	Same as usual	Less alert than usual	Much less alert
16. been feeling full of energy?	Better than usual	Same as usual	Less energy than usual	Much less energetic
17. had difficulty in getting off to sleep?	Not at all	No more than usual	Rather more than usual	Much more than usual
18. had difficulty in staying asleep once you are off?	Not at all	No more than usual	Rather more than usual	Much more than usual

Exhibit 5.15 *(Continued)*

227

Exhibit 5.15 *(Continued)*

19. *been having frightening or unpleasant dreams?*	Not at all	No more than usual	Rather more than usual	Much more than usual
20. *been having restless, disturbed nights?*	Not at all	No more than usual	Rather more than usual	Much more than usual
21. *been managing to keep yourself busy and occupied?*	More so than usual	Same as usual	Rather less than usual	Much less than usual
22. *been taking longer over the things you do?*	Quicker than usual	Same as usual	Longer than usual	Much longer than usual
23. *tended to lose interest in your ordinary activities?*	Not at all	No more than usual	Rather more than usual	Much more than usual
24. *been losing interest in your personal appearance?*	Not at all	No more than usual	Rather more than usual	Much more than usual
25. *been taking less trouble with your clothes?*	More trouble than usual	About same as usual	Less trouble than usual	Much less trouble
26. *been getting out of the house as much as usual?*	More than usual	Same as usual	Less than usual	Much less than usual
27. *been managing as well as most people would in your shoes?*	Better than most	About the same	Rather less well	Much less well
28. *felt on the whole you were doing things well?*	Better than usual	About the same	Less well than usual	Much less well
29. *been late getting to work, or getting started on your housework?*	Not at all	No later than usual	Rather later than usual	Much later than usual
30. *been satisfied with the way you've carried out your task?*	More satisfied	About same as usual	Less satisfied than usual	Much less satisfied
31. *been able to feel warmth and affection for those near to you?*	Better than usual	About same as usual	Less well than usual	Much less well
32. *been finding it easy to get on with other people?*	Better than usual	About same as usual	Less well than usual	Much less well
33. *spent much time chatting with people?*	More time than usual	About same as usual	Less than usual	Much less than usual
34. *kept feeling afraid to say anything to people in case you made a fool of yourself?*	Not at all	No more than usual	Rather more than usual	Much more than usual
35. *felt that you are playing a useful part in things?*	More so than usual	Same as usual	Less useful than usual	Much less useful
36. *felt capable of making decisions about things?*	More so than usual	Same as usual	Less so than usual	Much less capable
37. *felt you're just not able to make a start on anything?*	Not at all	No more than usual	Rather more than usual	Much more than usual

228

	Not at all	No more than usual	Rather more than usual	Much more than usual
38. felt yourself dreading everything that you have to do?	Not at all	No more than usual	Rather more than usual	Much more than usual
39. felt constantly under strain?	Not at all	No more than usual	Rather more than usual	Much more than usual
40. felt you couldn't overcome your difficulties?	Not at all	No more than usual	Rather more than usual	Much more than usual
41. been finding life a struggle all the time?	Not at all	No more than usual	Rather more than usual	Much more than usual
42. been able to enjoy your normal day-to-day activities?	More so than usual	Same as usual	Less so than usual	Much less than usual
43. been taking things hard?	Not at all	No more than usual	Rather more than usual	Much more than usual
44. been getting edgy and bad-tempered?	Not at all	No more than usual	Rather more than usual	Much more than usual
45. been getting scared or panicky for no good reason?	Not at all	No more than usual	Rather more than usual	Much more than usual
46. been able to face up to your problems?	More so than usual	Same as usual	Less able than usual	Much less able
47. found everything getting on top of you?	Not at all	No more than usual	Rather more than usual	Much more than usual
48. had the feeling that people were looking at you?	Not at all	No more than usual	Rather more than usual	Much more than usual
49. been feeling unhappy and depressed?	Not at all	No more than usual	Rather more than usual	Much more than usual
50. been losing confidence in yourself?	Not at all	No more than usual	Rather more than usual	Much more than usual
51. been thinking of yourself as a worthless person?	Not at all	No more than usual	Rather more than usual	Much more than usual
52. felt that life is entirely hopeless?	Not at all	No more than usual	Rather more than usual	Much more than usual
53. been feeling hopeful about your own future?	More so than usual	About same as usual	Less so than usual	Much less hopeful
54. been feeling reasonably happy, all things considered?	More so than usual	About same as usual	Less so than usual	Much less than usual
55. been feeling nervous and strung-up all the time?	Not at all	No more than usual	Rather more than usual	Much more than usual
56. felt that life isn't worth living?	Not at all	No more than usual	Rather more than usual	Much more than usual
57. thought of the possibility that you might make away with yourself?	Definitely not	I don't think so	Has crossed my mind	Definitely have
58. found at times you couldn't do anything because your nerves were too bad?	Not at all	No more than usual	Rather more than usual	Much more than usual
59. found yourself wishing you were dead and away from it all?	Not at all	No more than usual	Rather more than usual	Much more than usual
60. found that the idea of taking your own life kept coming into your mind?	Definitely not	I don't think so	Has crossed my mind	Definitely has

Exhibit 5.16   Abbreviated Versions of the General Health Questionnaire

Note: Using the item numbers from Exhibit 5.15 the contents of the shortened versions are as follows:

GHQ-12

  7. able to concentrate
14. lost sleep over worry
35. playing a useful part
36. capable of making decisions
39. constantly under strain
40. couldn't overcome difficulties

42. enjoy normal activities
46. face up to problems
49. unhappy and depressed
50. losing confidence in yourself
51. thinking of yourself as worthless
54. feeling reasonably happy

GHQ-20

In addition to the 12 items above, the 20-item version includes:

21. busy and occupied
26. getting out of house as usual
28. doing things well
30. satisfied with carrying out task

43. taking things hard
47. everything on top of you
55. nervous and strung-up
58. nerves too bad

Note: Item 30 is replaced by item 15 for use in the United States (3, p19).

GHQ-30

In addition to the 20 items above, the 30-item version includes:

20. restless, disturbed nights
27. managing as well as most people
31. feel warmth and affection
32. easy to get on with others
33. much time chatting

41. life a struggle all the time
45. scared or panicky
52. life entirely hopeless
53. hopeful about your future
56. life not worth living

Note: Item 33 is replaced by item 16 for use in the United States (3, p19).

GHQ-28

The 28-item version is as follows:

Scale A Somatic Symptoms	Scale B Anxiety and Insomnia
1. feeling perfectly well	14. lost sleep over worry
2. in need of a good tonic	18. difficulty staying asleep
3. run down	39. constantly under strain
4. felt that you are ill	44. edgy and bad-tempered
5. pains in head	45. scared or panicky
6. pressure in your head	47. everything on top of you
9. hot or cold spells	55. nervous and strung-up

Scale C Social Dysfunction	Scale D Severe Depression
21. busy and occupied	51. thinking of yourself as worthless
22. taking longer over things	52. life entirely hopeless
28. doing things well	56. life not worth living
30. satisfied with carrying out task	57. make away with yourself
35. playing a useful part	58. nerves too bad
36. capable of making decisions	59. dead and away from it all
42. enjoy normal activities	60. idea of taking your life

Adapted from Goldberg DP. The detection of psychiatric illness by questionnaire. London: Oxford University Press, 1972, Appendix 6.

rather than what is normal for this respondent. Therefore they proposed an alternative scoring system for the GHQ-30 that treats the response "no more than usual" as an indicator of a health problem for negatively worded items (e.g., "been having restless, disturbed nights"). The "no more than usual" response for positive items was taken as indicating a healthy response (7, p56). This score is termed the Corrected GHQ, or CGHQ (8). Some authors have found this score an improvement: it appeared to avoid the floor effect of the overall GHQ score, providing less skewed responses (7, Table III; 8). The correlation with the Zung depression scale was 0.50 for the GHQ and 0.59 for the CGHQ (7, Table IV). Sensitivity and specificity may be improved (7, p57; 9, Table III). Other reviews, by contrast, have found little difference between the GHQ and the CGHQ (10, p1012; 11; 12, p94).

Scores can be interpreted as indicating the severity of psychological disturbance on a continuum; as a screening test the score expresses the probability of being a psychiatric case. Any 12 positive answers on the GHQ-60 identify a probable case. Cutting points for the other versions are as follows: 5 positive answers for the GHQ-30 and GHQ-28, and 4 for the GHQ-20. At the cutting point the probability of being a case is 0.5. A cutting point of 2/3 has been tested for the GHQ-12 (5). These threshold scores may have to be altered depending on the expected prevalence of disorder and according to the purpose of the study: prevalence surveys versus detection of severe disorders, for example. Cutting points of 9/10, 10/11 or 11/12 have been used for the GHQ-60 (3).

Reliability

The test–retest coefficient after six months was 0.90 (N = 20) when the stability of the patient's condition was confirmed by repeating a standard psychiatric examination (3, p15). For another 65 patients who judged their own condition as having remained "about the same," the retest coefficient was 0.75 (3).

Split-half reliability on the 60-item version was 0.95 for 853 respondents (3). The equivalent value for the GHQ-30 was 0.92; for the GHQ-20, 0.90; and for the GHQ-12, 0.83 (1, Table 27). Chan and Chan reported an alpha of 0.85 for a clinical version of the GHQ-30 (13, Table 1).

Inter-rater reliability for 12 interviews showed a disagreement on only 4% of symptom scores (14, p 410).

Internal consistency estimates include split-half figures of 0.95 for the GHQ-60, 0.92 for the GHQ-30, 0.90 for the GHQ-20, and 0.83 for the GHQ-12 (15, p75).

Alpha coefficients for the GHQ-12 ranged from 0.82 to 0.90 in four studies (15, p75).

Validity

The General Health Questionnaire is probably the most thoroughly tested of the methods that we review in this book. Validation studies have been undertaken in many different countries and most have used directly comparable procedures. Because of the size of this literature we have been strictly selective in our presentation; the review article by Hedlund and Vieweg presents several pages of validity results (15, pp75–78).

Goldberg provided a table summarizing five studies that compared the GHQ-60 with a standardized psychiatric interview that he developed, the Clinical Interview Schedule (CIS) (3, 8). Results from studies in England, Australia, and Spain were very consistent, with correlations between the two scales ranging from 0.76 to 0.81. Sensitivity values ranged from 81% to 91%; specificity results in four of the studies ranged between 88% and 94%, while in the remaining study it was 73% (3, Table 4.1). Subsequent studies have also given comparable results: Hobbs et al. reported a correlation of 0.72 with the CIS and sensitivity results between 84% and 96% at specificities from 70% to 91% (16, Table IV). Slightly lower figures were obtained by Nott and Cutts with postpartum women (14).

Somewhat less adequate results were obtained by Benjamin et al., who applied the GHQ-60 to 92 women aged 40 to 49 years (17). They obtained a sensitivity of 54.5% at a specificity of 91.5%, and a Spearman correlation of 0.63 with the CIS (17). On further examination, the false negatives proved to be those who had long-standing disorders (see Commentary). Comparisons of the GHQ and the Present State Examination were made in England and India, giving correlations between 0.71 and 0.88 (3, Table 4.1).

Turning to the abbreviated versions of the GHQ, four studies of the 30-item scale have shown sensitivity values between 71%

and 91%, at specificities in the same range (3, 11). Sensitivity for the GHQ-28 was 85.6% at a specificity of 86.8% (3, p22). Studying general practice patients in Sydney, Australia, Tennant reported sensitivities ranging from 86.6% to 90% and specificities ranging from 90% to 94.4% (18, Table 1). Rather lower figures were obtained comparing GHQ-30 scores with the Schedule for Affective Disorders and Schizophrenia—a sensitivity of 68% and a specificity of 81% (19, Table 3). A comparison of the GHQ-28, -30 and -12 administered to young respondents showed the GHQ-28 was superior when compared with the Present State Examination (5). Correlations among the three abbreviated GHQ scales fell between 0.85 and 0.97 (5, Table 3). We present comparative data on the sensitivity and specificity of four versions of the GHQ in Table 5.4 (from 1, Table 27). Slightly lower figures were reported by Banks (5, Table 2). The GHQ-28 was found to remain sensitive to depression even when used with patients with dementia (9). The area under the ROC curve for the GHQ-12 was 0.87 in a Brazilian sample; the result was comparable to that obtained using Harding's 20-item Self Report Questionnaire (20).

Tarnopolovsky et al. examined the sensitivity and specificity of the 30-item GHQ as compared with the CIS, producing results that appear to be at odds with those reviewed above. The sensitivity results varied according to the prevalence of the disor-der in the study population. When half of the population scored above the cutting point, the sensitivity was 78%. Using statistical manipulations, Tarnopolovsky estimated that the sensitivity would fall to 54% as the ratio of high to low scoring cases falls to 22%. Kendall's tau correlations with the interview schedule ranged from 0.34 to 0.45 (21, Table V).

The validity results of the GHQ may be compared with those obtained using rival screening tests. Goldberg provided a table summarizing the results from which we drew the comparisons shown in Table 5.5 (1, Table 32). In other studies, the GHQ-28 performed somewhat less well than the Hospital Anxiety and Depression Scale, but somewhat better than the Rotterdam Symptom Checklist in a study of cancer patients (22, Table 1).

The correlation of the GHQ-30 with the Hopkins Symptom Checklist of physical and psychological symptoms was 0.78 (23, p65); the GHQ showed slightly higher sensitivity and specificity values (3). The Rand Mental Health Inventory had higher sensitivity and specificity than the GHQ-30: the area under the ROC curve was 0.76 for the MHI and 0.68 for the GHQ in detecting any disorder; the figures were 0.76 and 0.73 for affective disorders and 0.70 compared to 0.65 for anxiety (24, Table 3). The validity of the GHQ-28 was reviewed by Goldberg and Hillier. The correlation of the overall score with the Clinical Interview Schedule was 0.76 (2, Table 5).

Table 5.4 A Comparison of the Sensitivity and Specificity Results for Four Versions of the General Health Questionnaire

Note: The patients completed the GHQ-60. Validity estimates for the shortened versions were calculated by analyzing subsets of questions from the 60-item version.

	General practice patients		Hospital outpatients	
	Sensitivity %	Specificity %	Sensitivity %	Specificity %
GHQ-60	95.7	87.8	80.6	93.3
GHQ-30	91.4	87.0	64.5	91.6
GHQ-20	88.2	86.0	64.5	96.7
GHQ-12	93.5	78.5	74.2	95.0

Table 5.5 Comparison of the Validity of the General Health Questionnaire with that of Other Scales

	Sensitivity %	Specificity %	Overall misclassification %
GHQ-60	95.7	87.8	10.3
GHQ-30	85.0	79.5	19.1
Cornell Index	73.5	81.7	17.8
HOS (Macmillian)	75–84	54–68	22–40
22–Item Scale (Langner)	73.5	81.7	17.8

A correlation of 0.73 was obtained with the clinical depression rating, and of 0.67 with the anxiety rating. Using a cutting point of 4/5, the sensitivity was 88%, the specificity 84.2%, and the overall misclassification rate was 14.5% (2). The results were less good in a small study of 56 pain patients; the Spearman correlation with the CIS was 0.47 and sensitivity was 71% at a specificity of 63% (25, p199).

Goldberg summarized data on the association between the GHQ and demographic variables. Females tended to show higher scores; there was little clear association between age and GHQ scores, although there was a significant tendency for lower social class respondents to have higher scores (3).

The factor structure of the GHQ was originally studied by Goldberg and used as a basis for abbreviating the scale. Several analyses produced relatively consistent factors: somatic symptoms, sleep disturbance (sometimes combined with anxiety), social dysfunction, and severe depression (3; 4, Table 5). In subsequent studies Hobbs extracted three factors, covering debility (failure to cope), depression, and somatic symptoms (16). The area under the ROC curve for the depressive factor scores compared to a clinical diagnosis of depression was 0.75; the areas under the curve for other factors ranged from 0.50 (sleep) to 0.70 (social function) (26, Table 5).

The factor structure of the 30-item version has been studied intensively; the results appear broadly comparable. One study identified factors covering depression and anxiety, insomnia and lack of energy, social functioning, and anhedonia (unhappiness) (23). Cleary et al. reported similar findings from analyses of 1,072 respondents in Wisconsin (19). Berwick et al. identified six factors (27), while Huppert's study of 6,317 respondents in Britain identified five factors, covering anxiety, feelings of incompetence, depression, difficulty in coping, and social dysfunction (28, p182). A Chinese study also identified five factors: anxiety, inadequate coping, depression, insomnia, and social dysfunction (13). Scales in the GHQ-28 (selected via factor analysis) measure somatic symptoms, anxiety and insomnia, social dysfunction, and severe depression. These scales are not independent of each other: correlations range from 0.33 to 0.58 (2, Table 9). A factor analysis of the GHQ-12 from an Australian sample provided three factors: anhedonia and sleep disturbance, social performance, and loss of confidence (4). The evidence available suggests that several of the GHQ factors are stable across samples and among different versions of the questionnaire.

Sensitivity to change was reviewed by Ormel et al., and was found to be good (10).

Alternative Forms

The GHQ was developed in England, but with the aim of making comparative studies of psychiatric illness in England and the United States. Several of the items are rephrased for American use (1, 3):

2. _____ been feeling in need of some medicine to pick you up?

18. _____ had difficulty staying asleep?

27. _____ been managing as well as most people would in your place?

47. _____ found everything getting too much for you?

55. _____ been feeling nervous and up-tight (or hung up) all the time?

57. _____ thought of the possibility that you might do away with yourself?

The GHQ has been used across the world and versions exist in a very large number of languages; many of these versions have been validated. Validated examples include Italian (29), Cambodian (30), Mexican Spanish (31), Japanese (32), and Chinese (13, 33, 34). A comparison of experience with the GHQ in India and in Brazil led Sen et al. to conclude that the GHQ taps "an inner core of human suffering which can be reliably detected by suitably modified instruments developed in the West." (35, p277)

Commentary

The General Health Questionnaire offers a leading example of how health measurement methods should be developed. It was well founded on a clear conceptual approach, the initial item selection and item analyses are fully documented, and the questions have not been revised by subsequent users. The validation studies have been thorough and extensive; they have used comparable approaches and have consistently indicated a high degree of validity, markedly higher than that of rival methods. The scale has been tested in numerous countries and shows remarkably consistent validity results. Goldberg's book (1) is a model of clarity and thoroughness; unfortunately, the manual of the GHQ does not contain copies of the questionnaire (3).

Most of the criticisms that have been raised over the GHQ reflect limitations imposed by the deliberate design of the instrument. The response categories ask whether each symptom is worse than usual, and if a person has suffered a symptom for a long time and has come to consider it "usual," the scale will not identify this as a problem. Benjamin et al. viewed this as a limitation of the scale, although Goldberg developed the GHQ to measure changes in a person's condition and not the absolute level of the problem (17). It screens, therefore, for acute rather than chronic conditions. This issue has been resolved, however, by the alternative scoring procedure proposed by Goodchild and Duncan-Jones called the Corrected GHQ (7).

There has also been some dispute over the suitability of the items in the GHQ-60 that reflect physical symptoms ("feeling of tightness or pressure in your head," "perspiring a lot"). The physical items were excluded from the abbreviated versions of the GHQ because they produced a number of false-positive responses, although the problem seems to be far less serious than it is with Macmillan's HOS. Tennant, however, noted that "all false positives were subjects with substantial physical illness" (18): the difficulty of using somatic questions to screen for psychiatric disorders may still not have been resolved. Other studies of patients with physical illness also suggest that the GHQ identifies false-positives (25). The main dissonant note in the validation studies comes from Tarnopolovsky's study, which obtained lower sensitivity rates than those obtained by Goldberg (21). However, Tarnopolovsky's study was small and used estimation procedures to model changes in sensitivity rather than actual empirical evidence, so it should be replicated before we accept that its results are valid. The GHQ is most useful as part of a medical consultation and has seen widespread use in general practice for screening for mental disorders. We highly recommend it for these applications.

REFERENCES

(1) Goldberg DP. The detection of psychiatric illness by questionnaire. London: Oxford University Press, 1972. (Maudsley Monograph No. 21).

(2) Goldberg DP, Hillier VF. A scaled version of the General Health Questionnaire. Psychol Med 1979;9:139–145.

(3) Goldberg D. Manual of the General Health Questionnaire. Windsor, England: NFER Publishing, 1978.

(4) Worsley A, Gribbin CC. A factor analytic study of the twelve item General Health Questionnaire. Aust NZ J Psychiatry 1977;11:269–272.

(5) Banks MH. Validation of the General Health Questionnaire in a young community sample. Psychol Med 1983;13:349–353.

(6) Surtees PG, Miller PM. The interval General Health Questionnaire. Br J Psychiatry 1990;157:679–685.

(7) Goodchild ME, Duncan-Jones P. Chronicity and the General Health Questionnaire. Br J Psychiatry 1985;146:55–61.

(8) Huppert FA, Gore M, Elliott BJ. The value of an improved scoring system (CGHQ) for the General Health Questionnaire in a representative community sample. Psychol Med 1988;18:1001–1006.

(9) O'Riordan TG, Hayes JP, O'Neill D, et al. The effect of mild to moderate dementia on the Geriatric Depression Scale and on the General Health Questionnaire. Age Ageing 1990;19:57–61.

(10) Ormel J, Koeter MWJ, van den Brink W, Giel R. Concurrent validity of GHQ-28 and PSE as measures of change. Psychol Med 1989;19:1007–1013.

(11) Newman SC, Bland RC, Orn H. A comparison of methods of scoring the General Health Questionnaire. Compr Psychiatry 1988;29:402–408.

(12) Vázquez-Barquero JL, Díez-Manrique JF, Peña C, et al. Two stage design in a community survey. Br J Psychiatry 1986;149:88–97.

(13) Chan DW, Chan TSC. Reliability, validity and the structure of the General Health Questionnaire in a Chinese context. Psychol Med 1983;13:363–371.

(14) Nott PN, Cutts S. Validation of the 30-item General Health Questionnaire in post-partum women. Psychol Med 1982;12(2):409–413.

(15) Vieweg BW, Hedlund JL. The General Health Questionnaire (GHQ): a comprehensive review. J Operat Psychiatry 1983;14:74–85.

(16) Hobbs P, Ballinger CB, Smith AHW. Factor analysis and validation of the General Health Questionnaire in women: a general practice survey. Br J Psychiatry 1983;142:257–264.

(17) Benjamin S, Decalmer P, Haran D. Community screening for mental illness: a validity study of the General Health Questionnaire. Br J Psychiatry 1982;140:174–180.

(18) Tennant C. The General Health Questionnaire: a valid index of psychological impairment in Australian populations. Med J Aust 1977;2:392–394.

(19) Cleary PD, Goldberg ID, Kessler LG, et al. Screening for mental disorder among primary care patients. Arch Gen Psychiatry 1982;39:837–840.

(20) Mari JJ, Williams P. A comparison of the validity of two psychiatric screening questionnaires (GHQ-12 and SRQ-20) in Brazil, using Relative Operating Characteristic (ROC) analysis. Psychol Med 1985;15:651–659.

(21) Tarnopolsky A, Hand DJ, McLean EK, et al. Validity and uses of a screening questionnaire (GHQ) in the community. Br J Psychiatry 1979;134:508–515.

(22) Ibbotson T, Maguire P, Selby P, et al. Screening for anxiety and depression in cancer patients: the effects of disease and treatment. Eur J Cancer 1994;30A:37–40.

(23) Goldberg DP, Rickels K, Downing R, et al. A comparison of two psychiatric screening tests. Br J Psychiatry 1976;129:61–67.

(24) Weinstein MC, Berwick DM, Goldman PA, et al. A comparison of three psychiatric screening tests using Receiver Operating Characteristic (ROC) analysis. Med Care 1989;27:593–607.

(25) Benjamin S, Lennon S, Gardner G. The validity of the General Health Questionnaire for first-stage screening for mental illness in pain clinic patients. Pain 1991;47:197–202.

(26) Vázquez-Barquero JL, Williams P, Díez-Manrique JF, et al. The factor structure of the GHQ-60 in a community sample. Psychol Med 1988;18:211–218.

(27) Berwick DM, Budman S, Damico-White J, et al. Assessment of psychological morbidity in primary care: explorations with the General Health Questionnaire. J Chronic Dis 1987;40:S71–S79.

(28) Huppert FA, Walters DE, Day NE, et al. The factor structure of the General Health Questionnaire (GHQ-30): a reliability study on 6317 community residents. Br J Psychiatry 1989;155:178–185.

(29) Piccinelli M, Bisoffi G, Bon MG, et al. Validity and test–retest reliability of the Italian version of the 12-item General Health Questionnaire in general practice: a comparison between three scoring methods. Compr Psychiatry 1993;34:198–205.

(30) Cheung P, Spears G. Reliability and validity of the Cambodian version of the 28-

item General Health Questionnaire. Soc Psychiatry Psychiatr Epidemiol 1994; 29:95–99.

(31) Medina-Mora ME, Padilla GP, Campillo-Serrano C, et al. The factor structure of the GHQ: a scaled version for a hospital's general practice service in Mexico. Psychol Med 1983;13:355–361.

(32) Kitamura T, Sugawara M, Aoki M, et al. Validity of the Japanese version of the GHQ among antenatal clinic attendants. Psychol Med 1989;19:507–511.

(33) Chong M-Y, Wilkinson G. Validation of 30- and 12-item versions of the Chinese Health Questionnaire (CHQ) in patients admitted for general health screening. Psychol Med 1989;19:495–505.

(34) Cheng T-A, Williams P. The design and development of a screening questionnaire (CHQ) for use in community studies of mental disorders in Taiwan. Psychol Med 1986;16:415–422.

(35) Sen B, Mari JJ. Psychiatric research instruments in the transcultural setting: experiences in India and Brazil. Soc Sci Med 1986;23:277–281.

CONCLUSION

The more recent measurements presented in this chapter show evidence of considerable refinement in a field that was initially beset by unclear objectives and methodological disputes. The conceptual basis of the more recent scales, their statement of purpose, and their interpretation are all far more clearly spelled out than was the case for the early methods. The newer methods have generally been used without changes to the question wording, thus enhancing the comparability of results across different studies.

The major lessons to be learned relate to the conceptual formulation of an index. This area of measurement is inherently less specific than that of physical disability, and immense effort has been expended on debating what the scales measure. While the results of validation studies show the HOS or the Langner scale capable of screening for clinically identifiable disorders, they do not offer differential diagnoses in the tradi-

tional way that psychiatrists classify mental disorders. As we noted earlier, they represent the psychological counterpart of Selye's notion of stress, the nonspecific element common to a variety of disorders that warn the observer that something is wrong without specifying what. This idea may have been clear to the originators of the early scales, but if so, it was not sufficiently explained to prevent subsequent users from misinterpreting or overinterpreting the scales. Newer measurements have provided more explicit definitions of how they should and should not be interpreted, and of what high scores do and do not indicate.

We have also seen that there are serious disadvantages to making piecemeal alterations to the questions in a scale. If changes become necessary, it would be well to indicate this by altering the title, perhaps by adding a version number, similar to the approach used by Goldberg. We would also wish to discourage premature publication of draft questionnaires. Because of the pressure to publish in academic circles, draft forms of a measurement are frequently published and it then becomes difficult to ensure that users apply the final, definitive version.

The current status of this area of general psychological measurement is best summarized in terms of the individual measurement methods. The Goldberg scale provides a good method for screening for general psychological and psychiatric disorder. It has been used internationally, and many validation studies have demonstrated its psychometric qualities. The field of more subjective feelings of well-being is currently represented by Dupuy's scale, although the Bradburn questions continue to see some use. This may be because of the unfortunate lack of published validation studies on Dupuy's scale. It is disappointing that a scale of the potential of the General Well-Being Schedule does not benefit from a manual such as that produced by Goldberg for the General Health Questionnaire. The gap in the field of subjective well-being covered for so many years by the Bradburn scale was only partially covered by the Goldberg and Dupuy methods. More recently, this gap has been filled by the Rand scale, which expands the scope of the General Well-Being Schedule with additional positive items. This provides a good example of the planned and systematic development of a measurement method that reflects the current state of conceptual development and builds deliberately on existing measurements.

6

Depression[1]

Depression scales are among the best-established of health measurements; as with the activities of daily living scales, some of the best measures are over 20 years old. Most of the scales have received rigorous testing and have been used in numerous studies spanning many countries. Our selection of depression scales was relatively simple for there is close agreement among review articles over the ten-or-so leading methods in this field. This chapter describes purpose-built depression scales. In addition to these, most of the psychological well-being scales reviewed in Chapter 5 and the general health measures in Chapter 9 contain items or brief subscales covering depression.

As with disability and pain, depression is a term whose familiar use in everyday language complicates the acceptance of a precise, clinical definition (1).

Depression as an affect or feeling tone is a ubiquitous and universal condition which as a human experience extends on a continuum from normal mood swings to a pathological state. Thus, depression as a word can be used to

describe: (1) an affect which is a subjective feeling tone of short duration; or (2) a mood, which is a state sustained over a longer period of time; or (3) an emotion, which is comprised of the feeling tones along with objective indications; or (4) a disorder which has characteristic symptom clusters, complexes, or configurations. (2, p330)

"Depression" covers a wide range of states, from feeling sad, helpless, or demoralized, to a major depressive episode. Whether these fall on a continuum or form qualitatively different states is debatable (3). Snaith noted that depression

is used to indicate quite different concepts . . . for some, clinical depression is an extension of grief, for some it is a set of self-defeating attitudes, and for others it is the inevitable result of adversity, while the medically oriented psychiatrist considers there is a state based upon malfunctions of neurotransmitter systems in the brain. (4, p293)

A depressed or sad mood is a normal reaction to disappointment or loss; indeed, in the past it may have held survival advantages. Most mammals seem capable of depression in reaction to loss, and sadness may reinforce the bonds between infant and mother by recalling the fear of separation; it may foster social communication

1. This chapter was written by Ian McDowell and Elizabeth Kristjansson, with the assistance of Claire Newell.

about negative experiences and thereby support social learning and group behavior. It may also serve more direct physiological or intrapsychic functions of conservation due to withdrawal (5). Such situational depression should not, however, be confused with *disorders* of mood, in which the person suffers intense mental, emotional, and physical anguish and substantial disability. The two probably differ in kind, and certainly differ in seriousness; the worst outcome of major depression is suicide.

There are many possible ways to classify any disease or disorder—for example, along etiological lines, in terms of its biology, or in terms of the presenting symptoms. These may lead to different classifications, as is illustrated in the case of psychiatric disorders. As may be expected, this has led to continuing debate over the best way to classify disorders such as depression, producing rival schools of thought. The British school based diagnostic criteria for depression largely on the World Health Organization's International Classification of Disease. These criteria have, however, been modified over the years, in general moving somewhat closer to the North American approach. The North American diagnostic school has been guided by the *Diagnostic and Statistical Manual of the American Psychological Association (DSM),* currently in its fourth edition (6). Indeed, the content of many of the depression measurement scales is judged in terms of coverage of the *DSM* criteria. The *DSM* tradition situates depression within the broader category of mood or affective disorder, whose common feature is the patient's disturbed mood (either depressed or elated). This is a classification by symptom, for mood disorders are biologically heterogeneous and do not share a common etiology (7). Mood disorders are subdivided into depressive disorders and bipolar disorders. The latter are characterized by the presence of mania, a mood that is elated, expansive, or irritable, associated with symptoms such as hyperactivity, rac-

ing thoughts, or distractibility (7, p320). Bipolar disorder implies cyclical mood swings in which the patient can present either in the manic or depressive phase; cyclothymia is a mild but chronic form of mood swings. Depressive disorders can be subdivided into major depression and dysthymia, each with subcategories. Both are characterized by a depressed mood, loss of interest or pleasure in usual activities, and associated symptoms such as changed appetite or sleep disturbance; the difference is one of degree and dysthymia describes a milder disorder that does not meet the criteria for major depression. Whether the two conditions form a continuum, whether dysthymia is a precursor of depression, or whether they are different conditions—all are issues for further investigation.

Much of the challenge in assessing depression lies in placing the boundaries between normal depressed mood, dysthymia, and major depression. Very much the same issue occurs with dementia, in which the distinctions between normal cognitive declines of aging, cognitive impairment, and full dementia are still matters of debate. In the case of depression, the occurrence of features such as delusions, marked loss of weight, and suicidal threats are commonly taken as boundary markers for major depression; several sets of criteria have been proposed (8). The criteria in the fourth edition of the *DSM (DSM-IV)* identify change in affect as the central feature, with a depressed mood for most of the day, or a markedly diminished interest in daily activities. Frequency and duration are also considered: these symptoms should have occurred nearly every day for at least two consecutive weeks. In addition, four or more further symptoms must be present to qualify for major depression; the *DSM-IV* provides detailed definitions. These further symptoms include significant change in weight, insomnia or hypersomnia, psychomotor agitation or retardation, fatigue, feelings of worthlessness or guilt, diminished ability to concentrate, and suicidal ideation (6, p327). Severe depression is present when the person shows nearly all the symptoms of depression, and it keeps him from participating in his regular activities; moderate depression is present when the person has many of the symptoms and the depression often keeps him from doing the things he needs to do. Mild depression implies that a person shows some of the symptoms of depression and doing regular activities takes extra effort.

These criteria have been criticized. For example, Boyd et al. commented on the requirement that decline be present for a diagnosis of depression, offering an anecdotal case of an elderly woman with virtually no social life, living in isolation who appeared depressed but did not meet the criteria because her low role performance could not be shown to have declined (9).

While anxiety and depression are comparable and may result from similar circumstances, there is general agreement that the two are distinguishable and that anxiety is not an aspect of depression. Anxiety is readily detected: the anxious patient appears apprehensive, sweats, and complains of nervousness, palpitations, and faintness; somatic signs include rapid breathing, tachycardia, and labile blood pressure. Identifying depression is more challenging and may require time-consuming interviews; it is rare that a depressed patient does not also exhibit signs of anxiety (10, p1).

There are several ways of classifying depression, including a distinction on etiological lines between endogenous and reactive depression, and a distinction between neurotic and psychotic depression that reflects severity (2). Other classifications consider the level of psychomotor effects and whether the depression is accompanied by behavioral disturbances. More relevant to the task of measurement, great attention has been paid to classifying symptoms of depression. These are generally grouped into affective (crying, sadness, apathy), cognitive (thoughts of hopelessness, helplessness, suicide, worthlessness, guilt), and somatic (sleep disturbance, change in en-

ergy level, appetite, sleep, elimination) (11, 12). Not all are present in every case. The structure of the syndrome complicates the scoring used in measurement methods. For example, more symptoms may not imply more severe depression, and for this reason, clinicians rarely consider depressive symptoms as linear and additive, but classify them into dimensions or categories (13). Hence, a more sophisticated scoring algorithm may be required in place of an additive summary score. This issue also arises in scoring screening tests for dementia, as seen in Chapter 7.

MEASUREMENT OF DEPRESSION

The coexistence of many measurement scales reflects the divergence of conceptual approaches to depression and also the fact that depression is a syndrome rather than a single entity. No one symptom is diagnostic of depression, and different people exhibit widely different symptoms. Hence, a measurement scale has to cover several dimensions, and it is the choice of coverage that distinguishes most rival scales. These differences in content in turn reflect underlying differences—for example, in the theory of etiology of depression (e.g., biological versus psychodynamic)—or differences in the response system monitored (e.g., cognitive, behavioral, physiologic, or affective) (14). Depression scales are divided into self-rating methods and clinician-rating scales, which correspond roughly to their use in epidemiological versus clinical studies. The basic approach is the clinical rating, with self-ratings as a less costly alternative. A formal diagnosis of depression requires the exclusion of alternative explanations for the symptoms, and this requires a clinical examination. The *DSM-IV,* for example, requires the exclusion of possible explanations such as the physiological effects of drugs or medications and medical conditions such as hypothyroidism or schizophrenia. As this requires a clinical assessment, it is widely accepted that self-assessed measures of depression can identify the syndrome of depression but, as with dementia, cannot be diagnostic devices.

Self-ratings naturally emphasize the subjective and affective elements: the experience of depression. The practical advantages of the self-report are speed and economy since they do not require professional observation. The disadvantages include the lack of specificity of self-report methods: they identify dysfunction but cannot distinguish depression from general malaise. Only a clinical rating can record nonverbal indicators of depression, and a clinical rating can handle distorting factors such as denial or exaggeration. Somatic symptoms are not accurately covered by self-assessment, producing false positives among medically ill and elderly persons (15, pp92,94), a difficulty that is easier to control in the clinical interview. This echoes the debate over the Health Opinion Survey described in Chapter 5.

Because patients (especially severely depressed ones) lack the clinical perspective required to rate the severity of their symptoms, self-rating methods also cannot accurately indicate severity (16, p361). Patients with milder, neurotic forms of depression may rate themselves as more depressed than do clinicians; the reverse seems true of patients with severe depression (14, p85). It may be more difficult to distinguish between moderate and severe depression than between mild and moderate because in severe patients the symptom patterns become broader and more complex (17, p385), and in such instances a clinical rating scale may prove superior. Hence, although depression is a subjective phenomenon, there are clear limits to assessing depression via self-report. Hamilton put it bluntly: "Self-rating scales are popular because they are easy to administer. Apart from the notorious unreliability of self-assessment, such scales are of little use for semiliterate patients and are no use for seriously ill patients who are unable to deal with them." (18, p56)

Certain issues in measurement that exist in other fields seem magnified in depression. The nature of the disorder complicates its measurement; patients with severe depression may be unable to communicate meaningfully (19) and may lack motivation to respond to questions. Assessing older people holds the added complication of a tendency among the elderly to deny depression (12), while the presence of cognitive impairments also complicates the assessment of depression. Somatic complaints due to physical illness or to medication use may falsely elevate scores on depression scales that have a somatic component (20). Characteristic biases in measuring depression include the apparent difference between men and women in the prevalence of depressive symptoms. Western cultures sanction greater expression of feeling among women than among men, so women score higher on depression questions (21, p976). Whether this indicates measurement bias or a real difference is debatable, and methods such as the signal detection analyses used in pain measurement might be applied to study response thresholds. There is also a confounding effect whereby those in lower socioeconomic groups are likely to suffer greater stresses and more depression but also to exhibit different response styles and admit to more problems than the more educated.

SCOPE OF THE CHAPTER

This chapter opens with reviews of five self-rating depression scales. The Beck and Zung scales were developed in the 1960s to measure severity of depression; they are among the most widely used of all health measures. They have been widely tested, and we have extensive information on their performance. Next we review two depression screening instruments. The Center for Epidemiologic Studies Depression Scale was designed for survey use, and the Geriatric Depression Scale was intended for use with elderly people. We then review Lubin's Depression Adjective Check Lists, which focus on mood and the affective aspects of depression. This is followed by reviews of the leading clinical rating method, the Hamilton Rating Scale for Depression, and of two scales derived from it: the Montgomery-Åsberg Depression Rating Scale, which is also administered by a clinician, and the Carroll Rating Scale for Depression, which is a self-administered version of the Hamilton scale The comparative strengths of the scales are summarized in Table 6.1.

REFERENCES

(1) Kendall PC, Hollon SD, Beck AT, et al. Issues and recommendations regarding use of the Beck Depression Inventory. Cognitive Ther Res 1987;11:289–299.

(2) Zung WWK. From art to science: the diagnosis and treatment of depression. Arch Gen Psychiatry 1973;29:328–337.

(3) Cooke DJ. The structure of depression found in the general population. Psychol Med 1980;10:455–463.

(4) Snaith P. What do depression rating scales measure? Br J Psychiatry 1993;163:293–298.

(5) Klerman GL. The nature of depression: mood, symptom, disorder. In: Marsella AJ, Hirschfeld RMA, Katz MM, eds. The measurement of depression. New York: Guilford Press, 1987:3–19.

(6) American Psychiatric Association. Diagnostic and statistical manual of mental disorders DSM—IV. 4th ed. Washington, DC: American Psychiatric Association, 1994.

(7) Weissman MM, Klerman GL. Depression: current understanding and changing trends. Annu Rev Pub Health 1992;13:319–339.

(8) Zisook S, Click M Jr, Jaffe K, et al. Research criteria for the diagnosis of depression. Psychiatr Res 1980;2:13–23.

(9) Boyd JH, Weissman MM, Thompson WD, et al. Screening for depression in a community sample: understanding the discrepancies between depression symptom and diagnostic scales. Arch Gen Psychiatry 1982;39:1195–1200.

(10) Wetzler S, Katz MM. Problems with the differentiation of anxiety and depression. J Psychiatr Res 1989;23:1–12.

(11) Brink TL, Yesavage JA, Lum O, et al. Screening tests for geriatric depression. Clin Gerontol 1982;1:37–43.

(12) Thompson LW, Futterman A, Gallagher D. Assessment of late-life depression. Psychopharmacol Bull 1988;24:577–586.

(13) Myers JK, Weissman MM. Use of a self-report symptom scale to detect depression in a community sample. Am J Psychiatry 1980;137:1081–1084.

(14) Hughes JR, O'Hara MW, Rehm LP. Measurement of depression in clinical trials: an overview. J Clin Psychiatry 1982;43:85–88.

(15) Beck AT, Steer RA, Garbin MG. Psychometric properties of the Beck Depression Inventory: twenty-five years of evaluation. Clin Psychol Rev 1988;8:77–100.

(16) Carroll BJ, Fielding JM, Blashki TG. Depression rating scales: a critical review. Arch Gen Psychiatry 1973;28:361–366.

(17) Biggs JT, Wylie LT, Ziegler VE. Validity of the Zung Self-rating Depression Scale. Br J Psychiatry 1978;132:381–385.

(18) Hamilton M. A rating scale for depression. J Neurol Neurosurg Psychiatry 1960; 23:56–62.

(19) Kearns NP, Cruickshank CA, McGuigan KJ, et al. A comparison of depression rating scales. Br J Psychiatry 1982;141:45–49.

(20) Zemore R, Eames N. Psychic and somatic symptoms of depression among young adults, institutionalized aged and noninstitutionalized aged. J Gerontol 1979; 34:716–722.

(21) Blumenthal MD. Measuring depressive symptomatology in a general population. Arch Gen Psychiatry 1975;32:971–978.

THE BECK DEPRESSION INVENTORY
(Aaron T. Beck, 1961, Revised 1978)

Purpose

The Beck Depression Inventory (BDI) was originally designed to measure the depth or intensity of depression in psychiatric patients (1, 2). It has subsequently been used as a community screening instrument and for clinical research (3).

Conceptual Basis

The content of the BDI was guided by clinical observations made during psychotherapy rather than on the basis of a particular theory of depression (4). Because Beck stressed the cognitive genesis of depression, the content of the BDI emphasizes the patient's attitudes toward herself. Beck defined depression as "an abnormal state of

Table 6.1 Comparison of the Quality of Depression Measurements*

Measurement	Scale	Number of items	Application	Administered by (time)	Studies using method	Reliability Thoroughness	Reliability Results	Validity Thoroughness	Validity Results
Beck Depression Inventory (Beck, 1961)	ordinal	21	clinical, screening	interviewer, self (10-15 min)	many	+ + +	+ + +	+ + +	+ + +
The Self-rating Depression Scale (Zung, 1965)	ordinal	20	clinical	self (10–15 min)	many	+ +	+ +	+ + +	+ +
Center for Epidemiologic Studies Depression Scale (National Institute for Mental Health, 1972)	ordinal	20	survey	self	many	+ +	+ +	+ + +	+ + +
Geriatric Depression Scale (Brink, 1982)	ordinal	30	clinical, screening	self (8–10 min)	many	+ + +	+ + +	+ + +	+ + +
Depression Adjective Check Lists (Lubin, 1965)	ordinal	32	research	self (3 min per list)	many	+ + +	+ +	+ +	+ +
Hamilton Rating Scale for Depression (Hamilton, 1960)	ordinal	21	clinical	expert (30 min)	many	+ + +	+ +	+ + +	+ +
Montgomery-Åsberg Depression Rating Scale (Montgomery, 1979)	ordinal	10	research	expert	several	+ +	+ +	+	+ + +
Carroll Rating Scale for Depression (Carroll, 1981)	ordinal	52	clinical, research	self	several	+	+	+ +	+ +

*For an explanation of the categories used, see Chapter 1, pages 6–7.

the organism manifested by signs and symptoms such as low subjective mood, pessimistic and nihilistic attitudes, loss of spontaneity and specific vegetative signs. . . . This particular variable may occur together with any combination of other psychopathological variables such as anxiety, obsessions, phobias, and hallucinations" (4, pp201–202). Beck argued for a broad content, seeing depression "as a complex disorder involving affective, cognitive, motivational, and behavioral components" (4, p187). Beck recorded attitudes, behaviors, and symptoms that were specific to clinically depressed patients and were consistent with psychiatric literature at the time. These were grouped into the 21 symptom categories that make up the BDI. Beck observed that as depression deepens, the number of symptoms increases, and there is also a progression in the frequency and intensity of each (4, p188; 5, p154). Hence the structure of the BDI includes graded levels of intensity of each symptom.

Description

The BDI evaluates 21 symptoms of depression, 15 of which cover emotions, four cover behavioral changes and six cover somatic symptoms. Each symptom is rated on a four-point intensity scale and scores are added to give a total ranging from 0 to 63; higher scores represent more severe depression. The BDI was revised in 1978; the revised version is recommended and two items from this are shown in Exhibit 6.1.[2] The 21 items cover sadness*, pessimism*, sense of failure*, dissatisfaction*, guilt*, expectation of punishment, self-dislike*, self-accusations, suicidal ideas*, crying, irritability, social withdrawal*, indecisiveness*, body image change*, work retardation*, insomnia, fatigability*, anorexia*, weight loss, somatic preoccupation and loss of libido. Asterisks indicate items included in an abbreviated version described below. The 1978 version differs from the original by referring to "the past week" rather than to "today" and by making minor changes to the wording of 15 of the response statements (3, pp80–81). Unfortunately, much of the validation was undertaken on the original version, and there is little information on the equivalence of the two versions. The reading level

2. Copyright prevents us from reproducing the complete scale, which is printed in Beck AT, et al. *Cognitive Therapy of Depression*. New York: Guilford Press, 1979, pages 398–399.

Exhibit 6.1 Two Items from the Beck Depression Inventory

On this questionnaire are groups of statements. Please read each group of statements carefully. Then pick out the one statement in each group which best describes the way you have been feeling the *PAST WEEK, INCLUDING TODAY*. Circle the number beside the statement you picked. If several statements in the group seem to apply equally well, circle each one.
Be sure to read all the statements in each group before making your choice.

1 (Sadness)
   0 I do not feel sad.
   1 I feel sad.
   2 I am sad all the time and I can't snap out of it.
   3 I am so sad or unhappy that I can't stand it.

12 (Social withdrawal)
   0 I have not lost interest in other people.
   1 I am less interested in other people than I used to be.
   2 I have lost most of my interest in other people.
   3 I have lost all of my interest in other people.

---

required for the revised version is at the fifth- or sixth-grade (3, p81).

The BDI was originally administered by a trained interviewer, while the patient read a copy (1, p562); it is more commonly self-administered, taking five to ten minutes. Administration instructions are in the Appendix of Beck's book (4, pp336–337). If the respondent selects more than one statement in any group, the higher value is recorded; if her feelings lie between two alternatives, the one that is closer is scored. Computerized forms of the BDI are available (3, p80).

Beck warns against rigid adherence to set cutting points; these should be chosen according to the application. The following guidelines are commonly given: scores of less than 10 indicate no or minimal depression, 10 to 18 indicate mild to moderate depression, 19 to 29 indicate moderate to severe depression, and scores of 30 or more indicate severe depression (3, p79). Moran and Lambert suggested that scores of 10 to 15 indicate mild and 16 to 19 indicate moderate depression (6, p270). For psychiatric patients, a screening cut-point of 12/13 is suitable, while 9/10 is appropriate in screening medical patients (5, p163). Further discussion of cutting points is given by Kendall et al. (7).

In 1972, Beck and Beck proposed a 13-item abbreviated BDI for use by family physicians as a rapid screening tool (8). Items were selected on the basis of their item-total correlations and of their agreement with a clinician's ratings. Total scores of 0 to 4 on the short form indicate no or minimal depression; 5 to 7 indicate mild depression; 8 to 15, moderate; and 16 or more, severe depression (5, p164; 8, Table 2).

Reliability

Beck's original paper reported a split-half reliability of 0.86, or 0.93 with the Spearman-Brown correction (1, p565; 4, p194). In their review article, Beck et al. cited ten studies of psychiatric patients which yielded alpha coefficients ranging from 0.76 to 0.95, with a mean of 0.86. In 15 nonpsychiatric samples, alpha coefficients ranged from 0.73 to 0.92, with a mean of 0.81. Three of these studies concurrently reviewed the short-form BDI where the alphas fell about 0.02 below those for the long form (3, Table 1). Subsequent studies confirmed these findings (see, for example, references 9 and 10). Gallagher reviewed reliability studies on older adults and found similar results (11, p152). Schaefer et al. reported coefficient alphas of 0.94 for the long form for 15 psychiatric patients and 0.88 for 15 chemically dependent patients (12, p416).

Beck reviewed ten reports of retest reliability of the BDI at varying time intervals; Pearson correlations between administrations ranged from 0.48 to 0.86 in five studies of psychiatric patients and from 0.60 to 0.83 in six nonpsychiatric populations (3, Table 2). Among elderly patients, test–retest reliability at six to 21 days was 0.79 in depressed patients and 0.86 in normal respondents (13, Table 1).

Validity

There is extensive information on the validity of the BDI. In terms of content validity, the BDI covers six of the nine *DSM-III* criteria directly, two partially (it omits increases in appetite and sleep), and omits agitation (6, p294).

Beck reviewed 11 studies that showed the BDI capable of discriminating between groups that contrasted in level of depression (3, p90). A further 35 concurrent validation studies compared the BDI to other ratings of depression (3, Table 3). Fourteen studies reported correlations between the BDI and clinical ratings; coefficients for psychiatric patients ranged from 0.55 to 0.96, with a mean of 0.72. In three samples of nonpsychiatric patients, correlations ranged from 0.55 to 0.73, and the mean was 0.60 (3, p89). Correlations with the Hamilton Rating Scale for Depression (HRSD) ranged from 0.61 to 0.86 (mean 0.73) in five studies of psychiatric patients; the results were 0.73 and 0.80 in two studies of nonpsychiatric populations (3, p89; 14). A correlation of 0.62 was reported with the Hopkins Symptom Checklist depression score (15, Table 2). Oliver and Simmons validated the BDI against the Diagnostic Interview Schedule in a sample of 298 community volunteers. At a cutting point of 9/10, sensitivity was 84.6% and specificity was 86.4% (16, Table 1). If respondents with dysthymic disorder were excluded from the sample, sensitivity rose to 100% and specificity was 86%. In a study of 102 elderly outpatients the BDI had a sensitivity of 93.3% at a specificity of 81.5% compared to the Schedule for Affective Disorders (17, p945). Compared to *DSM-III* diagnoses made by clinical psychologists, sensitivity was 83% and specificity was 82% at a cut-point of 12/13 (18, Table 1). However, Whiffen warned that the BDI may miss cases of postpartum depression: in her small study, sensitivity was only 47.6% at a cutting point of 9/10 (19, Table 1). Kearns et al. found that the BDI discriminated poorly between levels of depression (20).

The BDI has been compared to most other depression measures. Compared to the Zung Self-rating Depression Scale, the mean correlation was 0.76 in eight studies of psychiatric populations and 0.71 in five nonpsychiatric samples (3, p89). Higher values of 0.89 (21, Table 4) and 0.86 (18, Table 2) have been reported. Compared to the Minnesota Multiphasic Personality Inventory Depression scale, the mean correlation was 0.76 in seven studies of psychiatric patients and 0.60 for three studies of nonpsychiatric samples (3, p89). Correlations with the Multiple Affect Adjective Checklist depression scale in three studies ranged from 0.59 to 0.66 (3, p89), while in Beck's original studies the correlations ranged from 0.40 to 0.66 in different samples (4, p199). The BDI had a correlation of 0.79 with the Geriatric Depression Scale (GDS) for 51 elderly volunteers (10, p1165) and one of 0.85 when used with medical outpatients (22, p994). The sensitivity and specificity of the BDI were slightly better than those of the GDS (22, Table 1). It also performed slightly better than the Center for Epidemiologic Studies Depression Scale in detecting depression among primary care patients (23, Table 2). In terms of divergent validity, the BDI correlated 0.14 with clinical ratings of anxiety, a lower association than that obtained for the depression scale of the Multiple Affect Adjective Checklist (4, pp200–201).

Reviews of the adequacy of the BDI as a measure of change are mixed. Moran and Lambert found the BDI to be more sensitive to change than other instruments (6, p294), while a more sophisticated meta-analysis of 19 studies with 1,150 respondents showed that the BDI was more conservative than the HRSD in estimating treatment change (14).

Beck et al. reviewed 13 factor analytic studies of the BDI and concluded that it contains one underlying factor which may be subdivided into three correlated components: negative attitudes toward self, performance impairment, and somatic disturbance (3, p92). Welch et al. compared analyses from five samples and identified a "large general factor that resulted in high internal reliability for the measure as a whole" (24, p825). Using a latent trait analysis, Clark et al. also found that a single dimension adequately described the data (25, p709). Their analysis suggested that the vegetative symptoms (sleep disturbance, weight loss, etc.) did not discriminate well between depressed and nondepressed subjects.

The validity of the short-form BDI has been tested in several studies. Turner and Romano found a sensitivity of 83% and a specificity of 89% at a cut-point of 7/8; at 3/4 sensitivity was 100% and specificity was 57% (18, Table 1). Scogin et al. found the sensitivity of the short form to be 98% and specificity 65%, using 4/5 as a cutting point. Raising the cutting point to 5/6 increased specificity to 77% (26, pp855–856). The short form has good internal consistency ($\alpha = 0.78$ to 0.86) (9, p1168; 27, p769). Correlations with the long form lie between 0.89 and 0.97 (3, p80; 9, p1168; 27, p769; 28, p1185); correlations with clinical ratings of depression lie between 0.55 and 0.67 (28, p1186). Factor analytic studies suggest that the short form measures somewhat different aspects of depression than the long form; its coverage of somatic components is weaker (27, 29). Steer and Beck stressed that the short form should not replace the long form; its intent was only to assist family practitioners in deciding whether their patients required more detailed psychological evaluation (30).

Alternative Forms

The BDI has been translated into many languages, including French, Spanish, German, Polish, Danish (3; 11, p154; 31, p127), Chinese (32, 33), and Turkish (34).

A 27-item self-report version of the BDI, the Child Depression Inventory, is available for school-aged children and adolescents (35). Steer et al. review the use of the BDI with children (31, pp133–134). A version designed for use with deaf persons is given by Leigh et al. (36).

Reference Standards

Scores have been reported from studies of general practice patients. Unfortunately, the proportions of patients scoring above commonly used cutting points varied widely in three reports (37, Table 2).

Commentary

The Beck Depression Inventory is an established and well-researched scale that is routinely included in psychological test batteries. Compared to the Zung and Lubin instruments reviewed in this chapter, the BDI has a broader coverage of the somatic aspects of depression and has been equally thoroughly tested.

As with all of the self-rating depression scales, however, there have been criticisms of the BDI. Most of the validation studies used the original version and we do not know how far these apply to the revised version. Several authors have argued that

the coverage of the BDI should be broadened. Items on increased weight, appetite and sleep (27), and psychomotor activity (6) have been proposed to make the BDI more congruent with *DSM-III* criteria. Vredenburg et al. tested such a version on 475 university students and concluded that it had "a better factor structure and somewhat higher reliability than the original scale" (27, p775). Beck and Steer responded that while increased appetite and sleep are symptoms of depression, they are nonspecific and their inclusion would lead to a high number of false-positives (3, p85; 30). It has been argued that the somatic content of the BDI may lead to false-positives among patients with physical problems; an illustration has recently been given for pain patients (38).

Several authors have found a social desirability response bias in which people respond on the basis of their judgment of the desirability or undesirability of the item content (3, p92; 39). The BDI correlates with other self-report measures of maladaptive functioning (40) and so may in part reflect general "negative affect" (7). Langevin and Stancer argued that this, together with the results of factor analytic studies, demonstrate that the BDI reflects a social undesirability response set rather than depression (41). Beck responded that people who are depressed tend toward low self-image; this indicates psychopathology and so the two are inherently confounded. He pointed to the agreement between the BDI and clinical ratings of depression to suggest that the validity of the scale is not reduced by the negative response set among depressed people (4, p207).

Some studies of college students have made much of the apparent instability of scores over time (42, 43), but the original BDI measured current state, and it is not surprising that a state measurement of depression finds mood changes over short periods. The intent of the revised version is to measure more stable characteristics; unfortunately, its success in this remains unknown.

The ease of completing the BDI has been debated: some suggest that the four-item response scales are difficult to administer (20); scales such as the GDS use a simpler yes/no response format that may require less concentration on the part of the respondent (11, p158; 22, p994).

As Beck never intended the BDI to be used for diagnosing depression, much of the extended debate over whether it can be used in this way is misplaced. Most commentators agree that although the BDI is sensitive, it may have low specificity, and that high scores on the BDI cannot be taken as diagnostic of depression (7). For example, Oliver and Simmons found that "the number of subjects scoring depressed on the BDI was about 2½ times the number diagnosed by the DIS" (16, pp893–894). Respondents who receive intermediate scores on the Beck should be considered dysphoric, and only with a fuller clinical interview should they be termed "depressed" (7, p297). With this caveat, the BDI is one of the best depression screening tools available.

Address

Copies of the Beck inventory are available from: The Psychological Corporation, 555 Academic Court, San Antonio, Texas, USA 78204-0952

REFERENCES

(1) Beck AT, Ward CH, Mendelson M, et al. An inventory for measuring depression. Arch Gen Psychiatry 1961;4:561–571.

(2) Bech P. Rating scales for affective disorders: their validity and consistency. Acta Psychiatr Scand 1981;64(suppl 295):1–101.

(3) Beck AT, Steer RA, Garbin MG. Psychometric properties of the Beck Depression Inventory: twenty-five years of evaluation. Clin Psychol Rev 1988;8:77–100.

(4) Beck AT. Depression: clinical, experimental, and theoretical aspects. New York: Harper & Row, 1967.

(5) Beck AT, Beamesderfer A. Assessment of depression: the Depression Inventory. Mod Probl Pharmacopsychiatry 1974;7:151–169.

(6) Moran PW, Lambert MJ. A review of current assessment tools for monitoring changes in depression. In: Lambert MJ, Christensen ER, DeJulio SS, eds. The measurement of psychotherapy outcome in research and evaluation. New York: Wiley, 1983:263–303.

(7) Kendall PC, Hollon SD, Beck AT, et al. Issues and recommendations regarding use of the Beck Depression Inventory. Cognitive Ther Res 1987;11:289–299.

(8) Beck AT, Beck RW. Screening depressed patients in family practice: a rapid technic. Postgrad Med 1972;52:81–85.

(9) Gould J. A psychometric investigation of the standard and short form Beck Depression Inventory. Psychol Rep 1982; 51:1167–1170.

(10) Gatewood-Colwell G, Kaczmarek M, Ames MH. Reliability and validity of the Beck Depression Inventory for a white and Mexican-American gerontic population. Psychol Rep 1989;65:1163–1166.

(11) Gallagher D. The Beck Depression Inventory and older adults. Review of its development and utility. Clin Gerontol 1986;5:149–163.

(12) Schaefer A, Brown J, Watson CG, et al. Comparison of the validities of the Beck, Zung, and MMPI depression scales. J Consult Clin Psychol 1985;53:415–418.

(13) Gallagher D, Nies G, Thompson LW. Reliability of the Beck Depression Inventory with older adults. J Consult Clin Psychol 1982;50:152–153.

(14) Edwards BC, Lambert MJ, Moran PW, et al. A meta-analytic comparison of the Beck Depression Inventory and the Hamilton Rating Scale for Depression as measures of treatment outcome. Br J Clin Psychol 1984;23:93–99.

(15) Winokur A, Guthrie MB, Rickels K, et al. Extent of agreement between patient and physician ratings of emotional distress. Psychosomatics 1982;23:1135–1146.

(16) Oliver JM, Simmons ME. Depression as measured by the DSM-III and the Beck Depression Inventory in an unselected adult population. J Consult Clin Psychol 1984;52:892–898.

(17) Gallagher D, Breckenridge J, Steinmetz J, et al. The Beck Depression Inventory and research diagnostic criteria: congruence in an older population. J Consult Clin Psychol 1983;51:945–946.

(18) Turner JA, Romano JM. Self-report screening measures for depression in chronic pain patients. J Clin Psychol 1984;40:909–913.

(19) Whiffen VE. Screening for postpartum depression: a methodological note. J Clin Psychol 1988;44:367–371.

(20) Kearns NP, Cruickshank CA, McGuigan KJ, et al. A comparison of depression rating scales. Br J Psychiatry 1982;141:45–49.

(21) Plutchik R, van Praag HM. Interconvertability of five self-report measures of depression. Psychiatr Res 1987;22:243–256.

(22) Norris JT, Gallagher D, Wilson A, et al. Assessment of depression in geriatric medical outpatients: the validity of two screening measures. J Am Geriatr Soc 1987;35:989–995.

(23) Zich JM, Attkisson CC, Greenfield TK. Screening for depression in primary care clinics: the CES-D and the BDI. Int J Psychiatry Med 1990;20:259–277.

(24) Welch G, Hall A, Walkey F. The replicable dimensions of the Beck Depression Inventory. J Clin Psychol 1990;46:817–827.

(25) Clark DC, Cavanaugh SA, Gibbons RD. The core symptoms of depression in medical and psychiatric patients. J Nerv Ment Dis 1983;171:705–713.

(26) Scogin F, Beutler L, Corbishley A, et al. Reliability and validity of the short form Beck Depression Inventory with older adults. J Clin Psychol 1988;44:853–857.

(27) Vredenburg K, Krames L, Flett GL. Reexamining the Beck Depression Inventory: the long and short of it. Psychol Rep 1985;56:767–778.

(28) Beck AT, Rial WY, Rickels K. Short form of Depression Inventory: cross-validation. Psychol Rep 1974;34:1184–1186.

(29) Berndt DJ. Taking items out of context: dimensional shifts with the short form of the Beck Depression Inventory. Psychol Rep 1979;45:569–570.

(30) Steer RA, Beck AT. Modifying the Beck Depression Inventory: reply to Vredenburg, Krames, and Flett. Psychol Rep 1985;57:625–626.

(31) Steer RA, Beck AT, Garrison B. Applications of the Beck Depression Inventory. In: Sartorius N, Ban T, eds. Assessment of depression. Berlin: Springer, 1986:123–142.

(32) Zheng Y, Wei L, Lianggue G, et al. Applicability of the Chinese Beck Depression Inventory. Compr Psychiatry 1988;29:484–489.

(33) Shek DTL. Reliability and factorial structure of the Chinese version of the Beck Depression Inventory. J Clin Psychol 1990;46:35–43.

(34) Karanci NA. Patterns of depression in medical patients and their relationship with causal attributions for illness. Psychother Psychosom 1988;50:207–215.

(35) Kovacs M. The Children's Depression Inventory (CDI). Psychopharmacol Bull 1985;21:995–998.

(36) Leigh IW, Robins CJ, Welkowitz J. Modification of the Beck Depression Inventory for use with a deaf population. J Clin Psychol 1988;44:728–732.

(37) Williamson HA, Williamson MT. The Beck Depression Inventory: normative data and problems with generalizability. Fam Med 1989;21:58–60.

(38) Williams AC, Richardson PH. What does the BDI measure in chronic pain? Pain 1993;55:259–266.

(39) Cappeliez P. Social desirability response set and self-report depression inventories in the elderly. Clin Gerontol 1989;9:45–52.

(40) Tanaka-Matsumi J, Kameoka VA. Reliabilities and concurrent validities of popular self-report measures of depression, anxiety, and social desirability. J Consult Clin Psychol 1986;54:328–333.

(41) Langevin R, Stancer H. Evidence that depression rating scales primarily measure a social undesirability response set. Acta Psychiatr Scand 1979;59:70–79.

(42) Burkhart BR, Rogers K, McDonald WD, et al. The measurement of depression: enhancing the predictive validity of the Beck Depression Inventory. J Clin Psychol 1984;40:1368–1372.

(43) Hatzenbuehler LC, Parpal M, Matthews L. Classifying college students as depressed or nondepressed using the Beck Depression Inventory: an empirical analysis. J Consult Clin Psychol 1983;51:360–366.

THE SELF-RATING DEPRESSION SCALE
(W.W.K. Zung, 1965)

Purpose

The Self-rating Depression Scale (SDS) was originally developed to quantify the severity of current depression in patients of all ages with a primary diagnosis of depressive disorder (1). It has subsequently been used in clinical studies to monitor changes following treatment, as a screening instrument in family practice, and in cross-cultural studies (2, p51). It is brief and simple to administer, yet comprehensive.

Conceptual Basis

Guided by previous literature and by factor analytic studies, Zung classified the symptoms of depression into affective, somatic, psychomotor, and psychological (3). Within each category, he identified numerous symptoms. For example, the affective or mood disorders include feelings and complaints of being depressed, sad, downhearted, and tearful; the physiological and somatic symptoms include tachycardia, constipation, fatigue, sleep disturbances, and decreases in appetite, weight, and libido. The psychomotor disturbances are either retardation or agitation, while the psychological disturbances include confusion, indecisiveness, irritability and feelings of emptiness, hopelessness, personal devaluation, dissatisfaction, and suicidal ruminations (4, p332). These subcategories

guided the content of the SDS, and Zung selected items to reflect them from verbatim records of patient interviews (1; 3, Table 21.1; 4).

Description

The SDS comprises 20 items; ten are worded positively and ten negatively. For each item, respondents indicate the frequency with which they experience the symptom or feeling, either at the time of testing (5) or in the previous week (3). The 1974 version of the scale (slightly modified from the original) is shown in Exhibit 6.2 (3, Table 21.2; 4, Table 3). Note that there is an error in item 13 in the version printed

Exhibit 6.2 The Zung Self-Rating Depression Scale

Note: The scores shown here are not included in the version presented to the respondent; they are replaced by boxes in which the respondent places check marks. The raw scores are summed and converted to a 25–100 scale by dividing the total by 0.8.

Please answer these items as they pertain to you now.

	None or a little of the time	Some of the time	Good part of the time	Most or all of the time
1. I feel down-hearted, blue, and sad	1	2	3	4
2. Morning is when I feel the best	4	3	2	1
3. I have crying spells or feel like it	1	2	3	4
4. I have trouble sleeping through the night	1	2	3	4
5. I eat as much as I used to	4	3	2	1
6. I enjoy looking at, talking to, and being with attractive women/men	4	3	2	1
7. I notice that I am losing weight	1	2	3	4
8. I have trouble with constipation	1	2	3	4
9. My heart beats faster than usual	1	2	3	4
10. I get tired for no reason	1	2	3	4
11. My mind is as clear as it used to be	4	3	2	1
12. I find it easy to do the things I used to	4	3	2	1
13. I am restless and can't keep still	1	2	3	4
14. I feel hopeful about the future	4	3	2	1
15. I am more irritable than usual	1	2	3	4
16. I find it easy to make decisions	4	3	2	1
17. I feel that I am useful and needed	4	3	2	1
18. My life is pretty full	4	3	2	1
19. I feel that others would be better off if I were dead	1	2	3	4
20. I still enjoy the things I used to do	4	3	2	1

Adapted from Zung WWK. How normal is depression? Kalamazoo, Michigan: The Upjohn Company, 1981:17. With permission.

in reference 3; the version shown in our exhibit is correct. The scale takes ten to 15 minutes to complete, according to the patient's age and condition (6, p364). Toner et al. found that only 43% of a sample of elderly patients could respond to all of the questions independently (7, p138). The exhibit also shows the response options; note the reverse scoring for the positive items. Item scores are added to form a total ranging from 20 to 80, with higher scores indicating increasing depression. The raw score is then converted to an index by dividing the total by 0.8, producing a range from 25 to 100 (1, Table 5). Most guidelines for interpreting results suggest that *index* scores of less than 50 are within the normal range, of 50 to 59 indicate minimal or mild depression, of 60 to 69 indicate moderate to marked depression, and above 70 indicate severe depression (2; 4, p335; 5). A cutoff of 54/55 is commonly used to identify depression in people aged over 60 (E.M. Zung, personal communication).

Reliability

Several studies have estimated the internal consistency of the SDS; sample sizes range from 100 to 225. Alphas ranging from 0.75 to 0.95 have been reported (7–9). Zung and Zung reviewed studies using the SDS with elderly people; in four such studies alphas ranged from 0.59 to 0.87 (10, Table 2). Split-half reliability was estimated at 0.73 (3, p225) and at 0.81 (11, Table 2). Mean item-total correlations were 0.36 in samples of New York drug addicts and Nigerian students; alphas were 0.75 and 0.79 (9, p28). The one-year test–retest correlation was 0.61 in 279 older subjects (12, p179).

Validity

The validity of the SDS has been extensively studied; review articles (2) and a meta-analysis summarize the results (13). The findings are mixed, however, giving an overall impression of modest validity.

Moran and Lambert commented on con-

tent validity. They rated the SDS third out of six scales in terms of coverage of the *DSM-III* criteria; it covers five criteria well, four partially, and overlooks one variable (14, pp286–287).

In Zung's early work the SDS identified significant differences among patients with depression, other psychiatric patients, and controls; it was also sensitive to treatment effects (1, Table 6; 5, Table 3). Biggs found the SDS to discriminate significantly among levels of depression (N = 26) (15, Table III). He noted, however, that it is easier for a self-rating scale to distinguish levels of depression than to discriminate between diagnostic groups (15, p382). Indeed, other studies have found the SDS to discriminate poorly among diagnostic groups (16, 17). Carroll found that, unlike the Hamilton Rating Scale for Depression, the SDS failed to distinguish between severely depressed inpatients, moderately depressed day patients, and mildly depressed general practice patients (6, Table 1). Moran and Lambert reviewed three discriminant validity studies and concluded that "The SDS is not a sensitive measure of depressive symptomatology" (14, p289). They also reviewed five drug trials and found that the SDS was consistently less sensitive than other instruments in detecting treatment effects (14, Table 9.4). Lambert's meta-analysis confirmed that the SDS showed smaller differences between treatment and control subjects than did the Hamilton Rating Scale for Depression (HRSD), and somewhat smaller than the Beck Depression Inventory (BDI) (13, pp54,57).

The SDS shows moderate to high correlations with other depression instruments. For example, Hedlund and Vieweg's review quotes five correlations between the SDS and the MMPI Depression Scale that ranged from 0.55 to 0.70 (2, Table 1); other studies found correlations of 0.59 (5) and 0.76 (18). Correlations between the SDS and the BDI ranged from 0.60 to 0.83 (14, Table 9.2); Turner and Romano reported a correlation of 0.86 (18, Table 1). Tanaka-Matsumi found the SDS correlated more highly with Spielberger's Trait Anxiety scale (0.74) than with the BDI (0.68) or the Lubin Depression Adjective Check Lists (0.54) (8, Table 2). Snow and Crapo found the SDS to correlate −0.53 with Bradburn's Affect Balance Scale, and −0.61 with the Life Satisfaction Index A (N = 205) (19, Table 2).

Zung's SDS has often been compared to clinical ratings using the HRSD; the findings vary widely. Hedlund and Vieweg quoted 18 such results, with correlations mainly falling in the range 0.38 to 0.80, but with outliers of 0.22 and 0.95 (2, Table 1). Zung and Zung quoted figures of 0.79 and 0.80 in elderly people (10, Table 2); Carroll obtained a correlation of 0.41 (6, Table 1). He noted that the agreement between the Hamilton and SDS was highest in mild depression; the self-assessed format of the SDS is a limitation with severely depressed patients. Biggs et al. obtained Spearman correlations with the Hamilton scale ranging from 0.45 to 0.76 in an intervention study followed over six weeks; the overall correlation was 0.80 (15, Table I). They noted that the lowest correlations were obtained at the start of the study, perhaps due to the narrower spread of depression scores before treatment. In a sample of 110 mentally retarded adults, Kazdin et al. obtained a correlation of only 0.14 with the Hamilton scale; the equivalent result for the Beck scale was 0.24 (20, p1042).

Toner et al. compared the SDS to the depression section of the abbreviated Comprehensive Assessment and Referral Evaluation (Short-CARE) and to physicians' ratings for a sample of 80 elderly outpatients. Only 65% of patients completed enough of the SDS to permit scoring. Agreement between the physician's rating of depression and the SDS (κ = 0.29) was lower than for the Short-CARE (κ = 0.46) (7, p138).

Correlations between the SDS and psychiatrists' ratings of severity in various studies include 0.20 and 0.69 (2, Table 1), 0.23 and 0.58 (21, p16). The SDS demon-strated adequate sensitivity and specificity for detecting depression in a sample of 40 chronic pain patients. At a cutoff of 50, sensitivity was 83% and specificity was 81%, results almost identical to those obtained for the BDI (18). In four studies of elderly people reviewed by Zung and Zung, sensitivity ranged from 58% to 82%, while specificity ranged from 80% to 87% (10, Table 2). The SDS had better sensitivity and specificity (76% and 96%) for detecting clinically diagnosed depression among 40 geriatric stroke patients than the Geriatric Depression Scale (GDS) or the Center for Epidemiologic Studies Depression Scale (22, Table 3). Yet, in another study, sensitivity (80%) and specificity (84%) results for the SDS were lower than those for the GDS and Hamilton scales (23).

Hedlund and Vieweg reviewed six factor analytic studies of the SDS, which identified between two and seven factors, with reasonable agreement over two or three of these dimensions, covering emptiness, agitation, and appetite change (2). Blumenthal found that 12 of the items loaded on four distinct subscales, which she labeled well-being, depressed mood, somatic symptoms, and optimism. She found that the subscales were not consistent across different population groups: some of the symptoms may reflect normal aging, thus altering their validity among the elderly. For example, the somatic symptoms may indicate depression in young people but physical problems in elderly people (24).

Alternative Forms

The SDS has seen extensive use in North America, the Far East, Australia, and Europe. It has been translated into at least 30 languages and has been used in cross-cultural studies.

Zung developed a clinician's rating scale version of the SDS, the Depression Status Inventory (DSI) (3, Table 21.7; 26, Table 1). The correlation between the DSI and SDS on 225 patients was 0.87, and the internal consistency of the DSI was 0.81

(3, p230; 26, p543). The DSI is rarely cited in the literature.

Snaith et al. described the Wakefield Self-assessment Depression Inventory, a modified version of the SDS which retains ten of the 20 items and adds two items covering anxiety (27). They also used response categories that blend frequency with severity: "Yes, definitely," "Yes, sometimes," "No, not much," and "No, not at all."

Reference Standards

Zung and Zung provided age-specific reference values from 938 normal controls (10, Table 3). Zung also summarized results from 11 countries that show mean scores for depressed and normal respondents (25, Tables 3 and 6).

Commentary

Zung's SDS is one of the most widely used of all health measurement scales but, as so often happens with older methods, the early tests of validity showed a promise that was not borne out. Evidence for the reliability of the scale is restricted to its internal consistency, which is adequate. Results of validity studies have been mixed; a few studies show good results; many show the SDS to be adequate; a few suggest weaknesses.

All self-rating depression scales encounter problems of denial and of poor motivation to respond among more severely depressed, withdrawn patients. The 1973 review by Carroll et al. pointed to limitations in self-rating methods in general, suggesting that they may be adequate to establish the presence of symptoms but not to quantify their severity, as patients lack the clinical perspective required to rate severity (6, p361). Specific criticisms of the SDS include its focus on assessing the frequency rather than the severity of symptoms, even though its intent was to assess the latter. Most clinical ratings of depression rate severity, and this may contribute to the low agreement between the Hamilton and Zung scales. The frequency response format does not suit items such as, "I notice that I am losing weight." Some authors have proposed changing to severity ratings to make the SDS more sensitive to the degree of depression (28, p987); Snaith's categories mentioned here are an example. The mix of positive and negative items may confuse some patients (7), and the negatively worded symptoms may measure a different construct than the positive items (29). Like the BDI, the SDS correlates highly with anxiety scales, suggesting that they may measure a broader state than depression (8).

With the exception of Zung's own studies, most research has shown that the SDS discriminates only moderately well between diagnostic groups (2). When used as a screening test, sensitivity and specificity seem adequate, although somewhat lower than for other self-rating scales. Recent reviews of the SDS are generally negative. Boyle and others view it as "a psychometrically crude instrument" that should not be used in research (2, p54; 6; 29, p54), while Rabkin and Klein state that it is not the instrument of choice for assessing depressive severity or change after treatment, although it may have a role as an adjunctive screening instrument (30).

REFERENCES

(1) Zung WWK. A Self-rating Depression Scale. Arch Gen Psychiatry 1965;12:63–70.

(2) Hedlund JL, Vieweg BW. The Zung Self-rating Depression Scale: a comprehensive review. J Operat Psychiatry 1979;10:51–64.

(3) Zung WWK. Zung Self-rating Depression Scale and Depression Status Inventory. In: Sartorius N, Ban T, eds. Assessment of depression. Berlin: Springer, 1986:221–231.

(4) Zung WWK. From art to science: the diagnosis and treatment of depression. Arch Gen Psychiatry 1973;29:328–337.

(5) Zung WWK. Factors influencing the Self-rating Depression Scale. Arch Gen Psychiatry 1967;16:543–547.

(6) Carroll BJ, Fielding JM, Blashki TG. Depression rating scales: a critical review. Arch Gen Psychiatry 1973;28:361–366.

(7) Toner J, Gurland B, Teresi J. Comparison of self-administered and rater-administered methods of assessing levels of severity of depression in elderly patients. J Gerontol 1988;43:P136–P140.

(8) Tanaka-Matsumi J, Kameoka VA. Reliabilities and concurrent validities of popular self-report measures of depression, anxiety, and social desirability. J Consult Clin Psychol 1986;54:328–333.

(9) Jegede RO. Psychometric properties of the Self-rating Depression Scale (SDS). J Psychol 1976;93:27–30.

(10) Zung WWK, Zung EM. Use of the Zung Self-rating Depression Scale in the elderly. Clin Gerontol 1986;5:137–148.

(11) Yesavage JA, Brink TL, Rose TL, et al. Development and validation of a geriatric depression screening scale: a preliminary report. J Psychiatr Res 1983;17:37–49.

(12) McKegney FP, Aronson MK, Ooi WL. Identifying depression in the old old. Psychosomatics 1988;29:175–181.

(13) Lambert MJ, Hatch DR, Kingston MD, et al. Zung, Beck, and Hamilton rating scales as measures of treatment outcome: a meta-analytic comparison. J Consult Clin Psychol 1986;54:54–59.

(14) Moran PW, Lambert MJ. A review of current assessment tools for monitoring changes in depression. In: Lambert MJ, Christensen ER, DeJulio SS, eds. The measurement of psychotherapy outcome in research and evaluation. New York: Wiley, 1983:263–303.

(15) Biggs JT, Wylie LT, Ziegler VE. Validity of the Zung Self-rating Depression Scale. Br J Psychiatry 1978;132:381–385.

(16) Schnurr R, Hoaken PCS, Jarrett FJ. Comparison of depression inventories in a clinical population. Can Psychiatr Assoc J 1976;21:473–476.

(17) Shanfield S, Tucker GJ, Harrow M, et al. The schizophrenic patient and depressive symptomatology. J Nerv Ment Dis 1970;151:203–210.

(18) Turner JA, Romano JM. Self-report screening measures for depression in chronic pain patients. J Clin Psychol 1984;40:909–913.

(19) Snow R, Crapo L. Emotional bondedness, subjective well-being, and health in elderly medical patients. J Gerontol 1982;37:609–615.

(20) Kazdin AE, Matson JL, Senatore V. Assessment of depression in mentally retarded adults. Am J Psychiatry 1983;140:1040–1043.

(21) Downing RW, Rickels K. Some properties of the Popoff Index. Clin Med 1972;79:11–18.

(22) Agrell B, Dehlin O. Comparison of six depression rating scales in geriatric stroke patients. Stroke 1989;20:1190–1194.

(23) Brink TL, Yesavage JA, Lum O, et al. Screening tests for geriatric depression. Clin Gerontol 1982;1:37–43.

(24) Blumenthal MD. Measuring depressive symptomatology in a general population. Arch Gen Psychiatry 1975;32:971–978.

(25) Zung WWK. How normal is depression? Kalamazoo, Michigan: The Upjohn Company, 1981.

(26) Zung WWK. The Depression Status Inventory: an adjunct to the Self-rating Depression Scale. J Clin Psychol 1972;28:539–543.

(27) Snaith RP, Ahmed SN, Mehta S, et al. Assessment of the severity of primary depressive illness: Wakefield Self-assessment Depression Inventory. Psychol Med 1971;1:143–149.

(28) Zinkin S, Birtchnell J. Unilateral electroconvulsive therapy: its effects on memory and its therapeutic efficacy. Br J Psychiatry 1968;114:973–988.

(29) Boyle GJ. Self-report measures of depression: some psychometric considerations. Br J Clin Psychol 1985;24:45–59.

(30) Rabkin JG, Klein DF. The clinical measurement of depressive disorders. In: Marsella AJ, Hirschfeld RMA, Katz MM, eds. The measurement of depression. New York: Guilford Press, 1987:30–83.

THE CENTER FOR EPIDEMIOLOGIC STUDIES DEPRESSION SCALE (CES-D) (National Institute of Mental Health, USA, 1972)

Purpose

The Center for Epidemiologic Studies Depression Scale (CES-D) is a 20-item, self-report depression scale developed to identify depression in the general population (1).

Conceptual Basis

The CES-D was designed to cover the major components of depression identified in the literature, with an emphasis on affective components: depressed mood, feelings of guilt and worthlessness, feelings of helplessness and hopelessness, psychomotor retardation, loss of appetite, and sleep disorders (1, p386). These symptoms can be experienced in the absence of depression, but Radloff argued that in people without depression they tend to be counterbalanced by positive affect (1, p391). The CES-D accordingly covers positive affect and this two-dimensional model of well-being reflects Bradburn's Affect Balance Scale. As with Bradburn's scale, there is empirical evidence that the positive items on the CES-D form a separate dimension rather than merely being the inverse of the negative items (2, p269).

Radloff recognized that there is considerable variation in the presentation of symptoms of depression. For example, lower socioeconomic groups report more physical symptoms while higher socioeconomic groups express depression affectively. The heterogeneity of response implies low intercorrelations among items, and also that cutting points are difficult to set.

Description

Items for the CES-D were selected from existing scales, including Beck's Depression Inventory (BDI), Zung's Self-rating Depression Scale (SDS), Raskin's Depression Scale, and the Minnesota Multiphasic Personality Inventory (1). The CES-D is normally self-administered, but may be used in an interview. Items refer to the frequency of symptoms during the past week (see Exhibit 6.3). Each question uses a 0-to-3 response scale; except for the four positive questions, a higher score indicates greater depression. Questions 4, 8, 12, and 16 were worded positively, in part to discourage a response set, and their scores are reversed by subtracting the score from 3. Question scores are then summed to provide an overall score ranging from 0 to 60. If more than five items on the scale are missing, a score is generally not calculated (3, p31). If one to five items are missing, scores on the completed items are summed (after reversal of the positive items); this total is divided by the number of items answered and multiplied by 20.

Scores of 16 or more are commonly taken as indicative of depression (4, p206). This is equivalent to experiencing six symptoms for most of the previous week, or a majority of the symptoms on one or two days. Several alternative cutting points have been suggested. Himmelfarb and Murrell proposed 19/20 for those aged over 55 (5, p339). Husaini et al. proposed 16/17 (one standard deviation below the mean score for acutely depressed outpatients) to indicate possible cases and 22/23 to indicate probable cases of depression (6). The validity results for the cutting points of 15/16 and 16/17 were virtually identical, so 15/16 is probably the most suitable.

Reliability

Radloff reported alpha coefficients of 0.85 for general population samples and of 0.90 for a patient sample; split-half reliability ranged from 0.76 to 0.85 (1, Table 3). Alphas of 0.85 were also reported by Roberts for Black and for White respondents (7, Table 3). Himmelfarb and Murrell reported alpha coefficients of 0.85 for a community sample (N = 235) and 0.91 for a clinical sample (N = 88) (5, Table 1). An alpha of 0.86 was obtained for frail elderly people (8, p161). A correlation of 0.76 (N = 24) was obtained between versions administered by a nurse and a research assistant (9, p242).

The concentration of the CES-D on recent symptoms may reduce test–retest reliability. Radloff reported low retest correlations, running from 0.32 to 0.67; most coefficients fell between 0.50 and 0.60 (1, Table 4).

Validity

Weissman et al. compared CES-D scores from a community sample, a group of depressed patients, and patients with other psychiatric conditions. Average scores were 38.1 for 148 acutely depressed patients, 14.9 for 87 recovered depressives, 13 for 50 schizophrenics, and 9.1 for 3,932 adults in the community (4, Table 3). The scale proved capable of distinguishing alcoholics and schizophrenics who were also depressed (as assessed by the Raskin Depression Scale) from others who were not; Weissman concluded that the CES-D was

Exhibit 6.3   The Center for Epidemiologic Studies Depression Scale (CES-D)

Note: Items 4, 8, 12, and 16 have their scores reversed before totalling.

Instructions for questions: Below is a list of the ways you might have felt or behaved. Please tell me how often you felt this way during the past week.

During the past week:	Rarely or none of the time (less than 1 day)	Some or a little of the time (1–2 days)	Occasionally or a moderate amount of the time (3–4 days)	Most or all of the time (5–7 days)
1. I was bothered by things that usually don't bother me	0	1	2	3
2. I did not feel like eating; my appetite was poor	0	1	2	3
3. I felt that I could not shake off the blues even with help from my family or friends	0	1	2	3
4. I felt that I was just as good as other people	0	1	2	3
5. I had trouble keeping my mind on what I was doing	0	1	2	3
6. I felt depressed	0	1	2	3
7. I felt that everything I did was an effort	0	1	2	3
8. I felt hopeful about the future	0	1	2	3
9. I thought my life had been a failure	0	1	2	3
10. I felt fearful	0	1	2	3
11. My sleep was restless	0	1	2	3
12. I was happy	0	1	2	3
13. I talked less than usual	0	1	2	3
14. I felt lonely	0	1	2	3
15. People were unfriendly	0	1	2	3
16. I enjoyed life	0	1	2	3
17. I had crying spells	0	1	2	3
18. I felt sad	0	1	2	3
19. I felt that people dislike me	0	1	2	3
20. I could not get "going"	0	1	2	3

Adapted from Radloff LS. The CES-D Scale: a self-report depression scale for research in the general population. Appl Psychol Measurement 1977;1:387, Table 1. Copyright 1977 West Publishing Co./Applied Psychological Measurement Inc. Reproduced by permission.

not merely measuring overall psychiatric impairment. The CES-D showed significant differences between respondents who reported needing help for an emotional problem and those who did not; mean scores also varied significantly with the presence of life events (1, Tables 7, 8).

Using the Raskin scale as a criterion, Weissman et al. reported high sensitivity for detecting depression in various patient groups. Sensitivity was 99% for acute depressives, 94% (at a specificity of 84%) for detecting depression among alcoholics, and 93% (specificity 86%) for schizophrenics (4, Table 7). Shinar et al. reported a sensitivity of 73% at a specificity of 100% for the cutting point of 16 or over (N = 27) (9, Table 4). Parikh et al. obtained a sensitivity of 86% at a specificity of 90% for the cutting point of 16 for 80 stroke patients (10, Table 3). Zich et al. tested the CES-D in a primary care setting; sensitivity was 100% and specificity 53% at the cutting point of 16 ($\kappa = 0.12$); at a cutting point of 27, specificity rose to 81% (κ = 0.34) (2, Table 2). They suggested that in a primary care setting with a low prevalence of depression, the cutting point should be raised above the conventional 16. A discrepant report is that of Myers and Weissman, who found a sensitivity of only 63.6% for detecting major depression, at a specificity of 93.9% in 482 community adults (11). Boyd et al. examined the discrepant cases from this study; the eight false-negative cases included four patients who denied their symptoms and three who had difficulty in completing the questionnaire (12).

Radloff reported a correlation of 0.56 with a clinical rating of severity of depression (1, p393). In a different sample, the CES-D scores correlated 0.44 with the Hamilton Rating Scale for Depression at admission and 0.69 after treatment (N = 35); the equivalent correlations with the Raskin scale were 0.54 at admission and 0.75 after treatment (1, p393). Weissman et al. reported correlations between the CES-D and other depression scales for five different patient groups. Correlations with the Hamilton scale ranged from 0.49 to 0.85 while those for the Symptom Check List-90 ranged from 0.72 to 0.87. Correlations with age, social class, and sex were almost all nonsignificant (4, Table 5). Shinar et al. reported correlations of 0.57 with the Hamilton scale, 0.65 with the SDS, and 0.77 with a depression categorization based on the *DSM-III* (9, Table 2). Virtually identical results were obtained by Parikh et al. (10, Table 2).

The CES-D has been compared to other measurements in several samples. Correlations with Bradburn's Affect Balance Scale ranged from 0.61 to 0.72; correlations with Langner's 22-item scale ranged from 0.54 to 0.60, and those with the Lubin Depression Adjective Check Lists were from 0.51 to 0.70 (1, Table 6).

Radloff reported consistent results of factor analyses across three samples during the early development of the CES-D. The analyses produced four factors, interpreted as depressed affect, positive affect, somatic symptoms and retarded activity, and interpersonal problems (1, p397). The same factor structure was obtained on samples of Black, White, and Chicano populations by Roberts (7), and it has been further replicated with minor variations (2, 8, 13, 14). A recent study of elderly people, however, found differences in the factor structures between race and gender groups (15). Liang et al. proposed a three-factor model that excluded the interpersonal problem factor and gave an extended discussion of the results of previous studies (16). While the results of factor analyses are relatively consistent, they should not be used as a basis for identifying subscores for the CES-D, for several reasons. The factors intercorrelate (8, Table 4); the scale as a whole has high internal consistency; and not all items load significantly on the factors.

Alternative Forms

Shrout and Yager argued that, owing to the high internal consistency of the CES-D, it could be shortened without substantial loss of reliability (14). Abbreviated versions of the CES-D have been proposed (16, Table 1; 17). A ten-item version for elderly people showed close agreement with the full version (κ = 0.97) and a test–retest reliability of 0.71 (18).

A Chinese version showed an alpha reliability of 0.92 (19).

An alternative approach to scoring the CES-D reflects the Research Diagnostic Criteria (RDC) for depression that specify six criteria to be met for a diagnosis (12; 20, p800). In place of an overall score, the CES-D responses indicate whether or not each of the criteria has been met; Boyd et al. indicated which CES-D questions correspond to the RDC criteria (12, Table 1).

Reference Standards

The CES-D was included in the HANES population survey in 1974–1975; norms were published for those aged 25–74 by age, sex, race, marital status, income and occupation (3). The average score for noninstitutionalized adults was 8.7; women had higher scores than men (3, p2). Eaton and Kessler further analyzed the HANES survey data for those who scored above the cutting point (21, Table 2). The results showed strong associations with employment status, educational level, income, and sex. Murrell et al. reported CES-D scores from a survey in Kentucky by gender, race, education, and income levels (22, Table 3). Golding et al. provide age-adjusted norms for samples of White and Mexican Americans (23, Tables 1–3). Vera et al. provide reference scores for two samples of Puerto Ricans by age, sex, and socioeconomic status (24, Table 2).

Commentary

The CES-D is one of the best-known survey instruments for identifying symptoms of depression. It has been extensively used in large studies and norms are available. It is applicable across age and sociodemographic groups; it has been used in cross-cultural research—for example, with elderly Puerto Ricans (25). It has often been used in studying the relationships between depressive symptoms and other variables.

As with other self-assessed depression scales, the CES-D should not be viewed as a diagnostic tool but rather as a screening test to identify groups at risk of depression. In clinical studies the CES-D has been shown capable of detecting depression in a variety of psychiatric patients, and results agree quite well with other, more detailed, instruments. It has limitations however. It cannot distinguish primary depression from that secondary to other diagnoses; this is relevant as the two types of condition may have differing courses and different treatment may be indicated (4, p213). Furthermore, it may fail to separate depression from generalized anxiety and may not distinguish past from present disorders: "many CES-D items are not essential symptoms of major depressive disorder, and serve equally well as symptoms of other syndromes or even of nonspecific demoralization" (26, p77). Finally, when applied in primary care or general population settings, it seems to generate a high number of false positives. Boyd et al. proposed that the CES-D should be administered before other questions, that the questions should be read to the respondent, and that a way should be found to deal with people who deny symptoms, such as interviewing their relatives (12, p1200).

The suitability of 16 as a cutting score has been discussed. While undue credence should never be placed in a single cutting point, 16 is most commonly used and seems adequate in clinical settings, although a higher point may be beneficial in primary care settings to reduce the number of false positives.

The CES-D performs comparably to other self-report scales, but there remains concern over its specificity. As a first screen it is adequate, but caution should be exercised in interpreting the nature of the disorder it detects.

REFERENCES

(1) Radloff LS. The CES-D Scale: a self-report depression scale for research in the general population. Appl Psychol Measurement 1977;1:385–401.
(2) Zich JM, Attkisson CC, Greenfield TK. Screening for depression in primary care clinics: the CES-D and the BDI. Int J Psychiatry Med 1990;20:259–277.
(3) Sayetta R, Johnson D. Basic data on depressive symptomatology, United States, 1974–75. Washington, DC: United States Government Printing Office, Public Health Services 1980. (DHEW (PHS) 80–1666).
(4) Weissman MM, Sholomskas D, Pottenger M, et al. Assessing depressive symptoms in five psychiatric populations: a validation study. Am J Epidemiol 1977;106:203–214.
(5) Himmelfarb S, Murrell SA. Reliability and validity of five mental health scales in older persons. J Gerontol 1983;38:333–339.
(6) Husaini BA, Neff JA, Harrington JB. Depression in rural communities: establishing CES-D cutting points. Nashville, Tennessee: Tennessee State University, 1979.
(7) Roberts RE. Reliability of the CES-D Scale in different ethnic contexts. Psychiatry Res 1980;2:125–134.
(8) Davidson H, Feldman PH, Crawford S. Measuring depressive symptoms in the frail elderly. J Gerontol 1994;49:P159–P164.

(9) Shinar D, Gross CR, Price TR, et al. Screening for depression in stroke patients: the reliability and validity of the Center for Epidemiologic Studies Depression Scale. Stroke 1986;17:241–245.

(10) Parikh RM, Eden DT, Price TR, et al. The sensitivity and specificity of the Center for Epidemiologic Studies Depression Scale in screening for post-stroke depression. Int J Psychiatry Med 1988;18:169–181.

(11) Myers JK, Weissman MM. Use of a self-report symptom scale to detect depression in a community sample. Am J Psychiatry 1980;137:1081–1084.

(12) Boyd JH, Weissman MM, Thompson WD, et al. Screening for depression in a community sample: understanding the discrepancies between depression symptom and diagnostic scales. Arch Gen Psychiatry 1982;39:1195–1200.

(13) Clark VA, Aneshensel CS, Fredrichs RR, et al. Analysis of effects of sex and age in response to items on the CES-D Scale. Psychiatry Res 1981;5:171–181.

(14) Shrout PE, Yager TJ. Reliability and validity of screening scales: effect of reducing scale length. J Clin Epidemiol 1989; 42:69–78.

(15) Callahan CM, Wolinsky FD. The effect of gender and race on the measurement properties of the CES-D in older adults. Med Care 1994;32:341–356.

(16) Liang J, Van Tran T, Krause N, et al. Generational differences in the structure of the CES-D Scale in Mexican Americans. J Gerontol 1989;44:S110–S120.

(17) Burnam MA, Wells KB, Leake B, et al. Development of a brief screening instrument for detecting depressive disorders. Med Care 1988;26:775–789.

(18) Andresen EM, Malmgren JA, Carter WB, et al. Screening for depression in well older adults: evaluation of a short form of the CES-D (Center for Epidemiologic Studies Depression Scale). Am J Prev Med 1994;10:77–84.

(19) Rankin SH, Galbraith ME, Johnson S. Reliability and validity data for a Chinese translation of the Center for Epidemiological Studies-Depression. Psychol Rep 1993;73:1291–1298.

(20) Schoenbach VJ, Kaplan BH, Grimson RC, et al. Use of a symptom scale to study the prevalence of a depressive syndrome in young adolescents. Am J Epidemiol 1982;116:791–800.

(21) Eaton WW, Kessler LG. Rates of symptoms of depression in a national sample. Am J Epidemiol 1981;114:528–538.

(22) Murrell SA, Himmelfarb S, Wright K. Prevalence of depression and its correlates in older adults. Am J Epidemiol 1983;117:173–185.

(23) Golding JM, Aneshensel CS, Hough RL. Responses to Depression Scale items among Mexican-Americans and non-Hispanic whites. J Clin Psychol 1991;47:61–75.

(24) Vera M, Alegria M, Freeman D, et al. Depressive symptoms among Puerto Ricans: island poor compared with residents of the New York City area. Am J Epidemiol 1991;134:502–510.

(25) Mahard RE. The CES-D as a measure of depressive mood in the elderly Puerto Rican population. J Gerontol 1988;43:P24–P25.

(26) Rabkin JG, Klein DF. The clinical measurement of depressive disorders. In: Marsella AJ, Hirschfeld RMA, Katz MM, eds. The measurement of depression. New York: Guilford Press, 1987:30–83.

THE GERIATRIC DEPRESSION SCALE
(T.L. Brink and
Jerome A. Yesavage, 1982)

Purpose

The Geriatric Depression Scale (GDS) was designed as a screening test for depression in elderly people (1). It is a self-rating scale intended primarily for clinical applications and was designed to be easily administered in an office setting.

Conceptual Basis

Brink and Yesavage argued that depression scales developed for younger people are inappropriate for the elderly (2). Symptoms indicative of depression in young people, such as sleep disturbance, weight loss, and pessimism about the future, may occur in the elderly as normal effects of aging or as the result of a physical illness. In the elderly, depression commonly coexists with dementia; cognitive problems compromise the accuracy of self-reports just as depression may mask cognitive abilities (1, p37). The GDS was designed as a simple, clear, and self-administered scale that does not rely on somatic symptoms.

Description

The Geriatric Depression Scale was developed from an initial pool of 100 items chosen by clinicians and researchers for their ability to distinguish elderly depressives from normal people. Questions that might elicit defensiveness were avoided and, for simplicity, a yes/no answer format was used for all items. The 30 items in the GDS were selected from the pool empirically, on the basis of high item-total correlations when administered to a mixed sample of 47 community residents and people hospitalized for depression, all of whom were over 55 years of age (1, p41).

The GDS is shown in Exhibit 6.4. The scale is normally self-administered in eight to ten minutes, but it can also be read in an interview (1, 3). If the scale is administered orally, the interviewer may have to repeat the question to get a response that is a clear yes or no. The time frame is the past week. One point is counted for each

Exhibit 6.4 The Geriatric Depression Scale

Note: N or Y indicates which answer is scored. The fifteen items marked with an asterisk form the abbreviated version.

Choose the best answer for how you felt over the past week

1. Are you basically satisfied with your life?	yes / no	N *
2. Have you dropped many of your activities and interests?	yes / no	Y *
3. Do you feel that your life is empty?	yes / no	Y *
4. Do you often get bored?	yes / no	Y *
5. Are you hopeful about the future?	yes / no	N
6. Are you bothered by thoughts that you just cannot get out of your head?	yes / no	Y
7. Are you in good spirits most of the time?	yes / no	N *
8. Are you afraid that something bad is going to happen to you?	yes / no	Y *
9. Do you feel happy most of the time?	yes / no	N *
10. Do you often feel helpless?	yes / no	Y *
11. Do you often get restless and fidgety?	yes / no	Y
12. Do you prefer to stay at home, rather than go out and do new things?	yes / no	Y *
13. Do you frequently worry about the future?	yes / no	Y
14. Do you feel that you have more problems with memory than most?	yes / no	Y *
15. Do you think it is wonderful to be alive now?	yes / no	N *
16. Do you often feel downhearted and blue?	yes / no	Y
17. Do you feel pretty worthless the way you are now?	yes / no	Y *
18. Do you worry a lot about the past?	yes / no	Y
19. Do you find life very exciting?	yes / no	N
20. Is it hard for you to get started on new projects?	yes / no	Y
21. Do you feel full of energy?	yes / no	N *
22. Do you feel that your situation is hopeless?	yes / no	Y *
23. Do you think that most people are better off than you are?	yes / no	Y *
24. Do you frequently get upset over little things?	yes / no	Y
25. Do you frequently feel like crying?	yes / no	Y
26. Do you have trouble concentrating?	yes / no	Y
27. Do you enjoy getting up in the morning?	yes / no	N
28. Do you prefer to avoid social gatherings?	yes / no	Y
29. Is it easy for you to make decisions?	yes / no	N
30. Is your mind as clear as it used to be?	yes / no	N

Reproduced from the Geriatric Depression Scale obtained from Dr. TL Brink. With permission.

depressive answer, as shown in the exhibit; points are added to form a total score ranging from 0 to 30, with higher values reflecting greater depression. Scores of 0 to 10 are considered within the normal range, 11 to 20 indicate mild depression and 21 to 30 indicate moderate to severe depression. A cutting point of 10/11 is generally used, although Kafonek used 13/14 (4) and others have used 14/15 (5).

Sheikh and Yesavage proposed an abbreviated version of the GDS to reduce problems of fatigue and lack of focus, especially among physically ill or demented patients (6). The 15 items are identified in the exhibit and take five to seven minutes to complete. Scores between 0 and 4 are considered normal; 5 to 9 indicate mild depression; and 10 to 15 indicate moderate to severe depression (3). Several authors have reported correlations between scores on the short and long forms: 0.84 (6, p169), 0.89 (7), and 0.66 in a sample of 81 without severely depressed individuals (3).

Reliability

Reflecting the manner in which the GDS was constructed, numerous studies show high internal consistency. Yesavage et al. reported an alpha coefficient of 0.94 in a mixed sample of normal and depressed elderly people (N = 100) (1, p43). Agrell and Dehlin found an alpha of 0.90 in 40 stroke patients (8, p1192) while Lyons et al. tested 69 hip fracture patients and reported alpha coefficients of 0.88 at admission and 0.93 at discharge (9, p205). Rule et al. obtained an alpha coefficient of 0.82 and a split-half reliability of 0.80 for 193 university students, higher than the figure for Zung's Self-rating Depression Scale (SDS) (10, Table 1). In a further study of 389 community residents, Cronbach's alpha ranged from 0.80 to 0.85 across five age groups of 29- to 99-year-olds (10, p40). Lesher reported an alpha coefficient of 0.99, a median item-total correlation of 0.34, and a split-half reliability of 0.84 for 52 nursing home residents (11, pp24–25).

The test–retest reliability of the GDS has also been shown to be high: 0.85 at one week (N = 20) (1, p44), 0.86 at one hour (12, Table 1), and 0.98 at ten to 12 days (9, p206). Brink et al. reported an inter-rater reliability of 0.85 in a sample of 54 nursing home residents (12, Table 1).

Validity

Several studies have compared the Geriatric Depression Scale to the Hamilton Rating Scale for Depression (HRSD), providing correlations of 0.78 (13, Table 2), 0.82 (2, p42), 0.62, and 0.81 (9, p206). Yesavage et al. found the GDS performed comparably to the Hamilton scale and that it was significantly better than the SDS in discriminating among 100 patients with different levels of depression, as defined by the Research Diagnostic Criteria. Scores on the GDS increased significantly with level of depression ($r = 0.82$). The equivalent correlation for the SDS was 0.69, while for the Hamilton scale it was 0.83 (1, pp44–45). Koenig et al. found the GDS correlated 0.82 with the Montgomery-Åsberg Depression Rating Scale (13, Table 2). For 67 veterans, the GDS correlated 0.85 with the Beck Depression Inventory; the Beck instrument showed slightly higher sensitivity and specificity (14, pp993–994).

In terms of sensitivity, the GDS may perform slightly better than the Zung and Hamilton scales; the GDS showed a sensitivity of 84% and specificity of 95% at a cutting point of 10/11 (2, Table 2). Compared to diagnoses based on the Diagnostic Interview Schedule in a sample of 128 hospitalized veterans, the GDS had a sensitivity of 92%, a specificity of 89%, a positive predictive value of 53%, and a negative predictive value of 99% at a cutoff of 10/11. The kappa agreement between the GDS and a structured psychiatric interview was 0.62 (15, Table 1). Lower validity was reported by Koenig et al., who found a sensitivity of 82% at a specificity of 67%. Among those with a positive GDS score, the likelihood of having a major depressive disorder was 27%; these results were comparable to those obtained using the Brief Carroll Rating Scale (16, Table 2).

Agrell and Dehlin compared the GDS to five other depression scales in a sample of 40 stroke patients. At a cutoff of 10/11, the GDS had the highest sensitivity (88%), but its specificity was low (64%). The GDS correlated 0.88 with the Zung SDS, 0.82 with the CES-D, and 0.77 with the HRSD (8, pp1192–1193). Lesher reported a sensitivity of 100% for detecting major depression and 69% for depressive disorders among 51 nursing home residents. Specificity was 74% (11, p25). Snowdon obtained a sensitivity of 93% at a specificity of 83%, using a cutting point of 10/11 (17).

The validity of the GDS among cognitively impaired patients has been reviewed extensively. Sheikh and Yesavage studied 43 demented patients and argued that the GDS distinguished successfully between those who were depressed and those who were not (6, p168). By contrast, others have found that the cognitive status of respondents heavily influences the validity of the GDS. Kafonek et al. found the GDS to be 75% sensitive in cognitively normal people but 25% sensitive in a group of cognitively impaired nursing home residents (4, p32). While Brink suggested that this might be an artefact of the unconventional cutoff or scoring method used (5), Kafonek argued that the results would have been the same with Brink's cutoff. Burke et al. tested the GDS on 70 cognitively intact people and 72 with mild dementia. Using the area under the receiver operating characteristic curve (AUC) as an indicator of test performance, the GDS was sensitive in detecting depression among those cognitively intact (AUC = 0.85) but performed no better than chance among those with dementia (AUC = 0.66, not significant) (18, p859). A recent nursing home study identified a Mini-Mental State Exam (MMSE) score of 14/15 as the threshold below which the GDS performs poorly. At 15 or over, sensitivity was 84% and specificity was 91%; the results were markedly less good at lower MMSE scores (19).

Lesher found the sensitivity of the standard and short forms of the GDS to be equal (7).

Weiss et al. assessed the suitability of six depression scales for people aged 75 or older, a group in which depression is often atypical. None of the scales studied, including the GDS, measured two-week persistence of symptoms as required by *DSM-III*. The GDS contains more items characteristic of depression in elderly people than other scales, but it nonetheless omits several relevant themes (20).

Cappeliez found that scores on the GDS were unrelated to a social desirability response set (21).

Alternative Forms

Cwikel and Ritchie translated the short version of the GDS for use in Israel. Sensitivity was 70% and specificity was 75% (22, p66); in commenting on this indifferent performance they suggested that some questions did not have equivalent meanings in different ethnic groups.

Commentary

Assessing depression among the elderly is challenging (23). There is empirical support for Brink and Yesavage's contention that somatic items are not useful indicators of depression among the elderly (24, 25), and so the GDS focuses on the affective aspects of depression. It is easily and quickly administered by non-physicians and is comprehensible to older persons (15). It has been tested in community and patient samples. Its reliability is good, and sensitivity and specificity have generally been high among cognitively intact elderly people. Indeed, as a screening test it appears to perform as well as the Hamilton scale, while it is briefer and more easily administered.

The GDS is less valid in assessing cognitively impaired patients. This is not surprising, for asking a person how she has felt in the past week is a recall task (18, p859). In such cases, self-report is commonly supplemented by evidence from an informant. The GDS has not been well validated on the very old. Although it may lack some items relevant to identifying depression, the GDS performs better than most self-rating scales when applied to elderly people. We recommend its use but, as with most self-rating depression scales, it should be followed by a psychiatric interview to confirm the classification.

REFERENCES

(1) Yesavage JA, Brink TL, Rose TL, et al. Development and validation of a geriatric depression screening scale: a preliminary report. J Psychiatr Res 1983;17:37–49.

(2) Brink TL, Yesavage JA, Lum O, et al. Screening tests for geriatric depression. Clin Gerontol 1982;1:37–43.

(3) Alden D, Austin C, Sturgeon R. A correlation between the Geriatric Depression Scale long and short forms. J Gerontol 1989;44:124–125.

(4) Kafonek S, Ettinger WH, Roca R, et al. Instruments for screening for depression and dementia in a long-term care facility. J Am Geriatr Soc 1989;37:29–34.

(5) Brink TL. Proper scoring of the Geriatric Depression Scale. J Am Geriatr Soc 1989;37:819–820.

(6) Sheikh JI, Yesavage JA. Geriatric Depression Scale (GDS): recent evidence and development of a shorter version. Clin Gerontol 1986;5:165–172.

(7) Lesher EL, Berryhill JS. Validation of the Geriatric Depression Scale—Short Form among inpatients. J Clin Psychol 1994;50:256–260.

(8) Agrell B, Dehlin O. Comparison of six depression rating scales in geriatric stroke patients. Stroke 1989;20:1190–1194.

(9) Lyons JS, Strain JJ, Hammer JS, et al. Reliability, validity, and temporal stability of the Geriatric Depression Scale in hospitalized elderly. Int J Psychiatry Med 1989;19:203–209.

(10) Rule BG, Harvey HZ, Dobbs AR. Reliability of the Geriatric Depression Scale for younger adults. Clin Gerontol 1989;9:37–43.

(11) Lesher EL. Validation of the Geriatric Depression Scale among nursing home residents. Clin Gerontol 1986;4:21–28.

(12) Brink TL, Curran P, Dorr ML, et al. Geriatric Depression Scale reliability: order, examiner and reminiscence effects. Clin Gerontol 1983;2:57–60.

(13) Koenig HG, Meador KG, Cohen HJ, et al. Depression in elderly hospitalized patients with medical illness. Arch Intern Med 1988;148:1929–1936.

(14) Norris JT, Gallagher D, Wilson A, et al. Assessment of depression in geriatric medical outpatients: the validity of two screening measures. J Am Geriatr Soc 1987;35:989–995.

(15) Koenig HG, Meador KG, Cohen HJ, et al. Self-rated depression scales and screening for major depression in the older hospitalized patient with medical illness. J Am Geriatr Soc 1988;36:699–706.

(16) Koenig HG, Meador KG, Cohen HJ, et al. Screening for depression in hospitalized elderly medical patients: taking a closer look. J Am Geriatr Soc 1992;40:1013–1017.

(17) Snowdon J. Validity of the Geriatric Depression Scale. J Am Geriatr Soc 1990;38:722–723.

(18) Burke WJ, Houston MJ, Boust SJ, et al. Use of the Geriatric Depression Scale in dementia of the Alzheimer type. J Am Geriatr Soc 1989;37:856–860.

(19) McGivney SA, Mulvihill M, Taylor B. Validating the GDS depression screen in the nursing home. J Am Geriatr Soc 1994;42:490–492.

(20) Weiss IK, Nagel CL, Aronson MK. Applicability of depression scales to the old old person. J Am Geriatr Soc 1986;34:215–218.

(21) Cappeliez P. Social desirability response set and self-report depression inventories in the elderly. Clin Gerontol 1989;9:45–52.

(22) Cwikel J, Ritchie K. The Short GDS: evaluation in a heterogeneous, multilingual population. Clin Gerontol 1988;8:63–71.

(23) Thompson LW, Futterman A, Gallagher D. Assessment of late-life depression. Psychopharmacol Bull 1988;24:577–586.

(24) Zemore R, Eames N. Psychic and somatic symptoms of depression among young adults, institutionalized aged and noninstitutionalized aged. J Gerontol 1979;34:716–722.

(25) Bolla-Wilson K, Bleecker ML. Absence of depression in elderly adults. J Gerontol 1989;44:53–55.

THE DEPRESSION ADJECTIVE CHECK LISTS
(Bernard Lubin, 1965)

Purpose

The Depression Adjective Check Lists (DACL) comprise seven scales which were developed as brief research instruments for measuring depressed mood (1). They are applicable to all ages and diagnostic groups. The seven forms of the DACL are designed to be equivalent and are intended for use where repeated assessments are to be made (2).

Conceptual Basis

Developed during the early 1960s in the context of a shift away from behaviorism, the DACL focused on the affective dimensions of depression. Lubin bypassed conceptual debates over the components of depression and concentrated on lowered mood but did not define exactly what aspects were to be covered. This may place the DACL within the European phenomenological tradition rather than the North American tradition. The adjective check list format was chosen as being suited to assessing mood, easy to administer, and acceptable to subjects.

Description

The DACL form one of a series of adjective check list scales. In 1960, Zuckerman published the Anxiety Adjective Check List; Lubin began developing the Depression Adjective Check Lists in 1963 and then collaborated with Zuckerman to incorporate the most discriminating items from the DACL into an expanded version of the anxiety check list, named the Multiple Affect Adjective Check List (MAACL), which was published in 1964 (3). As well as anxiety and depression, this scale covers hostility, positive affect, and sensation-seeking. Subsequently, Zuckerman, Lubin and Rinck collaborated to publish a revised version of the MAACL in 1983 (4).

The Depression Adjective Check Lists were derived from item analyses of 171 adjectives which connoted varying degrees of depression and elation (1, p5). The item analyses selected adjectives that distinguished depressed patients from normal people. The instrument was originally developed for a study of postpartum depression, so the initial analyses used female

subjects and identified 128 adjectives. The adjectives were grouped into lists A, B, C, and D, each containing 22 positive (i.e., indicative of depression) and ten negative adjectives. These lists are known as set 1. Subsequently, the initial 171 adjectives were tested on a sample of 100 normal and 47 depressed males. The 102 most discriminating adjectives were assigned to lists E, F, and G. These lists, known as set 2, each contain 22 positive and 12 negative adjectives. Lists A to D have no items in common and nor have lists E to G, but some adjectives are common to the two sets. The instrument is available in state and trait forms. The same adjective lists are used in each, but the instruction for the state form reads, "How do you feel now—today?" while that for the trait form reads, "How do you generally feel?" This is intended to cover "longer-enduring, more pervasive depressive mood" (2). The complete instrument, scoring templates, and a manual, which includes complete instructions and shows normative data (1), are available from Psychological Assessment Resources (Address section). Exhibit 6.5

Exhibit 6.5   Selected Items from the Depression Adjective Check Lists, Form E

Directions: Below you will find words which describe different kinds of moods and feelings. Check the words which describe *HOW YOU GENERALLY FEEL.* Some of the words may sound alike, but we want you to *check all the words that describe your feelings.* Work rapidly and check *all* of the words which describe how you *generally feel.*

1. ☐ Unhappy	18. ☐ Well
2. ☐ Active	19. ☐ Apathetic
6. ☐ Composed	23. ☐ Awful
7. ☐ Distressed	24. ☐ Glum
16. ☐ Vigorous	33. ☐ Criticized
17. ☐ Peaceful	34. ☐ Fit

Reproduced from an original provided by Dr. Lubin. The complete scale may be obtained from Psychological Assessment Resources Inc., PO Box 998, Odessa, Florida, USA 33556 shows part of list E as an illustration of the DACL.

The DACL are self-administered but may be read to the subject if needed. Normal subjects take about two and a half minutes to complete a list; psychiatric patients take longer. Scores for each list count the positive adjectives that are checked, plus the number of negative adjectives that are not checked: high scores indicate depressed mood. The maximum score is 32 for lists A to D and 34 for lists E to G. Scoring is simplified by a transparent overlay that indicates which responses are counted for each list. A cutting point of 13 or above (one standard deviation above the population mean score obtained by Lubin) has been used to indicate mild depression, and 16 or above (+2 SD) to indicate severe depression (5).

Reliability

Lubin reviewed the equivalence of the seven lists. Correlations among them range from 0.80 to 0.93 (1, Table 15). Several studies have found no significant differences in total scores among the lists in set 1 or in set 2 (1, p11).

Internal consistency estimates for individual lists, based on analyses of variance, have ranged from 0.79 to 0.90 (1, Table 12); Byerly and Carlson reported Kuder-Richardson 20 reliabilities for different patient groups ranging from 0.59 to 0.72 (6, p801). Beckingham and Lubin reported mean coefficient alpha scores for the trait form lists of 0.84 with elderly subjects. Split-half reliability averaged 0.76 (7, p407). Alphas of 0.85 and 0.87 (8, p419) and 0.91 (9, Table 2) have been reported for list E. Split-half reliability estimates for the state form range from 0.82 to 0.93 for normals and from 0.86 to 0.93 for patients (1, p10). The positive and negative adjectives in the lists correlate between −0.75 and −0.82 (1, Table 14).

Test–retest reliability of the state form lists ranged from 0.19 to 0.24 after a one-week interval in a sample of 75 subjects (1, p10). Lomranz reported retest reliability results of 0.45 for the state form after one week, and 0.59 after three weeks, in two studies using a Hebrew version of the DACL (10, p1313).

Lubin et al. examined the relationship between reading difficulty of the adjectives and reliability of the trait form of the DACL. Results were lower for subjects with lower reading ability, but overall reliability was reduced when adjectives above the grade eight level were excluded, as the benefit of eliminating the difficult words was offset by losses due to abbreviating the scale (11, Table 4).

Validity

Moran and Lambert rated the DACL fifth out of six depression scales in terms of its coverage of the *DSM-III* criteria because the lists tap only three variables directly. They argued that because the instrument focuses on the affective aspects of depression, it needs major additions to conform to *DSM-III* criteria (12, p295).

Analyses of variance showed significant differences between the DACL responses of 625 normals, 174 nondepressed patients, and 128 depressed patients (1, Table 20). Byerly and Carlson found that depressed patients received significantly higher scores on list E of the DACL than patients who were not depressed (6). Christenfeld et al. also found that mean scores on list E increased as a psychiatrist's rating of depressed mood increased (13). In Byerly and Carlson's discriminant analysis, the DACL correctly classified 75% of depressed and of non-depressed patients (1, Table 38). In a series of such analyses, the DACL performed slightly better than the Beck Depression Inventory (BDI) (1, p18).

Correlations with other instruments are moderate to high. For example, correlations with the BDI ranged from 0.38 to 0.50 in psychiatric patients (1, Table 22); the correlation was 0.41 in normal subjects (13, Table 1). Byerly and Carlson found correlations between list E and the BDI ranging from 0.42 to 0.73 (6, p801); other results include a correlation of 0.60 between list B and the BDI (9, Table 2) and of 0.69 in a mixed sample of healthy people and patients. The correlation with the Hamilton Rating Scale for Depression was 0.72 in the same study (14, Table 1). Correlations with Zung's SDS are lower, perhaps because it covers more physiological symptoms than the other instruments. Correlations ranged from 0.27 to 0.38 in a psychiatric sample (1, Table 22) and from 0.44 (13, Table 1) to 0.54 in normal samples (9, Table 2). Other results of correlating the DACL and Zung scales include 0.62 (10, p1313) and a range between 0.53 and 0.64 (1, Table 25). In two studies of psychiatric inpatients, correlations between lists E, F, and G and the MMPI depression scale ranged from 0.54 to 0.60 (1, Table 26). List E of the DACL correlated 0.77 with the CES-D in a sample of 48 normals (1, Table 29). Correlations with the Bradburn scale included −0.37 for normals and −0.47 for psychiatric patients (1, Table 28).

Correlations between the DACL and global ratings of depression lie mainly between 0.3 and 0.5 (15, 16). An exception was a study by Fogel, in which the DACL correlated 0.71 with a psychiatric rating (1).

Lubin, Hornstra, and Love found that list E was sensitive to change in depressive mood in users of a mental health center. They found a significant drop in DACL scores over a three-month treatment period, but no change after the end of treatment (1). Other studies have found the DACL sensitive to change in intervention studies (17, 18).

A factor analysis of list E placed the positive and negative adjectives on separate factors (1, Table 32). However, when factoring the DACL items along with those from the Zung and Beck instruments, Giambra found that the DACL adjectives loaded on one factor, which he labeled affective malaise (19). There is also some indication that the positive and negative items may not merely be the inverse of each other, but may reflect different phenomena (20, p391). This recalls the discussions of the dimensions of affect generated by the Bradburn scale that were discussed in Chapter 5.

Alternative Forms

Lubin created 14 briefer check lists by treating each column of adjectives in lists A through G as a separate instrument. He reported that internal consistency, alternate-form reliability, and concurrent and discriminant validity of the brief lists are high, although somewhat lower than for the full lists (1, pp23–27).

The check lists have been translated into many languages, including Hebrew, French, Spanish, Arabic, Chinese, Dutch, and Portuguese; most studies find their reliability comparable to that of the English version (1, p22; 10; 21–23). A version for adolescents has been developed (2).

Reference Standards

The DACL manual presents norms based on U.S. data by sex and age group (1, Tables 2–10). Means and standard deviations are also presented for depressed and nondepressed patient samples. A 1993 revision of the manual presents norms and percentile scores for community subjects, adolescents, and the elderly.

Commentary

The Depression Adjective Check Lists are widely used: a bibliography compiled by Lubin listed more than 500 citations by 1989, and a more recent one lists 99 more. The DACL are acceptable to respondents and are simple to administer. Other advantages include the existence of normative data and the alternative versions, which are useful when repeated assessments have to be made, as in longitudinal studies (20). Furthermore, Lubin has extensively studied the psychometric properties of the scales, examining issues rarely considered in other health indices, such as response set, alternative response modes, and readability (which lies between the fourth- and eighth-grade levels) (11, 15, 24, 25). Although separate lists were developed for the two sexes, this is commonly ignored. There is some evidence that the lists are not equally valid for both genders. In one study only lists E through G showed significant differences between normal males and nondepressed patients (1, Table 20). Lists A through D appear more suitable for females, and lists E through G seem to better suit males (26).

The lists have adequate internal consistency; the agreement between the alternative forms is a strong feature (12, p273). Evidence for the stability of the measurement, however, is sparse and the available retest results are low. At present, they are limited to the state form; data on the reliability of the trait forms are needed (8).

Commentaries on the validity of the DACL give conflicting impressions. This seems to reflect reviewers' differing expectations of the method and their different reactions to its comparatively narrow scope. Lubin intentionally focused on mood, a major, but not the only, symptom of depression. The DACL do not include *DSM* criteria such as the inability to think or concentrate, thoughts of suicide, or changes in appetite, sleep, or psychomotor activity and other behavioral manifestations (12, p286; 27, p421). Reflecting this focus, concurrent validity is moderate: correlations with psychiatric ratings of depression are somewhat lower than those of other self-rating instruments. Correlations between the DACL and other self-report depression measures are low to moderate (20); the low correlations between the DACL and the somatic items in the Zung and Beck instruments are to be expected (1, Tables 23, 24). While the check lists can be used to screen for depression, they must not be viewed as diagnostic. Lubin is, however, developing a brief Depression Extender Check List (DECL) which samples additional aspects of depression to form a diagnostic instrument (B. Lubin, personal communication, 1992).

The validation of the DACL took a psychometric rather than an epidemiologic approach. We know more about its correlations with other instruments than about its sensitivity in identifying depression. This may be weak: data from Byerly and Carlson's study show that the DACL correctly identified only 75% of depressives. The manual of the DACL pays little attention to cutting points for defining depression, and the discriminant validity of the DACL has not been well investigated (27). The issue of specificity has also been raised: the original item analysis selected adjectives that distinguished depressed patients from normals. This does not ensure specificity and the DACL may reflect a range of feelings broader than depression (28). This may limit their usefulness as a screening test or as an outcome measurement. Because of the large standard deviations in DACL scores and the resulting overlaps between group scores, several commentators suggest that the DACL may be adequate to detect group differences in depression but not to identify depressed individuals (20, p389; 29; 30, p217). McNair recommended that the DACL be restricted to research uses (28) and Moran and Lambert's review concluded that there were not adequate data to support their use as an outcome measure with patient populations (12, p295).

Address

Psychological Assessment Resources, Inc., PO Box 998, Odessa, Florida, USA 33556

REFERENCES

(1) Lubin B. Manual for the Depression Adjective Check Lists. Odessa, Florida: Psychological Assessment Resources, 1981.

(2) Lubin B. Citation Classic. Measuring depressive affect with an adjective checklist. Curr Contents 1991;6:16.

(3) Zuckerman M, Lubin B, Vogel L, et al. Measurement of experimentally induced affects. J Consult Psychol 1964;28:418–425.

(4) Zuckerman M, Lubin B, Rinck CM. Construction of new scales for the Multiple Affect Adjective Check List. J Behav Assess 1983;5:119–120.

(5) Davis TC, Nathan RG, Crouch MA, et al. Screening depression in primary care: back to the basics with a new tool. Fam Med 1987;19:200–202.

(6) Byerly FC, Carlson WA. Comparison among inpatients, outpatients, and normals on three self-report depression inventories. J Clin Psychol 1982;38:797–804.

(7) Beckingham AC, Lubin B. Reliability and validity of the trait form of set 2 of the Depression Adjective Check Lists with Canadian elderly. J Clin Psychol 1991; 47:407–414.

(8) DeSouza ER, Lubin B, van Whitlock R. Preliminary report on reliability and validity of the trait form of the Depression Adjective Check List in a representative community sample. J Clin Psychol 1991; 47:418–420.

(9) Tanaka-Matsumi J, Kameoka VA. Reliabilities and concurrent validities of popular self-report measures of depression, anxiety, and social desirability. J Consult Clin Psychol 1986;54:328–333.

(10) Lomranz J, Lubin B, Eyal N, et al. Measuring depressive mood in elderly Israeli: reliability and validity of the Depression Adjective Check Lists. Psychol Rep 1991; 68:1311–1316.

(11) Lubin B, Collins JF, Seever M, et al. Relationships among readability, reliability, and validity in a self-report adjective check list. Psychol Assess 1990;2:256–261.

(12) Moran PW, Lambert MJ. A review of current assessment tools for monitoring changes in depression. In: Lambert MJ, Christensen ER, DeJulio SS, eds. The measurement of psychotherapy outcome in research and evaluation. New York: Wiley, 1983:263–303.

(13) Christenfeld R, Lubin B, Satin M. Concurrent validity of the Depression Adjective Check List in a normal population. Am J Psychiatry 1978;135:582–584.

(14) Fitzgibbon ML, Cella DF, Sweeney JA. Redundancy in measures of depression. J Clin Psychol 1988;44:372–374.

(15) Razavi D, Delvaux N, Farvacques C, et al. Screening for adjustment disorders and major depressive disorders in cancer inpatients. Br J Psychiatry 1990;156:79–83.

(16) Cresswell DL, Lanyon RI. Validation of a screening battery for psychogeriatric assessment. J Gerontol 1981;36:435–440.

(17) Cutler NR, Cohen HB. The effect of one night's sleep loss on mood and memory in normal subjects. Compr Psychiatry 1979;20:61–66.

(18) Davis GR, Armstrong HE, Donovan DM, et al. Cognitive-behavioral treatment of depressed affect among epileptics: preliminary findings. J Clin Psychol 1984; 40:930–935.

(19) Giambra LM. Independent dimensions of depression: a factor analysis of three self-report depression measures. J Clin Psychol 1977;33:928–935.

(20) Mayer JM. Assessment of depression. In: McReynolds P, ed. Advances in psychological assessment. Vol. 4. San Francisco: Jossey-Bass, 1977:358–425.

(21) Chu CRL, Lubin B, Sue S. Reliability and validity of the Chinese Depression Adjective Check Lists. J Clin Psychol 1984; 40:1409–1413.

(22) Lubin B, Collins JF. Depression Adjective Check Lists: Spanish, Hebrew, Chinese and English versions. J Clin Psychol 1985; 41:213–217.

(23) DeSouza ER, Lubin B, Zanelli J. Norms, reliability, and concurrent validity measures of the Portuguese version of the Depression Adjective Check Lists. J Clin Psychol 1994;50:208–215.

(24) Lubin B, Collins JF, Seever M, et al. Readability of the Depression Adjective Check Lists (DACL) and the Multiple Affect Adjective Check List-Revised (MAACL-R). J Clin Psychol 1991;47:91–93.

(25) Caplan M, Lubin B, Collins JF. Response manipulation on the Depression Adjective Check List. J Clin Psychol 1982;38:156–159.

(26) Goodstein LD. Review of "Depression Adjective Check Lists". In: Burros O, ed. Seventh mental measurements yearbook. Highland Park, New Jersey: Gryphon Press, 1974:132–133.

(27) Carson TP. Assessment of depression. In: Ciminero AR, Clahoun KS, Adams HE, eds. Handbook of behavioral assessment. 2nd ed. New York: Wiley, 1986:404–445.

(28) McNair DM. Review of "Depression Adjective Check Lists". In: Burros O, ed. Seventh mental measurements yearbook. Highland Park, New Jersey: Gryphon Press, 1974:133–134.

(29) Lewinsohn PM, Hoberman HM. Depression. In: Bellack AS, Hersen M, Kazdin AE, eds. International handbook of behavior modification and therapy. New York: Plenum, 1990.

(30) Petzel TP. Depression Adjective Check Lists. In: Keyser DJ, Sweetland RC, eds. Test critiques. 3rd ed. Kansas City, Mis-

souri: Test Corporation of America, 1985:215–220.

THE HAMILTON RATING SCALE FOR DEPRESSION
(Max Hamilton, 1960)

Purpose

The Hamilton Rating Scale for Depression (HRSD) is completed by a clinician to indicate the severity of depression in patients already diagnosed with a depressive disorder; it is not a diagnostic instrument (1, 2). It covers depressive state rather than trait and is intended primarily as a research tool to be used in "quantifying the results of an interview" (1, p56).

Conceptual Basis

Hamilton wanted a reliable scale which was appropriate for patients with mental illness, which could be used with semi-literate or severely ill patients, which could give information about symptoms, and which was clearly related to diagnosis (3). Items were selected on the basis of the medical literature and clinical experience of the symptoms most frequently presented by patients (4).

Description

The HRSD contains 21 ratings, 17 of which are measured on three (0 to 2)- or five (0 to 4)-point scales and are used in scoring the instrument (summarized in Exhibit 6.6). The final four items provide more detail on the clinical characteristics of the depression and Hamilton did not include these in the score, although others have done so.

The HRSD is administered through a semi-structured clinical interview; there are no specified questions. Hamilton originally provided only a brief outline of the content of the interview, preferring not to constrain the freedom of the clinician. Subsequently he published a four-page guide to making ratings (2, pp291–295) and ten years later gave some further guidelines (3, pp148–151). An adequate interview requires a minimum of 30 minutes; interviewers should have good clinical experience. Hamilton recommended that two raters be used; one interviews the patient and the other adds questions where appropriate (2, p291). The two then complete rating forms independently and later compare scores and discuss differences (3, p147). To obtain the most complete information possible, near relatives or significant others should also be interviewed. The ratings cover depressive symptoms during the past few days or week. Intensity and frequency of symptoms are considered; ratings are based on a synthesis of both. Themes that are difficult to quantify are rated coarsely on a 0-to-2 scale: 0 = symptom absent, 1 = slight or doubtful, and 2 = clearly present. Other items are graded more finely on a 0-to-4 scale in terms of increasing intensity: 0 = symptom absent, 1 = doubtful or trivial, 2 = mild, 3 = moderate, and 4 = severe. Half-points may be used.

A total score sums the item responses and ranges from 0 to 52 points with rising severity of depression. Hamilton did not specify cutting points, but it is generally agreed that scores lower than 7 indicate an absence of depression; scores of 7 to 17 represent mild depression; 18 to 24, moderate; and 25 or above represent severe depression. Alternative cutting points were suggested by Bech et al.: 0 to 7 = no depression, 8 to 15 = minor, and 16 or more = major depression (5, p10). Scores of 17 or more are often used as a threshold for including patients in drug trials (6).

Unfortunately, there are many variants of the Hamilton scale, several of which are described in the Alternative Forms section. Of these, the 11-item abbreviation called the Bech-Rafaelsen Melancholia Scale (BRMS) is mentioned here because it is used as a comparison in the reliability and validity studies described in the following sections.

Reliability

Alpha internal consistency was reported from a WHO study in five countries and

Exhibit 6.6 The Hamilton Rating Scale for Depression

Item No.	Range of Scores	Symptom

1	0–4	*Depressed Mood*
		Gloomy attitude, pessimism about the future
		Feeling of sadness
		Tendency to weep
		   Sadness, etc 1
		   Occasional weeping 2
		   Frequent weeping.................... 3
		   Extreme symptoms................. 4

2	0–4	*Guilt* Self-reproach, feels he has let people down Ideas of guilt Present illness is a punishment Delusions of guilt Hallucinations of guilt
3	0–4	*Suicide* Feels life is not worth living Wishes he were dead Suicidal ideas & half-hearted ideas Attempts at suicide
4	0–2	*Insomnia, initial* Difficulty in falling asleep
5	0–2	*Insomnia, middle* Patient restless and disturbed during the night Waking during the night
6	0–2	*Insomnia, delayed* Waking in early hours of the morning and unable to fall asleep again

7	0–4	*Work and Interests*
		Feelings of incapacity
		Listlessness, indecisions and vacillation
		Loss of interest in hobbies
		Decreased social activities
		Productivity decreased
		Unable to work
		   Stopped working because of present illness only 4
		   (Absence from work after treatment or recovery may rate a lower score.)

8	0–4	*Retardation*
		Slowness of thought, speech, and activity
		Apathy
		Stupor
		   Slight retardation at interview 1
		   Obvious retardation at interview 2
		   Interview difficult.................... 3
		   Complete stupor 4

9	0–4	*Agitation* Restlessness associated with anxiety Figitiness at interview 1

Item No.	Range of Scores	Symptom
		Obvious restlessness picking at hands & clothes .... 2 Patient has to get up .... 3 Patient paces, picks at face and hair—tears at clothes........... 4
10	0–4	*Anxiety, psychic* Tension and irritability Worrying about minor matters Apprehensive attitude Fears
11	0–4	*Anxiety, somatic* Gastrointestinal, wind, indigestion Cardiovascular, palpitations, headache Respiratory, genito-urinary, etc.
12	0–2	*Somatic Symptoms, Gastrointestinal* Loss of appetite Heavy feelings in abdomen Constipation
13	0–2	*Somatic Symptoms, General* Heaviness in limbs, back, or head Diffuse backache Loss of energy and fatiguability
14	0–2	*Loss of libido* Pathological change
15	0–4	*Hypochondriasis* Self-absorption (bodily) Preoccupation with health Querulous attitude Strong conviction of organic disease Hypochondriacal delusions
16	0–2	*Loss of Weight*

17	2–0	*Insight*
		   Loss of insight......................... 2
		   Partial or doubtful loss 1
		   No loss.................................... 0
		   (Insight must be interpreted in terms of patient's understanding and background.)

18	0–2	*Diurnal Variation* Symptoms worse in morning or evening (Note which it is.)
19	0–4	*Depersonalization and Derealization* Feelings of unreality Nihilistic ideas
20	0–4	*Paranoid Symptoms* Suspicious Ideas of reference } Not with a Delusions of reference } depressive and persecution } quality Hallucinations, persecutory
21	0–2	*Obsessional Symptoms* Obsessive thoughts and compulsions against which the patient struggles

showed figures of $\alpha = 0.48$ at baseline, rising to 0.85 after 11 days of treatment (7, Table 2). Figures from a Spanish study ranged from $\alpha = 0.70$ to 0.76, according to diagnostic group (8, Table 5). Other estimates include 0.76 (9, p35), 0.83, 0.94, and 0.95 (10, Table 1). Carroll et al. obtained a median item-total correlation of 0.54 (range 0.19 to 0.78) (11, p198).

Maier et al. applied Rasch analyses to the HRSD and other depression ratings to evaluate the internal consistency and the consistency of interrelations among items in different samples. The results showed clear deviations from the assumptions of the model (12, pp7–8; 13; 14). Bech et al. confirmed these findings, showing that the hierarchical ranking of items varied from sample to sample (15). Maier explained: "The consequence of the insufficient Rasch model fitting is that the HAM-D scores cannot be compared across different samples or within a sample across different conditions (e.g. pre- and post-treatment)" (13, p70). These concerns led Bech et al. to propose a revised version of the HRSD (described in Alternative Forms section).

Inter-rater reliability for the HRSD total score is generally high. Hamilton originally reported a correlation of 0.90 between pairs of ratings for 70 patients (1). Montgomery and Åsberg found an inter-rater correlation of 0.89 before treatment (16). Hedlund and Vieweg reviewed ten reliability studies; in only one very small study did the inter-rater correlation fall below 0.84; most coefficients fell above 0.88 (10, Table 1). Intraclass coefficients include 0.70 to 0.72 (12, Table 2), 0.83 (17, Table 3), 0.85 (18, p1137), and 0.91 (19, Table 3). Reliability results for individual items are much less adequate. Maier et al. found that three items on the Hamilton scale had unacceptably low inter-rater reliability (intraclass coefficients of 0.19 to 0.40) and that five other items had only fair or poor reliability (12, p6). Rehm and O'Hara reported inter-rater reliabilities for individual items (across different raters and different studies) ranging from −0.07 to 0.95, while

overall reliabilities ranged from 0.78 to 0.96 (9, Table 1).

Intraclass test–retest reliability at three weeks was 0.72 for the 17-item version, 0.70 for the 21-item version, and 0.69 for an abbreviated five-item version (13, Table 1).

Validity

The content validity of the HRSD has been criticized on the grounds of being restricted and of covering more than just the severity of depression. In terms of its restrictiveness, it neglects cognitive and affective symptoms in favor of somatic symptoms which are indicative of more severe depression (20). It includes only four of the eight melancholia symptoms in *DSM-III* (21) and does not cover nonreactivity of mood, reduction of concentration, or anhedonia (22). Another criticism holds that the content is mixed: some items cover severity while others serve to classify depression rather than measure its severity (23, p130). This last criticism has stimulated the development of abbreviated forms of the HRSD (see below).

As a measure of the severity of depression, the Hamilton scale has frequently been compared to clinical ratings of severity. The results are generally good, although variable. The total score of the 17-item version was significantly related to globally assessed severity of depression on the Raskin three-item rating scale for depression ($r = 0.65$); correlations for the Montgomery-Åsberg Depression Rating Scale (MADRS) (0.71) and BRMS (0.70) were slightly higher (22, Tables 1–3). Four items in the Hamilton were not significantly related to the global rating. Other figures include a correlation of 0.81 between the HRDS and the Raskin and −0.86 between the HRDS and overall severity rated by the Global Assessment Scale (GAS); correlations between individual items and the global ratings ranged from 0.10 to 0.86 (9, Table 3). Hedlund and Vieweg's review cited correlations of 0.84, 0.89, and 0.90 with clinical ratings of severity; they also listed one correlation of

0.67 for a study that included depressed and nondepressed patients (10, p152). Other low correlations with a clinical severity rating include 0.68 (13, Table 3). The HRSD may be limited in its ability to discriminate between moderate and severe depression (13, 24), and the results given here indicate that not all of the items correlate with global assessments.

Many compare the HRSD to self-report scales; a consistent finding is that agreement improves following treatment. The pre-treatment correlations, for example, between the Hamilton and the Beck Depression Inventory (BDI) in seven studies ranged from only 0.21 to 0.82, with a median of 0.58; post-treatment correlations ranged from 0.68 to 0.80 (25, p152). In nine similar studies, correlations between the HRSD and Zung's Self-rating Depression Scale ranged from 0.22 to 0.95 (10, Table 2). The wide range of results depends partly on the differing types of patients included, but the reasons are not fully clear. Correlations with a range of other depression scales covered in Hedlund and Vieweg's review ranged from 0.63 to 0.87; correlations with the MMPI Depression Scale, however, were lower, at 0.27 and 0.34 (10, p156). We conclude that, compared to clinician ratings, the HRSD consistently performs better than the SDS (26, Table 1; 27; 28), about as well as the BDI (10, 24), but less well than the BRMS (24, 29).

Hamilton had a strong personal interest in factor analysis and identified four main factors: a general factor, a second factor that contrasted agitated and retarded depression, a third that covered insomnia and fatiguability, and a fourth factor that included other symptoms (1, pp58–59; 2, pp288–289). Many subsequent authors have reported factor analyses of the HRSD and review articles have been produced (8, 10, 30). One review of 12 studies shows that the number of factors extracted ranges from three to seven and most commonly is six (8, Table 6). Hedlund and Vieweg described two consistent factors: a general

severity of depression factor and a bipolar factor that distinguishes reactive from endogenous depression (10, p157).

Hedlund and Vieweg summarized over 30 studies that reviewed the HRSD as an indicator of change in clinical trials; they comment: "The HRSD is consistently reported to reflect clinically observed treatment changes . . . the HRSD and BDI tend to be about equally sensitive to severity of illness, while the SDS tends to be somewhat less reliable and sensitive" (10, p156). A meta-analysis of 36 studies compared effect sizes for the HRSD, the Zung Self-rating Depression Scale, and the Beck Depression Inventory (31). A second review compared effect sizes for BDI and HRSD in 19 studies (32). In both, the Hamilton scale was found consistently to provide the largest index of change. Compared to other clinician ratings, however, the Hamilton may not be superior. Change scores on the HRSD were compared to a clinician's classification of 35 patients under treatment into improved or not improved; the point biserial correlation was 0.59, comparing unfavorably to a figure of 0.70 for the MADRS (16, p385). Maier et al. have compared the discriminatory power of the HRSD and MADRS in two studies; in one the Hamilton was superior (12, p8) and in the other the MADRS proved superior (14). Eight of the HRSD items were not sensitive to change. Montgomery and Åsberg found correlations between their MADRS and a clinical judgment of improvement (0.70) to be superior to that of the Hamilton scale (0.59) (16, p385).

Alternative Forms

Although Hamilton regarded the 17-item version of the HRSD as definitive, the four extra items are sometimes scored to form a 21-item version; there is also a 24-item version which includes items on helplessness, hopelessness, and worthlessness (30). The 17- and 21-item versions correlated 0.94 in one study (22, p15).

Hamilton's hesitancy to publish precise details of rating procedures stimulated others to attempt this. A Structured Interview Guide developed by Williams, the SIGH-D, suggests open-ended questions for each item and indicates how to translate replies into ratings; use of the guide improved reliability of ratings (33, Table 2). Potts et al. developed a Structured Interview Guide for use in the Medical Outcomes Study, the SI-HDRS, which can be used by lay interviewers (34). The SI-HDRS has an alpha reliability of 0.82 (34, p344). Rehm and O'Hara also provided guidelines for standardizing the ratings (9).

Difficulties with certain items led to revisions to the content of the scale. Bech, Maier, and others showed that the items did not all measure severity of depression and Bech et al. identified six items that more specifically measure severity. These were items 1 (depressed mood), 2 (guilt), 7 (work and interests), 8 (retardation), 10 (psychic anxiety), and 13 (general somatic symptoms) (24, p168). These formed a psychometrically more adequate severity scale, showing a more monotonic relationship with clinical judgments of severity of depression than did the overall scale. Bech et al. referred to these six items as the melancholia subscale of the HRSD (35). Later, Bech and Rafaelsen included this subset in their Bech-Rafaelsen Melancholia Scale (BRMS), which is an abbreviated and more closely structured version of the HRSD containing 11 items (23, 36, 37). The scale properties of the BRMS are superior to those of the Hamilton scale; inter-rater reliability is generally higher, and the BRMS seems more sensitive to clinical change (12).

There are many other variants of the HRSD; some are reviewed by Zitman et al. who also found that less than half of the 37 researchers they interviewed had actually used the version of the HRSD that they cited (38). In North America, a version was published through the U.S. Department of Health, Education, and Welfare and has been widely used, although it is different from Hamilton's own guidelines (39). Hedlund and Vieweg present a further variant

of the HRSD (10, pp163–164). Miller et al. added items related to cognitive and melancholic symptoms and deleted items with low reliability and validity. They modified rating points and used a structured interview guide (21, pp137–142). Other modifications of the HRSD have reduced its overlap with anxiety measurements, increasing specificity (40). A self-rating version of the HRSD, the Carroll Rating Scale for Depression, is described in a separate review.

The Hamilton scale has been translated and tested in numerous languages, including French (41), Spanish (8, 42), Dutch (38), Russian, Japanese, and Hindi (7). A Brazilian version correlated 0.89 with the MADRS (43).

Commentary

For 35 years the HRSD has remained the most frequently used clinical rating scale for depression; one review reported its use in at least 500 published studies in the past ten years (44).

Since its initial publication, the HAM-D has emerged as the most widely used scale for patient selection and follow-up in research studies of treatments for depression.... Undoubtedly, the success of this scale is due to its comprehensive coverage of depressive symptoms and related psychopathology, as well as its strong psychometric properties. (33, p48)

The literature on the HRSD has reached a size such that there are several major reviews (10, 45). Validity appears adequate: the HRSD generally correlates well with global ratings of depression severity, although the correlations may be lower than those obtained for other rating scales. The HRSD is generally held to be sensitive to change in depression following treatment. Inter-rater reliability is generally good, although inter-rater agreement at the item level is less satisfactory. Despite criticisms, the HRSD is often used as a criterion against which self-report scales are validated; the various attempts to improve the Hamilton scale have not led to its displacement as the mainstay of depression rating scales.

Although the Hamilton scale appears successful, it has been criticized on a number of grounds. Indeed, Hamilton, who was obviously deeply respected by many of his critics, parried some of the criticism with wry and modest humor:

I went around with my scale and it created a tremendous wave of apathy. They all thought I was a bit mad. Eventually it got published in the *Journal of Neurology, Neurosurgery and Psychiatry*. It was the only one that would take it. And now everyone tells me the scale is wonderful. I always remember when it had a different reception. This makes sure I don't get a swollen head. (8, p90)

The issues regarding the HRSD include its content: it covers more behavioral and somatic symptoms of depression than do other scales (26, p361); indeed, it has been criticized for omitting affective symptoms such as nonreactivity of mood, reduction of concentration, and anhedonia (22, p18). This criticism should be considered carefully: the HRSD is not intended as a diagnostic instrument, so it may not need to cover every aspect of depression (8, p81). But the criticism is important if the emphasis on somatic items, indicators of more severe depression, means that the scale cannot discriminate among milder levels of depression (20). It is also curious that the HRSD contains a section on anxiety.

Several authors have criticized its lack of description of item content and item scores (12). Hamilton himself stated that the value of the scale "depends entirely on the skill of the interviewer in eliciting the necessary information" (1, p56). Considerable interpretation is necessary for rating items, and consistency across settings is questionable (21). Other criticisms involve its heterogeneous factor structure and the mixing of frequency and severity of symptoms. Because it covers several facets of depression, patients with low scores on several symptoms can receive the same scores as patients with a few high scoring symptoms; it is not clear whether these are equivalent in terms of severity (14). This raises questions about the internal structure of the HRSD. Having been developed empirically from reports made by patients, the scale is heterogeneous in content and does not meet the criteria for internal construct validity laid down by the Rasch approach to test development. Whether or not this is a limitation depends on one's philosophy; the debate between theoreticians and pragmatists is reminiscent of that surrounding the Health Opinion Survey, another scale from the same era that appears to meet its objectives despite far from perfect psychometric properties.

The case of Hamilton's depression scale holds an important lesson for the development of the field in general. From the outset there was general agreement that the scale was basically sound but that it required some refinement and clarification. Unfortunately, however, no one assumed stewardship of the scale by developing a manual, answering points raised, and issuing revisions as appropriate. Development of a good first edition of a scale is only half the battle: maintenance is equally important.

Hedlund and Vieweg concluded that the HRSD is a valid scale for its purpose, and Rabkin and Klein state that "we are confident that the Hamilton is an accurate index of depressive severity in patients diagnosed with a depressive disorder" (30, p52). It is suitable for determining the severity of depression in depressed patients, if proper caution is used. It cannot be used to diagnose depression and so is not suitable for unselected populations (46). Care should be taken in reporting which version of the scale is used and whether any changes are made. Thorough training is required on the instrument, as well as inter-rater reliability checks before and after training.

REFERENCES

(1) Hamilton M. A rating scale for depression. J Neurol Neurosurg Psychiatry 1960;23:56–62.

(2) Hamilton M. Development of a rating scale for primary depressive illness. Br J Soc Clin Psychol 1967;6:278–296.

(3) Hamilton M. The Hamilton Rating Scale

for Depression. In: Sartorius N, Ban T, eds. Assessment of depression. Berlin: Springer-Verlag, 1986:143–152.

(4) Lyerly SB. Handbook of psychiatric rating scales. 2nd ed. Rockville, Maryland: National Institute of Mental Health, 1978.

(5) Bech P, Kastrup M, Rafaelsen OJ. Mini-compendium of rating scales for states of anxiety, depression, mania, schizophrenia with corresponding DSM-III syndromes. Acta Psychiatr Scand 1986;73(suppl 326):1–37.

(6) Paykel ES. The Hamilton Rating Scale for Depression in general practice. In: Bech P, Coppen A, eds. The Hamilton scales. New York: Springer-Verlag, 1990:40–47.

(7) Gastpar M, Gilsdorf U. The Hamilton Depression Rating Scale in a WHO collaborative program. In: Bech P, Coppen A, eds. The Hamilton scales. New York: Springer-Verlag, 1990:10–19.

(8) Berrios GE, Bulbena-Villarasa A. The Hamilton Depression Scale and the numerical description of the symptoms of depression. In: Bech P, Coppen A, eds. The Hamilton scales. New York: Springer-Verlag, 1990:80–92.

(9) Rehm LP, O'Hara MW. Item characteristics of the Hamilton Rating Scale for Depression. J Psychiatr Res 1985;19:31–41.

(10) Hedlund JL, Vieweg BW. The Hamilton Rating Scale for Depression: a comprehensive review. J Operat Psychiatry 1979;10:149–165.

(11) Carroll BJ, Feinberg M, Smouse PE, et al. The Carroll Rating Scale for Depression. I. Development, reliability and validation. Br J Psychiatry 1981;138:194–200.

(12) Maier W, Philipp M, Heuser I, et al. Improving depression severity assessment—I. Reliability, internal validity and sensitivity to change of three observer depression scales. J Psychiatr Res 1988;22:3–12.

(13) Maier W. The Hamilton Depression Scale and its alternatives: a comparison of their reliability and validity. In: Bech P, Coppen A, eds. The Hamilton scales. New York: Springer-Verlag, 1990:64–71.

(14) Maier W, Philipp M. Comparative analysis of observer depression scales. Acta Psychiatr Scand 1985;72:239–245.

(15) Bech P, Allerup P, Maier W, et al. The Hamilton Scales and the Hopkins Symptom Checklist (SCL-90): a cross-national validity study in patients with panic disorders. Br J Psychiatry 1992;160:206–211.

(16) Montgomery S, Åsberg M. A new depression scale designed to be sensitive to change. Br J Psychiatry 1979;134:382–389.

(17) Kørner A, Nielsen BM, Eschen F, et al. Quantifying depressive symptomatology: inter-rater reliability and inter-item correlations. J Affect Disord 1990;20:143–149.

(18) Winokur A, Guthrie MB, Rickels K, et al. Extent of agreement between patient and physician ratings of emotional distress. Psychosomatics 1982;23:1135–1146.

(19) Endicott J, Cohen J, Nee J, et al. Hamilton Depression Rating Scale extracted from regular and change versions of the Schedule for Affective Disorders and Schizophrenia. Arch Gen Psychiatry 1981;38:98–103.

(20) Raskin A. Sensitivity to treatment effects of evaluation instruments completed by psychiatrists, psychologists, nurses, and patients. In: Sartorius N, Ban T, eds. Assessment of depression. Berlin: Springer, 1986:367–376.

(21) Miller IW, Bishop S, Norman WH, et al. The Modified Hamilton Rating Scale for Depression: reliability and validity. Psychiatry Res 1985;14:131–142.

(22) Maier W, Heuser I, Philipp M, et al. Improving depression severity assessment—II. Content, concurrent and external validity of three observer depression scales. J Psychiatr Res 1988;22:13–19.

(23) Bech P, Rafaelsen OJ. The use of rating scales exemplified by a comparison of the Hamilton and the Bech-Rafaelsen Melancholia Scale. Acta Psychiatr Scand 1980;62(suppl 285):128–131.

(24) Bech P, Gram LF, Dein E, et al. Quantitative rating of depressive states: correlation between clinical assessment, Beck's self-rating scale and Hamilton's objective rating scale. Acta Psychiatr Scand 1975;51:161–170.

(25) Shumaker SA, Anderson R, Hays R, et al. International use, application and performance of health related quality of life instruments. Qual Life Res 1993;2:367–487.

(26) Carroll BJ, Fielding JM, Blashki TG. Depression rating scales: a critical review. Arch Gen Psychiatry 1973;28:361–366.

(27) Schnurr R, Hoaken PCS, Jarrett FJ. Comparison of depression inventories in a clinical population. Can Psychiatr Assoc J 1976;21:473–476.

(28) Biggs JT, Wylie LT, Ziegler VE. Validity of the Zung Self-rating Depression Scale. Br J Psychiatry 1978;132:381–385.

(29) Kearns NP, Cruickshank CA, McGuigan KJ, et al. A comparison of depression rating scales. Br J Psychiatry 1982;141:45–49.

(30) Rabkin JG, Klein DF. The clinical measurement of depressive disorders. In: Marsella AJ, Hirschfeld RMA, Katz MM, eds. The measurement of depression. New York: Guilford Press, 1987:30–83.

(31) Lambert MJ, Hatch DR, Kingston MD, et al. Zung, Beck, and Hamilton rating scales as measures of treatment outcome: a meta-analytic comparison. J Consult Clin Psychol 1986;54:54–59.

(32) Edwards BC, Lambert MJ, Moran PW, et al. A meta-analytic comparison of the Beck Depression Inventory and the Hamilton Rating Scale for Depression as measures of treatment outcome. Br J Clin Psychol 1984;23:93–99.

(33) Williams JBW. Structured interview guides for the Hamilton Rating Scales. In: Bech P, Coppen A, eds. The Hamilton scales. New York: Springer-Verlag, 1990:48–63.

(34) Potts MK, Daniels M, Burnam MA, et al. A structured interview version of the Hamilton Depression Rating Scale: evidence of reliability and versatility of administration. J Psychiatr Res 1990;24:335–350.

(35) Bech P, Allerup P, Gram LF, et al. The Hamilton Depression Scale: evaluation of objectivity using logistic models. Acta Psychiatr Scand 1981;63:290–299.

(36) Bech P, Rafaelsen OJ. The Melancholia Scale: development, consistency, validity, and utility. In: Sartorius N, Ban T, eds. Assessment of depression. Berlin: Springer, 1986:259–269.

(37) Bech P. Rating scales for affective disorders: their validity and consistency. Acta Psychiatr Scand 1981;64(suppl 295):1–101.

(38) Zitman FG, Mennen MFG, Griez E, et al. The different versions of the Hamilton Depression Rating Scale. In: Bech P, Coppen A, eds. The Hamilton scales. New York: Springer-Verlag, 1990:28–34.

(39) ECDEU assessment manual for psychopharmacology. Rockville, Maryland: Department of Health, Education & Welfare, 1976. (Pub No ADM 76–336).

(40) Riskind JH, Beck AT, Brown G, et al. Taking the measure of anxiety and depression: validity of the reconstructed Hamilton scales. J Nerv Ment Dis 1987;175:474–479.

(41) Pull CB. French experiences with the Hamilton scales in comparison with other scales for depression and anxiety. In: Bech P, Coppen A, eds. The Hamilton scales. New York: Springer-Verlag, 1990:35–39.

(42) Ramos-Brieva JA, Cordero-Villafafila A. A new validation of the Hamilton Rating Scale for Depression. J Psychiatr Res 1988;22:21–28.

(43) Dratcu L, da Costa Ribeiro L, Calil HM. Depression assessment in Brazil: the first application of the Montgomery-Åsberg Depression Rating Scale. Br J Psychiatry 1987;150:797–800.

(44) Hooijer C, Zitman FG, Griez E, et al. The Hamilton Depression Rating Scale (HDRS): changes in scores as a function of training and version used. J Affect Disord 1991;22:21–29.

(45) Bech P, Coppen A, eds. The Hamilton scales. New York: Springer-Verlag, 1990.

(46) Mayer JM. Assessment of depression. In: McReynolds P, ed. Advances in psychological assessment. Vol. 4. San Francisco: Jossey-Bass, 1977:358–425.

THE MONTGOMERY-ÅSBERG DEPRESSION RATING SCALE
(Stuart A. Montgomery and Marie Åsberg, 1979)

Purpose

The Montgomery-Åsberg Depression Rating Scale (MADRS) is used by clinicians to assess the severity of depression among patients in whom a diagnosis of depressive illness has been made. It is designed to be sensitive to change resulting from treatment (1, 2).

Conceptual Basis

Psychiatric rating scales are commonly used to evaluate drug treatment effects. While most are able to distinguish between active drugs and placebos, Montgomery and Åsberg noted that few have been able to differentiate between various active drugs. Standard rating scales such as the Hamilton Rating Scale for Depression (HRSD) do not seem sensitive enough to detect these differences; this is probably because they have been developed for diagnosis and classification (3). The major goal in developing the Montgomery-Åsberg scale was to provide an instrument sensitive to change that was also practical to apply in a clinical setting.

Description

The items selected for the MADRS were the most frequently checked and the most sensitive to change among the items in Åsberg's Comprehensive Psychopathological

Rating Scale, which was designed to evaluate psychiatric treatment (3, 4). The ten MADRS ratings are completed during a clinical interview, which moves "from broadly phrased questions about symptoms to more detailed ones which allow a precise rating of severity" (1, p387). Ratings may blend patient responses with information from observation or interviews with other informants. The MADRS is used by clinicians such as psychiatrists, general practitioners, psychologists, or nurses. Interviews take 20 to 60 minutes. The ten ratings use 0-to-6 severity scales, with higher scores reflecting more severe symptoms. The topic of each rating is described, and definitions are provided for key scale steps (see Exhibit 6.7).

An overall score (range 0 to 60) is formed by adding the rating scores; no weights are used. Snaith et al. proposed the following cutting points: scores of 0 to 6 indicate an absence of symptoms; 7 to 19 represent mild depression; 20 to 34, moderate; and 35 to 60 indicate severe depression (5). Other proposed cut-points include 12 for mild depression, 24 for moderate, and 35 for severe (6, p88).

Reliability

An alpha of 0.86 was found in a study of 151 depressed patients (7). The consistency of fit of the MADRS scores to a Rasch measurement model across different subgroups of patients was assessed by Maier et al. and showed clear deviations from the assumptions of the model (8, pp7,8).

As with any rating scale, inter-rater reliability is an important concern, and it has been frequently examined. Montgomery and Åsberg reported inter-rater reliability ranging from 0.89 to 0.97 for various combinations of raters in small samples of 12 to 30 patients (1, Table III). Davidson et al. reported Spearman inter-rater correlations of 0.76 for the total score, while correlations for individual items ranged from 0.57 to 0.76 (2, Table 2). Intraclass coefficients for the MADRS fell between 0.66 and 0.82 (8, Table 2). An equivalent

figure of 0.86 was reported by Kørner et al. (9, Table 3).

Validity

In terms of content validity, the MADRS covers the core symptoms of depression with the exception of motor retardation (1, 10).

The MADRS has been compared to other depression rating scales, especially the Hamilton scale. Compared to a clinical rating of depression severity, the MADRS discriminated significantly between five levels of depression; its performance was about equal to that of the Hamilton scale and clearly superior to that of the Beck Depression Inventory (BDI) (11, p47). Maier et al. compared the MADRS and HRSD with clinical assessments of severity of depression; the correlation for the MADRS was 0.71, slightly higher than that for the HRSD (0.65) (10, Tables 1, 2). Equivalent figures from a second study were 0.75 for the MADRS and 0.68 for the HRSD (12, Table 3). All items on the MADRS were significantly associated with severity ratings. In addition, the MADRS correlated more highly with the global assessment of depression severity than with that of anxiety, was able to discriminate major depression with and without melancholia, and was significantly associated with psychosocial impairment (10). The MADRS has also been shown to be more successful at distinguishing between endogenous and nonendogenous depression than the Hamilton scale (2, Table 4).

Snaith and Taylor reported convergent and discriminant validity: MADRS scores correlated 0.81 with the depression score of the Hospital Anxiety and Depression Scale and 0.37 with its anxiety score, (13, Table 1). Two items, psychic anxiety and insomnia, showed correlations in excess of 0.5 with the anxiety score, and omitting these items from the MADRS reduced the discriminant correlation from 0.37 to 0.31 while leaving the correlation with the depression score unchanged (13, Table 1). Davidson et al. reported Spearman correla-

Exhibit 6.7   The Montgomery-Åsberg Depression Rating Scale (MADRS)

The rating should be based on a clinical interview moving from broadly phrased questions about symptoms to more detailed ones which allow a precise rating of severity. The rater must decide whether the rating lies on the defined scale steps (0, 2, 4, 6) or between them (1, 3, 5).

It is important to remember that it is only on rare occasions that a depressed patient is encountered who cannot be rated on the items in the scale. If definite answers cannot be elicited from the patient all relevant clues as well as information from other sources should be used as a basis for the rating in line with customary clinical practice.

The scale may be used for any time interval between ratings, be it weekly or otherwise but this must be recorded.

---

1. Apparent Sadness

Representing despondency, gloom and despair, (more than just ordinary transient low spirits) reflected in speech, facial expression, and posture. Rate by depth and inability to brighten up.

0 No sadness.
1
2 Looks dispirited but does brighten up without difficulty.
3
4 Appears sad and unhappy most of the time.
5
6 Looks miserable all the time. Extremely despondent.

---

2. Reported sadness

Representing reports of depressed mood, regardless of whether it is reflected in appearance or not. Includes low spirits, despondency or the feeling of being beyond help and without hope.

Rate according to intensity, duration and the extent to which the mood is reported to be influenced by events.

0 Occasional sadness in keeping with the circumstances.
1
2 Sad or low but brightens up without difficulty.
3
4 Pervasive feelings of sadness or gloominess. The mood is still influenced by external circumstances.
5
6 Continuous or unvarying sadness, misery or despondency.

---

3. Inner tension

Representing feelings of ill-defined discomfort, edginess, inner turmoil, mental tension mounting to either panic, dread or anguish.

Rate according to intensity, frequency, duration and the extent of reassurance called for.

0 Placid. Only fleeting inner tension.
1
2 Occasional feelings of edginess and ill-defined discomfort.
3
4 Continuous feelings of inner tension or intermittent panic which the patient can only master with some difficulty.
5
6 Unrelenting dread or anguish. Overwhelming panic.

---

4. Reduced sleep

Representing the experience of reduced duration or depth of sleep compared to the subject's own normal pattern when well.

0 Sleeps as usual.
1
2 Slight difficulty dropping off to sleep or slightly reduced, light or fitful sleep.
3
4 Sleep reduced or broken by at least two hours.
5
6 Less than two or three hours sleep.

---

5. Reduced appetite

Representing the feeling of a loss of appetite compared with when well. Rate by loss of desire for food or the need to force oneself to eat.

0 Normal or increased appetite.
1
2 Slightly reduced appetite.
3
4 No appetite. Food is tasteless.
5
6 Needs persuasion to eat at all.

6. Concentration difficulties

Representing difficulties in collecting one's thoughts mounting to incapacitating lack of concentration.

Rate according to intensity, frequency, and degree of incapacity produced.

0 No difficulties in concentrating.
1
2 Occasional difficulties in collecting one's thoughts.
3
4 Difficulties in concentrating and sustaining thought which reduces ability to read or hold a conversation.
5
6 Unable to read or converse without great difficulty.

7. Lassitude

Representing a difficulty getting started or slowness initiating and performing everyday activities.

0 Hardly any difficulties in getting started. No sluggishness.
1
2 Difficulties in starting activities.
3
4 Difficulties in starting simple routine activities which are carried out with effort.
5
6 Complete lassitude. Unable to do anything without help.

8. Inability to feel

Representing the subjective experience of reduced interest in the surroundings, or activities that normally give pleasure. The ability to react with adequate emotion to circumstances or people is reduced.

0 Normal interest in the surroundings and in other people.
1
2 Reduced ability to enjoy usual interests.
3
4 Loss of interest in the surroundings. Loss of feelings for friends and acquaintances.
5
6 The experience of being emotionally paralysed, inability to feel anger, grief or pleasure and a complete or even painful failure to feel for close relatives and friends.

9. Pessimistic thoughts

Representing thoughts of guilt, inferiority, self-reproach, sinfulness, remorse and ruin.

0 No pessimistic thoughts.
1
2 Fluctuating ideas of failure, self-reproach or self-depreciation.
3
4 Persistent self-accusations, or definite but still rational ideas of guilt or sin. Increasingly pessimistic about the future.
5
6 Delusions of ruin, remorse or unredeemable sin. Self-accusations which are absurd and unshakable.

Exhibit 6.7 *(Continued)*

279

Exhibit 6.7   *(Continued)*

10. Suicidal thoughts

Representing the feeling that life is not worth living, that a natural death would be welcome, suicidal thoughts, and preparations for suicide.

Suicidal attempts should not in themselves influence the rating.

0 Enjoys life or takes it as it comes.

1

2 Weary of life. Only fleeting suicidal thoughts.

3

4 Probably better off dead. Suicidal thoughts are common, and suicide is considered as a possible solution, but without specific plans or intention.

5

6 Explicit plans for suicide when there is an opportunity. Active preparations for suicide.

Adapted from Montgomery SA, Åsberg M. A new depression scale designed to be sensitive to change. Br J Psychiatry 1979;134:387–389. With permission.

tions averaging only 0.46 between HRSD ratings and the MADRS (2, Table 3). However, this seems the exception. Other coefficients are higher, including Spearman correlations with the HRSD of 0.82 and with the Bech-Rafaelsen Melancholia Scale (BRMS) of 0.92 (9, Table 4), and Pearson correlations of 0.85 with the HRSD, 0.89 with the BRMS, and 0.71 with the Raskin Depression Scale (10, pp15,16).

As a goal of the MADRS was to evaluate change in depression, sensitivity to change has been reported in several studies. Change scores on the MADRS were compared to a clinician's classification of 35 patients under treatment into improved or not improved; the point biserial correlation was 0.70, while the equivalent correlation for the HRSD was lower, at 0.59 (1, p385). Maier and Phillipp found that MADRS had higher mean discriminatory power (coefficient = 0.60) than the Hamilton (coefficient = 0.39) (7). By contrast, in two other studies the MADRS had slightly lower correlations with global assessments of change (0.61 and 0.63) than did the HRSD or the BRMS (8, p8; 12, Table 3).

Alternative Forms

English and Swedish versions of the MADRS were developed concurrently. A Brazilian version showed a correlation of 0.89 with the Hamilton scale (14). A French version has been validated (15).

Since the items on psychic anxiety and insomnia were reported to correlate highly with an anxiety scale (13), some users have omitted these from an abbreviated version of the MADRS (16).

Commentary

The MADRS was developed largely in response to the criticism that established methods such as the Hamilton Rating Scale for Depression were insensitive to clinically important changes in level of depression. It has been used widely in Britain and Europe. Most evaluations of the MADRS compare it to the Hamilton, and it makes a generally favorable impression. Compared to the Hamilton scale, the MADRS is easily administered and provides clearer guidelines to the rater. In turn, however, the Bech-Rafaelstan modification of the Hamilton scale seems to offer further improvement. In terms of general validity and reliability the MADRS performs comparably to, or slightly better than, the HRSD. Studies give varying impressions of whether the MADRS is, in fact, more sensitive to change; overall, there seems little difference between the MADRS and the Hamilton. The main contrast between the two scales is that the MADRS omits psychomotor symptoms. Focusing only on psychic symptoms of depression, the MADRS is valuable for assessing depression in physically ill people (5), whereas if the application calls for a broad assessment of the psychic, behavioral, and somatic features of depression, the Hamilton scale is more suitable (11, p48).

REFERENCES

(1) Montgomery SA, Åsberg M. A new depression scale designed to be sensitive to change. Br J Psychiatry 1979;134:382–389.

(2) Davidson J, Turnbull CD, Strickland R, et al. The Montgomery-Åsberg Depression Scale: reliability and validity. Acta Psychiatr Scand 1986;73:544–548.

(3) Åsberg M, Montgomery SA, Perris C, et al. A comprehensive psychopathological rating scale. Acta Psychiatr Scand 1978;58(suppl 271):5–27.

(4) Cronholm B. The Comprehensive Psychopathological Rating Scale (CPRS). In: Helgason T, ed. Methodology in evaluation of psychiatric treatment. Cambridge: Cambridge University Press, 1983:163–169.

(5) Snaith RP, Harrop FM, Newby DA, et al. Grade scores of the Montgomery-Åsberg Depression and the Clinical Anxiety Scales. Br J Psychiatry 1986;148:599–601.

(6) Wilkin D, Hallam L, Doggett MA. Measures of need and outcome for primary health care. Oxford: Oxford University Press, 1992.

(7) Maier W, Philipp M. Comparative analysis of observer depression scales. Acta Psychiatr Scand 1985;72:239–245.

(8) Maier W, Philipp M, Heuser I, et al. Improving depression severity assessment—I. Reliability, internal validity and sensitivity to change of three observer depression scales. J Psychiatr Res 1988;22:3–12.

(9) Körner A, Nielsen BM, Eschen F, et al. Quantifying depressive symptomatology: inter-rater reliability and inter-item correlations. J Affect Disord 1990;20:143–149.

(10) Maier W, Heuser I, Philipp M, et al. Improving depression severity assessment—II. Content, concurrent and external validity of three observer depression scales. J Psychiatr Res 1988;22:13–19.

(11) Kearns NP, Cruickshank CA, McGuigan KJ, et al. A comparison of depression rating scales. Br J Psychiatry 1982;141:45–49.

(12) Maier W. The Hamilton Depression Scale and its alternatives: a comparison of their reliability and validity. In: Bech P, Coppen A, eds. The Hamilton scales. New York: Springer-Verlag, 1990:64–71.

(13) Snaith RP, Taylor CM. Rating scales for depression and anxiety: a current perspective. Br J Clin Pharmacol 1985;19:17S-20S.

(14) Dratcu L, da Costa Ribeiro L, Calil HM. Depression assessment in Brazil: the first application of the Montgomery-Åsberg Depression Rating Scale. Br J Psychiatry 1987;150:797–800.

(15) Peyre F, Martinez R, Calache M, et al. New validation of the Montgomery and Åsberg Depression Scale (MADRS) on a sample of 147 hospitalized depressed patients. Ann Medicopsychol 1989;147:762–767.

(16) Bramley PN, Easton AME, Morley S, et al. The differentiation of anxiety and depression by rating scales. Acta Psychiatr Scand 1988;77:133–138.

THE CARROLL RATING SCALE FOR DEPRESSION
(Bernard J. Carroll, 1981)

Purpose

The Carroll Rating Scale (CRS) is a self-administered version of the Hamilton Rating Scale for Depression (HRSD) (1). It is intended to measure severity of diagnosed depression. It can also be used as a screening instrument and is used in research and clinical applications.

Conceptual Basis

The CRS closely follows the item content of the HRSD (1). The major difference between the HRSD and most of the self-rating scales lies in its coverage of somatic and behavioral symptoms of depression. To avoid falsely classifying physical illness as symptomatic of depression, most self-rating scales focus on subjective thoughts and feelings, leaving physical symptoms to a clinician to elicit through clinical examination. However, since feelings may indicate general malaise rather than specifically depression, a self-rating scale oriented toward the behavioral and somatic features of depression may be advantageous (2).

Description

Like the Hamilton scale, the Carroll Rating Scale covers 17 symptoms of depression and provides a 0-to-52 severity score.

Where Hamilton used a 0-to-2 rating for a symptom, the CRS includes two items and where Hamilton used a 0-to-4 rating, Carroll uses four items, giving a total of 52 yes/no statements (1, p194). The items are presented in a randomized order, as shown in Exhibit 6.8, which indicates the response that is scored for each item. Each depressive response counts one point toward the total score. The 17 Hamilton symptoms of depression and the corresponding Carroll items are as follows (1, pp198–199):

1. Depression 16, 32, 34, 48
2. Guilt 14, 20, 24, 44
3. Suicide 12, 17, 29, 46
4. Initial insomnia 9, 22
5. Middle insomnia 19, 27
6. Delayed insomnia 11, 35
7. Work and interests 3, 7, 25, 42
8. Retardation 21, 28, 30, 47
9. Agitation 6, 10, 37, 43
10. Psychic anxiety 8, 23, 31, 38
11. Somatic anxiety 13, 18, 33, 41
12. Gastrointestinal somatic symptoms 36, 50
13. General somatic symptoms 1, 51
14. Libido 4, 15
15. Hypochrondriasis 5, 39, 45, 49
16. Loss of weight 2, 52
17. Loss of insight 26, 40.

Carroll proposed that a cutoff of 10 should be used when the CRS is applied as a screening instrument (1, p195).

Reliability

Split-half reliability was 0.87 based on multiple ratings of a mixed sample of patients (1, p197). Item-total correlations ranged from 0.05 to 0.78 with a median of 0.55 (1, p198), similar to those for the HRSD.

Validity

Correlations of the CRS and the HRSD include 0.71 and 0.80 (1, p197), 0.75 (3, Table Ib), and 0.79 (4, p167). The correlation may, however, be lower for adolescents: Robbins obtained a figure of 0.46 for 81 adolescents aged 13–18 (5, p124). Feinberg et al. provided some evidence that

the CRS may prove more sensitive to a global clinical rating of depression than the HRSD (3, Figure 1). The CRS correlated 0.67 with a global rating of depression applied to a sample of 232 outpatients (3, Table Ib). It correlated −0.68 with a visual analogue mood scale phrased, "How are you feeling today?" (3, Table Ib) and 0.86 with the Beck Depression Inventory (BDI) (1, p197). Using partial correlations, Feinberg and Carroll showed that the BDI did not contain information in the HRSD beyond that also included in the CRS; the CRS did, however, contain information in the HRSD that was not covered by the BDI. Furthermore, the CRS and the BDI were significantly correlated (0.77) after their intercorrelations with the HRSD were partialled out. This suggests that the self-rating scales have access to a subjective dimension of depression not covered by the clinical rating method (6, p197).

Koenig et al. tested the Brief Carroll Depression Rating Scale as a screen for depression on 64 older medically ill hospital patients; a cutoff of 6 was optimal, giving a 100% sensitivity for detecting clinically diagnosed *DSM-III* depression at a specificity of 93%. Kappa agreement with the clinician's rating was 0.76 (7, Table 2). In a separate study, however, they reported less adequate results: sensitivity and specificity were 73% and 79%, respectively; among those who tested positive, the likelihood of a diagnosis of major depressive disorder was 28% (8, Table 2).

Smouse et al. compared the factor structure of the CRS and HRSD (N = 278). A strong first factor underlay both instruments, and they concluded that use of subscores (e.g., symptom scores) for either instrument holds no advantage over using the total scores (9).

Alternative Forms

There are French, Italian, and Chinese translations of the CRS (6, p189). A 12-item abbreviation of the CRS, the Brief Carroll Depression Rating Scale (BCDRS), has been used as a depression screening

Exhibit 6.8 The Carroll Rating Scale for Depression

Note: An asterisk indicates the response that is scored. These are not shown on the version presented to the respondent.

Complete *ALL* the following statements by *CIRCLING YES or NO*, based on how you have felt during the *past few days.*

1. I feel just as energetic as always	Yes	No*
2. I am losing weight	Yes*	No
3. I have dropped many of my interests and activities	Yes*	No
4. Since my illness I have completely lost interest in sex	Yes*	No
5. I am especially concerned about how my body is functioning	Yes*	No
6. It must be obvious that I am disturbed and agitated	Yes*	No
7. I am still able to carry on doing the work I am supposed to do	Yes	No*
8. I can concentrate easily when reading the papers	Yes	No*
9. Getting to sleep takes me more than half an hour	Yes*	No
10. I am restless and fidgety	Yes*	No
11. I wake up much earlier than I need to in the morning	Yes*	No
12. Dying is the best solution for me	Yes*	No
13. I have a lot of trouble with dizzy and faint feelings	Yes*	No
14. I am being punished for something bad in my past	Yes*	No
15. My sexual interest is the same as before I got sick	Yes	No*
16. I am miserable or often feel like crying	Yes*	No
17. I often wish I were dead	Yes*	No
18. I am having trouble with indigestion	Yes*	No
19. I wake up often in the middle of the night	Yes*	No
20. I feel worthless and ashamed about myself	Yes*	No
21. I am so slowed down that I need help with bathing and dressing	Yes*	No
22. I take longer than usual to fall asleep at night	Yes*	No
23. Much of the time I am very afraid but don't know the reason	Yes*	No
24. Things which I regret about my life are bothering me	Yes*	No
25. I get pleasure and satisfaction from what I do	Yes	No*
26. All I need is a good rest to be perfectly well again	Yes*	No
27. My sleep is restless and disturbed	Yes*	No
28. My mind is as fast and alert as always	Yes	No*
29. I feel that life is still worth living	Yes	No*
30. My voice is dull and lifeless	Yes*	No
31. I feel irritable or jittery	Yes*	No
32. I feel in good spirits	Yes	No*
33. My heart sometimes beats faster than usual	Yes*	No
34. I think my case is hopeless	Yes*	No
35. I wake up before my usual time in the morning	Yes*	No
36. I still enjoy my meals as much as usual	Yes	No*
37. I have to keep pacing around most of the time	Yes*	No
38. I am terrified and near panic	Yes*	No
39. My body is bad and rotten inside	Yes*	No
40. I got sick because of the bad weather we have been having	Yes*	No
41. My hands shake so much that people can easily notice	Yes*	No
42. I still like to go out and meet people	Yes	No*
43. I think I appear calm on the outside	Yes	No*
44. I think I am as good a person as anybody else	Yes	No*
45. My trouble is the result of some serious internal disease	Yes*	No
46. I have been thinking about trying to kill myself	Yes*	No
47. I get hardly anything done lately	Yes*	No
48. There is only misery in the future for me	Yes*	No
49. I worry a lot about my bodily symptoms	Yes*	No
50. I have to force myself to eat even a little	Yes*	No
51. I am exhausted much of the time	Yes*	No
52. I can tell that I have lost a lot of weight	Yes*	No

Adapted from Carroll BJ, Feinberg M, Smouse PE, Rawson SG, Greden JF. The Carroll Rating Scale for Depression. I. Development, reliability and validation. Br J Psychiatry 1981;138;198–200. With permission.

tool for older adults (7). It requires about two minutes to complete.

Commentary

The Carroll scale accurately reflects information contained in the HRSD and, with the possible exception of adolescents, the agreement between the two scales is high. The available evidence suggests that the CRS is reliable and the available validity results are promising. By saving the clinician's time, the CRS offers an economical alternative in regular monitoring of patients or in routine practice to identify patients who need more extensive follow-up (10). Its adequacy as a screen for depression needs more study. As with any self-rating scale, some patients may be unable to complete the CRS due to illiteracy or severe illness (4).

The scoring system of the CRS assumes that patients who endorse the more severe items in a symptom category will also endorse those less severe, thus giving a high score to that area in a manner equivalent to the higher weight assigned by a clinician using the HRSD (10, p70). This seems fair for most categories, with the possible exception of the "somatic anxiety" and "loss of insight" symptoms. The random ordering of items in the form used by patients may also generate some inconsistencies. The evidence from two studies suggests that the lowest agreement between self-ratings and clinicians' judgments lies in the scales on weight loss, retardation and agitation (1, p196; 4, p167).

Hamilton's Rating Scale for Depression has many strong points and has been extremely widely used; a good self-administered version therefore holds considerable potential utility. Carson says that "it appears to be a promising measure, potentially superior to other self-report depression scales" (11, p420).

REFERENCES

(1) Carroll BJ, Feinberg M, Smouse PE, et al. The Carroll Rating Scale for Depression. I. Development, reliability and validation. Br J Psychiatry 1981;138:194–200.

(2) Carroll BJ, Fielding JM, Blashki TG. Depression rating scales: a critical review. Arch Gen Psychiatry 1973;28:361–366.

(3) Feinberg M, Carroll BJ, Smouse PE, et al. The Carroll Rating Scale for Depression. III. Comparison with other rating instruments. Br J Psychiatry 1981;138:205–209.

(4) Nasr SJ, Altman EG, Rodin MB, et al. Correlation of the Hamilton and Carroll Depression Rating Scales: a replication study among psychiatric outpatients. J Clin Psychiatry 1984;45:167–168.

(5) Robbins DR, Alessi NE, Colfer MV, et al. Use of the Hamilton Rating Scale for Depression and the Carroll Self-rating Scale in adolescents. Psychiatry Res 1985; 14:123–129.

(6) Feinberg M, Carroll BJ. The Carroll Rating Scale for Depression. In: Sartorius N, Ban T, eds. Assessment of depression. Berlin: Springer, 1986:188–199.

(7) Koenig HG, Meador KG, Cohen HJ, et al. Self-rated depression scales and screening for major depression in the older hospitalized patient with medical illness. J Am Geriatr Soc 1988;36:699–706.

(8) Koenig HG, Meador KG, Cohen HJ, et al. Screening for depression in hospitalized elderly medical patients: taking a closer look. J Am Geriatr Soc 1992;40:1013–1017.

(9) Smouse PE, Feinberg M, Carroll BJ, et al. The Carroll Rating Scale for Depression. II. Factor analyses of the feature profiles. Br J Psychiatry 1981;138:201–204.

(10) Rabkin JG, Klein DF. The clinical measurement of depressive disorders. In: Marsella AJ, Hirschfeld RMA, Katz MM, eds. The measurement of depression. New York: Guilford Press, 1987:30–83.

(11) Carson TP. Assessment of depression. In: Ciminero AR, Clahoun KS, Adams HE, eds. Handbook of behavioral assessment. 2nd ed. New York: Wiley, 1986:404–445.

CONCLUSION

The scope of any review has to be restricted, and many other depression measures could have been included in this chapter. Some are closely related to those we have reviewed. The Wakefield Depression Inventory (1), for example, is a variant of Zung's scale and Max Hamilton was involved in its development; the Cronholm-

Ottosson Depression Rating Scale (2) was developed by a team that also involved Marie Åsberg. Other measures are more broad-ranging; we focused on scales that measure depression alone. We did not review combined scales such as the Hospital Anxiety and Depression Scale (3) or other more general assessments that include depression such as the Middlesex Hospital Questionnaire (4), Åsberg et al.'s Comprehensive Psychopathological Rating Scale (5), or the Schedule for Affective Disorders and Schizophrenia (6). Our omission of combined instruments does not imply any limitations in these methods; on the contrary, they may prove very suitable for many applications and readers who wish to measure general psychopathology may find them useful. There are also many other purpose-built depression scales that might be considered. The Popoff Index of Depression, for example, is a 15-item screening questionnaire for use in the family physician's office (7). There are many reviews of depression scales to which the reader can turn for descriptions of methods we did not review (8–13).

In trying to select a measurement, the reader will have noted that no instrument covers all the symptoms of depression. For an outcome measure or an instrument that measures severity, this may not matter if symptoms are carefully selected as markers of depression; for screening instruments, however, there may be stronger arguments for more comprehensive coverage. The choice between self- and clinician-rating methods is complex but some guidelines can be given. Self-rating methods are economical and do not require a skilled administrator. They cannot provide diagnostic information but serve well as screening instruments. For this, the Beck, GDS, and Zung instruments are suitable. The main difficulty with self-ratings lies in the respondent's lack of skill and experience: having a limited perspective on the range of severity of depression, she can only rely on her own experience as a basis for judging frequency or severity of symptoms, so

self-rating methods are limited as measures of intensity of depression (11, p408). Self-ratings assume, of course, that accurate information will be reported; this may be problematic as a depressed patient may not be aware of feelings, or may be unable or unwilling to reveal them. The cost of clinician-rating methods will be a consideration, but may be secondary if the depressed patient cannot judge and rate symptoms accurately. Self- and clinician-ratings probably reflect different aspects of depression and cannot be expected to have identical results:

The BDI, for example, emphasizes the subjective experience of depression including pessimism and self-punitive wishes. On the other hand, the HRS-D seems to emphasize symptoms reflecting the intensity of depression and its behavioral manifestations. Whereas 29% of a BDI score may be attributable to a physiological factor, 50% to 80% of the total score on the HRS-D is made up of behavioral and physiological (somatic) components. (14, p57)

This leads to different screening applications for each type of measure: "Since cognitive disturbances are prominent in mild or 'neurotic' depressions and physiologic disturbances are prominent in severe or 'psychotic' disturbances, a self-report scale like the BDI may be a more accurate measure in the neurotically depressed while the HRS may be more accurate in the psychotically depressed" (15, p85). However, if the purpose is to rate severity, it remains possible that patients with neurotic depression may exaggerate their symptoms compared to a clinician's rating (11, p408). Aside from cost, the most commonly cited limitation to clinical ratings is the possibility of bias in the rater; Hamilton proposed that two independent raters should compare their impressions, an approach that must rarely be feasible in practice. As an outcome indicator, the Hamilton scale seems to be more sensitive to change than either the Beck or Zung scale, but certain instruments may be more appropriate to certain types of treatment: the difference in effect sizes between the Zung Self-rating Depression Scale and the Hamilton Rating Scale for Depression was significantly larger for psychotherapy than for drug treatments (14, p58).

While many will continue to search for the more perfect mousetrap, the range of depression measures we currently have seems adequate for most purposes. The measurement of depression thus does not seem a priority for expansion within the field.

REFERENCES

(1) Snaith RP, Ahmed SN, Mehta S, et al. Assessment of the severity of primary depressive illness: Wakefield Self-assessment Depression Inventory. Psychol Med 1971;1:143–149.

(2) Cronholm B, Schalling D, Åsberg M. Development of a rating scale for depressive illness. Mod Probl Pharmacopsychiatry 1974;7:139–150.

(3) Zigmond AS, Snaith RP. The Hospital Anxiety and Depression Scale. Acta Psychiatr Scand 1983;67:361–370.

(4) Crown S, Crisp AH. A short clinical diagnostic self-rating scale for psychoneurotic patients. The Middlesex Hospital Questionnaire (M.H.Q.). Br J Psychiatry 1966;112:917–923.

(5) Åsberg M, Montgomery SA, Perris C, et al. A Comprehensive Psychopathological Rating Scale. Acta Psychiatr Scand 1978;58(suppl 271):5–27.

(6) Endicott J, Spitzer RL. A diagnostic interview for affective disorders and schizophrenia. Arch Gen Psychiatry 1978;35:837–844.

(7) Downing RW, Rickels K. Some properties of the Popoff Index. Clin Med 1972;79:11–18.

(8) Shaw BF, Vallis TM, McCabe SB. The assessment of the severity and symptom patterns in depression. In: Beckham EE, Leber WR, eds. Handbook of depression: treatment, assessment and research. Homewood, Illinois: Dorsey Press, 1985:372–407.

(9) Carson TP. Assessment of depression. In: Ciminero AR, Calhoun KS, Adams HE, eds. Handbook of behavioral assessment. 2nd ed. New York: Wiley, 1986:404–445.

(10) Rabkin JG, Klein DF. The clinical measurement of depressive disorders. In: Marsella AJ, Hirschfeld RMA, Katz MM, eds. The measurement of depression. New York: Guilford Press, 1987:30–83.

(11) Mayer JM. Assessment of depression. In: McReynolds P, ed. Advances in psychological assessment. Vol. 4. San Francisco: Jossey-Bass, 1977:358–425.

(12) Attkisson CC, Zich JM, eds. Depression in primary care: screening and detection. New York: Routledge, 1990.

(13) Moran PW, Lambert MJ. A review of current assessment tools for monitoring changes in depression. In: Lambert MJ, Christensen ER, DeJulio SS, eds. The measurement of psychotherapy outcome in research and evaluation. New York: Wiley, 1983:263–303.

(14) Lambert MJ, Hatch DR, Kingston MD, et al. Zung, Beck, and Hamilton rating scales as measures of treatment outcome: a meta-analytic comparison. J Consult Clin Psychol 1986;54:54–59.

(15) Hughes JR, O'Hara MW, Rehm LP. Measurement of depression in clinical trials: an overview. J Clin Psychiatry 1982;43:85–88.

7

Mental Status Testing[1]

Measures of mental status and cognitive functioning have long formed part of clinical practice, especially in geriatrics. They are now seeing increasing application in epidemiological studies and health surveys to assess the natural history of cognitive decline, to study need for care and the capacity for independent living, and to evaluate treatment. The growing interest is due to increased longevity, to the high prevalence of cognitive problems in the elderly, and to the destructive effect impaired cognition has on independence. The definition of cognition remains elusive; phrases such as "the use or handling of knowledge" and the "overall functioning of mental abilities" seem unsatisfying, so cognitive function is often defined operationally, in terms of success on cognitive tests (1). Cognition problems form a spectrum, beginning with mild declines—in recall and memory, or in other areas of functioning, such as concentration, or reasoning, or in finding the appropriate word—that may be a normal part of the aging process. At the other end of the spectrum lies dementia, the most ex-treme form of cognitive deterioration. Dementia affects 5% to 8% of all those aged over 65; it affects one-third of those aged 85 or over (2, 3); it is the most common psychiatric disorder of old age. An excellent review of the varying definitions of dementia is given by Huppert and Tym (2). Roth defined dementia in nontechnical language in terms of "the global deterioration of an individual's intellectual, emotional and cognitive faculties in a state of unimpaired consciousness" (4). Three elements in this definition hold implications for the measurement of dementia. First, the condition involves a decline from a previously higher level of function and so excludes, for example, those people who have been mentally retarded since birth. A measurement should therefore record alterations in state, rather than merely current state. Second, several functions are implied in "global deterioration." While memory loss is the central feature, most operational definitions of dementia hold that there must also be limitations in other cognitive functions (5). These include aphasia (disorders of language, generally due to left hemisphere lesions), apraxia (disorders in performing purposeful movements, of which constructional apraxia reflects a disorder of

1. This chapter was written by Ian McDowell and Elizabeth Kristjansson, with the assistance of Claire Newell.

287

visual and motor integration), and agnosia (disorders of recognition). Hence, dementia is a symptom complex rather than a single condition; memory loss is sensitive but not specific to dementia, and a screening test for dementia should have a broad content. Third, Roth's reference to unimpaired consciousness requires that the cognitive testing be fair and that any deficits observed not be due to intoxication, delirium, or to other acute confusional states. Delirium is associated with an alteration in the level of consciousness that leads to confusion and an inability to focus or sustain attention. This accordingly affects performance on cognitive tests and so must be excluded before dementia can be diagnosed. As with assessing depression, excluding these rival explanations implies the need for a clinical assessment; thus, self-administered tests may suffice for screening, but they are not adequate for full identification of dementia. A clinical assessment is required to differentiate between dementia and depression or acute confusional states, both of which can mimic the early stages of dementia. There are many possible causes of dementia, including reversible factors such as the effects of medications, of depression, and of metabolic or nutritional deficiencies; among the irreversible causes are Alzheimer's disease and strokes.

Alzheimer's disease accounts for up to two-thirds of dementias and is characterized by abnormal brain cells containing tangles of fibers (neurofibrillary tangles) and clusters of degenerating nerve endings (neuritic plaques) in the cerebral cortex (6). Alzheimer's disease can only be definitively diagnosed at autopsy. Its clinical diagnosis in patients presenting with characteristic symptoms requires a process of excluding rival possible explanations, such as vascular disease, metabolic disorders, systemic illnesses, brain tumors, and deficiency states (7, Table 5). Criteria for the clinical diagnosis of Alzheimer's disease have been established (8). The criteria require formal mental status testing; a history; physical, neurological, and psychiatric examinations; laboratory tests and a CT scan (6).

The clinical diagnosis has roughly a 90% to 95% accuracy when compared to subsequent pathological examination.

MEASUREMENTS OF COGNITION, COGNITIVE IMPAIRMENT, AND DEMENTIA

Tests of cognitive function may be divided into three main categories: intelligence tests, clinical neuropsychological tests, and laboratory tests (1). Of these, our review focuses on the middle category, which includes simple mental status screening examinations and detailed tests of specific cognitive functions. The distinction between the former· and the latter is that screening tests are broad, whereas neuropsychological tests of cognition provide in-depth appraisals of particular functions, such as memory, orientation, and praxis. We do not review complete neuropsychological tests; the tests that we review briefly evaluate a range of cognitive functions in order to provide a clinical overview of mental status. This is relevant in assessing cognitive impairment, which is not a specific mental disorder, but, rather, gathers together conceptually a wide range of conditions that are often encountered in combination. Mental status tests are used *(i)* to broadly assess cognitive performance or *(ii)* to screen for cognitive impairment or *(iii)* to screen for dementia. The distinction between these three goals is often not made precisely clear, and tests designed for each purpose often share items in common. Most mental status tests include assessment of orientation to time and place, concentration and attention tests, and memory tests for short- and long-term recall.

There are many mental status scales designed to identify dementia—the major clinical syndrome in the field of cognition. Dementia requires the assessment of several forms of cognitive deficit. Measurement instruments tend to one of two forms: either they combine existing single-purpose cognitive tests to form a "battery," or purpose-built mental status tests may be constructed. The components of purpose-built tests are mainly elements from neuropsychological instruments that are routinely used in clinical neuropsychological practice to assess specific aspects of cognitive functioning. Historically, these tests originated as bedside ratings intended to assess cognitive function objectively; they were subsequently adapted for use as screening tests for cognitive impairments and dementia. The emphasis was on practicality, and many of the instruments we review were developed by physicians in reaction to difficulties experienced in administering full neuropsychological test batteries to elderly patients. This focus on simplicity in designing tests has stimulated criticisms, and several themes recur in the reviews that follow. First, the tests are often narrow in their scope. They may be insensitive to the early stages of cognitive decline and fail to distinguish between normal senescent decline in cognitive function and the early stages of pathological decline. Second, they may not distinguish among the more severe levels of dementia. Third, test scores have to be interpreted in light of the respondent's educational level. Most tests tend to confuse lack of education with presence of cognitive impairment. Finally, and as with depression, the screening tests only give a general indication of the presence of a disorder and clinical evaluation remains essential in evaluating the individual patient (9, pp133–134). Hence such measures must be used with extreme caution as outcome indicators.

COMBINATIONS OF TESTS FOR ASSESSING DEMENTIA

Because dementia is a syndrome with several characteristic features, all assessment instruments include separate components. Further, few tests are capable of discriminating across all levels and types of dementia; tests that are useful in distinguishing mild impairment from normal cognitive functioning generally are not suited to differentiating among more advanced stages of dementia, and vice versa. Accordingly, both types of test may be applied in combination. For example, Katzman suggested using the Blessed Test or Short Blessed Test supplemented by the Mini-Mental State Examination (MMSE), which covers a broader range of functions (10). Eastwood used a combination of the Mental Status Questionnaire (MSQ), the Physical Health Questionnaire, the Present State Examination, the Face-Hand Test, a test of developmental reflexes, the Hachinski Scale, focal neurologic signs, and the Dementia Rating Scale (11). The Consortium to Establish a Registry for Alzheimer's Disease (CERAD) at Duke University used the Short Blessed Test; assessments of insight, depression, calculation ability, and language; clinical history; and the Blessed Dementia Scale (12). Shore et al. in the National Institutes of Mental Health longitudinal study of Alzheimer's disease, used the MMSE, the MSQ, the Extended Rating Scale for Dementia, the London Psychogeriatric Rating Scale, and the Hachinski Scale (13).

Several formal batteries of tests have been developed for assessing dementia: that proposed by Branconnier (14), Pfeffer's Mental Function Index (15), the approach of Ferris and Crook (16), the Storandt Battery (17), and the Eslinger Battery (18) are examples.

SCOPE OF THE CHAPTER

The profusion of cognitive screening questionnaires, diagnostic instruments, and neuropsychological tests has made selection for this chapter necessary and difficult. To narrow our review we excluded neuropsychological tests such as the Benton tests or the Wechsler Adult Intelligence Tests, for these generally require clinical training to administer and interpret. The test marketing companies that distribute them can provide extensive information on validity, reliability, and scoring procedures. Nor did we review the very large clinical diagnostic procedures—such as the Present State Examination (PSE); the Diagnostic Interview Schedule (DIS); the Geriatric Mental State Examination (GMS), which was derived from the PSE; and the Canberra Interview for the Elderly. The only exception in this category is the Cambridge Mental Disorders of the Elderly Examination (CAMDEX) which is reviewed because its components are used as stand-alone instruments in epidemiological surveys and in evaluating outcomes of care. Overall, the result of our selection process has been to include older scales, many at least 20 years old. As in other chapters, these older instruments are frequently used, and reviewing them forms an important introduction to this field.

The chapter opens with reviews of several assessments that were designed for clinical use. The Mattis Dementia Rating Scale was devised for seriously ill patients who could not complete standard neuropsychological test batteries. The Cognitive Capacity Screening Examination was intended as a cognitive screening test for use with general medical patients. The Alzheimer's Disease Assessment Scale was designed to measure behavioral and affective deficits in patients with Alzheimer's disease. The Clock Drawing Test originated as a brief bedside screen but has seen recent application as a community screening instrument. We then review two instruments developed by Gary Blessed: the Information-Memory-Concentration Test and the Dementia Scale. Both were developed for use with patients but can also be used in community screening. Next, we review the Mental Status Questionnaire and its revised version, the Short Portable Mental Status Questionnaire. The former is similar to the Blessed tests, while the latter is intended for community screening. The Mini-Mental State Examination that follows is the screening test most widely used in North American studies; we also describe some modified versions that appear to improve on the original. Finally, we review two broader-ranging clinical assessment tools—the Clifton Assessment Procedures for the Elderly and the Cambridge Mental Disorders of the Elderly Examination. A tabular comparison of these instruments is shown in Table 7.1.

REFERENCES

(1) Colsher PL, Wallace RB. Epidemiologic considerations in studies of cognitive function in the elderly: methodology and nondementing acquired dysfunction. Epidemiol Rev 1991;13:1–27.

(2) Huppert FA, Tym E. Clinical and neuropsychological assessment of dementia. Br Med Bull 1986;42:11–18.

(3) Canadian Study of Health and Aging Working Group. The Canadian Study of Health and Aging: study methods and prevalence of dementia. Can Med Assoc J 1994;150:899–913.

(4) Roth M. The diagnosis of dementia in late and middle life. In: Mortimer JA, Schuman LM, eds. The epidemiology of dementia. New York: Oxford University Press, 1980:24–61.

(5) American Psychiatric Association. Diagnostic and statistical manual of mental disorders DSM—IV. 4th ed. Washington, DC: American Psychiatric Association, 1994.

(6) Katzman R. Alzheimer's disease. N Engl J Med 1986;314:964–973.

(7) Ramsdell JW, Rothrock JF, Ward HW, et al. Evaluation of cognitive impairment in the elderly. J Gen Intern Med 1990;5:55–64.

(8) McKhann G, Drachman D, Folstein M, et al. Clinical diagnosis of Alzheimer's disease: report of the NINCDS-ADRDA Work Group under the auspices of Department of Health and Human Services Task Force on Alzheimer's disease. Neurology 1984;34:939–944.

(9) Davis PB, Morris JC, Grant E. Brief screening tests versus clinical staging in senile dementia of the Alzheimer type. J Am Geriatr Soc 1990;38:129–135.

(10) Katzman R. Differential diagnosis of dementing illnesses. Neurol Clin 1986;4:329–340.

(11) Eastwood MR, Lautenschlaeger E, Corbin S. A comparison of clinical methods for assessing dementia. J Am Geriatr Soc 1983;31:342–347.

(12) Welsh K, Butters N, Hughes J, et al. Detection of abnormal memory decline in mild cases of Alzheimer's disease using CERAD neuropsychological measures. Arch Neurol 1991;48:278–281.

(13) Shore D, Overman CA, Wyatt RJ. Improving accuracy in the diagnosis of Alzheimer's disease. J Clin Psychiatry 1983;44:207–212.

(14) Branconnier RJ. A computerized battery for behavioral assessment in Alzheimer's

Table 7.1 Comparison of the Quality of Mental Status Tests*

Measurements	Scale	Number of items	Application	Administered by (time)	Studies using method	Reliability		Validity	
						Thoroughness	Results	Thoroughness	Results
Dementia Rating Scale (Mattis, 1973)	ordinal	22	research	expert	several	+ +	+ +	+ +	+ +
Cognitive Capacity Screening Examination (Jacobs, 1977)	ordinal	30	clinical	expert (5–15 min)	several	+	+ +	+ +	+ +
Clock Drawing Test (Various authors, 1986)	ordinal	1†	clinical, screening	self	many	+ +	+ +	+ +	+ +
Alzheimer's Disease Assessment Scale (Rosen, 1983)	ordinal	21	screening	expert	several	+	+ + +	+ +	+ +
Information-Memory-Concentration Test (Blessed, 1968)	ordinal	29	clinical, survey	staff (10 min)	many	+	+ + +	+ +	+ + +
Dementia Scale (Blessed, 1968)	ordinal	22	research	interviewer	several	+	+	+ +	+
Mental Status Questionnaire (Kahn, 1960)	ordinal	10	clinical, survey	interviewer (5–10 min)	several	+	+ +	+ +	+ +
Short Portable Mental Status Questionnaire (Pfeiffer, 1975)	ordinal	10	screening, survey	interviewer (2 min)	many	+	+ +	+ +	+ +
Mini-Mental Status Examination (Folstein, 1975)	ordinal	30	clinical, screening	interviewer (5–10 min)	many	+ + +	+ +	+ + +	+ + +
Clifton Assessment Procedures for the Elderly (Pattie, 1975)	ordinal	12	clinical	staff	several	+ +	+ +	+ +	+ +
Cambridge Mental Disorders of the Elderly Examination (CAMDEX) (Roth, 1986)	ordinal	57	research, clinical	expert (80 mins)	many	+	+ + +	+ +	+ + +

*For an explanation of the categories used, see Chapter 1, pages 6–7.

†The Clock Test may include clock drawing, clock setting, and clock reading.

disease. In: Poon LW, ed. Handbook for clinical memory assessment of older adults. Washington, DC: American Psychological Association, 1986:189–196.

(15) Pfeffer RI, Kurosaki TT, Harrah CH, et al. A survey diagnostic tool for senile dementia. Am J Epidemiol 1981;114:515–527.

(16) Ferris SH, Crook T. Cognitive assessment in mild to moderately severe dementia. In: Crook T, Ferris S, Bartus R, eds. Assessment in geriatric psychopharmacology. New Canaan, Connecticut: Mark Powley, 1983:177–186.

(17) Storandt M, Botwinick J, Danziger WL, et al. Psychometric differentiation of mild senile dementia of the Alzheimer type. Arch Neurol 1984;41:497–499.

(18) Eslinger PJ, Damasio AR, Benton AL, et al. Neuropsychologic detection of abnormal mental decline in older persons. JAMA 1985;253:670–674.

THE DEMENTIA RATING SCALE
(Steven Mattis, 1973)

Purpose

The Dementia Rating Scale (DRS) was intended to identify cognitive deficits caused by neurological disease and was developed for research on cerebral blood flow in dementia (1). It was intended for use with severely affected institutionalized patients who would not be able to complete standard neuropsychological tests.

Conceptual Basis

Mattis noted that instruments such as the Wechsler Adult Intelligence Scale (WAIS) discriminate dementia patients from normal but are often too demanding for use in discriminating among dementia patients. He therefore developed the Dementia Rating Scale to identify presenile and senile dementia by recording behavior that corresponds to preschool-age development (2, p99).

Description

The DRS covers attention, perseveration (in the sense of uncontrollable repetition—verbal and motor), construction, conceptu-alization, and memory (verbal and nonverbal). It is a rating scale administered by a clinician; there are 36 items and items in each section are presented in a hierarchical order starting with the most difficult so that once the patient passes an item it is assumed that he will pass simpler items on that section (an approach also used in Cole's Hierarchic Dementia Scale). Applying the test to normal elderly patients takes ten to 15 minutes; for Alzheimer's patients, 30 to 45 minutes are required (2, p99). The complete scale is too long to present here; its content is summarized in Exhibit 7.1, and the complete scale is shown in the Appendix to Mattis's book chapter (2, pp108–121). Administration instructions are available (3).

Scores range from 0 to 144. Normal individuals over 65 years of age are expected to score 140 or above; a score of 100 or below "is often not consonant with survival over the next 20 months" (2, p99). Subsequent authors have used scores of 130 or more as indicating normality (4); the DRS manual recommends that scores below 123 be interpreted as representing impairment (3).

Reliability

A one-week test–retest reliability of 0.97 was reported in the original study of 30 Alzheimer's patients (1, Table 1). Reliability for subsections ranged from 0.61 on the attention section to 0.94 on the conceptualization section. Retest reliability at a mean of 16 months was reported as $r = 0.75$ (5, Table 3).

Split-half reliability was 0.90 in a sample of 25 nursing-home residents (6, p273). Alpha internal consistency coefficients were 0.95 for attention, 0.87 for perseveration, 0.95 for conceptualization, 0.75 for memory (7, p748), and 0.87 for the overall score (8, p212).

Validity

Several studies have validated the DRS against physiological indicators of brain function. The correlation between DRS

Exhibit 7.1   Content of the Dementia Rating Scale

Scales and items	Example of test items
I. Attention	
Digit span	Repeat three random digit strings forwards and backwards
Respond to successive commands	Open your mouth and close your eyes
Respond to single command	Stick out tongue
Imitate	Raise your right hand
II. Initiation and perseveration	
Verbal	Name things a person can buy at the supermarket
Motor—double alternating movement	Left palm up, right palm down, then switch simultaneously several times
Graphomotor functions	Copy four geometric figures
III. Construction	
Geometric figures	Copy six figures
IV. Conceptualization	
	Multiple choice:
Similarities—verbal	In what way are an apple and a banana alike?
Primary inductive reasoning	Name three things people eat. How are [the items named by patient] alike?
Differences	Which does not belong: dog, cat, car?
Similarities	Apple, banana. Are they both animals, fruit or green?
Identities and oddities	Which 2 figures are the same? Which one is different?
V. Memory	
Verbal recall	Recall a simple sentence after distraction
Create sentence	Make up a sentence using the words man and car
Orientation	Awareness of time, place, president
VI. Recall	
Sentence recall	Repeat the simple sentence and the sentence involving man and car
Verbal recognition	Forced choice format: select which word in a pair you have read on previous page
Design recognition	Forced choice format: select which design in pair you saw on previous page

Adapted from Mattis S. Mental status examination for organic mental syndrome in the elderly patient. In: Bellak L, Karasu TB, eds. Geriatric psychiatry: a handbook for psychiatrists and primary care physicians. New York: Grune & Stratton, 1976:108–121.

scores and cerebral blood flow was 0.86 (1, Figure 3; 2, p99; 6, p272). A positron emission tomography (PET) study of 17 patients with Alzheimer's disease and five controls gave correlations ranging from 0.50 to 0.69 between DRS scores and metabolism at various sites in the left hemisphere (9, Table 3). These correlations were similar to those obtained for the WAIS—a performance IQ test.

The DRS was validated against clinical diagnoses of 111 patients admitted to a neuropsychology clinic. As reported by Nelson et al., Montgomery and Costa found that the DRS correctly identified 62% of patients with clinically diagnosed dementia at a cutting point of 123 (10, Table 1). The DRS showed a clear association with a clinical rating of severity of Alzheimer's dementia (4, Table 3). All of the cognitively normal control group scored 136 or above; 83% of the "mild" Alzheimer's group fell in the range 103 to 130, and 71% of the "moderate" group scored 102 or below (4, p20); DRS scores provided a better discrimination of severity levels than did an activities of daily living scale, although in combination the two instruments approximated the accuracy of the clinical staging of dementia.

DRS scores correlated 0.75 with full-scale WAIS IQ scores (1, p300). Correlations with the Boston Naming Test were 0.35 and 0.49 in two samples differing in severity of dementia (7, Table 8). The correlation with the Mini-Mental State Examination was 0.78, comparable to a previous finding of 0.82 (8, p210).

Alternative Forms

The Extended Rating Scale for Dementia uses 14 items from the DRS, supplemented with a further nine items to assess the severity of dementia in patients with advanced disease (11). A result of 0.94 was obtained for both test–retest reliability and internal consistency (11, p350). Sensitivity was 89% at a specificity of 96%, rising to a sensitivity of 97% and a specificity of 100% for patients aged over 80 years (12, p851). In the group of patients under 65 years, sensitivity was only 75% and specificity was 95% (12, Table 8). Scores correlated significantly with total EEG change ($r = -0.77$) and with computerized tomography ratings of ventricular diameter ($r = -0.58$) (13, Table 2).

Commentary

The DRS is appropriate where a clinical rating scale is required for severely ill patients; it does not seem suitable as a screening instrument, although it is occasionally described as one (8). It is principally a research instrument that may offer a compromise between extensive instruments such as the WAIS or the Halstead-Reitan Battery and briefer screening instruments such as the Mini-Mental State Examination. Although most of the studies that have tested the DRS are small, reliability results seem good, and the main evidence for validity comes from studies that link the DRS with neurological and physiological findings; we have little information on its value as a diagnostic instrument.

REFERENCES

(1) Coblentz M, Mattis S, Zingesser LH, et al. Presenile dementia: clinical aspects and evaluation of cerebrospinal fluid dynamics. Arch Neurol 1973;29:299–308.

(2) Mattis S. Mental status examination for organic mental syndrome in the elderly patient. In: Bellak L, Karasu TB, eds. Geriatric psychiatry: a handbook for psychiatrists and primary care physicians. New York: Grune & Stratton, 1976:77–121.

(3) Mattis S. Dementia Rating Scale: professional manual. Odessa, Florida: Psychological Assessment Resources, 1988.

(4) Shay KA, Duke LW, Conboy T, et al. The clinical validity of the Mattis Dementia Rating Scale in staging Alzheimer's dementia. J Geriatr Psychiatry Neurol 1991; 4:18–25.

(5) Uhlmann RF, Larson EB, Buchner DM. Correlations of Mini Mental State and modified Dementia Rating Scale to measures of transitional health status in dementia. J Gerontol 1987;42:33–36.

(6) Gardner R Jr, Oliver-Muñoz S, Fisher L, et al. Mattis Dementia Rating Scale: internal reliability study using a diffusely impaired population. J Clin Neuropsychol 1981; 3:271–275.

(7) Vitaliano PP, Breen AR, Russo J, et al. The clinical utility of the Dementia Rating Scale for assessing Alzheimer patients. J Chronic Dis 1984;37:743–753.

(8) Bobholz JH, Brandt J. Assessment of cognitive impairment: relationship of the Dementia Rating Scale to the Mini-Mental State Examination. J Geriatr Psychiatry Neurol 1993;6:210–213.

(9) Chase TN, Foster NL, Fedio P, et al. Regional cortical dysfunction in Alzheimer's disease as determined by positron emission tomography. Ann Neurol 1984; 15(suppl):S170–S174.

(10) Nelson A, Fogel BS, Faust D. Bedside cognitive screening instruments: a critical assessment. J Nerv Ment Dis 1986;174:73–83.

(11) Hersch EL. Development and application of the Extended Scale for Dementia. J Am Geriatr Soc 1979;27:348–354.

(12) Lau C, Wands K, Merskey H, et al. Sensitivity and specificity of the Extended Scale for Dementia. Arch Neurol 1988;45:849–852.

(13) Merskey H, Ball MJ, Blume WT, et al. Relationships between psychological measurements and cerebral organic changes in Alzheimer's disease. Can J Neurol Sci 1980;7:45–49.

THE COGNITIVE CAPACITY SCREENING EXAMINATION (John W. Jacobs, 1977)

Purpose

The Cognitive Capacity Screening Examination (CCSE) is a 30-item test designed to assist the clinician in identifying organic mental syndromes, particularly delirium, among medical patients (1).

Conceptual Basis

Jacobs noted that busy clinicians often restrict their cognitive testing to orientation to time, place, and person; these, he argued, are the least sensitive indicators of organic mental syndromes. They may not distinguish between functional and organic syndromes and they may falsely classify depressed or anxious patients. Jacobs also noted that several cognitive tests discriminate against patients with low education, and that patients may resent questions that imply that they are ignorant (1, pp40–41). The CCSE was based on the concept that organic mental syndromes could be identified by requiring the subject to shift rapidly from one task to another, often with interposed distracting tasks.

Description

Addressing these limitations, the CCSE covers judgment, mental speed, and sustained effort. Jacobs argued that rapid shifts in thinking are relevant to diagnosing delirium, so he mixed the order of items. The 30 items, shown in Exhibit 7.2, are based on previous questionnaires and are administered by a physician, psychologist, or other health professional in five to 15 minutes. An overall score counts the number of questions answered correctly; 19/20 was recommended as the cutting point (1, p45).

Reliability

Two psychiatrists applied the CCSE twice within 24 hours to 50 consecutive patients. The Pearson correlation was 0.92 (κ = 0.62) (2, p322). In another case, there was complete agreement among three examiners of six subjects, three of whom were demented (1, p41). However, correction was not made for length of time between examinations or for other intervening variables.

Internal consistency alpha was 0.97 for 63 patients (3, p218).

Exhibit 7.2   The Cognitive Capacity Screening Examination

Instructions: Check items answered correctly. Write incorrect or unusual answers in space provided. If necessary, urge patient once to complete task.

Introduction to patient: "I would like to ask you a few questions. Some you will find very easy and others may be very hard. Just do your best."

1. What day of the week is this? _____
2. What month? _____
3. What day of month? _____
4. What year? _____
5. What place is this? _____
6. Repeat the numbers 8 7 2. _____
7. Say them backwards. _____
8. Repeat these numbers 6 3 7 1. _____
9. Listen to these numbers 6 9 4. Count 1 through 10 out loud, then repeat 6 9 4. (Help if needed. Then use numbers 5 7 3.) _____
10. Listen to these numbers 8 1 4 3. Count l through 10 out loud, then repeat 8 1 4 3. _____
11. Beginning with Sunday, say the days of the week backwards. _____
12. 9 + 3 is _____
13. Add 6 (to the previous answer or "to 12"). _____
14. Take away 5 ("from 18"). Repeat these words after me and remember them. I will ask for them later: HAT, CAR, TREE, TWENTY-SIX. _____
15. The opposite of fast is slow. The opposite of up is _____
16. The opposite of large is _____
17. The opposite of hard is _____
18. An orange and a banana are both fruits. Red and blue are both _____
19. A penny and a dime are both _____
20. What were those words I asked you to remember? (HAT) _____
21. (CAR) _____
22. (TREE) _____
23. (TWENTY-SIX) _____
24. Take away 7 from 100, then take away 7 from what is left and keep going: 100 − 7 is _____
25. Minus 7 _____

Exhibit 7.2   *(Continued)*

Exhibit 7.2   *(Continued)*

26. Minus 7 (write down answers; check correct subtraction of 7)	_____
27. Minus 7	_____
28. Minus 7	_____
29. Minus 7	_____
30. Minus 7	_____
Total Correct (maximum score = 30)	_____

Adapted from Jacobs JW, Bernhard MR, Delgado A, Strain JJ. Screening for organic mental syndromes in the medically ill. Ann Intern Med 1977;86:45.

Validity

Several studies have examined the sensitivity and specificity of the CCSE. For 24 patients undergoing psychiatric consultation, sensitivity was 94% and specificity was 71% (1, Table 1). The mean scores for schizophrenics and for patients with depression fell above the cutting point, suggesting that these patients were not falsely classified as having cognitive disorders (1, p42). As a comparison, the questions were administered to the ward doctors and nurses; reassuringly, none scored below 20 (1, p43). Compared to a full neurological examination, sensitivity was 62% for all cognitive deficits at a specificity of 90% with a cutting point of 19/20 (4, Tables 1, 2). Beresford reported a sensitivity of 84% and a specificity of 94% using a cutting point of 19/20 (2, p324). In a study of 65 elderly hospitalized patients, the CCSE correctly identified 100% of patients diagnosed with organic mental syndrome and 78% of CVA patients; specificity was 82% (5, Table 1). In a study of 62 patients from teaching hospitals, Webster found a sensitivity of 49% for detecting brain impairment and a specificity of 90% (6, Table 1). Schwamm et al. found a false-negative rate of 53% for the CCSE compared to 43% for the Mini-Mental State Examination (7, p486). For 66 general medical and surgical patients the CCSE had a sensitivity and specificity of 100% (3, Table 2).

Foreman reported correlations of 0.63 with the Short Portable Mental Status Questionnaire, 0.83 with the Dementia Rating Scale, and 0.88 with the Mini-Mental State Examination (3, Table 3). Scores on the CCSE varied by educational level (1, pp42–43).

Commentary

The CCSE has been quite widely tested over a number of years, showing variable and somewhat indifferent validity results. The variation may reflect the diverse populations on which it has been tested. Jacobs et al. were "forced to conclude from these findings that our stated goals had not been fully achieved" (1, p43). The CCSE was shown not to distinguish successfully between mental retardation and organic mental syndromes. Responses were influenced by educational level and by language comprehension; conversely, mental deficits may be obscured in people of higher intelligence. Jacobs concluded that the test does identify patients with diminished cognitive capacity arising from organic syndromes or mental retardation but also identifies people with low levels of intelligence or education or a background of cultural deprivation. Kaufman et al. noted that the CCSE detected cognitive deficits due to Alzheimer's disease and metabolic problems but did not identify deficits due to structural problems such as tumors or the aftermaths of stroke, and it often failed to detect mild dementia. Schwamm et al. commented that the items in the CCSE (like those in the MMSE) are comparatively undemanding, so mild impairments may be missed; they also noted that patients may fail all of the memory items and yet remain within the unimpaired range in the overall score (7, pp489–490).

The CCSE is a broad-spectrum screening instrument that can reasonably well identify cognitive impairments due to a range of conditions. We know little about its performance as a community screening test; if the purpose is to screen for dementia, one of the other instruments will prove superior.

REFERENCES

(1) Jacobs JW, Bernhard MR, Delgado A, et al. Screening for organic mental syndromes in the medically ill. Ann Intern Med 1977;86:40–46.

(2) Beresford TP, Holt RE, Hall RCW, et al. Cognitive screening at the bedside: usefulness of a structured examination. Psychosomatics 1985;26:319–324.

(3) Foreman MD. Reliability and validity of mental status questionnaires in elderly hospitalized patients. Nurs Res 1987; 36:216–220.

(4) Kaufman DM, Weinberger M, Strain JJ, et al. Detection of cognitive deficits by a brief mental status examination: the Cognitive Capacity Screening Examination, a reappraisal and a review. Gen Hosp Psychiatry 1979;1:247–255.

(5) Omer H, Foldes J, Toby M, et al. Screening for cognitive deficits in a sample of hospitalized geriatric patients: a re-evaluation of a brief mental status questionnaire. J Am Geriatr Soc 1983;31:266–268.

(6) Webster JS, Scott RR, Nunn B, et al. A brief neuropsychological screening procedure that assesses left and right hemispheric function. J Clin Psychol 1984;40:237–240.

(7) Schwamm LH, Van Dyke C, Kiernan RJ, et al. The Neurobehavioral Cognitive Status Examination: comparison with the Cognitive Capacity Screening Examination and the Mini-Mental State Examination in a neurosurgical population. Ann Intern Med 1987;107:486–491.

THE CLOCK DRAWING TEST
(Various authors, 1986 onward)

Purpose

Clock drawing has long been used as a test of cognitive function and has recently been proposed as a screening test for dementia.

Conceptual Basis

Clock drawing was introduced in the early 1900s as an indicator of constructional apraxia. Disorder in clock drawing ability was originally attributed to focal lesions of the occipital or parietal lobes, as demonstrated by studies of World War I soldiers with head wounds (1, p1238). More recently, disturbance of visuospatial skills has been shown to be an early sign of dementia. Distortions in placing the numbers on a clock face and drawing the hands to indicate specified times reveal and characterize deficits in visuospatial abilities and abstract thinking. In patients with advanced dementia, the clock drawing task may prove easier to administer than the normal, verbally mediated memory tasks (2). Clock drawing may also identify particular types of deficit; patients with left unilateral spatial neglect, for example, may place all 12 numbers on the right half of the clock (3). Errors in clock drawing may reflect constructional apraxia, while abnormal clock setting may reflect the conceptual difficulties seen in demented people (4). Rouleau et al. illustrate a number of clocks that reveal different types of cognitive deficit (5, Figures 1–4).

Description

The clock task may take the form of clock drawing, clock setting, or clock reading. For clock drawing, a predrawn circle is generally supplied and the respondent is asked to place the numbers in the appropriate places; alternatively, a blank sheet is used, and the respondent is asked to draw the circle and add the numbers. The clock setting task involves drawing hour and minute hands to specified times—such as ten minutes to two, or 7:45. In clock reading, the subject is typically shown a circle without numbers, but with marks indicating the locations of numbers and with hands drawn in to depict the time (4).

While the distorted clock drawn by someone with severe dementia can be immediately recognized, the creation of a reliable numerical score for the distortions is complex. Scoring varies in different studies; generally scores evaluate omissions of numbers, errors in placing the numbers, rotations, perseverations, switching numbers, and the spacing between the numbers. Examples of scoring approaches include the following:

1. Wolf-Klein et al. used a partially ordered classification of ten categories, of which six appeared to correspond to dementia and four to cognitive normality (6).

2. Sunderland et al. asked six raters to place 150 completed clocks into ten ordered categories running from "the *best* representation of a clock" to "the *worst* representation of a clock." From this they derived descriptive criteria with which to rank clocks on a 1-to-10 scale; examples of criteria are: "5. Crowding of numbers at one end of the clock or reversal of numbers" and "7. Placement of hands is significantly off course" (2, Table 1). They also provided drawings representing the ten scale points (2, Figure 1).

3. Rouleau et al. reported limitations in Sunderland's scoring system and proposed a modification in which a maximum of two points are awarded for drawing the clock-face circle, four points are given for correct placement of the numbers, and four points are won for setting the hands correctly. Criteria for awarding points were specified (5, Table 2).

4. Shulman et al. rank ordered the severity of errors in clock drawing along a five-point scale (7).

5. Ishiai et al. awarded a maximum of four points, giving one point each for the correct placement of the 3, the 6 and the 9 relative to the 12, and one point for correctly placing the remaining numbers (3).

6. A score that placed greater emphasis on clock setting than on drawing was proposed by Ganguli et al. The respondent receives two points for drawing a reasonable circle, two for putting the numbers in correctly (deleting one point for any numbers in the wrong place), and four points for drawing the appropriate length and position of the hands (8, pp50–51).

7. Watson et al. specified ten categories of errors and counted scores within each of these. Categories included, for example, omissions, rotations, and reversals of digits. They also counted the recognizability of the digits, the number of marks not representing digits, and inconsistent sizes of digits (1, p1236). They provided succinct scoring rules and mused about computerized scoring (1, Table 4 and p1239). Interestingly, they found that weighting errors made in the fourth quadrant of the clock (between 9 and 12) by a factor of four improved sensitivity and specificity (1, p1237).

8. Tuokko et al. developed a combined procedure that provides quantitative and qualitative ratings (9). Separate scores are derived for omissions, perseverations, rotations, misplacements, distortions, substitutions, and additions; within each of these, subtypes of error are defined (4, Table 1). A transparent overlay with lines indicating zones of acceptable positions for the numbers is used to enhance accuracy in judging the misplacement of numbers. For clock setting, one point is awarded for the correct placement of each hand and a further point for the correct relative lengths of the hands (maximum = three points) (4, p580).

Reliability

Ainslie and Murden tested the inter-rater reliability of various scoring methods; reliability for the Shulman and Wolf-Klein methods was good (κ = 0.74 and 0.73) but only fair for the Sunderland method (κ = 0.48) (10, p250). Sunderland et al. reported intraclass correlations for various subgroups of patients and normals ranging from 0.62 to 0.97; the agreement for the complete sample was 0.98 (2, pp727–728). Tuokko et al. reported inter-rater reliability coefficients ranging from 0.90 to 0.95 for their scoring system. Four-day test–retest reliability was 0.70 (4, p581). Test–retest reliability reported by Watson et al. was ρ = 0.76 (1, p1238). Inter-rater reliability for scoring the clocks ranged from ρ =

0.85 to $\rho = 0.95$ according to the identity of the rater (1, Table 5).

Validity

Ainslie and Murden compared the sensitivity and specificity of three scoring methods for a sample of 187 elderly people; sensitivity varied from 48% to 87% while specificity varied from 93% to 54% (10, Table 2). Sensitivity for Alzheimer's disease was 75% at a specificity of 94% (6, p733). At an arbitrary cutting point of 6, Sunderland et al. reported a sensitivity of 78% at a specificity of 96%. Adjusting the cutting point would not greatly improve these figures, for some Alzheimer patients received nearly perfect scores on the clock drawing task (2, p728). Tuokko et al. reported sensitivity of 92% and specificity of 86% for clock drawing; 87% and 97%, respectively, for clock setting; and 92% and 85% for clock reading (4, p579). Watson et al. reported sensitivity at 87% and specificity at 82% (1, Table 3).

Clock drawing scores showed significant differences between Alzheimer patients and controls and correlated 0.56 with the Global Deterioration Score, 0.51 with the Blessed Dementia Rating Scale, and 0.59 with the Short Portable Mental Status Questionnaire (2, pp727–728). A correlation of 0.30 with Katzman's Orientation-Memory-Concentration Test was reported (11, p143). Clock drawing did not correlate with other tests of unilateral spatial neglect, but clock scores correlated 0.75 with verbal WAIS scores (3, Table 1). Tuokko et al. reported correlations with other tests, showing higher coefficients for clock setting than for clock reading and drawing (9, Table 5.3).

Reference Standards

Tuokko et al. provide reference standards and show typical profiles for Alzheimer's disease and depression (9, Chapters 3, 4).

Commentary

The clock drawing test offers a rapid screening method that respondents find more interesting than the grade-school type of memory and arithmetic tasks found in other instruments. Clock drawing should be applicable across most cultures and language groups, although it is evidently unsuitable for people with visual impairments. The validity results reinforce the argument that visuospatial skills offer a useful screening approach for dementia, although arguably as a supplement to other methods rather than a stand-alone test.

The correlations between clock results and those of other screening instruments are only moderate, and the sensitivity and specificity results range from modest to comparable levels with other screening instruments. Clock drawing, like other tests, appears to be affected by educational level, although the extent varies according to the scoring system used (10, p251). Intelligence may compensate for spatial deficits in the clock-drawing task, for with planning the person may first insert the 3, 6, 9, and 12 and then fill the other numbers around these (3).

The clock test is attractive; Salvador Dali's famous 1931 painting of distorted clocks was entitled *The Persistence of Memory* and gave a surrealist representation of distorted time, memory, and perception that may depict more than an artist's view of the world. The challenge, however, lies in moving from clock drawing as a simple bedside assessment distinguishing normal from abnormal to developing a numerical rating method. Grossly abnormal clock drawings readily identify dementia, but it is difficult to quantify moderate impairment in clock drawing. Different approaches give differing results; reviews of scoring issues are contained in the report by Watson et al. (1) and Mendez et al. (12). Ainslie and Murden concluded that "if clock-drawing is to become a screening test that can be used by primary care physicians in a busy office practice, future study would need to focus on devising a standard set of instructions for the patient and on devising an educationally neutral standard scoring system" (10, p252). Although quantitative scores on the clock test may fail to distinguish between different diagnoses, qualitative review of the clock drawing errors may succeed. Rouleau et al., for example, found that their qualitative analysis of clocks distinguished between Alzheimer's and Huntington's disease patients when their scoring procedure did not (5).

Clock drawing offers an adjunct to other, verbal tests of memory and orientation; it is unlikely to suffice as a screen for dementia. Luckily most people whom we assess for cognitive impairments are still familiar with analogue clocks; as our children raised with digital watches grow old, the clock test may have to be replaced by something more appropriate to the times, such as a test in programming a VCR or surfing the internet.

REFERENCES

(1) Watson YI, Arfken CL, Birge SJ. Clock completion: an objective screening test for dementia. J Am Geriatr Soc 1993; 41:1235–1240.

(2) Sunderland T, Hill JL, Mellow AM, et al. Clock drawing in Alzheimer's disease: a novel measure of dementia severity. J Am Geriatr Soc 1989;37:725–729.

(3) Ishiai S, Sugishita M, Ichikawa T, et al. Clock-drawing test and unilateral spatial neglect. Neurology 1993;43:106–110.

(4) Tuokko H, Hadjistavropoulos T, Miller JA, et al. The clock test: a sensitive measure to differentiate normal elderly from those with Alzheimer disease. J Am Geriatr Soc 1992;40:579–584.

(5) Rouleau I, Salmon DP, Butters N, et al. Quantitative and qualitative analyses of clock drawings in Alzheimer's and Huntington's disease. Brain Cognition 1992; 18:70–87.

(6) Wolf-Klein GP, Silverstone FA, Levy AP, et al. Screening for Alzheimer's disease by clock drawing. J Am Geriatr Soc 1989; 37:730–734.

(7) Shulman K, Shedletsky R, Silver IL. The challenge of time: clock drawing and cognitive functioning in the elderly. Int J Geriatr Psychiatry 1986;1:135–140.

(8) Ganguli M, Ratcliff G, Huff FJ, et al. Effects of age, gender, and education on cognitive tests in a rural elderly community sample: norms from the Monongahela Valley Independent Elders Survey. Neuroepidemiology 1991;10:42–52.

(9) Tuokko H, Hadjistavropoulos T, Miller JA, et al. The clock test: administration and scoring manual. Toronto: Multi-Health Systems Inc, 1995.

(10) Ainslie NK, Murden RA. Effect of education on the clock-drawing dementia screen in non-demented elderly persons. J Am Geriatr Soc 1993;41:249–252.

(11) Huntzinger JA, Rosse RB, Schwartz BL, et al. Clock drawing in the screening assessment of cognitive impairment in an ambulatory care setting: a preliminary report. Gen Hosp Psychiatry 1992;14:142–144.

(12) Mendez MF, Ala T, Underwood KL. Development of scoring criteria for the clock drawing task in Alzheimer's disease. J Am Geriatr Soc 1992;40:1095–1099.

THE ALZHEIMER'S DISEASE ASSESSMENT SCALE
(Wilma G. Rosen and Richard C. Mohs, 1983)

Purpose

The Alzheimer's Disease Assessment Scale (ADAS) is a brief screening test that evaluates the severity of cognitive, affective, and behavioral deficits in patients with Alzheimer's disease (AD) and gives an index of the overall severity of dementia.

Conceptual Basis

Rosen and Mohs classified the major clinical characteristics of Alzheimer's disease into cognitive and noncognitive dysfunctions. The former include memory, language, and praxis, while the latter include mood state and behavioral changes (1, p1357).

Description

The ADAS assesses the clinical symptoms most frequently reported in patients with neuropathologically confirmed AD (2, Table 1). The items were drawn from existing scales or written by the authors. Initial testing shortened the ADAS from 40 to 21 items by selecting those with the highest inter-rater and test–retest reliabilities. Nine items assess cognitive performance via tests done by the patient; there are two memory tasks, and ten items cover noncognitive functioning obtained from observational ratings of behavior during testing or from an interview with an informant. The complete scale is too long to reproduce here, so we present a summary of the scale content in Exhibit 7.3. The scale and scoring procedures are shown in the Appendices to the article by Rosen et al. (1, pp1361–1364). They did not present the words used in the word recall and word recognition tasks (items 10 and 11) but they were listed by Zec et al., who also provided further information on administration (3, pp168–169).

Exhibit 7.3 Alzheimer's Disease Assessment Scale: Summary of Items

Item	Scale range
Cognitive Behavior	
1. Spoken language ability	(0–5)
2. Comprehension of spoken language	(0–5)
3. Recall of test instructions	(0–5)
4. Word-finding difficulty	(0–5)
5. Following commands	(0–5)
6. Naming objects and fingers	(0–5)
7. Constructions—copying forms	(0–5)
8. Ideational praxis	(0–5)
9. Orientation to time, place, and person	(0–8)
10. Word recall memory test	(0–10)
11. Word recognition memory test	(0–12)
Noncognitive behavior	
12. Tearful appearance	(0–5)
13. Appears or reports depressed mood	(0–5)
14. Concentration, distractibility	(0–5)
15. Lack of cooperation in testing	(0–5)
16. Delusions	(0–5)
17. Hallucinations	(0–5)
18. Pacing	(0–5)
19. Increased motor activity	(0–5)
20. Tremors	(0–5)
21. Increased or decreased appetite	(0–5)

Adapted from Rosen WG, Mohs RC, Davis KL. A new rating scale for Alzheimer's disease. Am J Psychiatry 1984:141:1361–1362, Appendix 2.

The ADAS is a rating scale in which the general content of each item (but not the precise wording) is specified; it is administered by a neuropsychologist or psychometrician who rates each item on a severity scale using the guidelines. For each severity scale, 0 signifies no impairment on a task or the absence of a particular behavior. A rating of 5 reflects severe impairment or high frequency of a behavior (1, p1362). Scores are generally calculated for the cognitive section (range 0 to 70) and for the noncognitive section (range 0 to 50); these may be combined to give a total score ranging from 0 to 120. Scores on the two memory items (range 0 to 22) are occasionally presented separately.

Reliability

Inter-rater reliability of the original, 40-item version was high: intraclass correlations were 0.99 for patients with dementia and 0.89 for normal elderly respondents (1, Table 1). One-month test–retest reliability was $\rho = 0.97$ for the Alzheimer patients, and 0.52 for the normal respondents, among whom there was a very narrow spread of scores (2, p42).

For the 21-item version, one-month test–retest reliability was 0.92 for the cognitive score (omitting the memory items), 0.59 for the noncognitive score, and 0.84 for the overall score. Inter-rater reliability was 0.99 for the cognitive and total scores and 0.95 for the noncognitive score (4, p297).

Validity

Rosen et al. assessed the criterion validity of the ADAS using a group of 15 Alzheimer patients and matched controls. The Sandoz Clinical Assessment—Geriatric score correlated 0.52 with the ADAS total score; the correlation with the nine-item cognitive scale was 0.67, and the correlation with the noncognitive scale was 0.25 (1, p1359). Equivalent correlations for the Blessed Memory-Information Test were higher, at −0.67 for the total score, and −0.78 and −0.42, respectively, for cognitive and noncognitive (1, p1359). In a study of 49 Alzheimer patients the ADAS total score correlated $\rho = 0.77$ with the Brief Cognitive Rating Scale and -0.71 with the Mini-Mental State Exam. The equivalent correlations for the cognitive section were 0.80 and -0.81 (5, Table 2). The ADAS total score correlated -0.63 with the concentration of acetylcholine in cerebrospinal fluid (used as a marker of cholinergic cell loss in Alzheimer's disease) (2, p43).

Compared with normal controls, Alzheimer patients were significantly more impaired on all of the cognitive items and the memory tasks, but on only three of the noncognitive items (1, Table 2). Comparing baseline scores with results one year later, total error scores increased significantly for the AD group but not for controls (1, Table 3). These analyses were replicated in another sample (4, Table 30–2). Eight Alzheimer patients were retested at 18 months and demonstrated continued decline (4, p299). Zec et al. showed that each of the cognitive items differentiated among Alzheimer patients of different levels of severity (3, pp170–172); not all of the noncognitive items, however, reflected level of dementia (3, Figure 2).

A factor analysis identified three factors: mental status, verbal fluency, and praxis; there was also an important common factor. The three factors had test–retest reliabilities of 0.83, 0.78, and 0.87; the common factor had a reliability of 0.90 (6). The cognitive and noncognitive scales correlated 0.59 in one study (4, p297) but only 0.20 in another (5, Table 2). Zec et al. reported no significant association between ADAS scores and educational level for a sample of cognitively normal subjects (3, p173).

Commentary

The ADAS is broad in scope and the early results suggest that it is valid as an indicator of severity of Alzheimer's disease. It has been used as an outcome measure in various drug trials and in longitudinal studies (3, 7). In clinical trials the cognitive subscale is commonly used alone.

There are some concerns over the ADAS. The original validation samples were small and did not show whether the scale discriminates between subtypes of dementia. Zec et al. raised a number of concerns. They found the naming and constructional praxis items to be less sensitive to mild dementia than the equivalent measures in other tests; this may limit the sensitivity of the ADAS to improvement (3, p177). They also noted that the cube drawing in item 7 produced false positive ratings from the control group, and they suggested various improvements to the test (3, pp178–180). Because the noncognitive items do not correlate either with the cognitive score on the ADAS or with other cognitive tests, the use of the overall summary score is not recommended (5, p103).

The ADAS nonetheless overcomes some of the shortcomings of earlier mental status tests and should be considered for use as a measure of severity and as a general screening device.

REFERENCES

(1) Rosen WG, Mohs RC, Davis KL. A new rating scale for Alzheimer's disease. Am J Psychiatry 1984;141:1356–1364.

(2) Mohs RC, Rosen WG, Greenwald BS, et al. Neuropathologically validated scales for Alzheimer's disease. In: Crook T, Ferris S, Bartus R, eds. Assessment in geriatric psychopharmacology. New Canaan, Connecticut: Mark Powley, 1983:37–45.

(3) Zec RF, Landreth ES, Vicari SK, et al, Alzheimer Disease Assessment Scale: a subtest analysis. Alzheimer Dis Assoc Disord 1992;6:164–181.

(4) Rosen WG, Mohs RC, Davis KL. Longitudinal changes: cognitive, behavioral, and affective patterns in Alzheimer's disease. In: Poon LW, Crook T, Davis KL, et al., eds. Handbook for clinical memory assessment of older adults. Washington, DC: American Psychological Association, 1986:294–301.

(5) Ihl R, Frölich L, Dierks T, et al. Differential validity of psychometric tests in dementia of the Alzheimer type. Psychiatry Res 1992;44:93–106.

(6) Kim YS, Nibbelink DW, Overall JE. Factor structure and reliability of the Alzheimer's Disease Assessment Scale in a multicenter

trial with linopirdine. J Geriatr Psychiatry Neurol 1994;7:74–83.

(7) Kluger A, Ferris SH. Scales for the assessment of Alzheimer's disease. Psychiatr Clin North Am 1991;14:309–326.

THE INFORMATION-MEMORY-CONCENTRATION TEST
(G. Blessed, 1968)

Purpose

The Information-Memory-Concentration Test (IMC) provides a quantitative estimate of the degree of intellectual and personality deterioration in senile dementia (1). It can be used in clinical practice and the community.

Conceptual Basis

A brief historical introduction may help clarify the relationship among several tests developed by Blessed, each of which has several different names.

As early as 1953 Roth and Hopkins published a test of orientation and information which they showed was capable of discriminating between organic mental illness (including the dementias) and functional illness such as affective disorders and schizophrenia (2). This was then expanded by Blessed, Tomlinson, and Roth to form a broad-ranging patient assessment, covering changes in ADL and performance on a range of cognitive and behavioral assessments suitable for people with dementia (1). The complete assessment, or "Blessed Test," comprises four scales: *(i)* A set of behavioral ratings that form the Dementia Scale, which we review next. This has several aliases, including the Blessed-Roth Dementia Scale, the Newcastle Dementia Scale (Blessed was working in Newcastle-upon-Tyne), and the Blessed Dementia Rating Scale (3). *(ii)* The "Information" Scale, which measures orientation to time and place. *(iii)* The Memory Scale. *(iv)* And last, the Concentration Scale (1). Scores on the last three are often combined to form the Blessed Information-Memory-Concentration Test (IMC), which we re-

view here; sometimes only two of the three are used, as in the Information-Concentration Test. The IMC is often referred to simply as The Blessed Test; it is occasionally named the Newcastle Memory, Information, and Concentration Test. Finally, as the Information subtest covers awareness of time and place, it is sometimes called the Orientation Test, so the overall scale can be called the Orientation-Memory-Concentration Test (OMC). We have followed Blessed's original phrase in this review, and refer to the IMC. This also helps to distinguish it from Katzman's modification, which is known as the OMC (see Alternative Forms, below).

Blessed developed the scales in the context of clinicopathological investigations of the links among cerebral pathology (notably the formation of plaques), intellectual deterioration, and the clinical syndrome of senile dementia. The scales were designed to quantify the degree of intellectual and personality deterioration.

Description

The IMC uses simple tests of orientation, remote and recent memory, and concentration to identify dementia and to estimate its severity (Exhibit 7.4). It is applied in a clinical interview with the patient, but personal memory information must be obtained from a collateral source to check the accuracy of the patient's report. Administration takes about ten minutes.

In this scale, a positive score is given to each item answered correctly, and overall scores range from 0 (complete failure) to 37 (full marks on the battery) (1, p799). Subsequent to Blessed's original work, many authors now count errors, thus reversing the direction of scoring. Using this approach, Katzman et al. took scores of 0 to 8 errors as indicating normality or minimal impairment; 9 to 19 errors as moderate impairment; and 20 or more errors as indicating severe impairment (4, p735; 5, p131). Fuld found that people making between 0 and 10 errors usually had good memory storage and retention, but might

Exhibit 7.4 The Information-Memory-Concentration Test

Note: Scores for correct responses shown; incorrect responses score 0.

Information Test

Name	1
Age	1
Time (hour)	1
Time of day	1
Day of week	1
Date	1
Month	1
Season	1
Year	1
Place—Name	1
Street	1
Town	1
Type of place (e.g., home, hospital, etc.)	1
Recognition of persons (cleaner, doctor, nurse, patient, relative; any two available)	2

Memory Test

1. Personal

Date of birth	1
Place of birth	1
School attended	1
Occupation	1
Name of sibs or Name of wife	1
Name of any town where patient had worked	1
Name of employers	1

2. Non-personal

Date of World War I[1]	1
Date of World War II[1]	1
Monarch[2]	1
Prime Minister[3]	1

3. Name and address (5-minute recall)

Mr. John Brown, 42 West Street, Gateshead	5

Concentration Test

Months of year backwards	2	1	0
Counting 1–20	2	1	0
Counting 20–1	2	1	0

[1] ½ point for approximation within 3 years

[2] President in U.S. version

[3] Vice President in U.S. version

Reproduced from Blessed G, Tomlinson BE, Roth M. The association between quantitative measures of dementia and of senile change in the cerebral grey matter of elderly subjects. Br J Psychiatry 1968;144:809. With permission.

have some difficulty with retrieval that could represent "benign senescent forgetfulness"; 17 or more errors may represent "malignant memory disorder."

Reliability

Two- to four-week test–retest reliability for 36 nursing-home residents was 0.88, and alpha was 0.93 (6, Table 1). Two-week retest reliability for 17 patients was $\rho = 0.96$ (7, p189) and 0.82 (8, Table 4). Thal et al. compared the reliabilities of the IMC and Mini-Mental State Exam at intervals ranging from one to six weeks. Results for the IMC ranged from 0.89 to 0.82, slightly higher than the equivalent figures for the MMSE (9, Table 2).

Validity

The IMC was originally developed for use in studies linking clinical symptoms of dementia with pathological findings. Blessed obtained a correlation of −0.59 with the count of senile plaques found in the brain cortex at autopsy (1, p803). A subsequent study by Blessed's group also showed associations with levels of choline acetyl transferase in the cerebral cortex at autopsy (10). Katzman et al. reported a correlation of 0.60 with brain plaque counts (4, p737).

The IMC correlated 0.81 with the Clinical Dementia Rating (5, Table 3). It correlated 0.94 with the Mental Status Questionnaire (4, p735). Correlations with the Mini-Mental State Examination include −0.83, −0.80, −0.73, 0.71 (a version of the IMC that used the reverse scoring) (8, Table 4), and −0.88 (11, Table 2). The IMC scores correlated 0.82 with scores on the Dementia Rating Scale (11, Table 2).

The sensitivity of the IMC to change was reported by Stern et al., who show tables estimating the required sample size for studies using the instrument (12, Table 4).

Alternative Forms

For use in the United States, "monarch" is replaced by "president," and "prime minister" by "vice president," presumably without claim of political equivalence. "Gateshead" is normally replaced with "Chicago," which someone presumably considered of equivalent salience.

There are various abbreviations of the IMC. Three items (recognition of persons, name of employers, and town where patient worked) have sometimes been deleted, yielding an overall score ranging from 0 to 33 rather than 37 (7,12). Katzman et al. developed a six-item version called the Orientation-Memory-Concentration test or the Short Blessed Test (SBT). The items are:

What year is it now?
What month is it now?
Repeat this phrase after me: John Brown, 42 Market Street, Chicago.
About what time is it?
Count backwards 20 to 1.
Say the months in reverse order.
Repeat the memory phrase. (4, p739)

The SBT correlated 0.94 with the complete test (4, p735) and 0.79 with the Clinical Dementia Rating (5, Table 3). Correlations with the Mini-Mental State Examination include 0.71 and −0.73 (due to reversed scoring in different versions of the OMC) (8, Table 4). Sensitivity was 88% at a specificity of 94% (13, Table 3).

A Chinese version of the IMC has been described (14).

Commentary

The Blessed IMC scales are among the oldest and most frequently used scales in the assessment of the severity of dementia, and they are frequently used as screening tests for dementia. They provide a good overall estimate of intellectual functioning that correlates well with clinical ratings of the severity of dementia. A major reason for the popularity of the IMC lies in its predictive validity as measured against subsequent autopsy findings; it can identify cognitive and behavioral symptoms typical of patients with Alzheimer's disease confirmed on autopsy. The content of the scale is simple and focuses on the practical tasks of daily life. The IMC was recommended by the NINCDS-ADRDA Work Group

(15, Table 1) and has been used in several large studies of dementia. Whereas other measurements we review have undergone many changes in content, the Blessed scales have the advantage that their original content has been retained (despite the various changes in title).

The validity findings for the six-item abbreviation suggest that it may serve as a good screening instrument that is briefer to administer and score; all items are applicable to patients whether in the home or in an institution, and it can be applied to patients with physical handicaps (e.g., blindness) (8, p926).

REFERENCES

(1) Blessed G, Tomlinson BE, Roth M. The association between quantitative measures of dementia and of senile change in the cerebral grey matter of elderly subjects. Br J Psychiatry 1968;114:797–811.

(2) Roth M, Hopkins B. Psychological test performance of patients over 60: senile psychosis and affective disorders. J Ment Sci 1953;101:281–301.

(3) Blessed G, Tomlinson BE, Roth M. Blessed-Roth Dementia Scale (DS). Psychopharmacol Bull 1988;24:705–708.

(4) Katzman R, Brown T, Fuld P, et al. Validation of a Short Orientation-Memory-Concentration Test of cognitive impairment. Am J Psychiatry 1983;140:734–739.

(5) Davis PB, Morris JC, Grant E. Brief screening tests versus clinical staging in senile dementia of the Alzheimer type. J Am Geriatr Soc 1990;38:129–135.

(6) Lesher EL, Whelihan WM. Reliability of mental status instruments administered to nursing home residents. J Consult Clin Psychol 1986;54:726–727.

(7) Fuld PA. Psychological testing in the differential diagnosis of the dementias. In: Katzman R, Terry RD, Bick KL, eds. Alzheimer's disease: senile dementia and related disorders. New York: Raven Press, 1978:185–192.

(8) Fillenbaum GG, Heyman A, Wilkinson WE, et al. Comparison of two screening tests in Alzheimer's disease: the correlation and reliability of the Mini-Mental State Examination and the modified Blessed Test. Arch Neurol 1987;44:924–927.

(9) Thal LJ, Grundman M, Golden R. Alzheimer's disease: a correlational analysis

of the Blessed Information-Memory-Concentration Test and the Mini-Mental State Exam. Neurology 1986;36:262–264.

(10) Perry EK, Tomlinson BE, Blessed G, et al. Correlation of cholinergic abnormalities with senile plaques and mental test scores in senile dementia. Br Med J 1978; 2:1457–1459.

(11) Salmon DP, Thal LJ, Butters N, et al. Longitudinal evaluation of dementia of the Alzheimer type: a comparison of 3 standardized mental status examinations. Neurology 1990;40:1225–1230.

(12) Stern RG, Mohs RC, Bierer LM, et al. Deterioration on the Blessed Test in Alzheimer's disease: longitudinal data and their implications for clinical trials and identification of subtypes. Psychiatry Res 1992; 42:101–110.

(13) Davous P, Lamour Y, Debrand E, et al. A comparative evaluation of the short Orientation Memory Concentration Test of cognitive impairment. J Neurol Neurosurg Psychiatry 1987;50:1312–1317.

(14) Jin H, Zhang MY, Qu OY, et al. Cross-cultural studies of dementia: use of a Chinese version of the Blessed-Roth Information-Memory-Concentration test in a Shanghai dementia survey. Psychol Aging 1989;4:471–479.

(15) McKhann G, Drachman D, Folstein M, et al. Clinical diagnosis of Alzheimer's disease: report of the NINCDS-ADRDA Work Group under the auspices of Department of Health and Human Services Task Force on Alzheimer's disease. Neurology 1984; 34:939–944.

THE DEMENTIA SCALE
(G. Blessed, 1968)

Purpose

Blessed's Dementia Scale (BLS-D) was developed as a research instrument to quantify the cognitive and behavioral symptoms typically seen in patients with dementia. It was originally used in studies linking manifestations of dementia with neuropathological findings in the brain.

Conceptual Basis

The Dementia Scale forms one of four tests developed by Blessed; the others are the Information Scale, the Memory Scale, and the Concentration Scale (1). These three

are often combined to form the Blessed Information-Memory-Concentration Test (IMC), which we review separately. The Dementia Scale is also known as the Blessed-Roth Dementia Scale, the Newcastle Dementia Scale, or the Blessed Dementia Rating Scale (2). We prefer the name "Dementia Scale," which distinguishes it from the Dementia Rating Scale developed by Mattis.

Blessed's scales were developed in the context of investigations of the links among cerebral pathology (notably the formation of plaques), intellectual deterioration, normal senescence, and the clinical syndrome of senile dementia. The scales were designed to quantify the extent of intellectual and personality deterioration.

Description

The BLS-D is a clinical rating scale with 22 items that measure changes in performance of everyday activities (eight items), self-care habits (three items), and changes in personality, interests and drives (11 items). Ratings are based on information from relatives or friends and concern behavior over the preceding six months (2).

Scores for each item are shown in Exhibit 7.5: total incompetence in an activity is rated 1 and partial, variable or intermittent incapacity is awarded a half-point. Overall scores range from 0 (normal) to 28 (extreme incapacity); a cognitive subscale omits questions 12–22 on personality, interests, and drives and has a range from 0 (normal) to 17 (severely demented).

Reliability

The inter-rater reliability for two raters was $r = 0.59$ (intraclass correlation = 0.30) (3, p329).

Validity

Dementia Scale scores correlated 0.77 with the count of plaques in the brains of 60 elderly patients (1, p802). The correlation with survival was -0.40 (1, p805). The Dementia Scale correlated 0.80 with the Clinical Dementia Rating; the equivalent

Exhibit 7.5   The Dementia Scale (Blessed)

Change in Performance of Everyday Activities

1. Inability to perform household tasks	1 ½ 0	
2. Inability to cope with small sums of money	1 ½ 0	
3. Inability to remember short list of items, e.g., in shopping	1 ½ 0	
4. Inability to find way about indoors	1 ½ 0	
5. Inability to find way about familiar streets	1 ½ 0	
6. Inability to interpret surroundings (e.g. to recognize whether in hospital, or at home, to discriminate between patients, doctors and nurses, relatives and hospital staff, etc.)	1 ½ 0	
7. Inability to recall recent events (e.g. recent outings, visits of relatives or friends to hospital, etc.)	1 ½ 0	
8. Tendency to dwell in the past	1 ½ 0	

Changes in Habits

9. Eating:

Cleanly with proper utensils	0
Messily with spoon only	2
Simple solids, e.g. biscuits	2
Has to be fed	3

10. Dressing:

Unaided	0
Occasionally misplaced buttons, etc.	1
Wrong sequence, commonly forgetting items	2
Unable to dress	3

11. Complete sphincter control

Complete sphincter control	0
Occasional wet beds	1
Frequent wet beds	2
Doubly incontinent	3

Changes in Personality, Interests, Drive

No change	0
12. Increased rigidity	1
13. Increased egocentricity	1
14. Impairment of regard for feelings of others	1
15. Coarsening of affect	1
16. Impairment of emotional control, e.g. increased petulance and irritability	1
17. Hilarity in inappropriate situations	1
18. Diminished emotional responsiveness	1
19. Sexual misdemeanour (appearing *de novo* in old age)	1
Interests retained	0
20. Hobbies relinquished	1
21. Diminished initiative or growing apathy	1
22. Purposeless hyperactivity	1

Reproduced from Blessed G, Tomlinson BE, Roth M. The association between quantitative measures of dementia and of senile change in the cerebral grey matter of elderly subjects. Br J Psychiatry 1968;144:808–809. With permission.

correlation for the cognitive subscale was 0.84 (4, Table 3). Scores differed significantly between patients with Alzheimer's disease and other forms of senile dementia and between different severities of Alzheimer's disease defined pathologically (5, Tables 3,4).

The Dementia Scale covers a wide range of topics, and a factor analysis identified four factors, covering cognitive problems, personality change, apathy or withdrawal, and performance in basic self-care (6, Table 2). Stern et al. showed that the pattern of decline over time in patients with dementia varied for the four factor scores in a plausible fashion. For example, deficits on the cognitive factor began early in the disease and continued to deteriorate, while deficits on the self-care factor only appeared after four or five years (6, p11).

Blessed noted that the scores for deterioration of personality were neither sensitive nor specific for dementia (7, p24).

Commentary

Assessing functional changes accompanying dementia is important in predicting the burden experienced by caregivers. Other scales that cover parts of this theme include the Dementia Behavior Disturbance scale (8). Blessed's Dementia Scale offers a broad-ranging method for achieving this, but care must be taken with selecting an appropriate scoring method. The overall score probably masks more subtle contrasts within dimensions of the scale, and the factor scores proposed by Stern et al. appear to offer an improvement on the overall score. Likewise, the emotional score cannot be used as an indicator of the severity of dementia, as the emotional changes it records do not necessarily accompany dementia, and more severely impaired patients may demonstrate fewer emotional changes (9, p311). The reliability figures are low, and Cole commented that vague scale items (e.g., impairment of emotional control) and items that call for complex judgment may have accounted for these low reliability figures (3, pp329–330). The

Dementia Scale may have clinical utility in estimating the level of care required; we recommend that users carefully balance the appropriateness of the scale for their purposes against the rather weak evidence for its reliability and validity. The BLS-D has been incorporated into the CAMDEX (reviewed separately).

REFERENCES

(1) Blessed G, Tomlinson BE, Roth M. The association between quantitative measures of dementia and of senile change in the cerebral grey matter of elderly subjects. Br J Psychiatry 1968;114:797–811.
(2) Blessed G, Tomlinson BE, Roth M. Blessed-Roth Dementia Scale (DS). Psychopharmacol Bull 1988;24:705–708.
(3) Cole MG. Interrater reliability of the Blessed Dementia Scale. Can J Psychiatry 1990;35:328–330.
(4) Davis PB, Morris JC, Grant E. Brief screening tests versus clinical staging in senile dementia of the Alzheimer type. J Am Geriatr Soc 1990;38:129–135.
(5) Blessed G. Clinical features and neuropathological correlations of Alzheimer type disease. In: Kay DWK, Burrows GD, eds. Handbook of studies on psychiatry and old age. Amsterdam: Elsevier, 1984:133–143.
(6) Stern Y, Hesdorffer D, Sano M, et al. Measurement and prediction of functional capacity in Alzheimer's disease. Neurology 1990;40:8–14.
(7) Blessed G. A clinical diagnosis of senile dementia of Alzheimer type in its early and established forms. In: Bès A, ed. Senile dementias: early detection. London: John Libbey Eurotext, 1986:22–32.
(8) Baumgarten M, Becker R, Gauthier S. Validity and reliability of the Dementia Behavior Disturbance scale. J Am Geriatr Soc 1990;38:221–226.
(9) Kluger A, Ferris SH. Scales for the assessment of Alzheimer's disease. Psychiatr Clin North Am 1991;14:309–326.

THE MENTAL STATUS QUESTIONNAIRE
(Robert L. Kahn, 1960)

Purpose

The Mental Status Questionnaire (MSQ) provides a brief, objective, and quantitative measurement of cognitive functioning of elderly people (1). It was intended for use with patient or community samples but results show it to be less appropriate in the community.

Conceptual Basis

No information is available.

Description

Ten questions cover orientation in time and place, remote memory, and general knowledge (see Exhibit 7.6). The ten items were selected as the most discriminating of 31 questions taken from existing mental status examinations and from clinical experience. The MSQ is generally administered by an interviewer and requires a few minutes. Some latitude is commonly allowed in the precision of responses, although this is rarely specified in reports on the scale. Typically, a latitude of three days in the date is permitted.

The number of errors is scored; omissions are counted as errors; a score of 0 is ideal. Milne et al. suggested a cutting point of 3 or more errors for identifying cases of chronic brain syndrome (2, Table 2). Zarit et al. grouped scores as 0 errors being ideal, 1 or 2 indicating a nonsignificant problem; 3 to 5 indicating mild to moderate impairment, and 6 to 10 indicating moderate to severe impairment (3, p60). Others have

Exhibit 7.6 The Mental Status Questionnaire

1. What is the name of this place?
2. Where is it located (address)?
3. What is today's date?
4. What is the month now?
5. What is the year?
6. How old are you?
7. When were you born (month)?
8. When were you born (year)?
9. Who is the president of the United States?
10. Who was the president before him?

Adapted from Kahn RL, Goldfarb AI, Pollack M, Peck A. Brief objective measures for the determination of mental status in the aged. Am J Psychiatry 1960;117:326.

altered the cutting point to allow one extra error for poorly educated people and for people from certain ethnic groups (4).

Reliability

Lesher and Whelihan obtained test–retest reliability of 0.87 at two to four weeks; split-half reliability was 0.82, and alpha was 0.81 (5, Table 1). Wilson and Brass reported an unpublished study in which, over four administrations of the MSQ at three-week intervals, scores changed one point or less in 75% of repeat administrations (6, p99).

Validity

Kahn et al. compared the MSQ to the Face-Hand Test and to psychiatric evaluations of 1,077 institutionalized patients. The results showed a strong association between MSQ scores and diagnoses of chronic brain syndrome (CBS). For example, of those scoring 10 MSQ errors, 95% had moderate or severe CBS; 75% were rated as moderate or severe CBS with psychosis. Conversely, of those scoring 0 errors, 94% were rated as having mild or no management problems (1, pp327–328).

In a community survey of 487 elderly people, the MSQ was 64% sensitive and 99% specific in detecting chronic brain syndrome, at a cutting point of 3 (2, Table 3). Using a sample of 83 community residents, Fillenbaum assessed the capability of the MSQ to discriminate between those subjects with psychiatric diagnoses of organic brain syndrome and normal subjects. At a cutting point of 3/4 errors, sensitivity of the MSQ was 45% and specificity was 98%. At a cutting point of 2/3 errors, the sensitivity was 55% and specificity was 96% (7, Table 2). In a multiple regression analysis, the MSQ items explained 46% of the variance in the diagnosis (7, Table 4).

Zarit et al. showed highly significant associations, adjusting for education, with a range of standard memory tests (3, Table 2). De Leon et al. compared MSQ scores to computerized tomography scan results for 43 outpatients with suspected senile dementia of the Alzheimer type. The MSQ correlated 0.46 with a CT scan rating of ventricular dilatation and 0.47 with cortical sulcal prominence; the equivalent correlations for the Global Deterioration Scale were higher, at 0.62 and 0.53 (8, p860). In a sample of psychogeriatric patients, the MSQ scores correlated 0.87 with a psychiatrist's rating of organicity (9, Table 1). Using a sample of 230 patients, Wilson and Brass obtained a correlation of 0.82 between the MSQ and a four-point clinical rating of severity of dementia (6, p95). They found that the questions on awareness of personal details and location (town, place, age, month born, and year born) served to differentiate moderate from severe dementia while the other five questions separated mild from moderate (6, p98). Fillenbaum reported correlations of 0.88 and 0.97 between the MSQ and the Short Portable MSQ in two studies (7, p381). A correlation of 0.60 was reported between the MSQ and the Dementia Rating Scale (10, p344). The MSQ correlated 0.92 with the Isaacs and Walkey Mental Impairment Measure (2, Table 1). MSQ scores correlated 0.80 with the Mini-Mental State Examination, 0.45 with the Storandt battery, and 0.57 with Blessed's Orientation-Memory-Concentration test (11, Table 4).

Alternative Forms

Readers should be cautioned that there are many minor variants of the MSQ and different cutting points are often used (see, for example, reference 4). The orientation scale, for example, is intended for patients in nursing homes and replaces items difficult for people in restricted environments (e.g., name of the president) with people more familiar (e.g., name of head nurse) (10, p343). When used in England or Canada, questions 9 and 10 are altered to "prime minister."

Whelihan et al. developed the Extended Mental Status Questionnaire with an additional 14 items (12). These cover recall of family names, orientation to immediate environment, recall of important cultural events and arithmetical operations. The Extended MSQ (EMSQ) was better at classifying dementia than was the Philadelphia Geriatric Center Delayed Memory Test, correctly classifying all 38 of the patients without dementia and 18 out of 20 moderately or severely demented cases. It did, however, falsely classify all 12 mildly demented patients as nondemented (12, p575). Test–retest reliability of the EMSQ was 0.88, and alpha was 0.85 (5, Table 1).

Pfeiffer developed the Short Portable MSQ (SPMSQ) in 1975; like the MSQ it has ten items, five of which are identical to those in the MSQ. The scoring procedures are, however, different. The SPMSQ is described in the following review.

Commentary

The MSQ is one of the first generation of brief rating scales for dementia. It has been widely used and was influential in the design of other scales, such as the SPMSQ dementia scale included in the Comprehensive Assessment and Referral Evaluation (CARE) reviewed in Chapter 9 (13). The MSQ is chiefly suited to institutional populations and appears to work less well in office or outpatient assessments: compared with other questionnaires, its sensitivity in community screening for dementia is low. Zarit showed only a modest difference in performance by educational level for most of the MSQ items with the exception of spelling, for which the differences were marked (3, Figure 1). Educational level does not appear to obscure the ability of the MSQ to identify impairment.

Among the shortcomings of the MSQ are its lack of clear justification for item content. It has been criticized for its omission of recent memory, which forms a critical indicator of the early dementing process (12). It offers a brief assessment that is easy to score, suited to assessing severe levels of cognitive impairment. The reader should consider the next review, which describes Pfeiffer's modification of the MSQ.

REFERENCES

(1) Kahn RL, Goldfarb AI, Pollack M, et al. Brief objective measures for the determination of mental status in the aged. Am J Psychiatry 1960;117:326–328.

(2) Milne JS, Maule MM, Cormack S, et al. The design and testing of a questionnaire and examination to assess physical and mental health in older people using a staff nurse as the observer. J Chronic Dis 1972;25:385–405.

(3) Zarit SH, Miller NE, Kahn RL. Brain function, intellectual impairment and education in the aged. J Am Geriatr Soc 1978; 26:58–67.

(4) Brink TL, Capri D, De Neeve V, et al. Senile confusion: limitations of assessment by the Face-Hand Test, Mental Status Questionnaire, and staff ratings. J Am Geriatr Soc 1978;16:380–382.

(5) Lesher EL, Whelihan WM. Reliability of mental status instruments administered to nursing home residents. J Consult Clin Psychol 1986;54:726–727.

(6) Wilson LA, Brass W. Brief assessment of the mental state in geriatric domiciliary practice: the usefulness of the Mental Status Questionnaire. Age Ageing 1973;2:92–101.

(7) Fillenbaum GG. Comparison of two brief tests of organic brain impairment, the MSQ and the Short Portable MSQ. J Am Geriatr Soc 1980;28:381–384.

(8) de Leon MJ, Ferris SH, Blau I, et al. Correlations between computerised tomographic changes and behavioral deficits in senile dementia. Lancet 1979;2:859–860.

(9) Cresswell DL, Lanyon RI. Validation of a screening battery for psychogeriatric assessment. J Gerontol 1981;36:435–440.

(10) Eastwood MR, Lautenschlaeger E, Corbin S. A comparison of clinical methods for assessing dementia. J Am Geriatr Soc 1983;31:342–347.

(11) Fillenbaum G, Heyman A, Williams K, et al. Sensitivity and specificity of standardized screens of cognitive impairment and dementia among elderly black and white community residents. J Clin Epidemiol 1990;43:651–660.

(12) Whelihan WM, Lesher EL, Kleban MH, et al. Mental status and memory assessment as predictors of dementia. J Gerontol 1984;39:572–576.

(13) Gurland B, Golden R, Challop J. Unidimensional and multidimensional approaches to the differentiation of depression and dementia in the elderly. In: Corkin S, Crowdon JH, Davis KL, Usdin E, eds. Alzheimer's disease: a report of progress. New York: Raven Press, 1982:119–125.

THE SHORT PORTABLE MENTAL STATUS QUESTIONNAIRE
(Eric Pfeiffer, 1975)

Purpose

The Short Portable Mental Status Questionnaire (SPMSQ) is intended to offer a rapid screen for cognitive deficit in the community-dwelling elderly (1, p120). It detects organic intellectual impairment and determines its degree (2).

Conceptual Basis

The SPMSQ was modeled on the Mental Status Questionnaire (MSQ), which is not successful in identifying mild to moderate cases and was modified for use in community settings. Accordingly, it was designed "as a somewhat more difficult but still brief test of cognitive functioning [that] could better discriminate among the more competent people living in the open setting" (1, p119). Pfeiffer sought a brief test that covered several aspects of intellectual functioning, that was simple to administer and score, and that was applicable to both community and institutional populations (2, p435).

Description

The ten questions were drawn from the MSQ and other tests and cover short- and long-term memory, orientation to surroundings, knowledge of current events, and ability to perform mathematical tasks (see Exhibit 7.7). Some MSQ questions were combined (e.g., month, day, and year today) and, to make the test more challenging, an answer is accepted as correct only if all parts of the answer are correct (1, p119). Administration instructions are given by Pfeiffer (2, p441). The SPMSQ is administered by a clinician in approximately two minutes.

Exhibit 7.7 Short Portable Mental Status
Questionnaire

*Instructions: Ask questions 1–10 in this list and
record all answers. Ask question 4A only if patient
does not have a telephone. Record total number of
errors based on ten questions.*

1. What is the date today?
    (Month _____ Day _____ Year _____)
2. What day of the week is it?
3. What is the name of this place?
4. What is your telephone number?
4A. What is your street address?
    *(Ask only if patient does not have a
    telephone)*
5. How old are you?
6. When were you born?
7. Who is the President of the U.S. now?
8. Who was President just before him?
9. What was your mother's maiden name?
10. Subtract 3 from 20 and keep subtracting 3
    from each new number, all the way down.

Adapted from Pfeiffer E. A Short Portable Mental Status
Questionnaire for the assessment of organic brain deficit in
elderly patients. J Am Geriatr Soc 1975;23:440.

The number of errors is counted, with
unanswered items treated as errors (3,
p383). As capacity to answer the questions
varies with race and education, the practice
in the United States has been to correct raw
scores to relate results for the respondent to
others of the same race and educational
level. For this, education is classified into
three levels: no more than grade school, no
more than high school, and beyond high
school. Race is divided into two categories:
Black and all others. An error score greater
than that made by about 90% of those in
the same race and educational combination
is considered to represent an impaired state
(3, p382). For White respondents with
some high school education, the following
criteria were established: 0 to 2 errors =
intact functioning, 3 to 4 errors = mild
impairment, 5 to 7 errors = moderate intellectual impairment, and 8 to 10 errors
= severe impairment. Pfeiffer took more
than four errors as indicative of "significant
impairment" (4, p435). One more error is

allowed if the respondent has only a grade
school education, and one less error is allowed for those with education beyond
high school. In each educational group, one
more error is allowed for Blacks (2, p441).
A similar approach, which produces
slightly different results, was given by Fillenbaum, who listed these error scores as
indicative of at least moderate cognitive
impairment (see Table 7.2). In other countries scores may or may not be adjusted for
educational level (5).

Reliability

Four-week test–retest reliabilities were
0.82 and 0.83 in two samples (2, p439); a
four-week test–retest intraclass correlations was 0.81 (6, Table 4). Lesher and
Whelihan examined reliability of the
SPMSQ on 36 nursing home residents
(mean age 85 years). Test–retest reliability
(at two to four weeks) was 0.85, and alpha
was 0.83 (7, Table 1).

Validity

The SPMSQ has been compared to clinical
ratings of dementia in numerous studies.
Pfeiffer compared the SPMSQ to a clinical
diagnosis of organic brain syndrome in institutional and community samples. The
sensitivity differed markedly in the two settings: 68% at a specificity of 96% in the
clinic sample versus 26% (specificity 98%)
in the survey sample (2, Tables 6,7). In a
further community study, with a cut-point
of 2 errors, sensitivity was 55% at a specificity of 96% for identifying cases of organic brain syndrome (3, p383). In the East

Table 7.2 Cutting Points for the Short
Portable Mental Status Questionnaire

	Educational level		
	Grade school	High school	Beyond high school
White	5	4	3
Black	6	5	4

Derived from Fillenbaum GG. Multidimensional functional
assessment of older adults: the Duke Older Americans Resources and Services procedures. Hillsdale, New Jersey: Lawrence Erlbaum Associates, 1988, p120.

Boston community study, sensitivity was 34% and specificity was 94% (8, p173). This compared adversely with the performance of the East Boston Memory Test (sensitivity 48%, specificity 95%). The sensitivity of the SPMSQ was particularly low with people aged 65 to 74 years (16%) and with those with more education (18%) (8, Table IV). In a Finnish study the sensitivity and specificity for detecting moderate to severe dementia in a community sample were 67% and 100%; for a sample of medical inpatients the figures were 86% and 99% (5, Table 5). In a mixed institutional and community sample, Smyer et al. present data from which a sensitivity of 85% and a specificity of 84% can be calculated (9, Table 5); compared to an ADL assessment of functioning, sensitivity was 82% and specificity 83% (9, Table 3). In a mixed clinical sample of 40 neurologic and psychiatric inpatients, the SPMSQ missed a large number of cases of organic brain syndrome, whether defined in terms of clinical diagnosis (sensitivity 27%) or neuropsychological diagnosis (sensitivity 27%) (10, Table 1). The positive predictive value of the SPMSQ for detecting organic brain syndrome among 95 consecutive admissions to a geriatric unit was 88%; the negative predictive value was 78% (11, p713).

Expressed as correlations with clinical ratings, SPMSQ scores correlated 0.63 with a psychiatric diagnosis of chronic brain syndrome (12, Table 3); the correlation was 0.79 with a clinical dementia rating, comparable to the 0.81 obtained for the Blessed Information-Memory-Concentration test (13, Table 3).

Correlations reported between the SPMSQ and MSQ include 0.88 (3, p381), 0.76 (14, Table 4), and 0.84 (12, Table 2). The SPMSQ has been compared to standard tests of cognitive performance; it correlated 0.66 with the Digit Span test, 0.60 with the Bender test, and 0.57 with the Basic Life Skills Assessment (11, p713). Scores correlated 0.69 with results of the MMSE (14, Table 4).

Reference Standards

Pfeiffer applied the SPMSQ to a community sample of 997 people aged 65 and over and reported error rates for each item by educational level and by racial group (2, Tables 3–5).

Commentary

The SPMSQ has been extensively used and has been incorporated, for example, into the OARS assessment (see Chapter 9). It has been tested in a number of studies and shows adequate reliability and validity in clinical samples that include people with more advanced dementia. However, the validity results for community samples are markedly lower, suggesting that the SPMSQ may not successful in correctly classifying people with mild levels of impairment. It may also fail to identify organic disorders in psychiatrically mixed populations. This may, of course, be the price paid by an instrument with only ten items. Dalton et al. argued that the test is "too simple in its task requirements, and, therefore, many patients with diagnosed brain damage were able to perform adequately on the SPMSQ" (10, p514). In their study, the cognitive deficits missed by the SPMSQ included impaired short-term memory, impaired learning, and inability to maintain and alternate between two sequences of thought. It is not clear whether the SPMSQ can distinguish between mild, moderate, and severe dementia because most validation studies combined all levels of severity (15); Pfeiffer's testing did not examine his stated objective of differentiating four levels of cognitive impairment. Somewhat at odds with these claims of low sensitivity to mild impairment, Davis et al. found a ceiling effect in which even at moderate dementia, scores on the SPMSQ approached their maximum (13, p133).

While it does not seem realistic to demand that a brief instrument cover a wide range of areas (Dalton et al. listed 16 or more areas that should be assessed), the omission of a learning task may have been critical in leading to false-negative classifications (10). There may also be practical difficulties in scoring the question on mother's maiden name (difficult to verify), and the question on knowing the address proved difficult for long-term institutional patients (10).

As with many other scales, scores vary by educational level, although this effect was less marked in the Finnish study (5, p414). Unlike other instruments, the developers of the SPMSQ tackled this problem from the outset, although the system of allowing an extra error here or denying one there has an air of improvisation.

The SPMSQ can serve well as a brief, perhaps narrow, instrument for use in assessing relatively severe levels of cognitive impairment. This differs from its original intended use as a community screen, for which other tests seem superior.

REFERENCES

(1) Fillenbaum GG. Multidimensional functional assessment of older adults: the Duke Older Americans Resources and Services procedures. Hillsdale, New Jersey: Lawrence Erlbaum Associates, 1988.

(2) Pfeiffer E. A Short Portable Mental Status Questionnaire for the assessment of organic brain deficit in elderly patients. J Am Geriatr Soc 1975;23:433–441.

(3) Fillenbaum GG. Comparison of two brief tests of organic brain impairment, the MSQ and the Short Portable MSQ. J Am Geriatr Soc 1980;28:381–384.

(4) Pfeiffer E, Johnson TM, Chiofolo RC. Functional assessment of elderly subjects in four service settings. J Am Geriatr Soc 1981;29:433–437.

(5) Erkinjuntti T, Sulkava R, Wikström J, et al. Short Portable Mental Status Questionnaire as a screening test for dementia and delirium among the elderly. J Am Geriatr Soc 1987;35:412–416.

(6) Cairl RE, Pfeiffer E, Keller DM, et al. An evaluation of the reliability and validity of the Functional Assessment Inventory. J Am Geriatr Soc 1983;31:607–612.

(7) Lesher EL, Whelihan WM. Reliability of mental status instruments administered to nursing home residents. J Consult Clin Psychol 1986;54:726–727.

(8) Albert M, Smith LA, Scherr PA, et al. Use of brief cognitive tests to identify individuals in the community with clinically diagnosed Alzheimer's disease. Int J Neurosci 1991;57:167–178.

(9) Smyer MA, Hofland BF, Jonas EA. Validity study of the Short Portable Mental Status Questionnaire for the elderly. J Am Geriatr Soc 1979;27:263–269.

(10) Dalton JE, Pederson SL, Blom BE, et al. Diagnostic errors using the Short Portable Mental Status Questionnaire with a mixed clinical population. J Gerontol 1987; 42:512–514.

(11) Wolber G, Romaniuk M, Eastman E, et al. Validity of the Short Portable Mental Status Questionnaire with elderly psychiatric patients. J Consult Clin Psychol 1984; 52:712–713.

(12) Haglund RMJ, Schuckit MA. A clinical comparison of tests of organicity in elderly patients. J Gerontol 1976;31:654–659.

(13) Davis PB, Morris JC, Grant E. Brief screening tests versus clinical staging in senile dementia of the Alzheimer type. J Am Geriatr Soc 1990;38:129–135.

(14) Fillenbaum G, Heyman A, Williams K, et al. Sensitivity and specificity of standardized screens of cognitive impairment and dementia among elderly black and white community residents. J Clin Epidemiol 1990;43:651–660.

(15) Ritchie K. The screening of cognitive impairment in the elderly: a critical review of current methods. J Clin Epidemiol 1988; 41:635–643.

THE MINI-MENTAL STATE EXAMINATION
(Marshal Folstein, 1975)

Purpose

The Mini-Mental State Examination (MMSE) gives a brief assessment of the person's orientation to time and place, recall ability, short-term memory, and arithmetic ability. It may be used as a screening test for cognitive loss or as a brief bedside cognitive assessment. It cannot be used to diagnose dementia (1).

Conceptual Basis

Evaluating the mental state of elderly psychiatric patients with formal psychological tests has become a routine part of the clinical examination. The tests are often too lengthy for elderly subjects and are based on theories rather than on the types of cognitive impairment that lead to practical difficulties in daily living (1, 2). Folstein designed the MMSE as a clinical aid in the cognitive assessment of elderly patients.

Description

Except for the language and motor skills items, the content of the MMSE was derived from existing instruments (2). The MMSE was termed "mini" because it concentrates only on the cognitive aspects of mental function, and excludes mood and abnormal mental functions that are covered, for example, in Blessed's Dementia Scale. It is administered by clinical or lay personnel after brief training and requires five to ten minutes for completion.

The MMSE includes 11 items, divided into two sections; the first requires verbal responses to orientation, memory, and attention questions. The second section requires reading and writing and covers ability to name, follow verbal and written commands, write a sentence, and copy a polygon (1) (see Exhibit 7.8). All questions are asked in the order listed and can be scored immediately by summing the points assigned to each successfully competed task; the maximum score is 30. Treating questions not answered as errors is probably the best approach (3). The issue of how to handle nonresponses due to illiteracy or blindness has not been well resolved and has been handled either by treating these as errors or by prorating the overall score, deleting such items from the numerator and denominator. The challenge of scoring the overlapping pentagon diagram was addressed in one study by computer digitizing (4).

The cutting point most commonly used to indicate cognitive impairment deserving further investigation is 23/24. Some authors recommend a cutting point of 24/25 to enhance sensitivity for mild dementia (5). The cutting point is commonly modulated according to educational level be-

cause a single cutting point may miss cases among more educated people and generate false positives among those with less education. Murden et al., for example, suggested that 23/24 was optimal for people with ninth-grade or higher education while 17/18 was optimal for those with less education (6, Table 4). Uhlmann and Larson refined this by proposing 20/21 for those with eight or nine years of schooling, 22/23 for those with ten to 12 years of schooling, and 23/24 for those with further education (7). A Finnish study suggested a sloping cutting point across age groups (8).

Reliability

Foreman reported an internal consistency alpha of 0.96 in a sample of 66 elderly hospitalized patients (9, p218). Kay et al. reported an alpha of 0.68 (5, p774).

Test–retest reliability has been examined in many studies; in a review of his original studies, Folstein reported that for samples of psychiatric and neurologic patients, the test–retest reliability "has not fallen below 0.89; inter-rater reliability has not fallen below 0.82" (10, p47). Results from other studies are summarized in Table 7.3, and more are cited in the review by Tombaugh and McIntyre (11, Table 1). With the exception of the study by Uhlmann, reliability declines as the time lapse increases. Thal's study compared the reliabilities of the Blessed IMC test and the MMSE, showing that at all testing intervals the results for the Blessed test (average 0.86) were slightly higher than those for the MMSE (average 0.80) (12, Table 2).

Inter-rater reliability has also been widely studied. Molloy et al. reported inter-rater reliability of 0.69 and 0.78 (13, Table 1). In a sample of 15 neurological inpatients, inter-rater reliability gave a Pearson correlation of 0.95 and a Kendall coefficient of 0.63 (14, p497). In a study by O'Connor et al., five coders rated taped interviews with 54 general practice patients. Kappas for individual items ranged from 0.88 to 1.00 with a mean kappa of 0.97 (15, p90).

Exhibit 7.8 The Mini-Mental State Examination

Items	Points
Orientation	
1. What is the Year?	1
Season?	1
Date?	1
Day?	1
Month?	1
2. Where are we? State?	1
County?	1
Town or city?	1
Hospital?	1
Floor?	1

Registration

3. Name three objects, taking one second to say each. Then ask the patient all three after you have said them. Give one point for each correct answer. Repeat the answers until the patient learns all three.   3

Attention and calculation

4. Serial sevens. Give one point for each correct answer. Stop after five answers. *Alternate:* Spell WORLD backwards.   5

Recall

5. Ask for names of three objects learned in Question 3. Give one point for each correct answer.   3

Language

6. Point to a pencil and a watch. Have the patient name them as you point.   2
7. Have the patient repeat "No ifs, ands, or buts."   1
8. Have the patient follow a three-stage command: "Take the paper in your right hand. Fold the paper in half. Put the paper on the floor."   3
9. Have the patient read and obey the following: "CLOSE YOUR EYES." (Write it in large letters.)   1
10. Have the patient write a sentence of his or her own choice. (The sentence should contain a subject and an object and should make sense. Ignore spelling errors when scoring.)   1
11. Enlarge the design printed below to 1–5 cm per side and have the patient copy it. (Give one point if all sides and angles are preserved and if the intersecting sides form a quadrangle.)   1

= Total 30

Reproduced from Folstein MF. The Mini-Mental State Examination. In: Crook T, Ferris S, Bartus R, eds. Assessment in geriatric psychopharmacology. New Canaan, Connecticut: Mark Powley, 1983:50–51. With permission.

Validity

In terms of content validity, the MMSE measures eight of the 11 main aspects of cognitive status; it omits abstraction, judgment, and appearance (9).

Group Differences. Folstein compared the mean MMSE scores for different groups of patients, obtaining 9.7 for patients with dementia, 19.0 for patients with depression and cognitive impairment, 25.1 for those with uncomplicated affective disorder or depression, and 27.6 for normals (1, p192). There was little variation in scores by age. Folstein also presented results indicating sensitivity to treatment (1, pp193–194).

Concurrent Validity. On small samples of elderly patients, the MMSE correlated 0.78 with the WAIS Verbal IQ scale and 0.66 with the WAIS Performance scale (20, p509). In 90 psychiatric inpatients, the MMSE had Spearman correlations of 0.41 with WAIS Verbal IQ and of 0.42 with Performance IQ (21, p129). It correlated 0.83 with the WAIS-Revised Version scores on a sample of 105 Alzheimer's disease patients (20, p510).

In a sample of 40 subjects, the MMSE and Reisberg's Global Deterioration Scale scores correlated −0.92 (22, Table 7). Correlations with Blessed's Dementia Rating Scale include 0.67 to 0.79 (19, Table 3). A correlation of 0.87 was reported with a separate Dementia Rating Scale developed by Lawson (9, Table 3). The MMSE showed modest correlations (ranging from 0.24 to 0.39) with verbal tests (18, Table 2). Correlations with other cognitive screening tests are higher: the MMSE scores correlated −0.88 with the Blessed Information-Memory-Concentration test and 0.82 with the Dementia Rating Scale (23, Table 2). Correlations with the Orientation-Memory-Concentration test include −0.77 (24, pP71) and −0.83 (17,

p925). Correcting the latter figure for unreliability of both tests gives an estimated correlation of −0.93 (17, p926). Tombaugh and McIntyre conclude that correlations with the Blessed test range from −0.66 to −0.93 (11, p927).

Predictive Validity. Mitrushina and Satz reported that all five respondents whose score decreased by more than seven points in three years were diagnosed with neurological deficits (18, p540). Faustman et al. found that the MMSE had limited utility in predicting the psychological functioning of 90 psychiatric inpatients (21).

The major focus in validating the MMSE has been on its sensitivity and specificity compared to clinical diagnoses. Representative results are shown in Table 7.4. Note that for the majority of studies, the criterion was a clinical assessment using *DSM-III* diagnoses of dementia. Again, a fuller list of results is contained in the review by Tombaugh and McIntyre (11, Table 2). Very few studies have presented validity findings in the form of ROC analyses; an exception is that of Kay et al., who showed that the MMSE performed very well in identifying moderate and severe cases of dementia, but less well in identifying mild cases (5, p779).

Several studies have commented on the effect of educational level on validity. Uhlmann and Larson reported sensitivity and

Table 7.3   Test-Retest Reliability for Mini-Mental State Examination

Study	Time lapse	Statistic*	Reliability
Anthony et al. (16)	24 hours	r	0.85–0.90
Folstein et al. (1)	24 hours	r	0.89
Dick et al. (14)	24 hours	r	0.92
Molloy et al. (13)	2 weeks	ICC	0.69
Fillenbaum et al. (17)	1 month	r	0.89
Thal et al. (12)	6 weeks	r	0.80
Mitrushina et al. (18)	1 year	r	0.45
Mitrushina et al. (18)	2 years	r	0.38
Uhlmann et al. (19)	16 months	r	0.86

*r = Pearson correlation, ICC = intraclass correlation

Table 7.4 Sensitivity and Specificity of the Mini-Mental State Examination in Detecting Dementia

Study	Sample	Cut-point	Sensitivity %	Specificity %
Anthony et al. (16)	97 hospital inpatients	23/24	87	82
Foreman (9)	66 hospital patients	23/24	82	80
Dick et al. (14)	143 neurological inpatients	23/24	76	96
van der Cammen et al. (26)	138 geriatric outpatients	24/25	88	82
Kafonek et al. (27)	70 chronic care patients	23/24	81	83
Kay et al. (5)	274 community residents	24/25	86	81
O'Connor et al. (15)	2,302 general practice patients	23/24	86	92
O'Connor et al. (15)	2,302 general practice patients	24/25	98	89
Weston (28)	98 general practice patients	23/24	83	100
Fillenbaum et al. (25)	164 community residents	23/24	100	78
Roth et al. (29)	92 hospital patients & community residents	23/24	94	85
Gagnon et al. (30)	2,792 community residents	23/24	100	78

specificity for various cutting points for three different educational groups; while the optimal cutting point varied by education, the area under the ROC curve was 0.95 or 0.96 for all educational groups. At the optimal cutting points, sensitivity was 82%, 79%, and 83% in the three educational groups. The corresponding specificity figures were 94%, 97%, and 100% (7, Table 1). Murden et al. found that education (but not race) was significantly related to MMSE scores. At 23/24, the MMSE had 93% sensitivity and 100% specificity in the high-education group and 98% sensitivity but only 75% specificity in the low education group. In the low-education group, using 17/18 as a cutoff resulted in a sensitivity of 81% and specificity of 100% (6, p152). Fillenbaum et al. showed that specificity was much lower in Blacks than in Whites, presumably a reflection of the education bias found in other studies (25).

Alternative Forms

There are variations in question wording, administration, and scoring. As the instrument was developed for hospital patients, the orientation questions refer to the name and floor of the hospital. These are altered for community residents. The choice of words for the recall question was originally left up to the examiner, but subsequently "apple," "penny," and "table" have been used, or else "shirt," "brown," and "honesty" (11, pp922–923). Finally, the MMSE included spelling the word "world" backwards as an alternative to counting by sevens, a move that gave rise to one of those occasionally fascinating backwaters of academic investigation: whole articles have addressed the issue. The intention had been to accept whichever alternative proved easiest for the respondent, but it turns out that the subtractive sevens is the more difficult task (31, 32), although perhaps not equally so for males and females (4). Some applications have used both items on the basis that the combination appears to predict the overall MMSE better than either item alone, giving a 12-item test and a maximum score of 35 points (5); others select the higher-scoring response (33, p79). It is clear that when using the MMSE the items used should be specified; as the MMSE is not sensitive to mild impairment, it may be advantageous to use the more difficult item.

Teng and Chui modified the MMSE by adding four items and refining the scoring system to provide a finer gradation (34).

They also provided clearer instructions for scoring, addressing, for example, the question of how to score the "world" item, which is often scored differently in different centers. The Modified Mini-Mental State Examination, or 3MS, was intended to improve discrimination among severe levels of dementia. Teng and Chui also provided clear instructions for applying the 3MS and developed interviewer training materials. The 3MS was used in a large study of dementia in Canada, and the sensitivity of the 3MS was 87% at a specificity of 89% (area under the ROC curve = 0.94) (35). These results were superior to those obtained using the MMSE. Teng et al. have subsequently developed the Cognitive Abilities Screening Instrument (CASI), which is an extension to the 3MS (36).

There have been a few abbreviations of the MMSE. For example, based on item analyses, Klein et al. proposed a five-item abbreviation, plus age, which retained high sensitivity and specificity (37).

Uhlmann et al. tested a written version among people with mild to moderate hearing loss. They found that verbal administration did not bias scores for people with mild or moderate hearing impairments; it also provided preliminary evidence that the written and standard MMSE are comparable (38).

Molloy et al. developed the Standardized Mini-Mental State Examination, which has expanded guidelines for administration and scoring, and time limits. They report that the Standardized MMSE was easier to administer, and intraclass inter-rater reliability improved from 0.69 for the MMSE to 0.92 for the standardized version (13, Table 1).

There are many translations of the MMSE, including French (30), Dutch (26), Spanish (39), Italian (40), Swedish (41), Chinese (42, 43), Finnish (8, 43), Korean (44), and Icelandic (4). The Chinese version showed a sensitivity of 77% and specificity of 70%, but varying the cutting points for different educational groups improved validity (42, Table 5).

Several issues have been noted in developing cross-culturally equivalent versions of the MMSE. Certain items appear to show particular variability across ethnic groups and should be modified (39). A trivial example is the orientation item "What county are we in?" which differs from country to country: a county in Britain is a very much more significant political entity than in the United States. The MMSE was modified for use in a West African setting; questions such as "How long does it take maize to ripen?" certainly seem to reverse the normal trend of questions being simpler for educated White people to answer! (45, 46).

Reference Standards

Folstein et al. presented scores from a population sample in Baltimore; 4.2% of those aged 18–64 scored 23 or less compared to 20.8% of those over 65 (2, Table 1). Bleecker et al. presented median and quartile scores by age for a small sample of healthy people (47). Heeran et al. presented norms from 532 healthy respondents over the age of 85. The median score was 28, and the lowest quartile cutoff was 26; they suggested that in this age group, scores below 25 warrant further testing (48, p1096). Holzer et al. provided norms for each item on the MMSE by age group (49, Table 3), and for the total scores by age, sex, and education (49, Tables 7 and 8). Brayne and Calloway provide some norms for British samples by age and socioeconomic status (50).

Commentary

The MMSE is brief and can be administered in a survey setting by a nonprofessional (51). It is a screening test only; diagnosis requires a full mental status examination, history, and physical examination. Validity results appear as good as, or slightly better than, those of other scales.

Various limitations to the MMSE have been identified. It may miss impairments resulting from right hemisphere lesions and may miss mild impairments (52). Many authors have reported that people with low education tend to give false-positive responses (11, p928). The major issue concerns whether this should be viewed as a bias in the test or as a risk factor. Kittner et al. provided a general discussion of adjusting cutting scores to remove the effect of education (53), while Berkman raised the challenge that, if low education is of etitological significance in dementia, then one should *not* adjust scores for educational attainment for fear of overadjusting (54). Both factors may be at work. As Tombaugh and McIntyre noted, "the prevalent view is that education introduces a psychometric bias leading to a misclassification of individuals from different educational backgrounds, and this bias should be corrected by employing norms stratified for education" (11, p928). Most norms are presented by educational level. Anthony et al. investigated an alternative approach, attempting to remove (rather than compensate for) the bias by deleting items that caused the false-positive responses. Unfortunately, each approach that improved specificity did so at the expense of sensitivity, and so no simple modification significantly improved the performance of the MMSE with less-educated persons (16, pp405–406). This was consonant with Katzman's results in the Chinese study.

The MMSE may not discriminate between moderate and severe cases of Alzheimer's disease but, more important in a screening instrument, data from Kay (5), from Huppert and Tym (51), and from Weston (28) suggest that the MMSE may miss many mild cases of dementia. This may be especially true among psychiatric patients (21). Schwamm also found that mild and moderate impairments are missed by the MMSE, as they are by most other cognitive screening instruments (55, 56). He and others propose that this is because the MMSE involves relatively simple tasks, has a limited number of test items within each cognitive domain, and combines results of performance in different domains into one overall score (51, 55, 56). Fillenbaum suggests that extreme caution should

be used when applying most instruments, including the MMSE, to minority groups, or groups with low education (25).

Perhaps reflecting its wide use and its apparent potential, various improvements have been proposed for the MMSE; these include altered cutting points by age and education, differential weighting of items, altering the content of the MMSE, and supplementing it with other tests. The first approach does not work well, for it usually trades gains in sensitivity for losses in specificity. The differential weighting has shown greater promise; for example, the scores assigned to each item appear somewhat arbitrary and not based on evidence of the relative contribution of each item in detecting dementia. Kay et al. showed that, when item scores were standardized, the internal consistency coefficient alpha rose from 0.68 to 0.80 (5, p774). Magaziner et al. showed that regression analyses could be used to reweight the individual items and thereby reduce the number of items required to achieve equally good discrimination (57). Altering the content MMSE was tested by the 3MS approach, which does appear to improve the validity findings compared to the original version; supplementing the MMSE with other tests to enhance its sensitivity to mild dementia remains a common recommendation, although there is little consensus over which test is the best supplement. The modifications made by Roth et al. for the Cambridge Mental Disorders of the Elderly Examination (CAMDEX) are described in our review of the CAMDEX.

The MMSE forms the leading screening instrument in North America but is somewhat less popular in Europe. It has known weaknesses as well as the great virtue of being well understood. The diversity of efforts to improve it demonstrate difficulties in developing the ideal dementia screening instrument.

REFERENCES

(1) Folstein MF, Folstein SE, McHugh PR. "Mini-Mental State": a practical method

for grading the cognitive state of patients for the clinician. J Psychiatr Res 1975; 12:189–198

(2) Folstein M, Anthony JC, Parhad I, et al. The meaning of cognitive impairment in the elderly. J Am Geriatr Soc 1985; 33:228–235.

(3) Fillenbaum GG, George LK, Blazer DG. Scoring nonresponse on the Mini-Mental State Examination. Psychol Med 1988; 18:1021–1025.

(4) Lindal E, Stefansson JG. Mini-Mental State Examination scores: gender and lifetime psychiatric disorders. Psychol Rep 1993;72:631–641.

(5) Kay DWK, Henderson AS, Scott R, et al. Dementia and depression among the elderly living in the Hobart community: the effect of the diagnostic criteria on the prevalence rates. Psychol Med 1985;15:771–788.

(6) Murden RA, McRae TD, Kaner S, et al. Mini-Mental State Exam scores vary with education in blacks and whites. J Am Geriatr Soc 1991;39:149–155.

(7) Uhlmann RF, Larson EB. Effect of education on the Mini-Mental State Examination as a screening test for dementia. J Am Geriatr Soc 1991;39:876–880.

(8) Ylikoski R, Erkinjuntti T, Sulkava R, et al. Correction for age, education and other demographic variables in the use of the Mini-Mental State Examination in Finland. Acta Neurol Scand 1992;85:391–396.

(9) Foreman MD. Reliability and validity of mental status questionnaires in elderly hospitalized patients. Nurs Res 1987; 36:216–220.

(10) Folstein MF. The Mini-Mental State Examination. In: Crook T, Ferris S, Bartus R, eds. Assessment in geriatric psychopharmacology. New Canaan, Connecticut: Mark Powley, 1983:47–51.

(11) Tombaugh TN, McIntyre NJ. The Mini-Mental State Examination: a comprehensive review. J Am Geriatr Soc 1992; 40:922–935.

(12) Thal LJ, Grundman M, Golden R. AlzHeimer's disease: a correlational analysis of the Blessed Information-Memory-Concentration Test and the Mini-Mental State Exam. Neurology 1986;36:262–264.

(13) Molloy DW, Alemayehu E, Roberts R. Reliability of a Standardized Mini-Mental State Examination compared with the traditional Mini-Mental State Examination. Am J Psychiatry 1991;148:102–105.

(14) Dick JPR, Guiloff RJ, Stewart A, et al. Mini-Mental State Examination in neurological patients. J Neurol Neurosurg Psychiatry 1984;47:496–499.

(15) O'Connor DW, Pollitt PA, Hyde JB, et al. The reliability and validity of the Mini-Mental State in a British community survey. J Psychiatr Res 1989;23:87–96.

(16) Anthony JC, LeResche L, Niaz U, et al. Limits of the 'Mini-Mental State' as a screening test for dementia and delirium among hospital patients. Psychol Med 1982;12:397–408.

(17) Fillenbaum GG, Heyman A, Wilkinson WE, et al. Comparison of two screening tests in Alzheimer's disease: the correlation and reliability of the Mini-Mental State Examination and the modified Blessed Test. Arch Neurol 1987;44:924–927.

(18) Mitrushina M, Satz P. Reliability and validity of the Mini-Mental State Exam in neurologically intact elderly. J Clin Psychol 1991;47:537–543.

(19) Uhlmann RF, Larson EB, Buchner DM. Correlations of Mini Mental State and modified Dementia Rating Scale to measures of transitional health status in dementia. J Gerontol 1987;42:33–36.

(20) Farber JF, Schmitt FA, Logue PE. Predicting intellectual level from the Mini-Mental State Examination. J Am Geriatr Soc 1988;36:509–510.

(21) Faustman WO, Moses JA Jr, Csernansky JG. Limitations of the Mini-Mental State Examination in predicting neuropsychological functioning in a psychiatric sample. Acta Psychiatr Scand 1990;81:126–131.

(22) Reisberg B, Ferris S, Anand R, et al. Clinical assessments of cognition in the aged. In: Shamoian LA, ed. Biology and treatment of dementia in the elderly. Washington, DC: American Psychiatric Press, 1984:16–37.

(23) Salmon DP, Thal LJ, Butters N, et al. Longitudinal evaluation of dementia of the Alzheimer type: a comparison of 3 standardized mental status examinations. Neurology 1990;40:1225–1230.

(24) Zillmer EA, Fowler PC, Gutnick HN, et al. Comparison of two cognitive bedside screening instruments in nursing home residents: a factor analytic study. J Gerontol 1990;45:P69–P74.

(25) Fillenbaum G, Heyman A, Williams K, et al. Sensitivity and specificity of standardized screens of cognitive impairment and dementia among elderly black and white community residents. J Clin Epidemiol 1990;43:651–660.

(26) van der Cammen TJ, van Harskamp F, Stronks DL, et al. Value of the Mini-Mental State Examination and informants' data for the detection of dementia in geriatric outpatients. Psychol Rep 1992;71:1003–1009.

(27) Kafonek S, Ettinger WH, Roca R, et al. Instruments for screening for depression

and dementia in a long-term care facility. J Am Geriatr Soc 1989;37:29–34.

(28) Weston WW. Screening for dementia in a family practice. Can Fam Physician 1987;33:2495–2500.

(29) Roth M, Tym E, Mountjoy CQ, et al. CAMDEX: a standardised instrument for the diagnosis of mental disorder in the elderly with special reference to the early detection of dementia. Br J Psychiatry 1986;149:698–709.

(30) Gagnon M, Letenneur L, Dartigues J-F, et al. Validity of the Mini-Mental State Examination as a screening instrument for cognitive impairment and dementia in French elderly community residents. Neuroepidemiology 1990;9:143–150.

(31) Watkins P, Gouvier WD, Callon E, et al. Equivalence of items on the Mini-Mental State. Arch Clin Neuropsychol 1989; 4:381–384.

(32) Ganguli M, Ratcliff G, Huff FJ, et al. Serial sevens versus world backwards: a comparison of the two measures of attention from the MMSE. J Geriatr Psychiatry Neurol 1990;3:203–207.

(33) O'Connor DW, Pollitt PA, Hyde JB, et al. A follow-up study of dementia diagnosed in the community using the Cambridge Mental Disorders of the Elderly Examination. Acta Psychiatr Scand 1990;81:78–82.

(34) Teng EL, Chui HC. The Modified Mini-Mental State (3MS) Examination. J Clin Psychiatry 1987;48:314–318.

(35) Canadian Study of Health and Aging Working Group. The Canadian Study of Health and Aging: study methods and prevalence of dementia. Can Med Assoc J 1994;150:899–913.

(36) Teng EL, Hasegawa K, Homma A, et al. The Cognitive Abilities Screening Instrument (CASI): a practical test for cross-cultural epidemiological studies of dementia. Int Psychogeriatr 1994;6:45–58.

(37) Klein LE, Roca RP, McArthur J, et al. Diagnosing dementia: univariate and multivariate analyses of the Mental Status Examination. J Am Geriatr Soc 1985;33:483–488.

(38) Uhlmann RF, Teri L, Rees TS, et al. Impact of mild to moderate hearing loss on mental status testing: comparability of standard and written Mini-Mental State Examinations. J Am Geriatr Soc 1989;37:223–228.

(39) Escobar JI, Burnam A, Karno M, et al. Use of the Mini-Mental Examination (MMSE) in a community population of mixed ethnicity: cultural and linguistic artifacts. J Nerv Ment Dis 1986;174:607–614.

(40) Mazzoni M, Ferroni L, Lombardi L, et al. Mini-Mental State Examination (MMSE): sensitivity in an Italian sample of patients with dementia. Ital J Neurol Sci 1992; 13:323–329.

(41) Grut M, Fratiglioni L, Viitanen M, et al. Accuracy of the Mini-Mental Status Examination as a screening test for dementia in a Swedish elderly population. Acta Neurol Scand 1993;87:312–317.

(42) Katzman R, Zhang M, Qu OY, et al. A Chinese version of the Mini-Mental State Examination: impact of illiteracy in a Shanghai dementia survey. J Clin Epidemiol 1988;41:971–978.

(43) Salmon DP, Riekkinen PJ, Katzman R, et al. Cross-cultural studies of dementia: a comparison of Mini-Mental State Examination performance in Finland and China. Arch Neurol 1989;46:769–772.

(44) Park JH, Kwon YC. Modification of the Mini-Mental State Examination for use in the elderly in a non-western society. Int J Geriatr Psychiatry 1990;5:381.

(45) Ogunniyi A, Osuntokun BO, Lekwauwa UG. Screening for dementia in elderly Nigerians: results of the pilot test of a new instrument. East Afr Med J 1991;68:448–454.

(46) Ogunniyi A, Lekwauwa UG, Osuntokun BO. Influence of education on aspects of cognitive functions in non-demented elderly Nigerians. Neuroepidemiology 1991; 10:246–250.

(47) Bleecker ML, Bolla-Wilson K, Kawas C, et al. Age-specific norms for the Mini-Mental State Exam. Neurology 1988;38:1565–1568.

(48) Heeren TJ, Lagaay AM, van Beek WCA, et al. Reference values for the Mini-Mental State Examination (MMSE) in octo- and nonagenarians. J Am Geriatr Soc 1990; 38:1093–1096.

(49) Holzer CE, Tischler GL, Leaf PJ, et al. An epidemiologic assessment of cognitive impairment in a community population. Res Community Ment Health 1984;4:3–32.

(50) Brayne C, Calloway P. The association of education and socioeconomic status with the Mini Mental State Examination and the clinical diagnosis of dementia in elderly people. Age Ageing 1990;19:91–96.

(51) Huppert FA, Tym E. Clinical and neuropsychological assessment of dementia. Br Med Bull 1986;42:11–18.

(52) Naugle RI, Kawczak K. Limitations of the Mini-Mental State Examination. Cleve Clin J Med 1989;56:277–281.

(53) Kittner SJ, White LR, Farmer ME, et al.

Methodological issues in screening for dementia: the problem of education adjustment. J Chronic Dis 1986;39:163–170.

(54) Berkman LF. The association between educational attainment and mental status examinations: of etiologic significance for senile dementias or not? J Chronic Dis 1986;39:171–174.

(55) Schwamm LH, Van Dyke C, Kiernan RJ, et al. The Neurobehavioral Cognitive Status Examination: comparison with the Cognitive Capacity Screening Examination and the Mini-Mental State Examination in a neurosurgical population. Ann Intern Med 1987;107:486–491.

(56) Nelson A, Fogel BS, Faust D. Bedside cognitive screening instruments: a critical assessment. J Nerv Ment Dis 1986;174:73–83.

(57) Magaziner J, Bassett SS, Hebel JR. Predicting performance on the Mini-Mental State Examination: use of age- and education-specific equations. J Am Geriatr Soc 1987;35:996–1000.

THE CLIFTON ASSESSMENT PROCEDURES FOR THE ELDERLY
(A.H. Pattie and C.J. Gilleard, 1975)

Purpose

The Clifton Assessment Procedures for the Elderly (CAPE) evaluates the presence and severity of impairment in mental and behavioral functioning. It was intended for elderly chronic psychiatric patients (1).

Conceptual Basis

The CAPE consists of two components: the Cognitive Assessment Scale (CAS) and the Behavior Rating Scale (BRS). The former was first published as the Clifton Assessment Schedule (2), while the latter was derived from the Stockton Geriatric Rating Scale (3).

This scale indicates the patient's likely level of dependency, suggesting the "degree of support typically provided by society in association with given levels of disability" (1, p10). It was designed to be brief enough for practical use with elderly patients and applicable across a wide range of abilities.

Description

The CAPE was named after the Clifton Hospital in York, England. The Cognitive Assessment Scale is a psychological test that assesses the degree of cognitive impairment. It is generally administered by nurses treating the patient. The complete schedule is shown in the manual of the CAPE (1, pp3–7); a summary of its content is given in Exhibit 7.9. It includes a 12-item information and orientation subtest (taking the form of questions such as, "What is your date of birth?"), a brief mental abilities test (e.g., "Will you count up from 1 to 20 for me—as quickly as you can?"), and a psychomotor performance test which involves tracing a line through a maze. The time taken for the psychomotor maze test and the number of errors on the other tests are converted into a score out of 12. The conversion is explained in the manual (1, p12). Pattie and Gilleard recommend a cutting point of 8, commenting that scores of 7 and below generally indicate dementia or acute organic brain syndrome.

The BRS is an 18-item rating scale completed by relatives or staff familiar with the patient's behavior. It covers physical disability including ADL performance, apathy, communication difficulties, and social disturbance. Scores range from 0 to 36, with higher scores indicating more disability (1, pp7–9).

Scores on the two instruments are transferred onto a report form that translates the raw scores into a five-category grading system that indicates the level of dependency associated with the impairments and hence the support the patient is likely to require (1, pp11–12). Grade A represents no mental impairment and no significant behavioral disability; grade B represents mild impairment in both areas that will require some support for people living in the community. Grade C includes medium levels of impairment requiring considerable support for community living. Grade D includes those with marked impairment and dependency; people in this category

Exhibit 7.9 Summary Content of the Clifton Assessment Procedures for the Elderly

COGNITIVE ASSESSMENT SCALE

Information and Orientation

Correct recall of:

Name:	Hospital/address:	Colour of British flag:
Age:	City:	Day:
D.o.B.:	P.M.:	Month:
Ward/place:	U.S. President:	Year:

Mental Ability

Ability to count 1 to 20 (timed)

Reciting alphabet (timed)

Write name

Reading a list of pre-selected words

Psychomotor

The patient is asked to draw around a pre-printed spiral maze, avoiding "obstacles" drawn in the pathway; performance is timed.

BEHAVIOR RATING SCALE

Physical Disability

Bathing and dressing

Walking ability

Continence

Staying in bed during the day

Confusion (unable to find way around, loses things)

Appearance

Apathy

Would need supervision if allowed outside

Helps out in the home or ward

Keeps occupied

Socializes

Accepts suggestions to do things

Communication Difficulties

Understands what is communicated to him/her

Able to communicate

Social Disturbance

Objectionable to others during day

Objectionable to others during night

Accuses others of wrongdoing

Hoards apparently meaningless items

Sleep pattern

Adapted from Pattie AH, Gilleard CJ. Manual of the Clifton Assessment Procedures for the Elderly (CAPE). Sevenoaks, Kent: Hodder and Stoughton, 1979:3–9.

are usually institutionalized. Grade E includes those with maximal impairment, typical of psychogeriatric patients requiring a great deal of nursing attention and care (1, p10).

Reliability

Pattie and Gilleard reported test–retest reliability results for the CAS scales from a number of studies. Results for the information/orientation (I/O) scale ranged from 0.79 to 0.90; for the mental ability scale results ranged from 0.61 to 0.89, and for the psychomotor test the results ranged from 0.56 to 0.79 (1, p21).

Inter-rater reliability for the BRS subscales were reported from five studies. Correlations for physical disability ranged from 0.70 to 0.91; apathy results ranged from 0.81 to 0.87; communication from 0.45 to 0.72; and social disturbance ranged from 0.69 to 0.88 (1, Table 7). Inter-rater agreement for the CAS was 0.99 in one study (4, Table 1).

Internal consistency of the CAPE has been reviewed in several ways. The intercorrelations among the subscale scores range from 0.30 to 0.78 (1, Table 14). Lesher and Whelihan tested reliability of the information/orientation section on 36 nursing home residents (mean age 85 years). Test–retest reliability at two to four weeks was 0.84, and alpha was 0.77 (5, Table 1). These results were lower than those obtained for the other scales included in Lesher and Whelihan's review.

Validity

All subscores showed clear distinctions between well elderly people, people under care in the community by the social services agencies, and psychiatric patients (1, Tables 3–5; 2, Table 1). Each subscore of the CAS predicted subsequent likelihood of discharge (1, Table 1). Predictive validity has also been tested by comparing CAPE scores with subsequent mortality. Total CAS scores and the mental ability score were associated with subsequent mortality

(6); in another sample, both cognitive and behavior scores predicted subsequent mortality (7).

The validity of the information/orientation subtest of the CAS has been studied separately. Comparing 33 dementia patients and 67 psychiatric patients, the I/O had a sensitivity of 91% and a specificity of 93% (2, Table II). Figures of 87% and 97% were reported at a cutting point of 7/8 for a general practice study (8, Table V). The mental ability subtest had lower sensitivity and specificity: 52% and 89%, respectively. A subsequent study replicated these results (9). A cutting point of 7/8 resulted in a sensitivity of 80% for discriminating patients with dementia from those with functional psychiatric disorders such as affective illness or schizophrenia (10, p458). Specificity was 85%. In the same study, scores on the CAS successfully predicted poor outcome at the end of the two-year study. Black et al. reported sensitivity and specificity of the I/O subtest as somewhat lower than those for the Mini-Mental State Exam (MMSE) or the CAMCOG (11, Table II). Further examination of this was undertaken by Jagger et al., who proposed altering the cutting point from 7/8 to 8/9 (12, p208).

Factor analyses of the BRS identified three main factors. The first combined the physical disability and communication scales; the second included the apathy items; and the third contained the social disturbance items (1, p27).

The information/orientation score of the CAS correlated 0.90 with the Wechsler Memory Scale (N = 33 patients) and gave an 84.5% correct classification into organic or functional disorders as rated by the Wechsler scale (1, p23). In three studies, correlations between the information/orientation test and the Wechsler Adult Intelligence Scale (WAIS) ranged from 0.22 to 0.37 with the WAIS Verbal scale and 0.51 to 0.74 with the Performance scale. Correlations for the psychomotor score were very similar, while those between the men-

tal ability scale and the WAIS Performance scale were lower, at 0.35 to 0.54 (1, p24).

Alternative Forms

An abbreviated version of the CAPE is designed for use in large-scale surveys. This includes the information/orientation scale from the CAS and the physical disability (PD) scale from the BRS. Scores are formed by subtracting the PD scores from the I/O (range $+12$ to -12) and converted into five categories (13). Test–retest reliability ranged from 0.82 to 0.89 in three studies (13, Table 2) and was 0.91 in another (14). Concurrent and predictive validity have also been demonstrated in several studies (13–15), although McPherson et al. found that the PD score added little beyond the I/O and that classification of patients by severity of dementia showed considerable overlap between groups in the middle of the severity spectrum (15, p9O).

Reference Standards

Normative data were reported in the CAPE manual, which shows mean scores, medians, and interquartile ranges on each subscale for well people in the community and for a range of patient types (1, Tables 3–5 and p29).

Commentary

The Clifton Assessment Procedures have been tested in a number of studies using large samples of patients. The results show good reliability and high sensitivity and specificity when used with psychiatric inpatients. It has mainly been tested on hospital populations and its performance on community samples is unknown.

The issue has been raised of how to score the CAPE when a patient, because of blindness or arthritic hands, cannot complete the maze test. The original approach, of awarding zero, may lead to falsely classifying physical difficulties as a cognitive problem; prorating the score based on scores in other parts of the CAPE does not work well (16). There have been extensive but rather fruitless discussions over the adequacy of the I/O subtest as a screening test compared to the MMSE as well as the best cutting points. These discussions would benefit greatly from reanalyses of the data using ROC analyses to summarize the performance of the tests across all cutting points. Furthermore, the debate over the CAPE versus the MMSE appears to concern adequacy in estimating the prevalence of dementia; this does not seem an appropriate application for a screening test.

The CAPE provide reliable estimates of cognitive and behavioral impairment for institutionalized elderly populations. As a screening test for community use, the CAPE would probably be less adequate than other available instruments such as the MMSE.

REFERENCES

(1) Pattie AH, Gilleard CJ. Manual of the Clifton Assessment Procedures for the Elderly (CAPE). Sevenoaks, England: Hodder and Stoughton, 1979:1–32.

(2) Pattie AH, Gilleard CJ. A brief psychogeriatric assessment schedule: validation against psychiatric diagnosis and discharge from hospital. Br J Psychiatry 1975; 127:489–493.

(3) Meer B, Baker JA. The Stockton Geriatric Rating Scale. J. Gerontol 1966;21:392–403.

(4) Smith AHW, Ballinger BR, Presly AS. The reliability and validity of two assessment scales in the elderly mentally handicapped. Br J Psychiatry 1981;138:15–16.

(5) Lesher EL, Whelihan WM. Reliability of mental status instruments administered to nursing home residents. J Consult Clin Psychol 1986;54:726–727.

(6) Gamsu CV, McLaren SM, McPherson FM. Prediction of survival in dementia by cognitive tests: a six-year follow-up. Br J Clin Psychol 1990;29:99–104.

(7) Moran SM, Cockram LL, Walker B, et al. Prediction of survival by the Clifton Assessment Procedures for the Elderly (CAPE). Br J Clin Psychol 1990;29:225–226.

(8) Clarke M, Jagger C, Anderson J, et al. The prevalence of dementia in a total population: a comparison of two screening instruments. Age Ageing 1991;20:396–403.

(9) Pattie AH, Gilleard CJ. The Clifton Assessment Schedule—further validation of a psychogeriatric assessment schedule. Br J Psychiatry 1976;129:68–72.

(10) Pattie AH, Gilleard CJ. The two-year predictive validity of the Clifton Assessment Schedule and the Shortened Stockton Geriatric Rating Scale. Br J Psychiatry 1978;133:457–460.

(11) Black SE, Blessed G, Edwardson JA, et al. Prevalence rates of dementia in an ageing population: are low rates due to the use of insensitive instruments? Age Ageing 1990;19:84–90.

(12) Jagger C, Clarke M, Anderson J, et al. Dementia in Melton Mowbray—a validation of earlier findings. Age Ageing 1992;21:205–210.

(13) Pattie AH. A survey version of the Clifton Assessment Procedures for the Elderly (CAPE). Br J Clin Psychol 1981;20:173–178.

(14) McPherson FM, Tregaskis D. The short-term stability of the survey version of CAPE. Br J Clin Psychol 1985;24:205–206.

(15) McPherson FM, Gamsu CV, Kiemle G, et al. The concurrent validity of the survey version of the Clifton Assessment Procedures for the Elderly (CAPE). Br J Clin Psychol 1985;24:83–91.

(16) McPherson FM, Gamsu CV, Cockram LL, et al. Use of the CAPE Pm test with disabled patients. Br J Clin Psychol 1986;25:145–146.

THE CAMBRIDGE MENTAL DISORDERS OF THE ELDERLY EXAMINATION
(Sir Martin Roth, 1986)

Purpose

The Cambridge Mental Disorders of the Elderly Examination (CAMDEX) is a clinical interview schedule that standardizes the information collected in a routine diagnostic interview for dementia. It "focuses on the diagnosis of dementia, with particular reference to its mild forms and to the identification of specific types of dementia" (1, p700).

Conceptual Basis

Roth argued that a complete picture of dementia requires three types of instrument: cognitive screening tests, dementia severity tests, and behavior rating scales that test problems in ADL. The CAMDEX incorporates these in a single instrument (1, p698). The procedure was developed from a review of weaknesses in existing scales and aims "to remedy gaps in the existing standardised interviews and scales of measurement." (1, p700)

Description

The CAMDEX includes three components: a clinical interview, a set of cognitive tests, and an interview with a relative to obtain independent information on the patient's past and present state. The cognitive tests include existing instruments such as the Mini-Mental State Examination (MMSE), the Blessed Dementia Score, and Hachinski's Ischemia Scale. The CAMDEX includes eight sections (1, pp701–702):

1. Section A covers symptoms of severe mental conditions, past history, and family history of mental disorders.
2. Section B is a cognitive examination, the "CAMCOG." This incorporates an extended version of the MMSE (19 items), as

> the MMSE does not sample certain cognitive functions e.g. abstract thinking and perception, which are relevant to diagnosis and are included in DSM-III operational criteria for primary degenerative dementia. Second, many functions are assessed by the MMSE in insufficient detail. For example, memory is assessed only by the repetition and recall of three words; we have added items covering remote and recent memory and the recall of new information. . . . [Thus the CAMCOG] assesses orientation, language, memory, praxis, attention, abstract thinking, perception and calculation. (1, p701)

Section B has a total of 57 items.

3. Section C includes the interviewer's observations on the patient's appearance, behavior, mood, and level of consciousness. It is completed at the end of the interview.

4. In section D a physical examination provides information to differentiate between primary and secondary dementias. It covers blood pressure, reflexes, gait, defects of hearing or sight, tremor, and Parkinsonism.
5. Section E covers laboratory tests: blood analyses and radiological investigations.
6. Section F lists current medications taken by the subject.
7. Section G records further information that arises spontaneously during the interview; it is likely to be of particular use in classifying atypical and difficult cases.
8. Section H includes a structured interview with a relative or caregiver who knows the person well. It incorporates the Blessed Dementia Score. The Hachinski Ischemia Score is also incorporated into the CAMDEX.

The complete CAMDEX is too long to reproduce here; it can be purchased from the Cambridge Department of Psychiatry (see Address section).

The CAMDEX is generally administered by a psychiatrist; the interview with the patient takes about 60 minutes, the informant interview takes about 20 minutes. At the end of the interview, the psychiatrist makes a diagnosis based on operational criteria. Eleven diagnostic categories are specified: four categories of dementia, two of clouding or delirium, and a range of other psychiatric states such as depression or paranoia. The severity of dementia and depression are graded on five-point scales (1, p702).

In addition to the clinician's diagnoses, several scores are derived from the CAMDEX. The CAMCOG scores cognitive impairment based on the 57 items in section B; it has a maximum score of 106 and Roth recommended a cutting point of 79/80 (1, p703). Scores for the Mental Status Questionnaire (2) can also be derived from the CAMCOG items. There is a scale representing organicity, composed of 18 items from the patient interviews, 14 from the relative interview, and two based on the interviewer's observations. A multi-infarct scale, designed to distinguish multi-infarct dementias, includes eight items from the relative's interview, two from the patient interview, and two from the interviewer's observations. Finally, a depression scale includes nine items from the patient interview and four from the relative's interview (3, p404).

Reliability

An inter-rater reliability among four psychiatrists, each interviewing 40 patients, showed median agreement phi coefficients of 0.94 for section A, 0.90 for section B, 0.83 for section C, and 0.91 for section H (1, p703). There was complete agreement among raters on the classification of patients as demented or as normal, but the phi coefficient of agreement was reduced to 0.63 when dementia was divided into four subcategories. Hendrie et al. calculated inter-rater reliabilities for 40 psychogeriatric patients and 15 controls who were interviewed by clinicians of varying backgrounds. Phi coefficients for the 69 individual items of the CAMCOG ranged from 0.50 to 1.00; the median was 0.86. The Pearson correlation between raters for total score on the CAMCOG was 0.88. Phi coefficients for the patient interview, interviewer's observations, and informant interview ranged from 0.50 to 1.00, and Pearson correlations between raters for total score on these sections ranged from 0.81 to 0.99 (3, Table 2).

Data on test–retest reliability are limited because of the difficulty in readministering such a lengthy test to elderly people.

Validity

Roth reported 92% sensitivity and 96% specificity for the CAMCOG, compared to a clinical diagnosis, although it appears from the text of the report that these figures may actually refer to positive and negative predictive values rather than sensitivity and specificity (1, p703). Mean scores for depressed patients did not differ significantly from those of the normals; mean scores for both groups were clearly different than those for the demented patients (1, Table III). Compared to Copeland's Geriatric Mental State Examination, the CAMCOG showed a sensitivity of 97% and a specificity of 91% (4, pp194–195). These results were considerably better than those obtained by the MMSE but were comparable to those obtained by the Clifton Assessment Procedures for the Elderly (CAPE), which had a sensitivity of 94% and a specificity of 91%. However, the CAMCOG missed 21% of cases meeting the *DSM-III* criteria for dementia: these were mostly mild cases. With a 79/80 cutoff, sensitivity and specificity were both 100% in one study of 28 psychogeriatric patients and 15 community controls (3, p405). The MMSE showed an 82% sensitivity and 100% specificity (with a 23/24 cutoff) in the same study. The organicity, multi-infarct dementia, and depression scales succeeded in distinguishing Alzheimer's disease, multi-infarct dementia, and depression, respectively, from all other conditions (3, Table 5).

O'Connor et al. reviewed predictive validity by reassessing 137 cases one year after an initial CAMDEX assessment. Very few errors in the original assessment were noted: 97% of the diagnoses were confirmed (5, p79). Depression had been missed in several minimally demented subjects, and four of 67 cases of mild dementia were altered on review (5, p81). A subsequent two-year follow-up assessment by the same team confirmed the appropriateness of the initial diagnoses; O'Connor provided case histories to illustrate the few apparently anomalous changes (6).

The CAMCOG correlated −0.70 with the Blessed Dementia Score and −0.78 with a clinical rating of severity of dementia (1, p704). The correlation with the Blessed score in another study was 0.75 (4, p195). CAMCOG scores correlated more highly with an organicity score (−0.63) than with a depression score (0.22) (1, Table V).

Commentary

The CAMDEX was designed to respond to limitations of the MMSE and other widely used scales. "It replicates a full clinical assessment ... in a structured, orderly fashion, but this breadth and depth of coverage make it an expensive instrument to use" (7, p218). The cognitive capacity component, known as the CAMCOG scale, appears superior to the MMSE: it covers a wider range of cognitive functions; it detects mild levels of impairment and avoids ceiling effects (1, p708).

The value of including assessments by relatives in addition to self-assessments was indicated by the finding that relatives were better able to assess cognitive ability although they were often unaware of the patient's depression. The information provided by informants generally agreed closely with the observations made by clinicians (8).

Because of its length and the need for a psychiatrist to lead the interview, the CAMDEX is generally applied following an initial screening test. However, it has been used in epidemiological studies in England, and the CAMCOG section might be used as a separate assessment instrument.

Address

Department of Psychiatry, Level 4, Addenbrooke's Hospital, Hills Rd, Cambridge CB2 2QQ, England

REFERENCES

(1) Roth M, Tym E, Mountjoy CQ, et al. CAMDEX: a standardised instrument for the diagnosis of mental disorder in the elderly with special reference to the early detection of dementia. Br J Psychiatry 1986; 149:698–709.

(2) Kahn RL, Goldfarb AI, Pollack M, et al. Brief objective measures for the determination of mental status in the aged. Am J Psychiatry 1960;117:326–328.

(3) Hendrie HC, Hall KS, Brittain HM, et al. The CAMDEX: a standardized instrument for the diagnosis of mental disorder in the elderly: a replication with a US sample. J Am Geriatr Soc 1988;36:402–408.

(4) Blessed G, Black SE, Butler T, et al. The diagnosis of dementia in the elderly. A comparison of CAMCOG (the cognitive section of CAMDEX), the AGECAT program, DSM-III, the Mini-Mental State Examination, and some short rating scales. Br J Psychiatry 1991;159:193–198.

(5) O'Connor DW, Pollitt PA, Hyde JB, et al. A follow-up study of dementia diagnosed in the community using the Cambridge Mental Disorders of the Elderly Examination. Acta Psychiatr Scand 1990;81:78–82.

(6) O'Connor DW, Pollitt PA, Jones BJ, et al. Continued clinical validation of dementia diagnosed in the community using the Cambridge Mental Disorder of the Elderly Examination. Acta Psychiatr Scand 1991;83:41–45.

(7) O'Connor DW. The contribution of CAMDEX to the diagnosis of mild dementia in community surveys. Psychiatr J Univ Ottawa 1990;15:216–220.

(8) O'Connor DW, Pollitt PA, Brook CPB, et al. The validity of informant histories in a community study of dementia. Int J Geriatr Psychiatry 1989;4:203–208.

CONCLUSION

The field of cognitive assessment has been very actively studied in recent years. Not only is there a proliferation of scales, but there has been continuing attention to the underlying conceptual and theoretical issues. Validation studies are generally well done; many of the instruments have received extensive validity and reliability testing. It will be good, however, to see the application of some of the more recent statistical procedures to summarizing the testing results; validity is commonly described in terms of sensitivity and specificity rather than in terms of ROC analyses, which simplify the comparison between scales.

In addition to the reviews in this chapter, scales in other chapters contain cognitive components that may be suitable for particular applications. These include the Comprehensive Assessment and Referral Evaluation (see Chapter 9), the Functional Activities Questionnaire (FAQ), and the Functional Status Rating System (both reviewed in Chapter 3). The FAQ is often used as a cognitive screening test, although it is expressed in the format of an instrumental activities of daily living questionnaire. This feature may make it more acceptable to respondents than the quiz format of memory questions and arithmetic tests that characterize most of the instruments described in the present chapter.

ADDITIONAL INSTRUMENTS

There are numerous other cognitive function tests that we have not included as full reviews, for reasons of space or of their early stages of development. They deserve mention here, to guide the reader who has not found a suitable method among the instruments that we review in this chapter.

Screening Tests

The first category of additional instruments includes several screening tests. The Cross-Cultural Cognitive Examination (CCCE) is a brief screening test designed to identify all forms of dementia; it can be applied in nonliterate populations by lay interviewers (1–3). As an innovative way to achieve validity in a brief instrument, the CCCE contains a five-minute screening test plus a 20-minute mental status examination applied to those who fail the screening component. The screen is intended to be sensitive; the examination, specific. Early results seem very good and interested readers should monitor the further development of this instrument. Another instrument designed for use in nonliterate groups is the ten-item Elderly Cognitive Assessment Questionnaire (ECAQ), which drew items from the MMSE and GMS. Sensitivity was reported as 85% at a specificity of 92% (4, p119). An eight-item screening test described by Kokmen et al. is called the Short Test of Mental Status (STMS) (5). It contains one item on each of orientation, attention, immediate recall, calculation, abstraction, construction (using the clock test), information, and delayed recall. The test takes about five minutes to administer and

some validity information is available (6).

Three brief batteries of existing neuropsychological tests are worthy of mention. First, Martha Storandt developed a brief battery of four tests to differentiate between persons in the early stages of Alzheimer's disease and normal older adults. The tests were selected through discriminant analysis in a case-control study. The discriminant function included the logical memory and mental control subtests of the Wechsler Memory Scale, form A of the Trailmaking Test and word fluency for letters S and P. This battery took approximately 10 minutes to complete and could be administered by research assistants. The initial validity figures presented by Storandt were outstanding: 98% correct classification in the challenging task of identifying early Alzheimer's disease (7). Replication confirmed that the battery did distinguish normal people from those with early dementia, but that it did not distinguish among different types of dementia (8). In a later report, Storandt retested the battery on a larger sample and again showed good discrimination ability, but the tests selected by the new discriminant analysis changed and Storandt recommended switching to the newly identified tests (9, p385). This approach is worth consideration in screening for the early stages of dementia. Second, Eslinger et al. also proposed a brief battery of tests to distinguish dementia from normal aging (10). The Eslinger battery includes the Benton Visual Retention Test (a test of short-term memory for designs), the Benton Controlled Oral Word Association Test (naming as many words that begin with a selected letter as possible in a set time) and the Benton Temporal Orientation Test (accuracy of recall of the month, day, year, and time of day). The battery takes ten to 15 minutes to complete. Validity is comparable to that of the Storandt battery (8). Finally, Pfeffer assembled three tests into a brief battery to serve as a population screen for mild dementia in community surveys (11, 12). This was named the Mental Function Index

(MFI) and is a weighted combination of scores from the Mini-Mental State Examination, the Smith Symbol Digit Modalities test, and the Raven matrices subtest B. Hence, it is an extension of the MMSE designed to overcome the MMSE's weaknesses. The instrument is applied by a nurse clinician in 15 to 25 minutes. Reliability results were very high: test–retest reliability was 0.97; sensitivity was 0.93 at a specificity of 0.80 (12, Table 4). Further validation results include a sensitivity of 71% and a specificity of 91% (13)—little different from the MMSE alone. Some commentators have been critical. Mowry and Burvill, for example, found that the MFI did not differentiate mild dementia from other diagnoses, and they concluded that "in its present form, the MFI cannot be recommended as a screening instrument for mild dementia." (14, p332)

The Short Test of Mental Status can be administered in five minutes and assesses orientation, attention, immediate recall, delayed recall, arithmetic, construction, and information (5). Preliminary validity results appear good (sensitivity 86%, specificity 94%) (6).

The East Boston Memory Test is a relatively recent instrument that has shown good validity (15). It consists of a brief story containing three sentences, each of which includes two ideas. The person retells the story immediately after hearing it and errors are scored. This test has been shown superior to the Short Portable Mental Status Questionnaire as a screen for dementia (16).

The Delayed Word Recall Test is a memory task designed to discriminate patients with dementia from normal elderly subjects in large-scale screening studies (13). Disturbance of recent memory is the most common deficit seen in early Alzheimer's disease, mainly learning new material and retrieving it with minimal cuing. The test requires the person to make up sentences that incorporate the words to be remembered, followed by a delay period, then a free recall phase. Early results suggest that the instrument is highly sensitive in discriminating those with mild Alzheimer's disease from normals, although it may not be suitable for patients with more severe dementia, because the requirement of making up a sentence may prove too difficult.

A recent test that is attracting considerable attention is the Cognitive Abilities Screening Instrument (CASI) developed by Evelyn Teng. This may be the Swiss army knife of the dementia field; it is designed to be cross-culturally applicable and serves as a screening test for dementia and as an indicator of disease progression; it also provides a profile of impairment among various cognitive domains (17). Items were drawn from the Modified Mini-Mental State Examination (3MS) and the Hasegawa Dementia Screening Scale and were tested simultaneously in the United States and in Japan. These early trials suggest that both sensitivity and specificity lie in the mid 90s, higher than the level achieved by the 3MS (17, Table 4). A feature of this scale and of Teng's 3MS is the availability of high-quality materials, including exam questions, for training interviewers. Careful attention has been paid to detail in these instruments, in a manner reminiscent of scales such as the Short-Form-36 Health Survey reviewed in Chapter 9. It will be interesting to see further information on reliability and validity over the coming years.

Instruments for Clinical Application

Several measures have been developed for use with patient samples. These include the Stroke Unit Mental Status Examination (SUMSE), which is a bedside evaluation of cognitive function following a stroke. It focuses on the types of deficit caused by strokes (e.g., language disorders, visuoperceptual deficits, and memory disorders). Evidence for validity and reliability are available (18). The Neurobehavioral Cognitive Status Examination (NCSE) assesses multiple domains of cognitive functioning in patient populations and presents these in profile form rather than as a summary score (19).

Reisberg has developed two measures of the severity of cognitive decline: the Brief Cognitive Rating Scale (BCRS) and the Global Deterioration Scale (20–22). The BCRS is a clinical rating scale that summarizes the extent of cognitive impairment on five clinical axes: concentration, recent memory, past memory, orientation and functioning, and self-care. Each is rated on a seven-point severity scale (20, pp29–31). The Global Deterioration Scale provides a seven-category overall rating of the progression of dementia, ranging from no cognitive decline to very severe decline. Clinical markers of each stage are provided (20, pp32–35).

Hachinski's Ischemic Score is a list of clinical signs that distinguish the degenerative dementias such as Alzheimer's disease from vascular or multi-infarct dementias (23). It has been extensively tested, criticized, and revised over the years (24–26) but remains one of the most widely used instruments of its kind.

The Information Questionnaire on Cognitive Decline in the Elderly (IQCODE) collects information on changes in cognitive functioning from an informant. The rationale is that to estimate cognitive decline, an accurate picture of previous function is required and people with dementia are unable to provide such information. The questionnaire contains 26 items covering daily tasks requiring memory (e.g., remembering things that have happened recently, understanding magazine or newspaper articles), and the informant is asked to compare the person's current performance with her performance ten years previously. Evidence for reliability and validity are available (27) and a 16-item short form has been tested (28).

Shader developed the Sandoz Clinical Assessment—Geriatric (SCAG) to assess change following treatment (29). This is an 18-item clinical rating scale that covers agitation, cognitive dysfunction, depressed mood, and withdrawal. It is widely used as an outcome measure in drug research (30), although it is not without criticism (31).

Cole and Dastoor developed the Hierarchic Dementia Scale to measure the severity of cognitive and behavioral symptoms of dementia. In a manner similar to that used by Katz in his Index of ADL, a reversal of the hierarchy of cognitive development during childhood was postulated for senile decline (32, p298; 33). For example, in declining language skills, nominal aphasia usually occurs before paraphasia, which precedes the appearance of word substitutions and then the use of deformed words. Within each of the 20 cognitive functions assessed, there is also a hierarchy of severity. If the response to the initial item in a list is incorrect, the interviewer keeps testing on consecutively lower items in the subscale until two sequential items are answered correctly. For more severely demented patients, the interviewer starts with easier items and proceeds up until two consecutive items are missed. Reliability appears good and there is some evidence for concurrent validity.

Diagnostic Instruments

Finally, there are several major clinical assessments that are used in diagnosing dementia. The Structured Interview for the Diagnosis of Dementia of the Alzheimer type (SIDAM) provides a differential diagnosis of dementias according to *DSM-III* and *International Classification of Disease–Tenth Revision* criteria. It comprises a brief clinical interview covering medical history, a standard cognitive performance test, and a series of diagnostic algorithms that guide differential diagnoses. Early results have shown satisfactory reliability and concordance with independent diagnoses (34). Other diagnostic instruments include the British Present State Examination (PSE), the American Diagnostic Interview Schedule (DIS), and the Geriatric Mental State Examination (GMS), which was derived from the PSE. In turn, the Canberra Interview for the Elderly (CIE) was based on the GMS and includes material from ADL scales and from the Comprehensive Assessment and Referral Evaluation

(CARE) instrument described in Chapter 9 (35–37). These instruments provide complete diagnostic algorithms and sometimes use computer scoring. They have often been examined for reliability and validity and extend the field of cognitive testing far beyond the scope of those instruments we have selected to review in this chapter.

REFERENCES

(1) Glosser G, Wolfe N, Albert ML, et al. Cross-Cultural Cognitive Examination: validation of a dementia screening instrument for neuroepidemiological research. J Am Geriatr Soc 1993;41:931–939.

(2) Glosser G, Wolfe N, Kliner-Krenzel L, et al. Cross-Cultural Cognitive Examination performance in patients with Parkinson's disease and Alzheimer's disease. J Nerv Ment Dis 1994;182:432–436.

(3) Wolfe N, Imai Y, Otani C, et al. Criterion validity of the Cross-Cultural Cognitive Examination in Japan. J Gerontol 1992; 47:P289–P296.

(4) Kua EH, Ko SM. A questionnaire to screen for cognitive impairment among elderly people in developing countries. Acta Psychiatr Scand 1992;85:119–122.

(5) Kokmen E, Naessens JM, Offord KP. A Short Test of Mental Status: description and preliminary results. Mayo Clin Proc 1987;62:281–288.

(6) Kokmen E, Smith GE, Petersen RC, et al. The Short Test of Mental Status: correlations with standardized psychometric testing. Arch Neurol 1991;48:725–728.

(7) Storandt M, Botwinick J, Danziger WL, et al. Psychometric differentiation of mild senile dementia of the Alzheimer type. Arch Neurol 1984;41:497–499.

(8) Tierney MC, Snow G, Reid DW, et al. Psychometric differentiation of dementia: replication and extension the findings of Storandt and coworkers. Arch Neurol 1987;44:720–722.

(9) Storandt M, Hill RD. Very mild senile dementia of the Alzheimer type: II. Psychometric test performance. Arch Neurol 1989;46:383–386.

(10) Eslinger PJ, Damasio AR, Benton AL, et al. Neuropsychologic detection of abnormal mental decline in older persons. JAMA 1985;253:670–674.

(11) Pfeffer RI, Kurosaki TT, Harrah CH, et al. A survey diagnostic tool for senile dementia. Am J Epidemiol 1981;114:515–527.

(12) Pfeffer RI, Kurosaki TT, Chance JM, et al. Use of the Mental Function Index in older adults: reliability, validity and measurement of change over time. Am J Epidemiol 1984;120:922–935.

(13) Knopman DS, Ryberg S. A verbal memory test with high predictive accuracy for dementia of the Alzheimer type. Arch Neurol 1989;46:141–145.

(14) Mowry BJ, Burvill PW. A study of mild dementia in the community using a wide range of diagnostic criteria. Br J Psychiatry 1988;153:328–334.

(15) Scherr P, Albert M, Funkenstein HH, et al. Correlates of cognitive function in an elderly community population. Am J Epidemiol 1988;128:1084–1101.

(16) Albert M, Smith LA, Scherr PA, et al. Use of brief cognitive tests to identify individuals in the community with clinically diagnosed Alzheimer's disease. Int J Neurosci 1991;57:167–178.

(17) Teng EL, Hasegawa K, Homma A, et al. The Cognitive Abilities Screening Instrument (CASI): a practical test for cross-cultural epidemiological studies of dementia. Int Psychogeriatr 1994;6:45–58.

(18) Hajek VE, Rutman DL, Scher H. Brief assessment of cognitive impairment in patients with stroke. Arch Phys Med Rehabil 1989;70:114–117.

(19) Schwamm LH, Van Dyke C, Kiernan RJ, et al. The Neurobehavioral Cognitive Status Examination: comparison with the Cognitive Capacity Screening Examination and the Mini-Mental State Examination in a neurosurgical population. Ann Intern Med 1987;107:486–491.

(20) Reisberg B. The Brief Cognitive Rating Scale and Global Deterioration Scale. In: Crook T, Ferris S, Bartus R, eds. Assessment in geriatric psychopharmacology. New Canaan, Connecticut: Mark Powley, 1983:19–35.

(21) Reisberg B, Ferris S, Anand R, et al. Clinical assessments of cognition in the aged. In: Shamoian LA, ed. Biology and treatment of dementia in the elderly. Washington, DC: American Psychiatric Press, 1984:16–37.

(22) Reisberg B, Schneck MK, Ferris SH, et al. The Brief Cognitive Rating Scale (BCRS): findings in primary degenerative dementia (PDD). Psychopharmacol Bull 1983; 19:47–51.

(23) Hachinski VC, Iliff LD, Zilhka E. Cerebral blood flow in dementia. Arch Neurol 1975;32:632–637.

(24) Huppert FA, Tym E. Clinical and neuropsychological assessment of dementia. Br Med Bull 1986;42:11–18.

(25) Small GW. Revised ischemic score for diagnosing multi-infarct dementia. J Clin Psychiatry 1985;46:514–517.

(26) Dening TR, Berrios GE. The Hachinski Ischaemic Score: a reevaluation. Int J Geriatr Psychiatry 1992;7:585–590.

(27) Jorm AF, Jacomb PA. The Informant Questionnaire on Cognitive Decline in the Elderly (IQCODE): socio-demographic correlates, reliability, validity and some norms. Psychol Med 1989;19:1015–1022.

(28) Jorm AF. A short form of the Informant Questionnaire on Cognitive Decline in the Elderly (IQCODE): development and cross-validation. Psychol Med 1994;24:145–153.

(29) Shader RI, Harmatz JS, Salzman C. A new scale for clinical assessment in geriatric populations: Sandoz Clinical Assessment—Geriatric (SCAG). J Am Geriatr Soc 1974;22:107–113.

(30) Venn RD. The Sandoz Clinical Assessment—Geriatric (SCAG) scale: a general purpose psychogeriatric rating scale. Gerontology 1983;29:185–198.

(31) Salzman C. The Sandoz Clinical Assessment—Geriatric scale. In: Crook T, Ferris S, Bartus R, eds. Assessment in geriatric psychopharmacology. New Canaan, Connecticut: Mark Powley, 1983:53–58.

(32) Cole MG, Dastoor DP. A new hierarchic approach to the measurement of dementia. Psychosomatics 1987;28:298–304.

(33) Cole MG, Dastoor DP, Koszycki D. The Hierarchic Dementia Scale. J Clin Exp Gerontol 1983;5:219–234.

(34) Zaudig M, Mittelhammer J, Hiller W, et al. SIDAM—a structured interview for the diagnosis of dementia of the Alzheimer type, multi-infarct dementia and dementias of other aetiology according to ICD-10 and DSM-III-R. Psychol Med 1991;21:225–236.

(35) Kay DWK, Henderson AS, Scott R, et al. Dementia and depression among the elderly living in the Hobart community: the effect of the diagnostic criteria on the prevalence rates. Psychol Med 1985;15:771–788.

(36) Henderson AS. The Canberra Interview for the Elderly: a new field instrument for the diagnosis of dementia and depression by ICD-10 and DSM-III-R. Acta Psychiatr Scand 1992;85:105–113.

(37) Mackinnon A, Christensen H, Cullen JS, et al. The Canberra Interview for the Elderly: assessment of its validity in the diagnosis of dementia and depression. Acta Psychiatr Scand 1993;87:146–151.

8

Pain Measurements

Several arguments have been raised to support the claim that pain measurement is the most challenging and difficult area of subjective health measurement. It has been argued that pain is a private and internal sensation that cannot be directly observed or measured, but whose measurement depends wholly on the subjective response of the person experiencing it. By contrast, the measurement of physical disability is more direct: we both define and measure it in terms of observable behaviors such as walking a given distance or climbing stairs. It is also clear that pain is multidimensional; a single assessment of intensity will not adequately reflect the contrast between, say, a pin prick, a toothache, and a burn. Finally, pain measurement is, par excellence, the area in which subjective reports represent a blend of the strength of the underlying pain and of the person's emotional response to it. The anxiety and fear that so often accompany pain are strongly influenced by cultural norms and values and seriously complicate its measurement.

These comments are true, and yet they do not quite capture the essence of the difficulty of measuring pain; indeed, they can also apply to other areas of measurement—depression, anxiety, patient satisfaction. Like pain, depression is also an inner state, private and only measurable indirectly. Like pain, it has several aspects, such as intensity and temporal variation, but measuring depression differs from measuring pain in that we consider depression as a response, whereas we normally talk of pain as a stimulus. This may be the nub of the problem in pain measurement; we try to infer pain (as a stimulus) from the sufferer's subjective response to it. However, the way the pain is reported is influenced by many factors, biological, social, and psychological. Biologically, there may not be a linear relationship between pain and the extent of tissue damage; minor damage may give rise to intense pain and vice versa. Numerous individual and cultural factors, including sex, upbringing, personality, and age, have been shown to influence a person's response to pain (1, 2). Psychological factors also modify the reaction to pain, and these may vary independently of the strength of the pain stimulus so that they cannot be predicted from it. Thus, more than is the case with other areas of subjective measurement, reports of pain reflect the combined influence of the pain stimulus, environmental circumstances, and the characteristics of the individual experiencing it.

The multidimensional assessment of pain began in the 1950s. For example, Beecher distinguished two components of pain: the original sensation, which he described in terms of its intensity and its temporal and spatial distribution, and the reactive component, which he considered to be a function of personality, emotional, and social factors (3). This distinction achieved widespread acceptance and later research identified physiological mechanisms underlying the variation in response to pain between different people. Melzack's gate control theory of pain, for example, accepts the relevance of psychological factors in mediating the pain response (4). Treatment for pain reflects these multiple influences on the pain experience; pain therapy may tackle either the physical pain stimulus or the patient's reaction to it. Psychological or behavioral approaches to therapy may be used to modify the response to intractable pain where the stimulus itself cannot be alleviated. Clinical experience also shows that the required dose of analgesics will vary according to the individual's pain threshold, larger doses being needed for those with lower thresholds.

A wide variety of pain measurement methods have been proposed to respond to the challenges of measuring pain. Historically, these have evolved from a straightforward approach in which pain is defined and measured in terms of the person's subjective response, to a series of more complex methods that attempt to disentangle the subjective element in the response from a more objective estimate of the underlying pain. The former approach has been long established and forms the basis for the majority of the current measurement techniques. As an example, Merskey's definition of pain speaks in terms of a single-dimensional subjective response: "Pain is an unpleasant experience which we primarily associate with tissue damage, or describe in terms of tissue damage . . . the presence of which is signalled by some form of visible or audible behavior."(5, p195)

Subjective measurements of pain usually concentrate on its sensation and intensity, although other dimensions include the emotional reaction to the pain experience, or its temporal fluctuation. Most authors concur that measurements can capture two dimensions of the pain experience: the sensory aspects of the pain and the person's emotional reaction to the pain experience (6, p296). Some measurement methods attempt to distinguish the stimulus strength from the subjective response, although these techniques are not yet widely used. They are mainly based on sensory decision theory, which was described in Chapter 2. In its application to pain measurement, this involves the repeated presentation of two stimuli: noise (e.g., a low level of electrical current) or experimentally induced pain, in random order. The respondent classifies each as painful or not, and from the resulting pattern of true- and false-positive responses, indices of discriminability and of response bias can be derived (7). The first shows how accurately the respondent can distinguish between various levels of a pain stimulus; this index of perceptual performance reflects the functioning of the neurosensory system. The second index shows the threshold at which the respondent applies the term "pain" in describing these stimuli; it is related to his attitudes toward pain. A high response threshold suggests stoicism; a low one indicates an individual who readily reports pain. This analytic technique has been used in experimental studies to determine whether analgesics work by influencing discriminability (i.e., by making the stimulus feel less noxious) or by shifting the response bias (making the respondent more or less willing to call the stimulus "painful"). Clark and Yang showed that a placebo worked as an analgesic principally by reducing the respondent's tendency to label the experimental stimulus as "painful" rather than by altering the person's ability to feel it: the placebo seems to alter the affective response, not the perception of the stimulus (7).

Although they offer exciting research possibilities, measurement methods based on sensory decision theory are seldom used in clinical applications, which employ far simpler, intensity scales. The present chapter describes a range of methods of both types, partly in the hope of encouraging a shift away from the current heavy reliance on simple intensity measurements.

SCOPE OF THE CHAPTER

The techniques for collecting data to measure pain fall into three main categories: *(i)* those that record verbal or written descriptions of pain, *(ii)* those that rate pain via its effect on the observable behavior of the person experiencing it, and *(iii)* analogue techniques, commonly used in laboratory studies, in which the respondent compares her pain with an experimentally induced pain stimulus of known intensity. Unfortunately, few studies have yet compared these different approaches, and the comparisons that have been made suggest a rather low agreement: they appear to be measuring different aspects of pain (8). General reviews of pain measurement techniques are given by Frederiksen et al. (1), Chapman (9), Reading (10), and Over (11).

QUESTIONNAIRE TECHNIQUES

The majority of pain questionnaires concentrate on intensity and use adjectives (mild, moderate, severe) or a numerical scale to represent the intensity continuum. A variant of this has been to use visual analogue scales that represent the intensity dimension by a plain line without verbal or numerical guides (see the review of Huskisson's measurement technique). Intensity ratings may be extended to add a time dimension by using diaries or pain charts that record variations in pain over the course of a day, and may show the medications taken. Cumulative scores representing the duration of pain at each intensity level may be derived from the chart (12). In clinical settings, verbal ratings, nu-merical scales, an the visual analogue scale seem to be interchangeable (13). All three methods appear highly intercorrelated, although the numerical and visual analogue correlate the most strongly. With less educated patients, numerical ratings may be more easily understood than the visual analogue scale (14), and the numerical scales can evidently be more easily administered to very sick patients. Hence, numerical scales have been endorsed for use in cancer clinical trials as easier to understand and easier to score (15).

Extending the questionnaire approach to cover more than the intensity and duration of pain, Melzack's McGill Pain Questionnaire gives a qualitative description of the pain and of the patient's affective response to pain. Subsequent refinements of the McGill method, such as Tursky's Pain Perception Profile, have sought to improve on its scale characteristics.

These methods concentrate on the sufferer's own pain level. Other questionnaires have been developed to assess the respondent's emotional response to pain other than her own as a way to indicate her affective response to pain, which is presumed to influence the reporting of pain severity. One method consists of a color film depicting increasingly severe levels of pain applied to a human hand. The viewer's emotional response to the scenes is graded (16).

BEHAVIORAL MEASUREMENTS OF PAIN

Because pain causes changes in behavior (often involuntarily), such changes can be used as indicators of pain levels. This is analogous to the behavioral rating scales used to measure functional disability (see, for example, the Kenny scale in Chapter 3). Fordyce has discussed the correspondence between verbal responses and overt pain behavior (17, 18). Whether recording behavior offers a more "objective" approach to measuring pain is open to debate; behavior could reflect the subjective response to pain as much as do verbal reports, but it may also be argued that pain behavior such as grimacing or wincing is involuntary and less influenced by attitudes than is answering questions. A critical review of the use of behavior as a basis for inferring pain is given by Turk and Flor (19).

There are several types of behavioral measurement of pain. An approach commonly used in clinical studies is to record reductions in functional performance due to pain, with the pain being graded according to how seriously it limits physical function. Examples of such scales are given by Kessler (20) and by Fields et al. (21) and are illustrated by Jette's index, which is described in Chapter 3. Alternatively, pain may be inferred from health care utilization, including taking medications. This is a common approach in research on headaches, although medication use reflects both the pain and the attitudes of the sufferer to drugs. In another approach, other behaviors (voluntary and involuntary) such as gasping, grimacing, panting, or rubbing parts of the body may be observed and recorded. An experimental procedure may be used in which the patient makes a series of body movements and the response is observed (22, 23). Observation should evidently be as unobtrusive as possible, although this may be hard to standardize and may prove costly. Craig and Prkachin list a number of behavioral measurements of this type (24), and examples include the University of Alabama in Birmingham (UAB) Pain Behavior Scale (25) and an observational method used with low back pain patients (26).

ANALOGUE METHODS

The analogue approach requires the person to match his "normal" pain with various levels of experimentally induced pain, typically radiant heat or an electric shock. Once a match is found, the clinical pain is described in terms of the strength of the stimulus used to induce the experimental pain. There are several alternative strate-

gies. The respondent may be asked to apply a physical effort (such as squeezing a pressure bulb) at an intensity that matches his pain level; Peck had patients match the intensity of their pain with the intensity of a sound produced by an audiometer (27). Smith et al. described the submaximal effort tourniquet method, in which the blood circulation in the arm is stopped by an inflated blood-pressure cuff; the respondent is then asked to squeeze a hand exerciser slowly 20 times. This produces an increasingly intense pain, and the time between squeezing the exerciser and the point at which the patient judges the experimental pain to match his "normal" pain gives a numerical indication of his clinical pain. The length of endurance until the pain becomes unbearable indicates the maximum pain tolerance level (9, 28). Clinical pain may be expressed as a percentage of the pain tolerance level. Sternbach has discussed the limitations of the tourniquet test. These include variability in strength between individuals and problems of representing pain on a linear time scale when arguably pain does not rise as a linear function of time in the test; there may also be a practice effect (29).

There has also been a more general discussion of the validity of the analogue methods as indicators of clinical pain (8). Many of the affective features of the pain response normally seen in clinical settings may be modified in laboratory experiments. Much of the fear and anxiety that accompanies normal pain are absent: the sufferer knows the experimental pain is of a fixed duration and under the control of the experimenter. Over (11) commented that while laboratory experiments studying pain responses may constitute good psychophysics, they may have little relevance to pain outside the laboratory.

We have chosen to review measurement scales that illustrate some of the themes we have introduced. We begin with visual analogue scales that measure pain intensity and follow this with the McGill Pain Questionnaire developed by Melzack as a multidimensional pain rating. Following this we review two recent scales that are derived from the McGill Questionnaire: the Brief Pain Inventory and the Medical Outcomes Study instrument. We then review two condition-specific instruments: Fairbank's Oswestry questionnaire for low back pain and the Leavitt's Back Pain Classification Scale. Leavitt's scale distinguishes between pain that reflects psychological disturbance and that based on organic causes, as does the next scale we review: Zung's Pain and Distress Scale. The final two methods we describe, the Illness Behavior Questionnaire developed by Pilowsky and the Pain Perception Profile by Tursky, both distinguish between the affective response to pain and its underlying physical intensity. Table 8.1 summarizes the characteristics of the scales reviewed.

REFERENCES

(1) Frederiksen LW, Lynd RS, Ross J. Methodology in the measurement of pain. Behav Ther 1978;9:486–488.

(2) Tursky B, Jamner LD, Friedman R. The Pain Perception Profile: a psychophysical approach to the assessment of pain report. Behav Ther 1982;13:376–394.

(3) Beecher HK. The measurement of pain: prototype for the quantitative study of subjective responses. Pharmacol Rev 1957;9:159–209.

(4) Melzack R. The puzzle of pain. New York: Basic Books, 1973.

(5) Bond MR. New approaches to pain. Psychol Med 1980;10:195–199.

(6) Cleeland CS. Pain assessment in cancer. In: Osoba D, ed. Effect of cancer on quality of life. Boca Raton, Florida: CRC Press, 1991:293–305.

(7) Clark WC, Yang JC. Applications of sensory decision theory to problems in laboratory and clinical pain. In: Melzack R, ed. Pain measurement and assessment. New York: Raven Press, 1983:15–25.

(8) Postlethwaite R, Grieve N, Santacroce T, et al. An analysis of pain produced by the submaximum effort tourniquet test. In: Peck C, Wallace M, eds. Problems in pain. Sydney, Australia: Pergamon Press, 1980:128–135.

(9) Chapman CR. Measurement of pain: problems and issues. In: Bonica JJ, Albe-Fessard DG, eds. Advances in pain research and therapy. Vol. I. New York: Raven Press, 1976:345–353.

(10) Reading AE. Testing pain mechanisms in persons in pain. In: Wall PD, Melzack R, eds. Textbook of pain. 2nd ed. Edinburgh: Churchill-Livingstone, 1989:269–280.

(11) Over R. Clinical and experimental pain. In: Peck C, Wallace M, eds. Problems in pain. Sydney, Australia: Pergamon Press, 1980:94–100.

(12) Elton D, Burrows GD, Stanley GV. Clinical measurement of pain. Med J Aust 1979;1:109–111.

(13) Jensen MP, Karloy P, Braver S. The measurement of clinical pain intensity: a comparison of six methods. Pain 1986;27:117–126.

(14) Ferraz MB, Quaresma MR, Aquino LRL, et al. Reliability of pain scales in the assessment of literate and illiterate patients with rheumatoid arthritis. J Rheumatol 1990;17:1022–1024.

(15) Moinpour CM, Feigl P, Metch B, et al. Quality of life end points in cancer clinical trials: review and recommendations. J Natl Cancer Inst 1989;81:485–495.

(16) Elton D, Burrows GD, Stanley GV. Apperception of pain. In: Peck D, Wallace M, eds. Problems in pain. Sydney, Australia: Pergamon Press, 1980:117–120.

(17) Fordyce WE. The validity of pain behavior measurement. In: Melzack R, ed. Pain measurement and assessment. New York: Raven Press, 1983:145–153.

(18) Fordyce WE, Lansky D, Calsyn DA, et al. Pain measurement and pain behavior. Pain 1984;18:53–69.

(19) Turk DC, Flor H. Pain > pain behaviors: the utility and limitations of the pain behavior construct. Pain 1987;31:277–295.

(20) Kessler HH. Disability—determination and evaluation. Philadelphia: Lea & Febiger, 1970.

(21) Fields HL, Florence D, Keefe F, et al. Measuring pain and dysfunction. In: Osterweis M, Kleinman A, Mechanic D, eds. Pain and disability: clinical, behavioral, and public policy perspectives. Washington, DC: National Academy Press, 1987:211–231.

(22) Waddell G, McCulloch J, Kummel E, et al. Nonorganic physical signs in low back pain. Spine 1980;5:117–125.

(23) Follick MJ, Ahern DK, Aberger EW. Development of an audiovisual taxonomy of pain behavior: reliability and discriminant validity. Health Psychol 1985;4:555–568.

(24) Craig KD, Prkachin KM. Nonverbal measures of pain. In: Melzack R, ed. Pain mea-

Table 8.1 Comparison of the Quality of Pain Scales*

Measurement	Scale	Number of items	Application	Administered by (time)	Studies using method	Reliability		Validity	
						Thoroughness	Results	Thoroughness	Results
Visual Analogue Pain Rating Scale (Various authors, 1974)	ratio	1	clinical	self (30 sec)	many	+ +	+ + +	+ +	+ +
McGill Pain Questionnaire (Melzack, 1975)	ordinal, interval	20	clinical	self (15–20 min)	many	+	+	+ +	+ +
Brief Pain Inventory (Cleeland, 1982)	ordinal	20	clinical	self (10-15 min)	several	+	+ +	+	+
Medical Outcomes Study Pain Measures (Sherbourne, 1992)	ordinal	12	survey	self	few	+	+ +	+	+ +
Oswestry Low Back Pain Disability Questionnaire (Fairbank, 1980)	ordinal	60	clinical	self (<5 min)	few	+	+ +	+	+
Back Pain Classification Scale (Leavitt, 1978)	interval	13	clinical	self (5–10 min)	several	+	+ +	+ +	+ +
Pain and Distress Scale (Zung, 1983)	ordinal	20	clinical	self	few	+	+ +	+	+ +
Illness Behavior Questionnaire (Pilowsky, 1975)	ordinal	52	clinical	self	many	+ +	+ +	+ + +	+ +
Pain Perception Profile (Tursky, 1976)	ratio	37	research	expert	few	+	0	+	0

*For an explanation of the categories used, see Chapter 1, pages 6–7.

surement and assessment. New York: Raven Press, 1983:173–179.

(25) Richards JS, Nepomuceno C, Riles M, et al. Assessing pain behavior: the UAB Pain Behavior Scale. Pain 1982;14:393–398.

(26) Keefe FJ, Block AR. Development of an observation method for assessing pain behavior in chronic low back pain patients. Behav Ther 1982;13:363–375.

(27) Peck RR. A precise technique for the measurement of pain. Headache 1967;7:189–194.

(28) Smith GM, Lowenstein E, Hubbard JH, et al. Experimental pain produced by the submaximal effort tourniquet technique: further evidence of validity. J Pharmacol Exp Ther 1968;163:468–474.

(29) Sternbach RA. The tourniquet pain test. In: Melzack R, ed. Pain measurement and assessment. New York: Raven Press, 1983:27–31.

VISUAL ANALOGUE PAIN RATING SCALES
(Various authors, from 1974 onward)

Purpose

Visual analogue rating scales (VAS) provide a simple way to record subjective estimates of pain intensity.

Conceptual Basis

Visual analogue measurements are normally used only to rate the overall severity of pain, although there is no reason why a VAS could not be applied in measuring other dimensions, such as levels of anxiety or the emotional responses associated with pain. Indeed, visual analogue scales have long been used in many areas of psychological measurement (1) and have recently been incorporated into health-related quality of life instruments.

Description

Visual analogue scales have been used in psychological assessment since the early years of the 20th century and are often used in measuring pain. The application of this approach to pain can be linked to the work of Huskisson, who popularized it during the 1970s (2). A visual analogue scale is a line that represents the continuum of the symptom to be rated. The scale, conventionally a straight line 10 cm long, is marked at each end with labels that indicate the range being considered: in measuring pain Huskisson used the phrases "pain as bad as it could be" and "no pain" (3, 4). Typical formats are shown in Exhibit 8.1. Alternative phrases that have been recommended for the extreme end include "agonizing pain" (5, Table 4) and "worst pain imaginable" (6). Patients are asked to place a mark on the line at a point representing the severity of their pain. The scale requires only about 30 seconds to complete.

Many alternative formats have been tested. For example, intermediate marks may be placed in the line, although a plain line is normally used; this may be printed either vertically or horizontally. Curved lines have been tried (with or without intermediate marks). Descriptive terms may be placed along the plain line, such as "severe," "moderate," or "mild." Some of the studies comparing these alternatives are reviewed, and we provide summary recommendations concerning alternative formats in the Commentary section.

There are several ways to score the VAS. The distance of the respondent's mark from the lower end of the scale, measured in millimeters, forms the basic score, ranging from 0 to 100. Alternatively, a 20-point grid may be superimposed over the line to give a categorical rating. Huskisson justified this approach by noting that it represents the maximal level of discrimination people can use in recording pain levels (2). The distribution of results is not normal, and transformations may be applied to normalize the data (2, p1128; 7). While nonparametric statistical analyses are generally considered appropriate (3), one study showed that VAS measures produced a measurement with ratio scale properties (8). Scoring procedures have been reviewed (1, pp1016–1017; 9).

In estimating pain relief, it may not be

Exhibit 8.1   Alternative Formats for Rating Scales Tested by Huskisson

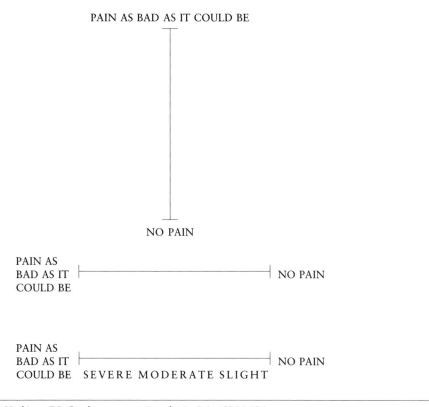

Adapted from Scott J, Huskisson EC. Graphic representation of pain. Pain 1976;2:176.

appropriate simply to compare scores before and after treatment, for the possible magnitude of this difference is determined by the initial score (2). Indeed, initial and subsequent pain ratings tend to be correlated; Huskisson reported coefficients of 0.62 and 0.63 (2, Figures 5,6). Rather than comparing ratings before and after treatment, therefore, Huskisson recommended using a rating of pain relief. This can take the form of a descriptive scale (such as none, slight, moderate, or complete relief) or a visual analogue scale ranging from no relief to complete relief of pain. Comparing the two methods, Huskisson showed that the simple descriptive scale gave better results when completed by patients without assistance (2). An advantage of a pain relief scale is that, whatever their initial pain

level, each respondent has the same magnitude of potential response (5, p239).

Reliability

Scott and Huskisson studied the repeatability of visual analogue pain scales and also compared scales printed vertically and horizontally. One hundred rheumatology patients were given a vertical and a horizontal scale in random order. The correlation was 0.99 between the scores, although scores on the horizontal scale were slightly, but not significantly, lower than on the vertical scale (mean 10.85 versus 11.05) (10, Table 1). A comparison of retest reliability with literate and nonliterate patients found the VAS to be more reliable (0.94) in literate than in nonliterate groups (0.71); equivalent figures for a numerical rating scale were 0.96 and 0.95, suggesting that the numerical rating scale was not affected by literacy level; results for a verbal rating scale were 0.90 and 0.82 (11, Table 2).

Validity

Huskisson reported a correlation of 0.75 between a visual analogue scale printed vertically and a four-point descriptive scale rating pain as slight, moderate, severe, or agonizing (4). The association was probably attenuated by the restricted number of categories on the descriptive scale. Similar analyses on samples of 100 and 104 rheumatic patients gave correlations ranging from 0.71 to 0.78 between four-point descriptive scales and visual analogue scales printed vertically or horizontally. Correlations between the vertical and horizontal scales ranged from 0.89 to 0.91 (12, Tables 1,2). A correlation of 0.81 was reported between a VAS and a five-point verbal rating scale using repeated measurements of six patients (13). The VAS was also more sensitive to change than the verbal rating scale. In an experimental study, Price et al. found that a VAS provided a better ratio scale indication of facial pain than did a numerical rating scale; a mechanically administered VAS provided similar results to a paper-and-pencil version (14).

Elton et al. obtained correlations from 0.60 to 0.63 between a visual analogue scale and Melzack's McGill Pain Questionnaire (MPQ), although the latter was scored in an unconventional manner (15, Table 1). In a second study, correlations with the MPQ ranged from 0.42 (affective score) to 0.57 (evaluative) (16, Table 1); a third study gave correlations that varied widely according to the type of patient being assessed: the correlation between the VAS and the Present Pain Index ranged from 0.21 to 0.76 (17, Tables 2,3). McCormack et al. reviewed 17 correlations between VAS pain measures and other pain assessments. Only two correlations were not significant and the coefficients ranged from 0.29 to 0.92 (1, Table 4).

Visual analogue scales are more sensitive to change than are verbal rating scales and so require smaller sample sizes in evaluative studies (5, p238). The comparison with numerical rating scales is less clear, however. Guyatt et al. showed that both methods showed similar responsiveness when standardized to the same scale range and so, given its greater simplicity, they recommended the numerical rating over the VAS (18).

Alternative Forms

Exhibits 8.1 and 8.2 illustrate some of the formats for the VAS. Other methods that have been tested include a computer animation, showing a scale with a moving marker which the respondent stops at the appropriate place while the computer calculates the score (19). A simpler mechanical device uses a 15-cm plastic slider that is moved by the respondent, revealing a bar of deepening red that indicates perceived intensity; a numerical-score is indicated on the back (14). Scales have also been presented as thermometers to try and clarify the metaphor and to underscore the links with health.

The correlation between vertical and horizontal scales is generally high. In measur-

Exhibit 8.2 Formats of the Numerical Rating (NRS) and Visual Analogue Scales (VAS) as Used by Downie et al.

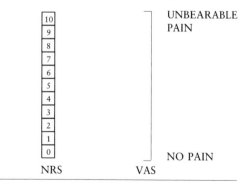

Reproduced from Downie WW, Leatham PA, Rhind VM, Wright V, Branco JA, Anderson JA. Studies with pain rating scales. Ann Rheum Dis 1978;37:378, Figure 1. With permission.

ing shortness of breath, for example, the correlation between vertical and horizontal scales was 0.97 (20). As discussed below, there may be reasons that favor the horizontal format.

In her study of children aged 3 to 15 years, McGrath et al. successfully used the VAS to provide numerical-scale weights for a pain measurement using pictures of faces expressing pain (21, p391).

Commentary

Huskisson summarized the advantages of visual analogue scales as follows:

Visual analogue scales provide the patients with a robust, sensitive, reproducible method of expressing pain severity. Results correlate well with other methods of measuring pain. The method is applicable to all patients regardless of language and can be used by children aged 5 or more years. (3, p768)

Most studies that compare VAS with numerical and verbal ratings conclude that the VAS or the numerical ratings are statistically preferable to the verbal rating scales (5). Some patients have difficulty with the VAS, however; these seem mainly to be elderly or less educated respondents who may have difficulty in grasping the metaphor of the continuum represented by the VAS (11). Frank et al. suggested that a scale showing faces that vary in their expression of pain may be better for nonliterate groups (22). Downie et al. compared a visual analogue scale with a ten-point numerical rating scale of the type shown in Exhibit 8.2 and argued that the latter "was to be preferred on the grounds of measurement error," perhaps because the visual analogue scale offers a confusingly wide range of choice (12). Of 100 patients assessed by Huskisson, seven were unable to understand the idea of the scale when it was first explained, though all could use a descriptive scale (2). Some patients cluster their scores at the midpoint of the scale or at either end, suggesting that they do not comprehend the idea of the continuum (1, p1014). Accordingly, Scott and Huskisson

recommended that patients complete a visual analogue scale under supervision before doing it on their own.

Several conclusions may be drawn from the studies that have compared different formats for the VAS. First, horizontal lines are generally preferred to vertical. Dixon and Bird warned that a distortion may arise in using a vertical scale from perspective when the page lies flat on a table (23). The failure rate may be higher in vertical than horizontal scales (1, p1008). Vertical scales give less normally distributed data (5, p238). An interesting exception to these results was obtained in a study of Chinese postoperative pain patients, who made fewer errors using the vertical format (which, of course, resembles the orientation of Chinese writing) (24). Second, a comparison of 5-, 10-, 15-, and 25-cm lines suggested that the 5-cm line provided less reliable results than other lengths (25). The conventional 10-cm line seems the most appropriate (6). Third, there seems little to gain by adding intermediate dividing marks along the line (5, p238). Fourth, a straight line seems adequate, although in one study some respondents found that a curved line had the benefit of familiarity by reminding them of an analogue dial (such as a speedometer or bathroom scale) (5, p238). Fifth, it is generally recommended that neither numbers nor verbal labels be placed along the length of the line (1, p1008). Scott and Huskisson tested many formats and concluded that scales with adjectives tended to produce a clustering of responses beside the adjectives (2, Figures 2,3). If adjectives are to be used, they should be printed so that they spread along the entire length of the line, as illustrated in the last example of Exhibit 8.1.

A debate has arisen over whether or not patients should be shown their initial pain ratings when reassessing pain on follow-up. Scott and Huskisson argued that, because increasing time between assessments may make it difficult to recall the initial pain, patients should see their previous scores when making subsequent judgments of pain severity (26). Other authors concur that recall of the initial ratings is inaccurate and perhaps biased (27, 28). Dixon and Bird disagreed: although patients may find it easier to rate their current pain level when shown previous scores, such ratings may not agree with other indices of disease progress (23). They also showed that the accuracy with which a person could reproduce marks on a visual analogue scale varied according to the placement of the original mark: not surprisingly, marks close to the ends or the center of the line were more accurately reproduced than marks in other positions (23).

Visual analogue scales give more sensitive and precise measurements than descriptive pain scales. They can also be used to record other ratings: intensity, frequency, etc. The choice between verbal rating scales and the VAS will depend upon the degree of sensitivity required: for research purposes, a categorical rating may be too crude, although it appears to be simpler for patients to complete. The data presented by Downie et al. suggest that a ten-point numerical scale may provide a compromise position between the four-point rating and the visual analogue methods.

REFERENCES

(1) McCormack HM, Horne DJdeL, Sheather S. Clinical applications of visual analogue scales: a critical review. Psychol Med 1988;18:1007–1019.

(2) Huskisson EC. Measurement of pain. Lancet 1974;2:1127–1131.

(3) Huskisson EC. Measurement of pain. J Rheumatol 1982;9:768–769.

(4) Scott J, Huskisson EC. Graphic representation of pain. Pain 1976;2:175–184.

(5) Sriwatanakul K, Kelvie W, Lasagna L, et al. Studies with different types of visual analog scales for measurement of pain. Clin Pharmacol Ther 1983;34:234–239.

(6) Seymour RA, Simpson JM, Charlton JE, et al. An evaluation of length and endphrase of visual analogue scales in dental pain. Pain 1985;21:177–185.

(7) Stubbs DF. Visual analogue scales. Br J Clin Pharmacol 1979;7:124.

(8) Price DD, McGrath PA, Rafii A, et al. The validation of visual analogue scales as ratio scale measures for chronic and experimental pain. Pain 1983;17:45–56.

(9) Maxwell C. Sensitivity and accuracy of the visual analogue scale: a psycho-physical classroom experiment. Br J Clin Pharmacol 1978;6:15–24.

(10) Scott J, Huskisson EC. Vertical or horizontal visual analogue scales. Ann Rheum Dis 1979;38:560.

(11) Ferraz MB, Quaresma MR, Aquino LRL, et al. Reliability of pain scales in the assessment of literate and illiterate patients with rheumatoid arthritis. J Rheumatol 1990;17:1022–1024.

(12) Downie WW, Leatham PA, Rhind VM, et al. Studies with pain rating scales. Ann Rheum Dis 1978;37:378–381.

(13) Ohnhaus EE, Adler R. Methodological problems in the measurement of pain: a comparison between the verbal rating scale and the visual analogue scale. Pain 1975;1:379–384.

(14) Price DD, Bush FM, Long S, et al. A comparison of pain measurement characteristics of mechanical visual analogue and simple numerical rating scales. Pain 1994;56:217–226.

(15) Elton D, Burrows GD, Stanley GV. Clinical measurement of pain. Med J Aust 1979;1:109–111.

(16) Ahles TA, Ruckdeschel JC, Blanchard EB. Cancer-related pain—II. Assessment with visual analogue scales. J Psychosom Res 1984;28:121–124.

(17) Perry F, Heller PH, Levine JD. Differing correlations between pain measures in syndromes with or without explicable organic pathology. Pain 1988;34:185–189.

(18) Guyatt GH, Townsend M, Berman LB, et al. A comparison of Likert and visual analogue scales for measuring change in function. J Chronic Dis 1987;40:1129–1133.

(19) Swanston M, Abraham C, Macrae WA, et al. Pain assessment with interactive computer animation. Pain 1993;53:347–351.

(20) Gift AG. Validation of a vertical visual analogue scale as a measure of clinical dyspnoea. Rehabil Nurs 1989;14:323–325.

(21) McGrath PA, de Veber LL, Hearn MT. Multidimensional pain assessment in children. In: Fields HL, Dubner R, Cervero F, eds. Advances in pain research and therapy. Vol. 9. New York: Raven Press, 1985:387–393.

(22) Frank AJM, Moll SMH, Hart JF. A comparison of three ways of measuring pain. Rheumatol Rehabil 1982;21:211–217.

(23) Dixon JS, Bird HA. Reproducibility along a 10 cm vertical visual analogue scale. Ann Rheum Dis 1981;40:87–89.

(24) Aun C, Lam YM, Collett B. Evaluation of the use of visual analogue scale in Chinese patients. Pain 1986;25:215–221.

(25) Revill SI, Robinson JO, Rosen M, et al. The reliability of a linear analogue for evaluating pain. Anaesthesia 1976;31:1191–1198.

(26) Scott J, Huskisson EC. Accuracy of subjective measurements made with or without previous scores: an important source of error in serial measurement of subjective states. Ann Rheum Dis 1979;38:558–559.

(27) Linton SJ, Gotestam KG. A clinical comparison of two pain scales: correlation, remembering chronic pain, and a measure of compliance. Pain 1983;17:57–65.

(28) Carlsson AM. Assessment of chronic pain. I. Aspects of the reliability and validity of the visual analogue scale. Pain 1983; 16:87–101.

THE McGILL PAIN QUESTIONNAIRE
(Ronald Melzack, 1975)

Purpose

The McGill Pain Questionnaire (MPQ) was designed to provide a quantitative profile of three aspects of pain (1). The method was originally used in evaluating pain therapies; its use as a diagnostic aid has also been described (2).

Conceptual Basis

Melzack's major contribution to pain measurement has been to emphasize that the pain experience comprises several distinct aspects. In 1973 he wrote:

The problem of pain, since the beginning of this century, has been dominated by the concept that pain is purely a sensory experience. Yet it has a unique, distinctively unpleasant, affective quality that differentiates it from sensory experiences such as sight, hearing or touch. . . .

The motivational-affective dimension of pain is brought clearly into focus by clinical studies on frontal lobotomy. . . . Typically, these patients report after the operation that they still have pain but it does not bother them. . . . the suffering, the anguish are gone. . . . Similarly, patients exhibiting "pain asymbolia" . . . after

lesions of portions of the parietal lobe or the frontal cortex are able to appreciate the spatial and temporal properties of noxious stimuli (for example, they recognize pin pricks as sharp) but fail to withdraw or complain about them. . . .

These considerations suggest that there are three major psychological dimensions of pain: sensory-discriminative, motivational-affective, and cognitive-evaluative. (3, pp93–95)

Melzack argued that these three aspects of the pain experience are subserved by distinct systems in the brain (3) and he attempted to measure these dimensions with the MPQ. Melzack stressed that the questionnaire represented a first attempt at developing a measurement reflecting his theory of pain, and he suggested that other investigators might ultimately refine it (1). Nonetheless, the method continues to be used in its original form.

Description

The complete MPQ comprises sections recording the patient's diagnosis, drug regimen, medical history concerning pain, present pain pattern, accompanying symptoms and modifying factors, effects of pain, and the list of words describing pain which is the part of the instrument most commonly used. The present discussion concerns only this latter section of the questionnaire.

Melzack and Torgerson selected 102 words describing pain from the literature and from existing questionnaires (4). They sorted these words into the three major classes proposed in Melzack's theory of pain: words concerned with the sensory qualities of pain (e.g., temporal, thermal), those covering affective qualities of pain (e.g., fear, tension), and "evaluative words that describe the subjective overall intensity of the total experience of pain" (4). Within the three major classes, Melzack and Torgerson grouped words that were qualitatively similar, as shown in Exhibit 8.3. The suitability of this a priori grouping was checked by 20 reviewers. At first there were 16 such subclasses, but four others were added to give a final questionnaire with 20 subclasses (1).

Exhibit 8.3 The McGill Pain Questionnaire

PRI: S _____ A _____ E _____ M(S) _____ M(AE) _____ M(T) _____ PRI(T) _____
(1–10) (11–15) (16) (17–19) (20) (17–20) (1–20)

1 FLICKERING
QUIVERING
PULSING
THROBBING
BEATING
POUNDING

2 JUMPING
FLASHING
SHOOTING

3 PRICKING
BORING
DRILLING
STABBING
LANCINATING

4 SHARP
CUTTING
LACERATING

5 PINCHING
PRESSING
GNAWING
CRAMPING
CRUSHING

6 TUGGING
PULLING
WRENCHING

7 HOT
BURNING
SCALDING
SEARING

8 TINGLING
ITCHY
SMARTING
STINGING

9 DULL
SORE
HURTING
ACHING
HEAVY

10 TENDER
TAUT
RASPING
SPLITTING

11 TIRING
EXHAUSTING

12 SICKENING
SUFFOCATING

13 FEARFUL
FRIGHTFUL
TERRIFYING

14 PUNISHING
GRUELLING
CRUEL
VICIOUS
KILLING

15 WRETCHED
BLINDING

16 ANNOYING
TROUBLESOME
MISERABLE
INTENSE
UNBEARABLE

17 SPREADING
RADIATING
PENETRATING
PIERCING

18 TIGHT
NUMB
DRAWING
SQUEEZING
TEARING

19 COOL
COLD
FREEZING

20 NAGGING
NAUSEATING
AGONIZING
DREADFUL
TORTURING

PPI
0 No pain
1 MILD
2 DISCOMFORTING
3 DISTRESSING
4 HORRIBLE
5 EXCRUCIATING

PPI _____ COMMENTS:

CONSTANT
PERIODIC
BRIEF

ACCOMPANYING
SYMPTOMS:
NAUSEA
HEADACHE
DIZZINESS
DROWSINESS
CONSTIPATION
DIARRHEA

COMMENTS:

SLEEP:
GOOD
FITFUL
CAN'T SLEEP

COMMENTS:

FOOD INTAKE:
GOOD
SOME
LITTLE
NONE

COMMENTS:

ACTIVITY:
GOOD
SOME
LITTLE
NONE

COMMENTS:

Reproduced from Melzack R. Psychologic aspects of pain. Pain 1980;8:145. With permission.

An equal-appearing interval scaling procedure was used to estimate the intensity of pain represented by the words in each subclass. Three groups of judges (140 students, 20 physicians, and 20 patients) rated each word on a seven-point scale (4). Where there was disagreement among the three groups of judges on the rank ordering of a word within a subclass, the word was deleted from the questionnaire; scale values for the remaining words were based on the ratings made by patients. These values are shown in Exhibit 8.4.

The words were originally read to the patient by an interviewer so that unfamiliar words could be explained. This took 15 to 20 minutes, reducing to five to 10 minutes for patients familiar with the method. Subsequent users have employed the check list in a written format. The respondent is asked to select the one word in each subclass that most accurately describes her pain at that time (1). If none of the words applies, none is chosen. Other instructions have been used: patients may be asked to describe their "average pain," their "most intense" pain (5), or how their pain "typically feels" (6).

Four scoring methods were proposed by Melzack:

1. The sum of the scale values for all the words chosen in a given category (sensory, etc.) or across all categories. This was called a Pain Rating Intensity Score using scale values: PRI(S). The scale

Exhibit 8.4   Scale Weights for Scoring the McGill Pain Questionnaire

1	Flickering	1.89	2	Jumping	2.60	3	Pricking	1.94
	Quivering	2.50		Flashing	2.75		Boring	2.05
	Pulsing	2.56		* Shooting	3.42		Drilling	2.75
	* Throbbing	2.68					* Stabbing	3.45
	Beating	2.70					Lancinating	3.50
	Pounding	2.85						
4	* Sharp	2.95	5	Pinching	1.95	6	Tugging	2.16
	Cutting	3.20		Pressing	2.42		Pulling	2.35
	Lacerating	3.64		* Gnawing	2.53		Wrenching	3.47
				* Cramping	2.75			
				Crushing	3.58			
7	* Hot	2.47	8	Tingling	1.60	9	Dull	1.60
	* Burning	2.95		Itchy	1.70		Sore	1.90
	Scalding	3.50		Smarting	2.00		Hurting	2.45
	Searing	3.88		Stinging	2.25		* Aching	2.50
							* Heavy	2.95
10	* Tender	1.35	11	* Tiring	2.42	12	* Sickening	2.75
	Taut	2.36		* Exhausting	2.63		Suffocating	3.45
	Rasping	2.61						
	* Splitting	3.10						
13	* Fearful	3.30	14	* Punishing	3.50	15	Wretched	3.16
	Frightful	3.53		Gruelling	3.73		Blinding	3.45
	Terrifying	3.95		* Cruel	3.95			
				Vicious	4.26			
				Killing	4.50			
16	Annoying	1.89	17	Spreading	3.30	18	Tight	2.25
	Troublesome	2.42		Radiating	3.38		Numb	2.10
	Miserable	2.85		Penetrating	3.72		Drawing	2.53
	Intense	3.75		Piercing	3.78		Squeezing	2.35
	Unbearable	4.42					Tearing	3.68
19	Cool		20	Nagging	2.25			
	Cold			Nauseating	2.74			
	Freezing			Agonizing	3.20			
				Dreadful	4.11			
				Torturing	4.53			

* Asterisks identify the words included in the short-form MPQ.

Adapted from Melzack R, Torgerson WS. On the language of pain. Anesthesiology 1971;34:54–55, Table 1.

weights are shown in Exhibit 8.4. (Note that no scale weights are available for category 19.) This score can also be modified by dividing the summed value for each dimension by the total possible score on that dimension, giving a score ranging from 0 to 1.00 (7, p45).

2. As above, but replacing the scale values by a code indicating the rank placement of each word selected within its subclass: PRI(R). This score can be modified by multiplying the rank placement by a weight for each of the 20 groups of words in order to reflect the differing severity represented by the groups. The 20 weights are shown by Melzack et al. (8, Table 1).

3. The Number of Words Chosen: NWC.

4. The Present Pain Intensity (PPI) score on a 0-to-5 scale from the pain description section of the questionnaire shown in Exhibit 8.3: PPI.

Reliability

Melzack reported a small test–retest study in which ten patients completed the questionnaire three times at intervals ranging from three to seven days; there was an average consistency of response of 70.3% (1, p287). The extent of correlation between sensory and affective scores varies according to the type of pain being considered: in one study the range was from 0.51 to 0.85 (9, Tables II, III).

Validity

Melzack reviewed the agreement among the four scoring methods (1). Correlations are presented in Table 8.2 and show that the PPI score is not closely reflected by the other scores.

Dubuisson and Melzack compared responses to the MPQ given by 95 patients suffering from one of eight distinct pain syndromes. Discriminant function analyses showed that 77% of patients could be correctly classified into diagnostic groups on the basis of their verbal description of pain (2, 10).

Correlations between MPQ scores and

Table 8.2 Pearson Correlations Among Four Scoring Procedures for the McGill Pain Questionnaire (N = 248)

	PRI(S)	PRI(R)	NWC	PPI
PRI(S)	. . .	0.95	0.97	0.42*
PRI(R)		. . .	0.89	0.42
NWC			. . .	0.32
PPI				. . .

* Melzack did not give a precise figure, but stated it was "virtually identical" to the 0.42 obtained between PPI and PRI(R).

Adapted from Melzack R. The McGill Pain Questionnaire: major properties and scoring methods. Pain 1975;1:285.

visual analogue scales for 40 patients ranged from 0.50 for the affective score to 0.65 for the PPI and for the total score (11, Table 2). Equivalent figures from another study were 0.42 for the affective score and 0.57 for the evaluative (12, Table I).

Several reviewers of the MPQ have addressed the question of whether Melzack's selection and grouping of words do indeed reflect the three dimensions he proposed. Studies in Canada (5), the United States (13), and Britain (14), each using different types of pain patient, have reviewed the factor structure of the MPQ. A critical review of factor analytic investigations is given by Prieto and Geisinger (15). Two studies extracted four factors (11, 13), two found five (5, 16), and one found six (17); there is some correspondence between the factors obtained, although this is not great. Accordingly, differing conclusions have been drawn concerning the structure of the MPQ: Reading concluded that "Factorial investigations of the questionnaire provide support for the distinction between affective and sensory dimensions, but not for a distinctive evaluative component" (14). Crockett et al. concluded that "the repeated demonstration that the MPQ assesses substantially more than the three components originally proposed suggests that considerable caution is warranted with respect to using the 'sensory-evaluative-affective' method of scoring this test" (16, p461). Turk et al., however, concluded that the factor analyses confirmed the three-factor structure (sensory, affective, evaluative), although these factors were intercorrelated (18). There is clearly continuing debate over the structure of the MPQ. The factors tend to intercorrelate highly (0.64 to 0.81) but Melzack argued that this does not contradict their use as separate scores (19).

Alternative Forms

Because of the nuances of the adjectives in the MPQ, translation is challenging. Nonetheless, there are versions in most European languages including French (20), Italian (21), German (22), Dutch (23, 24), Danish (25), Norwegian (26), and Finnish (27). There is an Arabic version (28). Many of these adapt, rather than translate, the original and include widely varying numbers of adjectives: results cannot be compared. A Swedish abbreviated version, for example, contains 15 items and appears to have adequate reliability and validity (29). At times the linguistic challenge of translating the MPQ seems too strong to resist: there are at least three French Canadian versions, as well as a French version for use in France.

There have been various extensions to the MPQ. One version, called the McGill Comprehensive Pain Questionnaire, covers details of the patient's illness, personality, milieu, and coping resources (30). The Dartmouth Pain Questionnaire adds questions on pain complaints, somatic pain symptoms, and reductions in function and in self-esteem; some validity evidence is available (31). Another version added computer-colored animation to illustrate categories such as pressure (picture of a clamp squeezing a ball), throbbing (a hammer falling from various heights), piercing (a needle), and burning (32).

A short-form MPQ has been developed which includes 15 words (11 sensory, four affective) (33). The 15 words are identified with an asterisk in Exhibit 8.4; note that Melzack presents hot and burning together, as "hot-burning," and likewise combines "tiring-exhausting" and "punishing-cruel."

Each word or phrase is rated on a four-point intensity scale—0 = none, 1 = mild, 2 = moderate, and 3 = severe. In addition, the six-point PPI rating is included (see Exhibit 8.3) as is a visual analogue scale for rating intensity (33, Fig.1).

Commentary

There can be no question that Melzack's McGill Pain Questionnaire is the leading instrument for describing the diverse dimensions of pain. It is used extensively in many countries and has taken on the status of gold standard against which other, newer instruments are compared. Nonetheless, Melzack originally presented the MPQ as a preliminary version of a measurement method, and variants have been used in several studies. A strong point is that the MPQ was based on a clear theory of pain. The extensive influence of the MPQ is shown by the incorporation of sections into other scales, such as the Brief Pain Inventory, the MOS Pain Measures, the Back Pain Classification Scale and the Pain Perception Profile. A limitation of verbal descriptions is that people's use of pain language is probably not sufficiently consistent for an instrument such as the MPQ to be used to diagnose types of pain. When patients are grouped, responses for different types of pain are distinguishable, but it is unlikely that an individual's responses can be used to diagnose the cause of pain (17). This is especially true in patients with psychological disturbance (34).

Discussions of the MPQ focus on four main issues: the constitution of subcategories within the questionnaire, the suitability of selecting only one word from each category, the choice of summary scores, and the question of whether the MPQ does, in fact, reflect Melzack's theory of pain. The approach of selecting only one word in each category assumes that the words in each category are homogeneous and differ only in intensity. Some of the early studies by Reading et al. suggest that Melzack's approach is suitable (35, p381), although this would appear to be a potential topic for latent trait analysis. In terms of scoring the MPQ, the 20 category scores proved superior to the three subscale scores in one study (35). Hand and Reading found no advantage in an alternative scoring approach that used 16 instead of 20 categories (36).

We may enquire whether the MPQ does, in fact, succeed in reflecting Melzack's theory of pain. Crockett et al. argued that the results of their factor analyses offered empirical validation of Melzack's *a priori* classification of pain descriptors and concurred with Melzack's emphasis on the need to describe pain in terms of several dimensions rather than as a single intensity score. However, there remains debate over the structure of the MPQ, and technical problems in examining how closely it reflects Melzack's theory have enraptured methodologists. For example, there are several problems in using factor analysis to assess the validity of the questionnaire. Melzack and Torgerson recognized that words from different components (e.g., affective, evaluative) may correlate with one another, while different subclasses in each component will not necessarily intercorrelate (4). If this is the case, one would not expect words in, say, the sensory component to load on a single factor. Evidently the conventional response procedure cannot be used whereby the respondent selects only one word in each subclass, for then the correlations among the words will be zero, and so the grouping of words into subclasses cannot be tested empirically. Furthermore, because each word reflects both a type and an intensity of pain, a factor analysis may extract type of pain or intensity of pain factors, or both. This was illustrated by a study that departed from normal usage and presented the MPQ words in random order, asking subjects to check every word that described their pain (6). The seven factors that were interpretable cut across Melzack's groupings and took words at similar levels of intensity from a wide range of subclasses.

Although it is hard to show that Mel-zack's questionnaire does reflect his conceptual definition of pain, the MPQ is still the leading pain measurement scale, and we recommend its continued use.

REFERENCES

(1) Melzack R. The McGill Pain Questionnaire: major properties and scoring methods. Pain 1975;1:277–299.

(2) Melzack R. Psychologic aspects of pain. Pain 1980;8:143–154.

(3) Melzack R, Wall PD. The challenge of pain. 2nd ed. New York: Penguin Books, 1988.

(4) Melzack R, Torgerson WS. On the language of pain. Anesthesiology 1971; 34:50–59.

(5) Crockett DJ, Prkachin KM, Craig KD. Factors of the language of pain in patient and volunteer groups. Pain 1977;4:175–182.

(6) Leavitt F, Garron DC, Whisler WW, et al. Affective and sensory dimensions of back pain. Pain 1978;4:273–281.

(7) Melzack R. The McGill Pain Questionnaire. In: Melzack R, ed. Pain measurement and assessment. New York: Raven Press, 1983:41–47.

(8) Melzack R, Katz J, Jeans ME. The role of compensation in chronic pain: analysis using a new method of scoring the McGill Pain Questionnaire. Pain 1985;23:101–112.

(9) Perry F, Heller PH, Levine JD. Differing correlations between pain measures in syndromes with or without explicable organic pathology. Pain 1988;34:185–189.

(10) Dubuisson D, Melzack R. Classification of clinical pain descriptions by multiple group discriminant analysis. Exp Neurol 1976;51:480–487.

(11) Taenzer P. Postoperative pain: relationships among measures of pain, mood, and narcotic requirements. In: Melzack R, ed. Pain measurement and assessment. New York: Raven Press, 1983:111–118.

(12) Ahles TA, Ruckdeschel JC, Blanchard EB. Cancer-related pain—II. Assessment with visual analogue scales. J Psychosom Res 1984;28:121–124.

(13) Prieto EJ, Hopson L, Bradley LA, et al. The language of low back pain: factor structure of the McGill Pain Questionnaire. Pain 1980;8:11–19.

(14) Reading AE. The internal structure of the McGill Pain Questionnaire in dysmenorrhoea patients. Pain 1979;7:353–358.

(15) Prieto EJ, Geisinger KF. Factor-analytic studies of the McGill Pain Questionnaire. In: Melzack R, ed. Pain measurement and assessment. New York: Raven Press, 1983:63–70.

(16) Crockett DJ, Prkachin KM, Craig KD, et al. Social influences on factored dimensions of the McGill Pain Questionnaire. J Psychosom Res 1986;30:461–469.

(17) Kremer EF, Atkinson JH Jr. Pain language: affect. J Psychosom Res 1984;28:125–132.

(18) Turk DC, Rudy TE, Salovey P. The McGill Pain Questionnaire reconsidered: confirming the factor structure and examining appropriate uses. Pain 1985;21:385–397.

(19) Melzack R. Discriminative capacity of the McGill Pain Questionnaire. Pain 1985;23:201–203.

(20) Boureau F, Luu M, Doubrère JF. Comparative study of the validity of four French McGill Pain Questionnaire (MPQ) versions. Pain 1992;50:59–65.

(21) DeBenedittis G, Massei R, Nobili R, et al. The Italian Pain Questionnaire. Pain 1988;33:53–62.

(22) Radvila A, Adler RH, Galeazzi RL, et al. The development of a German language (Berne) pain questionnaire and its application in a situation causing acute pain. Pain 1987;28:185–195.

(23) Vanderiet K, Adriaensen H, Carton H, et al. The McGill Pain Questionnaire constructed for the Dutch language (MPQ-DV). Preliminary data concerning reliability and validity. Pain 1987;30:395–408.

(24) Vermote R, Ketelaer P, Carton H. Pain in multiple sclerosis patients. A prospective study using the McGill Pain Questionnaire. Clin Neurol Neurosurg 1986;88:87–93.

(25) Drewes AM, Helweg-Larsen S, Petersen P, et al. McGill Pain Questionnaire translated into Danish: experimental and clinical findings. Clin J Pain 1993;9:80–87.

(26) Strand LI, Wisnes AR. The development of a Norwegian pain questionnaire. Pain 1991;46:61–66.

(27) Ketovuori H, Pontinen PJ. A pain vocabulary in Finnish—the Finnish Pain Questionnaire. Pain 1981;11:247–253.

(28) Harrison A. Arabic pain words. Pain 1988;32:239–250.

(29) Burckhardt CS, Bjelle A. A Swedish version of the short-form McGill Pain Questionnaire. Scand J Rheumatol 1994; 23:77–81.

(30) Monks R, Taenzer P. A comprehensive pain questionnaire. In: Melzack R, ed. Pain measurement and assessment. New York: Raven Press, 1983:233–237.

(31) Corson JA, Schneider MJ. The Dartmouth Pain Questionnaire: an adjunct to the McGill Pain Questionnaire. Pain 1984; 19:59–69.

(32) Swanston M, Abraham C, Macrae WA, et al. Pain assessment with interactive computer animation. Pain 1993;53:347–351.

(33) Melzack R. The short-form McGill Pain Questionnaire. Pain 1987;30:191–197.

(34) Atkinson JH Jr, Kremer EF, Ignelzi RJ. Diffusion of pain language with affective disturbance confounds differential diagnosis. Pain 1982;12:375–384.

(35) Reading AE, Hand DJ, Sledmore CM. A comparison of response profiles obtained on the McGill Pain Questionnaire and an adjective checklist. Pain 1983;16:375–383.

(36) Hand DJ, Reading AE. Discriminant function analysis of the McGill Pain Questionnaire. Psychol Rep 1986;59:763–770.

THE BRIEF PAIN INVENTORY
(Formerly the Wisconsin Brief Pain Questionnaire)
(Charles S. Cleeland, 1982)

Purpose

The Brief Pain Inventory (BPI) measures the severity of cancer pain and its impact on the patient's functioning; it can also be used for other diseases.

Conceptual Basis

Cleeland argued that effective intervention for cancer must control the intensity of pain and restore function that was limited because of pain. Accordingly, the Brief Pain Inventory measures the intensity of pain (the "sensory" dimension) and functional limitations due to pain (the "reactive" dimension) (1). While these are conceptually distinct, they are expected to intercorrelate. Cleeland's interest focused on cancer patients but his intention was to develop an instrument that could be used with other conditions.

Description

Cleeland's studies of cancer were the impetus for developing an instrument to measure the severity and impact of pain. The McGill Pain Questionnaire was considered but rejected as being too long and difficult, and limited by its omission of pain history and interference with activities (2). Some of the pain descriptors and the diagram showing the location of pain were, however, retained. Cleeland originally called his scale the Wisconsin Brief Pain Questionnaire (3); tests of validity led to the deletion of redundant items from the total of 17. The BPI also includes ratings of the intensity of pain and the impact of pain. The 20 items are shown in Exhibit 8.5. Intensity is recorded on numerical scales running from 0 (no pain) to 10 ("pain as bad as you can imagine"). As pain may vary during a day, the intensity is rated at the time of completing the questionnaire (pain now), and also at its worst, least, and average over the past day or week, the choice depending on the context of the study. Final intensity scores may represent the worst pain or the average of the four ratings for each item. Cleeland denotes "significant pain" as pain that is rated higher than the midpoint on the pain intensity scales (1, p298).

The impact of the pain is recorded in terms of how much it interferes with mood, walking and other physical activity, work, social activity, relations with others, and sleep (1). These six ratings are made on 0-to-10 numeric scales running from "no interference" to "interferes completely." The mean of these six scores is used to indicate the level of pain interference.

The BPI also records the location of the pain on a diagram of a human figure (1). Finally, patients are asked to select words (taken from the McGill Pain Questionnaire) which best describe their pain, and they indicate the extent and duration of pain relief obtained from analgesics (4). The instrument takes ten to 15 minutes to complete. Comparable results are obtained from self- and interviewer-administered versions (1).

Reliability

Reliability data for four language versions of the BPI have been collected. Coefficient alpha values for the four pain intensity items were 0.87 for the English version (N = 1106), 0.85 for the French version (N = 324), 0.86 for the Mandarin Chinese version (N = 200), and 0.80 for the Filipino version (N = 267). Alphas for the interference scale include 0.91 (English), 0.90 (French), 0.91 (Chinese), and 0.86 (Filipino) (C.S. Cleeland, personal communication, 1995).

Validity

The BPI detected expected differences in severity of pain between groups of patients who differed in the site of their disease, in their requirements for analgesics, and in the presence of metastases (1, p299). Reports of pain severity increased with increased reports of disturbed sleep, activity limitations, and reliance on medications (5). In a discriminant analysis, the BPI items distinguished between groups of patients receiving different types of analgesia; the intensity scales were more discriminative than the interference items (4, Table 3).

The correlations among the pain intensity ratings (now, least, worst, average) fell in the range 0.57 to 0.80, while correlations among the interference scales ranged from 0.44 to 0.83 (4, Table 1). Correlations between the intensity and interference ratings ran from 0.27 to 0.63. Factor analysis confirmed the separation of severity and interference factors, and this has been replicated in studies in Vietnam, Mexico, and the Philippines (1, Table 2; 4, Table 2).

The internal structure of the BPI appears logically consistent: as ratings of pain intensity increase, the interference items are endorsed in a sequence running from work, to mood, sleep, activity, walking, and, finally, relations with others (1, Table 1).

Alternative Forms

A short form, the BPI-SF, was developed for clinical trials where multiple assessments of pain were required.

Translations into French, Spanish, Vietnamese (4), and Mandarin Chinese have been validated. The scale has also been translated into other languages, including

Exhibit 8.5 The Brief Pain Inventory

1. Throughout our lives, most of us have had pain from time to time (such as minor headaches, sprains, and toothaches). Have you had pain *other* than these everyday kinds of pain during the *last week*?

   1. ☐ Yes   2. ☐ No

   IF YOU ANSWERED YES TO THIS QUESTION, PLEASE GO ON TO QUESTION 2 AND FINISH THIS QUESTIONNAIRE. IF NO, YOU ARE FINISHED WITH THE QUESTIONNAIRE. THANK YOU.

2. On the diagram, shade in the areas where you feel pain. Put an X on the area that hurts the most.

Right   Left | Left   Right

3. Please rate your pain by circling the one number that best describes your pain at its *worst* in the last week.

   | 0 | 1 | 2 | 3 | 4 | 5 | 6 | 7 | 8 | 9 | 10 |

   No Pain   Pain as bad as you can imagine

4. Please rate your pain by circling the one number that best describes your pain at its *least* in the last week.

   | 0 | 1 | 2 | 3 | 4 | 5 | 6 | 7 | 8 | 9 | 10 |

   No Pain   Pain as bad as you can imagine

5. Please rate your pain by circling the one number that best describes your pain on the *average*.

   | 0 | 1 | 2 | 3 | 4 | 5 | 6 | 7 | 8 | 9 | 10 |

   No Pain   Pain as bad as you can imagine

6. Please rate your pain by circling the one number that tells how much pain you have *right now*.

   | 0 | 1 | 2 | 3 | 4 | 5 | 6 | 7 | 8 | 9 | 10 |

   No Pain   Pain as bad as you can imagine

7. What kinds of things make your pain feel better (for example, heat, medicine, rest)?

   _____

   _____

8. What kinds of things make your pain worse (for example, walking, standing, lifting)?

_____

_____

9. What treatments or medications are you receiving for your pain?

_____

_____

10. In the last week, how much relief have pain treatments or medications provided? Please circle the one percentage that most shows how much relief you have received.

    0%   10%   20%   30%   40%   50%   60%   70%   80%   90%   100%
    No   Complete
    Relief   Relief

11. If you take pain medication, how many hours does it take before the pain returns?

☐ 1. Pain medication doesn't help at all.   ☐ 5. Four hours.

☐ 2. One hour.   ☐ 6. Five to twelve hours.

☐ 3. Two hours.   ☐ 7. More than twelve hours.

☐ 4. Three hours.   ☐ 8. I do not take pain medication.

12. Circle the appropriate answer for each item.

I believe my pain is due to:

Yes ☐ No ☐ 1. The effects of treatment (for example, medication, surgery, radiation, prosthetic device).

Yes ☐ No ☐ 2. My primary disease (meaning the disease currently being treated and evaluated).

Yes ☐ No ☐ 3. A medical condition unrelated to primary disease (for example, arthritis).

13. For each of the following words, check yes or no if that adjective applies to your pain.

Aching	☐ Yes	☐ No
Throbbing	☐ Yes	☐ No
Shooting	☐ Yes	☐ No
Stabbing	☐ Yes	☐ No
Gnawing	☐ Yes	☐ No
Sharp	☐ Yes	☐ No
Tender	☐ Yes	☐ No
Burning	☐ Yes	☐ No
Exhausting	☐ Yes	☐ No
Tiring	☐ Yes	☐ No
Penetrating	☐ Yes	☐ No
Nagging	☐ Yes	☐ No
Numb	☐ Yes	☐ No
Miserable	☐ Yes	☐ No
Unbearable	☐ Yes	☐ No

14. Circle the one number that describes how, during the past week, _pain_ has interfered with your:

A. General Activity

    0   1   2   3   4   5   6   7   8   9   10
    Does not   Completely
    interfere   interferes

Exhibit 8.5 *(Continued)*

Exhibit 8.5   *(Continued)*

B. Mood

0	1	2	3	4	5	6	7	8	9	10

Does not   Completely
interfere   interferes

C. Walking ability

0	1	2	3	4	5	6	7	8	9	10

Does not   Completely
interfere   interferes

D. Normal work (includes both work outside the home and housework)

0	1	2	3	4	5	6	7	8	9	10

Does not   Completely
interfere   interferes

E. Relations with other people

0	1	2	3	4	5	6	7	8	9	10

Does not   Completely
interfere   interferes

F. Sleep

0	1	2	3	4	5	6	7	8	9	10

Does not   Completely
interfere   interferes

G. Enjoyment of life

0	1	2	3	4	5	6	7	8	9	10

Does not   Completely
interfere   interferes

Adapted from an original provided by Dr. CS Cleeland. With permission.

Arabic, German, Italian, Norwegian, and Russian.

Commentary

Like the Medical Outcomes Study Pain Measures, the BPI was based on the Wisconsin Brief Pain Questionnaire. The BPI offers a brief rating method that lies between simple, visual analogue ratings and more complex methods such as McGill Pain Questionnaire. Although the intensity and interference ratings intercorrelate, they are rated somewhat independently and so are not redundant. The consistency of findings between studies suggests that the scales are robust. The cross-cultural work with the BPI has led to some interesting comparisons of pain experience in different cultures and indicates that the scale would be suitable for international trials of analgesia and cancer treatment. The instrument has been used in a multicenter study of pain in the United States (6). The BPI was carefully formulated on the basis of a critical review of previous measures; it incorporates components that have been tested and is based on a conceptual theory. We hope that further validation information will shortly be published.

REFERENCES

(1) Cleeland CS. Pain assessment in cancer. In: Osoba D, ed. Effect of cancer on quality of life. Boca Raton, Florida: CRC Press, 1991:293–305.
(2) Cleeland CS. Measurement and prevalence of pain in cancer. Semin Oncol Nurs 1985;1:87–92.
(3) Daut RL, Cleeland CS, Flanery RC. Development of the Wisconsin Brief Pain Questionnaire to assess pain in cancer and other diseases. Pain 1983;17:197–210.
(4) Cleeland CS, Ladinsky JL, Serlin RC, et al. Multidimensional measurement of cancer pain: comparisons of U.S. and Vietnamese

patients. J Pain Symptom Manag 1988;3:23–27.

(5) Daut RL, Cleeland CS. The prevalence and severity of pain in cancer. Cancer 1982;50:1913–1918.

(6) Cleeland CS, Gonin R, Hatfield AK, et al. Pain and its treatment in outpatients with metastatic cancer. N Engl J Med 1994;330:592–596.

THE MEDICAL OUTCOMES STUDY PAIN MEASURES
(Cathy D. Sherbourne, 1992)

Purpose

The Medical Outcomes Study (MOS) Pain Measures cover severity in terms of the intensity, frequency, and duration of pain and record the impact of pain on behavior and moods (1, p223). They are intended for use as outcome measures and in population surveys.

Conceptual Basis

From a review of many ways of classifying pain, Sherbourne selected intensity, frequency, duration, and impact of pain on behavior as the most relevant outcome indicators for evaluating pain treatment (1). "For those concerned with the return of the patient to normal functioning and the assessment of pain relief, it seems important to measure not only the intensity of the pain experience but the effects of pain on normal functional abilities" (1, p221). Sherbourne termed these the "sensory and the performance aspects of the pain experience" (1, p223). The intention was to develop pain measures that were not specific to a condition or disease. Pain measures have not typically been included in health surveys and Sherbourne wished to compare pain scores to other aspects of health.

Description

The MOS pain measurement was based largely on the Wisconsin Brief Pain Questionnaire. Twelve self-report items cover the severity of pain over the past 4 weeks and its effect on mood and behaviors.

When the questions are used in a survey, a skip question—"Did you experience any bodily pain during the past 4 weeks?"—may be added to identify those for whom the pain questions need not be asked (1, p224,225). Those who skip the questions are given a score of 1 (no interference) on the effects of pain measure. People who experienced more than one pain during this time are asked to describe their feelings of pain in general (1, p225). The 12 questions are shown in Exhibit 8.6.

A principal components analysis identified two factors, corresponding to severity and pain effects. The question on the number of days that pain interfered with activities loaded on both factors, so Sherbourne suggested three scores: effects of pain (items 4a through 4f), pain severity (items 1–3, 6, and 7), and days pain interfered (item 5). In addition, an overall score can be calculated (1, p228). The pain effects score is calculated by averaging across all six items, giving a score from 1 to 5; this is transformed to a 0-to-100 scale. For the pain severity scale, each item is first standardized to a mean of 0 and standard deviation of 1; then the items are averaged. The range of scores in the validation study ran from -1.17 to $+2.26$ (1, Table 13-5). The overall score is calculated by first standardizing each item to a mean of 0 and a standard deviation of 1 and then averaging all items (1, p231). High scores indicate more pain.

Reliability

The items included on the severity and effects of pain scales all correlated 0.57 or greater with their scale scores (1, Table 13-3). Internal consistency for the overall score was 0.93; for the effects score it was 0.91 and for the severity score 0.86 (1, Table 13-5).

Validity

Sherbourne presented correlations of the four pain measures with 15 criterion scores

Exhibit 8.6 The Medical Outcomes Study Pain Measures

The following questions are about the pain or pains you experienced in the *past 4 weeks*. If you had more than one pain, answer the questions by describing your feelings of pain in general.

1. How much *bodily* pain have you generally had during the *past 4 weeks?*

(Circle One)

None..1
Very mild...2
Mild...3
Moderate 4
Severe 5
Very severe 6

2. During the *past 4 weeks,* how often have you had pain or discomfort?

(Circle One)

Once or twice 1
A few times 2
Fairly often 3
Very often..4
Every day or almost every day 5

3. When you had pain during the *past 4 weeks,* how long did it usually last?

(Circle One)

A few minutes 1
Several minutes to an hour..2
Several hours 3
A day or two 4
More than two days...5

4. During the *past 4 weeks,* how much did pain interfere with the following things?

(Circle One Number on Each Line)

	Not At All	*A Little Bit*	*Moderately*	*Quite A Bit*	*Extremely*
a. Your mood	1	2	3	4	5
b. Your ability to walk or move about	1	2	3	4	5
c. Your sleep	1	2	3	4	5
d. Your normal work (including both work outside the home and housework)	1	2	3	4	5
e. Your recreational activities	1	2	3	4	5
f. Your enjoyment of life	1	2	3	4	5

5. During the *past 4 weeks,* how many days did pain interfere with the things you usually do? (Your answer may range from 0 to 28 days.)

WRITE IN # OF DAYS: _____

6. Please circle the one number that best describes your pain on the *average* over the *past 4 weeks.*

No Pain

Pain As Bad As You Can Imagine

0 1 2 3 4 5 6 7 8 9 10 11 12 13 14 15 16 17 18 19 20

7. Please circle the one number that best describes your pain *at its worst* over the *past 4 weeks.*

No Pain

Pain As Bad As You Can Imagine

0 1 2 3 4 5 6 7 8 9 10 11 12 13 14 15 16 17 18 19 20

From Stewart AL, Ware JE Jr. Measuring functioning and well-being: the Medical Outcomes Study approach. Durham, North Carolina: Duke University Press, 1992:374,378–379. With permission.

drawn from the Medical Outcomes Study (N = 3,053). Correlations with a physical symptoms score ranged from 0.52 (for days pain interfered) to 0.68 (for the overall pain score); correlations with a health distress score ranged from 0.43 to 0.57 (1, Table 13-7). No correlations with other pain measurement scales are available.

Commentary

The MOS pain instrument offers a brief measure suitable for surveys or for clinical settings when the goal is to assess the impact of pain on daily living, rather than to provide a detailed assessment of the nature of the pain. While little information on validity is yet available, the method seems potentially valuable as a midsized measure, falling between the visual analogue scales and the longer scales described in this chapter. If the MOS instrument is to gain acceptance, it will have to be compared with other pain assessments and be tested for sensitivity to change. The 20-point rating scales should have adequate sensitivity to change in pain levels, although Sherbourne does suggest that asking directly about pain relief may be valuable (1, p234). Finally, we suggest that the development of alternative versions of the MOS scales be resisted and that the questions be used in their present form so that evidence for the adequacy of the instrument can cumulate.

REFERENCE

(1) Sherbourne CD. Pain measures. In: Stewart AL, Ware JE Jr, eds. Measuring functioning and well-being: the Medical Outcomes Study approach. Durham, North Carolina: Duke University Press, 1992:220–234.

THE OSWESTRY LOW BACK PAIN DISABILITY QUESTIONNAIRE
(Jeremy Fairbank, 1980, Revised 1986)

Purpose

The Oswestry questionnaire indicates the extent to which a person's functional level is restricted by back or leg pain. It was intended for clinical use and is completed by the patient.

Conceptual Basis

No information is available.

Description

The Oswestry Low Back Pain Disability Questionnaire includes ten six-point scales. The first section rates the intensity of pain and the remaining nine cover the disabling effect of pain on typical daily activities: personal care, lifting, walking, sitting, standing, sleeping, sex life, social life, and traveling. This questionnaire therefore concentrates on the effects, rather than the nature, of pain.

The patient marks the statement in each section that most accurately describes the effect of her pain; if two items are marked, the more severe is scored. Each section is scored on a 0-to-5 scale, with higher values representing greater disability. The sum of the ten scores is expressed as a percentage of the maximum score; this is termed the Oswestry Disability Index (ODI). If the patient fails to complete a section, the percentage score is adjusted (i.e., the score is expressed as a percentage of 45 rather than 50). ODI scores from 0 to 20 represent minimal disability, 20 to 40 represent moderate disability, 40 to 60 represent severe disability, while scores of 60 and over indicate that the patient is severely disabled by pain in several areas of life (1).

When self-administered, the questionnaire takes less than five minutes to complete and one minute to score; if the questions are read to a patient, it requires about ten minutes. The questionnaire is shown in Exhibit 8.7. (Note that this is a revision of the version shown in our first edition.)

Reliability

Twenty-two patients with low back pain completed the questionnaire twice, on consecutive days. A test–retest correlation of 0.99 was obtained (1, p273). Fairbank also reported "a good internal consistency," but offered no statistical summary of this (1).

Exhibit 8.7   The Oswestry Low Back Pain Disability Questionnaire

This questionnaire has been designed to give us information as to how your back or leg pain has affected your ability to manage in everyday life. Please answer every section and mark in each section ONLY THE ONE BOX which applies to you. We realise you may consider that two of the statements in any one section relate to you, but PLEASE JUST MARK THE BOX WHICH MOST CLEARLY DESCRIBES YOUR PROBLEM.

Section 1—Pain Intensity

☐ I have no pain at the moment.

☒ The pain is very mild at the moment.

☐ The pain is moderate at the moment.

☐ The pain is fairly severe at the moment.

☐ The pain is very severe at the moment.

☐ The pain is the worst imaginable at the moment.

Section 2—Personal Care (washing, dressing, etc.)

☒ I can look after myself normally without causing extra pain.

☐ I can look after myself normally but it is very painful.

☐ It is painful to look after myself and I am slow and careful.

☐ I need some help but manage most of my personal care.

☐ I need help every day in most aspects of self care.

☐ I do not get dressed, wash with difficulty and stay in bed.

Section 3—Lifting

☒ I can lift heavy weights without extra pain.

☐ I can lift heavy weights but it gives extra pain.

☐ Pain prevents me from lifting heavy weights off the floor but I can manage if they are conveniently positioned, e.g. on a table.

☐ Pain prevents me from lifting heavy weights but I can manage light to medium weights if they are conveniently positioned.

☐ I can lift only very light weights.

☐ I cannot lift or carry anything at all.

Section 4—Walking

☒ Pain does not prevent me walking any distance.

☐ Pain prevents me walking more than 1 mile.

☐ Pain prevents me walking more than 1/4 mile.

☐ Pain prevents me walking more than 100 yards.

☐ I can only walk using a stick or crutches.

☐ I am in bed most of the time and have to crawl to the toilet.

Section 5—Sitting

☐ I can sit in any chair as long as I like.

☐ I can sit in my favorite chair as long as I like.

☒ Pain prevents me from sitting for more than 1 hour.

☐ Pain prevents me from sitting for more than 1/2 hour.

☐ Pain prevents me from sitting for more than 10 minutes.

☐ Pain prevents me from sitting at all.

Section 6—Standing

☒ I can stand as long as I want without extra pain.

☐ I can stand as long as I want but it gives me extra pain.

☐ Pain prevents me from standing for more than 1 hour.

☐ Pain prevents me from standing for more than 1/2 hour.

☐ Pain prevents me from standing for more than 10 minutes.

☐ Pain prevents me from standing at all.

Section 7—Sleeping

☒ My sleep is never disturbed by pain.

☐ My sleep is occasionally disturbed by pain.

☐ Because of pain I have less than 6 hours sleep.

☐ Because of pain I have less than 4 hours sleep.

☐ Because of pain I have less than 2 hours sleep.

☐ Pain prevents me from sleeping at all.

Section 8—Sex Life (if applicable)

☒ My sex life is normal and causes no extra pain.

☐ My sex life is normal but causes some extra pain.

☐ My sex life is nearly normal but is very painful.

☐ My sex life is severely restricted by pain.

☐ My sex life is nearly absent because of pain.

☐ Pain prevents any sex life at all.

Section 9—Social Life

☒ My social life is normal and causes me no extra pain.

☐ My social life is normal but increases the degree of pain.

☐ Pain has no significant effect on my social life apart from limiting my more energetic interests, e.g. sport, etc.

☐ Pain has restricted my social life and I do not go out as often.

☐ Pain has restricted social life to my home.

☐ I have no social life because of pain.

Section 10—Travelling

☐ I can travel anywhere without pain.

☒ I can travel anywhere but it gives extra pain.

☐ Pain is bad but I manage journeys over two hours.

☐ Pain restricts me to journeys of less than one hour.

☐ Pain restricts me to short necessary journeys under 30 minutes.

☐ Pain prevents me from travelling except to receive treatment.

From an original provided by Dr. J Fairbank. With permission.

Validity

In a study of 25 patients suffering from a first attack of low back pain, expected to remit spontaneously, scores on the questionnaire showed a significant improvement over a three-week period (1).

The Oswestry questionnaire has been compared to the St. Thomas's pain questionnaire; unfortunately, no statistical summary of the association was given (2, p177).

In a receiver operating characteristic curve validity analysis, the area under the curve was 0.78, a result very similar to that obtained for the Roland Morris Pain Questionnaire (3).

Alternative Forms

A computerized version has been described (2, Appendix 12.2). Scores on this version correlated 0.89 with the conventional version (2, p176).

An alternative version was developed for use in studies of chiropractice which omitted the section on sex life, altered the remaining sections, and added a section on changes in level of pain (4). Fairbank, however, does not recommend this version (personal communication, 1989).

Commentary

This questionnaire has been included because it represents a measurement of disability and handicap due to pain, rather than of pain as impairment. As such, it provides potentially valuable information in addition to that offered by the measurements developed by Huskisson and Melzack. The British Medical Research Council and the journal *Spine* have recom-

mended that the Oswestry questionnaire be used as a standard measurement for assessing back pain. The preliminary nature of the validity and reliability tests indicates that further analyses need to be carried out to assess the quality of this measurement.

REFERENCES

(1) Fairbank JCT, Couper J, Davies JB, et al. The Oswestry Low Back Pain Disability Questionnaire. Physiotherapy 1980;66: 271–273.

(2) Baker DJ, Pynsent PB, Fairbank JCT. The Oswestry Disability Index revisited: its reliability, repeatability and validity, and a comparison with the St Thomas's Disability Index. In: Roland MO, Jenner JR, eds. Back pain: new approaches to rehabilitation and education. Manchester, England: Manchester University Press, 1989:174–186.

(3) Stratford PW, Binkley J, Solomon P, et al. Assessing change over time in patients with low back pain. Phys Ther 1994;74:528–533.

(4) Hudson-Cook N, Tomes-Nicholson K, Breen A. A revised Oswestry Disability Questionnaire. In: Roland MO, Jenner JR, eds. Back pain: new approaches to rehabilitation and education. Manchester, England: Manchester University Press, 1989:187–204.

THE BACK PAIN CLASSIFICATION SCALE
(Frank Leavitt and David C. Garron, 1978)

Purpose

The Back Pain Classification Scale (BPCS) is a screening device that distinguishes low back pain due to psychological disturbance from that due to organic disease (1). It was principally intended as a clinical tool to identify patients with low back pain who would benefit from a more thorough psychological evaluation.

Conceptual Basis

Leavitt and Garron noted that for many patients with low back pain organic pathology cannot be demonstrated, and that the pain may reflect psychological distress: "People in psychological distress are assumed to develop physical symptoms as a means of communicating and/or managing emotional or interpersonal difficulties" (1, p149). Diagnosis of such problems is hard: "Patients are habitually silent about psychological problems, and even the most astute of physicians are by their training poorly equipped to evaluate these highly complex processes with any degree of sophistication" (2, p79). Because of the difficulty in diagnosis, the existence of a psychological basis for pain is commonly inferred from the absence of organic pathology, rather than being positively demonstrated in its own right (1). Addressing this problem, several studies have used MMPI scales to identify an emotional basis for pain complaints; the MMPI Low Back Scale identifies consistent response patterns apparently reflecting pain of a psychosomatic origin (1). The MMPI, however, has a high misclassification rate, and its length is not readily accepted by pain patients. Leavitt therefore developed the BPCS as an alternative means to distinguish between organic and psychological bases for low back pain.

Description

The BPCS was derived from the observation that patients whose pain reflected psychological disturbance used verbal pain descriptors differently than did patients whose pain had an organic basis (3). Patients with pain attributable to a psychological cause (termed "functional pain") described their pain as more variable, diffuse, and intense. They used a wider variety of words to describe their pain, typically endorsing more of the affective and skin pressure types of pain descriptor (2, 3).

The BPCS forms one component of the longer Low Back Pain Symptom Checklist shown in Exhibit 8.8. This comprises 103 adjectives taken from the McGill Pain Questionnaire and other sources. The 103 words include 71 that may be scored to provide seven pain scales and the 13 words that form the Back Pain Classification Scale. These are randomly distributed through the questionnaire, and all 103 items are normally asked even if only the 13 words comprising the BPCS are to be analyzed. The results reported below refer only to the Classification Scale, which is shown in Exhibit 8.9. The seven scales derived from the Symptom Checklist were identified via factor analyses and describe various aspects of the pain experience. The first factor describes emotional discomfort, while the second is a mixed emotional and sensory factor. The remaining five cover sensory aspects of pain (4). The Low Back Pain Symptom Checklist is self-administered and takes between five and ten minutes to complete.

The BPCS was developed empirically from a comparison of the responses of 62 patients whose back pain was explained organically and 32 patients whose pain was judged (via a battery of mental and psychological tests) to have a psychological origin (1). A discriminant analysis identified the 13 words that distinguished between the two types of patient (1, p152). The BPCS is scored using weights derived from the discriminant function analyses, shown in Exhibit 8.9. The weights for the items selected by the respondent are added, and a positive total implies pain of psychological origin, whereas a negative score reflects pain of organic origin. The higher the score (in either direction) the more likely is the diagnosis.

Reliability

A test–retest reliability of 0.86 after 24 hours was obtained from a hospitalized

Exhibit 8.8   The Low Back Pain Symptom Checklist

What does your pain usually feel like?

Directions: The words below describe different qualities of pain. Place an X in the boxes beside the words that best describe how your pain typically feels. You may check as many boxes as you wish that describe your typical pain **this last week.**

☐ squeezing	☐ splitting	☐ continuous
☐ aching	☐ torturing	☐ transient
☐ gruelling	☐ pricking	☐ pulling
☐ periodic	☐ troublesome	☐ tender
☐ nagging	☐ throbbing	☐ intermittent
☐ quivering	☐ numb	☐ suffocating
☐ radiating	☐ nauseating	☐ taut
☐ heavy	☐ drilling	☐ frightful
☐ boring	☐ jumping	☐ crushing
☐ miserable	☐ dreadful	☐ pinching
☐ cutting	☐ drawing	☐ flashing
☐ cruel	☐ rasping	☐ killing
☐ penetrating	☐ blinding	☐ fearful
☐ annoying	☐ spreading	☐ beating
☐ exhausting	☐ tearing	☐ cramping
☐ wrenching	☐ rhythmic	☐ lacerating
☐ pounding	☐ shooting	☐ wretched
☐ momentary	☐ hurting	☐ intense
☐ dull	☐ hot	☐ pins and needles
☐ pulsing	☐ punishing	☐ superficial
☐ stinging	☐ burning	☐ deep
☐ brief	☐ sharp	☐ localized
☐ cold	☐ tiring	☐ unlocalized
☐ flickering	☐ scalding	☐ spasms
☐ unbearable	☐ gnawing	☐ diffuse
☐ tugging	☐ stabbing	☐ surface
☐ agonizing	☐ tingling	☐ stiff
☐ piercing	☐ freezing	☐ skin pain
☐ smarting	☐ tight	☐ muscle pain
☐ steady	☐ itchy	☐ bone pain
☐ constant	☐ pressing	☐ joint pain
☐ lancinating	☐ sore	☐ moving pain
☐ terrifying	☐ sickening	☐ electrical
☐ vicious	☐ searing	☐ shock-like
☐ cool		

Reproduced from the Low Back Pain Symptom Checklist, obtained from Dr. Frank Leavitt. With permission.

363

Exhibit 8.9 The Back Pain Classification Scale, Showing Discriminant Function Coefficients

Note: Words with positive coefficients reflect pain of psychological origin, those with negative coefficients indicate organic pain.

Pain variables	Unstandardized coefficients
Squeezing	0.67
Nagging	−0.67
Exhausting	0.50
Dull	−0.49
Sickening	0.69
Troublesome	0.47
Throbbing	−0.33
Tender	0.66
Intermittent	−0.51
Numb	0.66
Shooting	−0.30
Punishing	−1.64
Tiring	0.49

Reproduced from Leavitt F, Garron DC. The detection of psychological disturbance in patients with low back pain. J Psychosom Res 1979;23;152, Table 2. With permission.

sample (N = 114). A split-half reliability of 0.89 was obtained from 158 patients hospitalized with low back pain (2, p83). A five-day retest gave a reliability of only 0.44 (5, p274).

Validity

Most of the validation studies have compared classifications by the BPCS with independent clinical assessments.

To check the discriminant analysis used to select the adjectives included in the BPCS, Leavitt and Garron carried out a cross-validation study on a different sample of pain patients. The scale correctly classified 132 out of 159 cases: a rate of 83% (1, p152).

A more exacting validation studied 174 patients who had clear organic pain; of these, 124 had no clinical evidence for psychological involvement, while 50 had organic disease plus psychological involvement (6). All but one of the organic patients were correctly classified (99.2%), while 86% of those with psychological sequelae were classified correctly (6, Table 2). However, to achieve this classification required 43 pain words, rather than the 13 in the BPCS. Indeed, seven of the 13 BPCS words were not among the 43 words (6, Table 5). A replication study used the same 43 words and showed a small decline in rates of correct classification (6, Table 4).

Leavitt studied 91 patients with low back pain that could not be attributed to organic disease. This group was divided into 59 patients with clinically manifest symptoms of psychological disorders and 32 patients without. The BPCS achieved a 78% correct classification of these two types of pain patient, compared with 64.5% for the MMPI scales measuring hypochondriasis and hysteria, and 37.4% for the MMPI Low Back Scale (7, pp302–303).

In a further examination of the discriminal ability of the BPCS, a sample of 120 patients with low back pain was divided into two groups on the basis of their BPCS scores: 79 patients whose pain apparently had an organic basis and 41 whose pain was classified as nonorganic (8). All patients were examined by a clinical psychologist who also administered the MMPI. The group identified by the BPCS as exhibiting pain of psychological origin gave higher scores on all ten clinical scales of the MMPI, eight of these differences being statistically significant ($p < 0.01$) (8, Table 2). The clearest differences were on the MMPI hypochondriasis and hysteria scales.

In a prospective study, 108 patients were divided into those for whom an organic basis could be identified clinically for their pain versus those for whom there was none (9). All were treated medically and were followed for 14 weeks after discharge. The BPCS scores at admission were used to classify the group without organic signs into two subgroups: those showing psychological symptoms and those showing none. Over a 14-week follow-up period the progress of the two latter groups differed, with the group exhibiting psychological symptoms showing less improvement (9). Patients with no organic basis for their pain reported as much pain on retesting 14 weeks after treatment as the organic group did prior to treatment (2). Sanders compared the classification made by the BPCS with one made on the basis of a medical record review. The BPCS correctly classified 80% of the low back pain patients, but only 60% of 50 headache patients; no better than would have been achieved by classifying all patients as psychopathological (10, Table II).

In an experimental study, Leavitt compared pain patients with healthy controls who were asked to reply to the Symptom Checklist as though trying to convince their doctor that they had a serious back problem (11). Using up to 17 words from the Symptom Checklist achieved a 66% correct identification of those faking pain and a 93% correct classification of those with pain. Using up to 54 words achieved 87% and 93% correct classifications, respectively (11, Table IV). In a replication study, the percentages classified correctly shrank by about 8% (Table V). These studies indicate that the pain words can be used to distinguish people in pain from those who are simulating pain.

Concurrent validity was evaluated by comparing the BPCS to the Pain Drawing Test, which includes a line drawing of a body on which respondents indicate the position and nature of their pain. The two scales agreed on classifying 76% of respondents into disturbed or nondisturbed (12, Table 2). The BPCS results predicted subsequent return to work: 72% of those classified as nondisturbed resumed work, compared to 46% of those with disturbance (12, p956).

Demographic variables including age, sex, education, religion, and race do not predict scores on the BPCS, so it can be used in comparing patients with different sociodemographic backgrounds (2). In a multiple regression study, Garron and Leavitt showed that the MMPI hypochondriasis scale explained 15.5% of the variance

in the BPCS (13, p62). Adding a battery of other tests and MMPI scales to the regression analysis raised the variance explained to 34%.

Alternative Forms

The reliability of a Spanish version, the Hispanic Low Back Pain Symptom Checklist, has been tested (14).

Commentary

The Back Pain Classification Scale performs a diagnostic and screening task similar to that of Zung's Pain and Distress Scale and Pilowsky's Illness Behavior Questionnaire. In early studies the scale seemed to succeed in positively identifying patients whose pain was due to psychological distress. It also shows that not all patients for whom no organic basis can be found for their pain do, in fact, suffer from psychological disorders. Thus, for example, Leavitt and Garron used the BPCS to classify patients into four categories according to the presence or absence of organic and psychological problems (3). The discriminal ability of the BPCS is high and appears to exceed that of the MMPI. Leavitt and Garron concluded that the BPCS provides a viable clinical alternative to the more cumbersome MMPI for distinguishing between pain of organic and of psychosomatic origin.

However, there are hazards in using discriminant analysis to identify subsets of questions. The results are often unstable, and testing on further samples may identify new sets of discriminating items. This was found by Storandt in the dementia field; she, like Leavitt, achieved remarkably good classification in two separate studies, but using different sets of items each time. Furthermore, the items chosen in this empirical manner often do not make conceptual sense; Leavitt was candid about this:

Why this particular set of verbal pain descriptors works as discriminators and others do not is unclear from research to date. The shared variance of pain words with MMPI items is only 21%, and does not seem to fit any particular pattern in terms of the sensory and affective divisions of pain experience. Much research is still needed to understand the apparently heterogeneous content of the scale as it reflects some pain experience and/or personal characteristics that are as of yet not apparent. . . . Although the BPCS indicates with a high degree of probability that a psychological disturbance exists, it does not identify the specific nature of the emotional problems. (2, pp83–84)

These comments echo those concerning the psychological screening scales such as the Health Opinion Survey or Langner's 22-item scale, reviewed in Chapter 5: they represent at best indicators of nonspecific distress and do not guide the user to any specific clinical interpretation of the nature of the psychological problem involved.

It is apparent that the 13 words in the BPCS are insufficient for some discrimination tasks and more of the words in the Symptom Checklist are required for some applications (6, 11). Of greater concern is the finding of the very modest overlap between the original 13 words and the discriminating words identified in these subsequent studies. Leavitt has shown good *post hoc* discrimination in a number of studies, but as the identity of the most discriminative words is not constant, it will be very difficult to derive a consistently efficient screening instrument to distinguish organic from functional reports of pain. The best compromise is probably to use the 13 words from the BPCS, although if these are used as a screening test, users will always retain the uneasy feeling that other words might have worked as well or better.

REFERENCES

(1) Leavitt F, Garron DC. The detection of psychological disturbance in patients with low back pain. J Psychosom Res 1979;23:149–154.
(2) Leavitt F. Detecting psychological disturbance using verbal pain measurement: the Back Pain Classification Scale. In: Melzack R, ed. Pain measurement and assessment. New York: Raven Press, 1983:79–84.
(3) Leavitt F, Garron DC. Psychological disturbance and pain report differences in both organic and non-organic low back pain patients. Pain 1979;7:187–195.
(4) Leavitt F, Garron DC, Whisler WW, et al. Affective and sensory dimensions of back pain. Pain 1978;4:273–281.
(5) Biedermann HJ, Monga TN, Shanks GL, et al. The classification of back pain patients: functional versus organic. J Psychosom Res 1986;30:273–276.
(6) Leavitt F. Use of verbal pain measurement in the detection of hidden psychological morbidity among low back pain patients with objective organic findings. Psychol Health 1987;1:315–326.
(7) Leavitt F. Comparison of three measures for detecting psychological disturbance in patients with low back pain. Pain 1982;13:299–305.
(8) Leavitt F, Garron DC. Validity of a Back Pain Classification Scale for detecting psychological disturbance as measured by the MMPI. J Clin Psychol 1980;36:186–189.
(9) Leavitt F, Garron DC. Validity of a Back Pain Classification Scale among patients with low back pain not associated with demonstrable organic disease. J Psychosom Res 1979;23:301–306.
(10) Sanders SH. Cross-validation of the Back Pain Classification Scale with chronic, intractable pain patients. Pain 1985; 22:271–277.
(11) Leavitt F. Pain and deception: use of verbal pain measurement as a diagnostic aid in differentiating between clinical and simulated low-back pain. J Psychosom Res 1985;29:495–505.
(12) McNeill TW, Sinkora G, Leavitt F. Psychologic classification of low-back pain patients: a prognostic tool. Spine 1986; 11:955–959.
(13) Garron DC, Leavitt F. Psychological and social correlates of the Back Pain Classification Scale. J Pers Assess 1983;47:60–65.
(14) Leavitt F, Gilbert NS, Mooney V. Development of the Hispanic Low Back Pain Symptom Check List. Spine 1994;19:1048–1052.

THE PAIN AND DISTRESS SCALE (William W.K. Zung, 1983)

Purpose

The self-rating Pain and Distress Scale was intended as a brief measurement of the mood and behavior changes that are associated with acute pain. It does not directly assess the severity of the pain itself.

Conceptual Basis

No information is available.

Description

Zung's Pain and Distress Scale (PAD) describes the physical and emotional sequelae of pain. These include limitations in activities of daily living and psychological responses such as agitation, depression, and decreased alertness. The PAD contains 20 items that were selected on clinical grounds and reflect problems (particularly psychological) that commonly accompany pain. Zung grouped the items on a conceptual basis: one item covers pain (item 18); six reflect mood changes (items 1, 2, and 16–19); the remaining 13 items cover behavioral changes (see Exhibit 8.10).

The PAD scale is self-administered, and the questions use four-point response scales indicating the frequency with which that symptom is experienced; higher scores denote more frequent symptoms. The time period to which the items refer is not fixed; any appropriate period, such as a week, may be used. The scores for each question are summed and are expressed as a percentage of the maximum attainable score.

Reliability

Zung reported an alpha internal consistency of 0.89 based on data from 122 pain patients and 195 controls (1, p892).

Validity

A comparison of pain patients and controls showed that each of the 20 items discriminated significantly ($p < 0.01$) between them (1). A discriminant function analysis

Exhibit 8.10 The Pain and Distress Scale

	None or a little of the time	Some of the time	Good part of the time	Most or all of the time
1. I feel miserable, low and down	☐	☐	☐	☐
2. I feel nervous, tense, and keyed up	☐	☐	☐	☐
3. I get tired for no reason	☐	☐	☐	☐
4. I can work for as long as I usually do	☐	☐	☐	☐
5. I am as efficient in my work as usual	☐	☐	☐	☐
6. I have trouble falling asleep	☐	☐	☐	☐
7. I have trouble sleeping through the night	☐	☐	☐	☐
8. I wake up earlier than I want to	☐	☐	☐	☐
9. I feel rested when I get out of bed	☐	☐	☐	☐
10. I am restless and can't keep still	☐	☐	☐	☐
11. I find it hard to do the things I usually do	☐	☐	☐	☐
12. I find it hard to think and remember things	☐	☐	☐	☐
13. My mind is foggy and I can't concentrate	☐	☐	☐	☐
14. I am as alert as I could be	☐	☐	☐	☐
15. I still enjoy the things I used to	☐	☐	☐	☐
16. I enjoy listening to the radio or watching TV	☐	☐	☐	☐
17. I enjoy visiting friends and relatives	☐	☐	☐	☐
18. I have aches and pains that bother me	☐	☐	☐	☐
19. I am more irritable than usual	☐	☐	☐	☐
20. Everything I do is an effort	☐	☐	☐	☐

was used to identify 11 items that discriminated with a sensitivity of 84.4% and a specificity of 99.5% (1, p893). These 11 items represented both mood and behavior changes. A factor analysis identified six factors that cut across the conceptual assignment of items described here, in that most of the factors included both behavioral and mood-change items.

Commentary

This pain rating scale differs from others in this chapter in that it concentrates more on the distress associated with pain than on evaluating the pain itself. Many of the items reflect general anxiety and depressive responses and are not phrased to refer specifically to pain as the source of the symptoms. Zung's method may be compared with two other scales we review: Pilowsky's Illness Behavior Questionnaire, which is designed to diagnose the psychological causes for an exaggerated pain response, and Leavitt's Back Pain Classification Scale, which also distinguishes pain of organic origin from that due to psychological causes. Zung's method, by contrast, covers psychological problems *associated with* pain, commonly as responses to the pain rather than as causes.

There is very little information available on the reliability and validity of the PAD scale. It is important to show how well the PAD scores correlate with those obtained from established pain measurement methods such as Melzack's MPQ, and also with depression scores. The validity testing used patients with acute, traumatic pain; the method has not been tested on chronic pain patients. Zung's method deliberately identifies separate aspects of pain, although the maneuver of combining these various dimensions into a single overall score would appear, to some extent, to vitiate his original purpose. It may be that future versions of the PAD scale will develop a more adequate scoring system that provides separate scores for different dimensions of the pain experience.

REFERENCE

(1) Zung WWK. A self-rating Pain and Distress Scale. Psychosomatics 1983;24:887–894.

THE ILLNESS BEHAVIOR QUESTIONNAIRE
(I. Pilowsky and N.D. Spence, 1975, Revised 1983)

Purpose

The Illness Behavior Questionnaire (IBQ) assesses maladaptive responses to illness. It covers hypochondriacal responses, denial, and changes in affect and was designed to indicate the extent to which such psychological states may explain apparently exaggerated responses to illness. Although it is applicable to any illness, it has been most widely used in studies of pain.

Conceptual Basis

Most people are aware of their body's state of health and respond to ill health in characteristic ways. In some cases, however, the person's psychological response to illness is exaggerated and this influences the way she reports symptoms. The IBQ is designed to identify psychological syndromes that may account for a discrepancy between the objective level of pathology and the patient's response to it, termed abnormal illness behavior. The IBQ was developed from a hypochondriasis questionnaire developed for this purpose, the Whiteley Index of Hypochondriasis, which is incorporated within the IBQ (1–3). The IBQ is a more general assessment tool which covers other syndromes in addition to hypochondriasis and is based on Mechanic's concept of illness behavior. Illness behavior refers both to overt actions, such as consulting a physician, and to the patient's emotional and psychological reaction to illness (3), covering "the ways in which symptoms may be differentially perceived, evaluated and acted (or not acted) upon by different kinds of persons" (4, p62). Illness behavior refers to "the patient's psychological trans-actions with his/her physical symptoms" (5, p222) and can take normal or abnormal forms. Pilowsky proposed that a number of common psychiatric syndromes such as hypochondriasis, conversion reaction, neurasthenia, and malingering may be viewed as forms of abnormal illness behav-ior. In each case, there is a discrepancy between the objective somatic pathology present and the patient's response to it. While this may occur in many conditions, it is well illustrated by reactions to pain:

patients with intractable pain may be described as displaying "abnormal" or "maladaptive" ill-ness behaviour in so far as their behaviour devi-ates from that regarded as appropriate to the degree of somatic pathology observed, and is not modified by suitable explanation and reas-surance provided by a doctor. (4, p62)

Pilowsky argued that experiencing intracta-ble pain may serve as a form of psychologi-cal atonement in response to guilt or it may permit denial or avoidance of conflicts. Pain may also occur in conjunction with chronic muscular activity, perhaps brought on for psychological reasons (4). The ques-tions in the IBQ are concerned with the attitudinal and emotional components of illness behavior rather than with overt be-havior.

Pilowsky has contributed to the further conceptual development of abnormal ill-ness behavior, adopting the term dysnosog-nosia (6). A classification scheme subdi-vides such behaviors into somatically focused and psychologically focused, each divided into illness affirming and illness denying (6, Figure 1).

Description

The IBQ is a self-administered question-naire that uses a yes/no response format. The original version contained 52 ques-tions, later expanded to the now-standard 62-item version shown in Exhibit 8.11. A 30-item abbreviation has also been used (7). Ten of the questions were taken from

the Whiteley Index of Hypochondriasis (2, 3). The IBQ is introduced to the patient as a survey containing "a number of questions about your illness and how it affects you" (7).

The 62 questions are grouped into seven dimensions identified empirically via factor analysis. Pilowsky describes these dimen-sions as follows (1, p3):

1. General Hypochondriasis. A general factor marked by phobic concern about one's state of health. Associated with a high level of arousal or anxiety and with some insight into inappropriateness of attitudes. A high score also suggests an element of interpersonal alienation, but one that is secondary to the patient's phobic concern.
2. Disease Conviction. Characterised by affirmation that physical disease exists, symptom preoccupation, and rejection of the doctor's reassurance.
3. Psychological vs. Somatic Perception of Illness. A high score indicates that the patient feels somehow responsible for (and in fact deserves) his illness, and perceives himself to be in need of psychi-atric rather than medical treatment. A low score indicates a rejection of such attitudes and a tendency to somatise concerns.
4. Affective Inhibition. A high score indi-cates difficulty in expressing personal feelings, especially negative ones, to others.
5. Affective Disturbance. Characterized by feelings of anxiety and/or sadness.
6. Denial. A high score indicates a ten-dency to deny life stresses, and to attri-bute all problems to the effects of illness.
7. Irritability. Assesses the presence of angry feelings, and interpersonal friction.

A total score for the questionnaire may be obtained by counting the responses that represent problems—these are indicated by asterisks in the exhibit. Alternatively, scores may be provided for the seven di-mensions; the numbers in the last column in Exhibit 8.11 show the scale on which the question is scored. High scores "suggest

Exhibit 8.11 The Illness Behavior Questionnaire, Showing the Response That Is Scored and the Factor Placement of 30 Items Which Loaded on One of Seven Factors

Note: The asterisks indicate the response that is scored. We have added these to the questionnaire presented by Pilowsky and Spence.

Here are some questions about you and your illness. Circle either YES or NO to indicate your answer to each question.

			Scale
1. Do you worry a lot about your health?	YES	NO	—
2. Do you think there is something seriously wrong with your body?	YES*	NO	2
3. Does your illness interfere with your life a great deal?	YES*	NO	2
4. Are you easy to get on with when you are ill?	YES	NO*	7
5. Does your family have a history of illness?	YES	NO	—
6. Do you think you are more liable to illness than other people?	YES	NO	—
7. If the doctor told you that he could find nothing wrong with you, would you believe him?	YES	NO*	2
8. Is it easy for you to forget about yourself and think about all sorts of other things?	YES	NO	—
9. If you feel ill and someone tells you that you are looking better, do you become annoyed?	YES*	NO	1
10. Do you find that you are often aware of various things happening in your body?	YES*	NO	2
11. Do you ever think of your illness as a punishment for something you have done wrong in the past?	YES*	NO	3
12. Do you have trouble with your nerves?	YES*	NO	5
13. If you feel ill or worried, can you be easily cheered up by the doctor?	YES	NO	—
14. Do you think that other people realise what it's like to be sick?	YES	NO	—
15. Does it upset you to talk to the doctor about your illness?	YES	NO	—
16. Are you bothered by many pains and aches?	YES	NO*	3
17. Does your illness affect the way you get on with your family or friends a great deal?	YES*	NO	7
18. Do you find that you get anxious easily?	YES*	NO	5
19. Do you know anybody who has had the same illness as you?	YES	NO	—
20. Are you more sensitive to pain than other people?	YES*	NO	1
21. Are you afraid of illness?	YES*	NO	1
22. Can you express your personal feelings easily to other people?	YES	NO*	4
23. Do people feel sorry for you when you are ill?	YES	NO	—
24. Do you think that you worry about your health more than most people?	YES*	NO	1
25. Do you find that your illness affects your sexual relations?	YES	NO	—
26. Do you experience a lot of pain with your illness?	YES	NO	—
27. Except for your illness, do you have any problems in your life?	YES	NO*	6
28. Do you care whether or not people realise you are sick?	YES	NO	—
29. Do you find that you get jealous of other people's good health?	YES*	NO	1
30. Do you ever have silly thoughts about your health which you can't get out of your mind, no matter how hard you try?	YES*	NO	1
31. Do you have any financial problems?	YES	NO*	6
32. Are you upset by the way people take your illness?	YES*	NO	1
33. Is it hard for you to believe the doctor when he tells you there is nothing for you to worry about?	YES	NO	—
34. Do you often worry about the possibility that you have got a serious illness?	YES	NO	—
35. Are you sleeping well?	YES	NO*	2
36. When you are angry, do you tend to bottle up your feelings?	YES*	NO	4
37. Do you often think that you might suddenly fall ill?	YES*	NO	1
38. If a disease is brought to your attention (through the radio, television, newspapers or someone you know) do you worry about getting it yourself?	YES*	NO	1

39. Do you get the feeling that people are not taking your illness seriously enough?	YES	NO	—
40. Are you upset by the appearance of your face or body?	YES	NO	—
41. Do you find that you are bothered by many different symptoms?	YES *	NO	2
42. Do you frequently try to explain to others how you are feeling?	YES	NO	—
43. Do you have any family problems?	YES	NO *	6
44. Do you think there is something the matter with your mind?	YES *	NO	3
45. Are you eating well?	YES	NO	—
46. Is your bad health the biggest difficulty of your life?	YES	NO *	3
47. Do you find that you get sad easily?	YES *	NO	5
48. Do you worry or fuss over small details that seem unimportant to others?	YES	NO	—
49. Are you always a co-operative patient?	YES	NO	—
50. Do you often have the symptoms of a very serious disease?	YES	NO	—
51. Do you find that you get angry easily?	YES *	NO	7
52. Do you have any work problems?	YES	NO	—
53. Do you prefer to keep your feelings to yourself?	YES *	NO	4
54. Do you often find that you get depressed?	YES *	NO	5
55. Would all your worries be over if you were physically healthy?	YES *	NO	6
56. Are you more irritable towards other people?	YES *	NO	7
57. Do you think that your symptoms may be caused by worry?	YES *	NO	3
58. Is it easy for you to let people know when you are cross with them?	YES	NO *	4
59. Is it hard for you to relax?	YES *	NO	5
60. Do you have personal worries which are not caused by physical illness?	YES	NO *	6
61. Do you often find that you lose patience with other people?	YES *	NO	7
62. Is it hard for you to show people your personal feelings?	YES *	NO	4

Derived from Pilowsky I, Spence ND. Manual for the Illness Behaviour Questionnaire (IBQ). 2nd ed. Adelaide, Australia: University of Adelaide, 1983, Appendix A. With permission.

maladaptive ways of perceiving, evaluating, or acting in relation to one's state of health" (4).

Reliability

Test–retest correlations for the seven scales of the 62-item version were reported for 42 cases. After a delay of one to 12 weeks, correlations ranged from 0.67 to 0.87, with only three coefficients below 0.84 (1, Appendix E). The ten hypochondriasis items previously tested showed a test–retest correlation of 0.81 (N = 71) (1, 3). Kappa coefficients for all 62 items were reported for a test–retest study; ten items yielded nonsignificant kappas (8, Table 1).

Internal consistency values (coefficient theta) for the seven scales ranged from 0.36 to 0.72 (8, Table 3).

Comparisons of patient scores and ratings made by their spouses on the seven scales provided correlations ranging between 0.50 and 0.78 for 42 patients (1, p37).

Validity

Pilowsky reported evidence for the validity of the ten questions on hypochondriasis from the Whiteley Index (3). The scores of 118 patients were compared with their spouse's perception of what the patient's response would have been. A correlation of 0.59, or 0.65 when corrected for attenuation, was obtained (3, p90). A factor analysis of the ten items provided three factors that reflected clinically relevant aspects of hypochondriasis: bodily preoccupation, disease phobia, and conviction of the presence of disease with refusal to be reassured (3).

Fifty-two Item Version. Much of Pilowsky and Spence's development work on the IBQ concerned factor analyses of the 52 items using an extremely small sample of only 100 patients with chronic pain of various types (1, 4, 9). Seven factors were identified, which accounted for 63% of the variance (5). Forty items loaded on these factors, as shown in Exhibit 8.11. This analysis has been replicated on other groups of pain patients with comparable results. Most applications of the IBQ report scale scores based on these seven factors.

Modest associations were reported between the IBQ factors and pain behaviors (such as guarding, bracing, rubbing, or grimacing). Using multiple regression, the overall variance explained by IBQ scores and other variables ranged from 6% to 22% (10, Table III).

Thirty-Item Version. Speculand et al. used the 30-item IBQ to compare 24 patients suffering from intractable facial pain with 24 age- and sex-matched dental patients. Two of the seven factor scores showed significant differences: disease conviction and psychological versus somatic perception of disease (7). Other studies have shown that certain of the factor scores discriminate between different types of pain patients (5, 11–14). Speculand et al. used a discriminant analysis to compare responses of dental patients with patients with chronic facial pain, and from their results a sensitivity of 87.5% at a specificity of 62.5% can be calculated (7, Table 3).

Sixty-two Item Version. Pilowsky et al. applied the 62-item version of the IBQ to patients who underwent coronary artery bypass surgery and used a discriminant function analysis to contrast those who showed relief of angina with those who did not (2). Six factor scores provided an 82% correct classification. In a cross-cultural study Pilowsky et al. developed a discriminant function equation from interviews with 100 pain patients and 78 general practice patients in Seattle, Washington, and applied the equation to equivalent groups of patients in Australia to evaluate its discriminal ability. The results showed a sensitivity of 97% at a specificity of 73.6% (15, p206). The IBQ has been used in distinguishing between organic and functional symptoms; it showed a clear distinction between psychiatric patients and patients with multiple, nonspecific symptoms (16, Table II).

The 62 items were analyzed using a numerical taxonomy procedure that groups items into classes that are internally consistent and distinct from other classes. Two classes comprised more than five items; the first of these described "patients who reject the possibility that their condition might be linked to psychological problems," and the second included those who "view their pain problem within a psychological and emotional framework" (17, p93). The authors note that patients whose responses place them in the first category may find somatic and behavioral treatment appropriate, while patients in the second category may be accessible to therapies involving cognitive strategies (17, p94).

Evidence for convergent and divergent validity may be obtained from correlations with the Center for Epidemiologic Studies Depression Scale (CES-D). Pearson correlations were high for affective disturbance (0.55), disease conviction (0.50), and hypochondriasis (0.47); they were low for affective inhibition (0.10) and denial (−0.19) (18, Table VIII). Correlations between the affective disturbance scale (factor 5) and the Zung Self-rating Depression Scale and the Levine-Pilowsky Depression Questionnaire were 0.54 and 0.56; it also correlated significantly with the Spielberger state anxiety (0.59) and trait anxiety (0.76) scales (1, p10). The affective disturbance scale also correlated 0.28 with the subsequent number of visits to general practitioners; other scales that predicted utilization were disease conviction (0.20), affective state (0.19), and disease affirmation (0.18) (19, Table III).

Alternative Forms

Twenty-one of the items distinguished between people told in an experiment to deliberately exaggerate their reports of pain and pain patients whose pain had a neurotic origin. These items were formed into a Conscious Exaggeration (CE) scale (20). This correlated 0.64 with psychiatric ratings of patients' exaggeration (21, p297). The CE scale scores correlated 0.77 with the hypochondriasis scale and 0.71 with the disease conviction scale (22, Table V).

A critical review of the IBQ was provided by Main and Waddell. Their item analyses led to an abbreviation to 37 items representing three scales; these predicted disability, distress, and pain reports more adequately than did the original seven scales (8).

Pilowsky et al. have described the Illness Behavior Assessment Schedule, which is a standardized clinical interview tool covering the same fields as the IBQ (23).

The validity of an Italian translation has been reported (18).

Reference Standards

The manual of the IBQ reports reference standards from samples of patients from pain clinics, general practice, and psychiatric and general hospitals (1, Appendix F).

Commentary

The Illness Behavior Questionnaire has been used in Australia, North America, Europe, and India, mostly in studies analyzing responses to illness through comparisons of different types of pain patients. The widespread use of the method suggests that it fills a gap in the range of measurements currently available. A strength of the IBQ is its foundation on an extensive conceptual analysis of pain responses (24). The IBQ has been used in many psychosomatic studies of the links among anxiety and depression and the presentation of illness (18, 20, 25).

While the IBQ has been extensively used, few studies have focused on its validity. The studies using the IBQ are important and interesting, but they often cannot be used for the secondary purpose of drawing conclusions on the performance of the measurement itself. Although it has been used with depression and anxiety scales, for example, correlations are generally not reported (25, 26). Several papers present multivariate analyses that incorporate the

IBQ but do not allow us to identify its unique association with the criterion variables (10, 25). We do not have a formal construct validation review, for example, reporting multitrait multimethod analyses. Some of the evidence for validity of the IBQ is methodologically weak. The factor analytic studies have used unacceptably small samples, often analyzing 52 questions with as few as 100 cases. Main and Waddell, in particular, were critical of the poor psychometric properties of the IBQ.

The IBQ covers a field similar to that of Zung's Pain and Distress Scale. They differ in that the IBQ is intended principally for explaining chronic, intractable pain which is not readily explicable in terms of the level of tissue damage observed, while Zung's method provides a simple description of the psychological sequelae of pain. Pilowsky's method is similar in intent to Leavitt's Back Pain Classification Scale but differs in being applicable to a far broader range of ailments. The IBQ has considerable potential; the manual provides good documentation and readers interested in using the method should consult recent literature to see whether additional validity data have been published.

REFERENCES

(1) Pilowsky I, Spence ND. Manual for the Illness Behaviour Questionnaire (IBQ). 2nd ed. Adelaide, Australia: University of Adelaide, 1983.
(2) Pilowsky I, Spence ND, Waddy JL. Illness behaviour and coronary artery by-pass surgery. J Psychosom Res 1979;23:39–44.
(3) Pilowsky I. Dimensions of hypochondriasis. Br J Psychiatry 1967;113:89–93.
(4) Pilowsky I, Spence ND. Illness behaviour syndromes associated with intractable pain. Pain 1976;2:61–71.
(5) Demjen S, Bakal D. Illness behavior and chronic headache. Pain 1981;10:221–229.
(6) Pilowsky I. Abnormal illness behaviour (dysnosognosia). Psychother Psychosom 1986;46:76–84.
(7) Speculand B, Goss AN, Spence ND, et al. Intractable facial pain and illness behaviour. Pain 1981;11:213–219.
(8) Main CJ, Waddell G. Psychometric con-

struction and validity of the Pilowsky Illness Behaviour Questionnaire in British patients with chronic low back pain. Pain 1987;28:13–25.

(9) Pilowsky I, Spence ND. Is illness behaviour related to chronicity in patients with intractable pain? Pain 1976;2:167–173.

(10) Keefe FJ, Crisson JE, Maltbie A, et al. Illness behavior as a predictor of pain and overt behavior patterns in chronic low back pain patients. J Psychosom Res 1986; 30:543–551.

(11) Chapman CR, Sola AE, Bonica JJ. Illness behavior and depression compared in pain center and private practice patients. Pain 1979;6:1–7.

(12) Pilowsky I, Spence ND. Pain and illness behaviour: a comparative study. J Psychosom Res 1976;20:131–134.

(13) Pilowsky I, Chapman CR, Bonica JJ. Pain, depression and illness behaviour in a pain clinic population. Pain 1977;4:183–192.

(14) Pilowsky I, Spence ND. Pain, anger and illness behaviour. J Psychosom Res 1976;20:411–416.

(15) Pilowsky I, Murrell TGC, Gordon A. The development of a screening method for abnormal illness behaviour. J Psychosom Res 1979;23:203–207.

(16) Singer A, Thompson S, Kraiuhin C, et al. An investigation of patients presenting with multiple physical complaints using the Illness Behaviour Questionnaire. Psychother Psychosom 1987;47:181–189.

(17) Pilowsky I, Katsikitis M. A classification of illness behaviour in pain clinic patients. Pain 1994;57:91–94.

(18) Fava GA, Pilowsky I, Pierfederici A, et al. Depression and illness behavior in a general hospital: a prevalence study. Psychother Psychosom 1982;38:141–153.

(19) Pilowsky I, Smith QP, Katsikitis M. Illness behaviour and general practice utilisation: a prospective study. J Psychosom Res 1987;31:177–183.

(20) Clayer JR, Bookless C, Ross MW. Neurosis and conscious symptom exaggeration: its differentiation by the Illness Behaviour Questionnaire. J Psychosom Res 1984;28:237–241.

(21) Clayer JR, Bookless-Pratz CL, Ross MW. The evaluation of illness behaviour and exaggeration of disability. Br J Psychiatry 1986;148:296–299.

(22) Mendelson G. Measurement of conscious symptom exaggeration by questionnaire: a clinical study. J Psychosom Res 1987; 31:703–711.

(23) Pilowsky I, Bassett D, Barrett R, et al. The Illness Behavior Assessment Schedule: reliability and validity. Int J Psychiatry Med 1983;13:11–28.

(24) Pilowsky I. A general classification of abnormal illness behaviours. Br J Med Psychol 1978;51:131–137.

(25) Joyce PR, Bushnell JA, Walshe JWB, et al. Abnormal illness behaviour and anxiety in acute non-organic abdominal pain. Br J Psychiatry 1986;149:57–62.

(26) Pilowsky I, Bassett DL. Pain and depression. Br J Psychiatry 1982;141:30–36.

THE PAIN PERCEPTION PROFILE
(Bernard Tursky, 1976)

Purpose

The Pain Perception Profile (PPP) offers quantitative estimates of the intensity, unpleasantness, and type of pain a person experiences. It was intended for clinical use by behavior therapists treating pain patients (1).

Conceptual Basis

Tursky's PPP was developed at about the same time as Melzack's McGill Pain Questionnaire and, like the MPQ, it tackles the problem of how best to devise numerical ratings for the words that people typically use to describe their pain. Unlike the category scaling used in the MPQ, however, Tursky used magnitude estimation procedures (see Chapter 2) to scale the characteristic pain response of each individual. Tursky argued that the MPQ is limited in its ability to provide quantitative pain information and that the use of categorical scales constrains the patient's ability to adequately rate her pain (1). However, to provide more adequate numerical estimates of pain, considerably more information must be collected from the respondent.

Description

The patient is given a pain diary which includes pain descriptors based on those used in the McGill Pain Questionnaire. Before the diary is completed, a set of optional experimental procedures may be applied to provide precise estimates of the way in which each respondent uses the adjectives to describe pain. These procedures identify the respondent's pain sensation and tolerance thresholds, her ability to judge reliably between differing levels of pain stimulation, and her characteristic use of the pain descriptors. The preliminary stages can be omitted; if used, the full profile comprises four measurement stages, described here.

The first part of the PPP establishes the respondent's pain sensation threshold. An experiment is performed in which gradually increasing levels of electrical stimulation are applied to the respondent, who is asked to indicate at what level she experiences sensation, discomfort, pain, and her limit of tolerance. The stimulation is applied through an electrode on the forearm; the equipment is portable and does not have to be used in a laboratory setting. Its major purpose is to provide the clinician with a better understanding of the patient's pain response and possible bias in rating pain; the level of electrical stimulation required to produce each response may be compared to reference standards to identify abnormal pain responses. The difference between pain threshold and pain tolerance indicates the patient's pain sensitivity range, a predictor of her ability to endure pain (1). This may be useful in prescribing treatment and may be used to study the effect of treatment, including psychological intervention.

The second part of the PPP uses magnitude estimation methods to examine the respondent's rating of the painfulness of a series of electrical stimuli and identifies the mathematical power function (see Chapter 2), which describes the relationship between the intensity of the experimental stimulus and the person's judgment of pain. These judgments and the power exponent can be compared to standards to evaluate the patient's ability to make normal judgments of pain stimulation.

A greater exponent may be indicative of hypersensitivity, a lesser exponent indicative of hyposensitivity, and a significantly non-linear relationship may indicate a possible neurologic malfunction or an attempt on the part of the patient to manipulate his self-report. Changes in the exponent or the intercept may reflect alterations in the patient's pain responsivity as a function of treatment intervention. (1, p383)

In the third part of the assessment, the patient uses a cross-modality matching procedure (see Chapter 2) to rate the intensity of pain represented by the descriptors that are part of the pain diary. The adjectives cover three dimensions of pain: 14 describe pain intensity, 11 cover the emotional reaction to pain (unpleasantness), and 13 describe the sensation of pain (see Exhibit 8.12). The words were selected primarily from the McGill Pain Questionnaire and were tested in preliminary scaling studies (1). Reference scale values are available for the words (1, Table 2).

The fourth and final phase in administering the PPP involves the use of the daily pain diary shown in Exhibit 8.12. Using the three categories of pain descriptors scaled previously, the patient records her pain at specified times of the day. The diary also records the source of the discomfort, its time of onset, its duration, and the medication taken for each reported pain period. Instructions for using the diary are given by Tursky et al. (1, p390).

Reliability

Some data on the reliability of the four parts of the PPP were provided by Tursky et al. The test–retest reliability for 20 pain patients in making judgments of pain thresholds and discomfort levels were reported as showing close agreement, although Tursky did not summarize the data statistically (1).

Validity

Jamner and Tursky examined the validity of the classification into intensity and affective pain descriptors using a classical

Exhibit 8.12   The Pain Perception Profile: Sample Page from a Pain Diary, Including Lists of Pain Descriptors

INTENSITY	UNPLEASANTNESS	FEELING
Moderate	Distressing	Stinging
Just Noticeable	Tolerable	Grinding
Mild	Awful	Squeezing
Excruciating	Unpleasant	Burning
Very Strong	Unbearable	Shooting
Very Intense	Uncomfortable	Numbing
Severe	Intolerable	Throbbing
Intense	Bearable	Stabbing
Very Weak	Agonizing	Itching
Strong	Miserable	Aching
Weak	Distracting	Cramping
Not Noticeable	Not Unpleasant	None
		Pressure

PRESCRIBED MEDICATION	HOW OFTEN	DOSE SIZE	HOW MANY

DATE ___7 - 28 - 77 Thursday___

Type of Discomfort	TIME		AVERAGE DISCOMFORT NUMBER 40				MEDICATION		
			DISCOMFORT RATING						
	Dur.	Begin	Intensity Word	Unpleasant Word	Feeling Word	Numb.	Name	How Many	Dose
headache		5:30 AM	strong	distracting	throbbing	80	all meds as prescribed		
same headache		12:45 PM	moderate	tolerable	throbbing	40			
same headache		6:45 PM	strong	distracting	throbbing	80			
RATING FOR THE DAY			strong	distracting	throbbing	80			

HOURS SLEPT LAST NIGHT ___5 hrs. (Intermittent) 12:30 AM to 5:30 AM___

STRESSFUL EVENTS AND COMMENTS ___Nausea, diarrhea, dizziness (morning). Went to sleep with headache (strong). Sweated___

Reproduced from Tursky B, Jamner LD, Friedman R. The Pain Perception Profile: a psychophysical approach to the assessment of pain report. Behav Ther 1982;13:389. With permission.

conditioning experiment. A skin conductance response was conditioned to the concept of pain intensity for one experimental group and to pain unpleasantness for another group (2). Following conditioning, there was a highly significant ($p < 0.001$) difference between the two groups in their response to affective and intensity adjectives, measured via skin conductance (2,

p280). "These results provide psychophysiological evidence for the distinctness of the concept of pain intensity from its associated affective features." (2, p281)

Commentary

The Pain Perception Profile differs from most other measurements in this book in that it lacks published validity and reliability data, and yet we have included it, as an example of a sophisticated rating technique that could illustrate the types of methodological development to be anticipated in future health measurement methods. Our description of the method does not provide sufficient information for the reader to apply the PPP; fuller details on its administration are contained in Tursky's report.

Although this method is the most detailed and mathematically complex of the pain measurement methods reviewed, Tursky argues that it is sufficiently simple to be used in a clinician's office by personnel with basic training in its administration. So far the method has not achieved widespread use. It is also necessary that validity data be collected to indicate how far the results of the magnitude estimation procedures produce results that differ from the simpler estimates obtained from the McGill Pain Questionnaire, which it incorporates.

REFERENCES

(1) Tursky B, Jamner LD, Friedman R. The Pain Perception Profile: a psychophysical approach to the assessment of pain report. Behav Ther 1982;13:376–394.
(2) Jamner LD, Tursky B. Discrimination between intensity and affective pain descriptors: a psychophysiological evaluation. Pain 1987;30:271–283.

CONCLUSION

The fascinating story of the development of pain measurements well illustrates several of the themes in our book. In many ways it has been one of the most successful areas of health measurement. For instance, there have been clear links between conceptual work on the definition of pain and the development of measurement scales, so the results obtained using these methods have led to refinements in the conceptual definitions of pain. The leading measurement methods have been widely used and have been used in consistent ways that permit direct comparisons between results ob-

tained in different studies. Close attention has been paid to reliability and validity in the development of the measurement methods and these have used advanced statistical and analytic techniques. Furthermore, the link between clinical interests in pain management and the measurement techniques has been closer in this field than in, say, physical disability. Pressure from clinicians eager to evaluate their interventions led to the development of methods that distinguish between the objective experience of pain and the subjective response to it, one of the few areas of measurement in which this has been attempted. There was even an attempt to coin a term, "analgesimetry," to refer to pain measurement (1, p237). Finally, the reader gains the impression that the many researchers working on the problem of pain measurement, who come from widely differing disciplines, benefit from the existence of a dedicated journal *(Pain)* that has published many of the leading articles on pain measurement. By contrast, other fields of measurement lack a clearly identifiable journal that deals comprehensively with measurement and conceptual issues.

New and often innovative pain measures continue to be developed. The 41-item Biobehavioral Pain Profile records cognitive, behavioral, and physiological reactions to pain (2). The seven-item Pain Disability Index describes pain-related disability in areas such as family life, occupation, recreation, self-care, and social activity (3). In the field of back pain, in which numerous measurements have been proposed, the Low Back Pain Rating Scale has built upon the design of previous scales and has undergone preliminary validity testing (4). In our first edition, we also described the SAD Index for the Clinical Assessment of Pain. This provides a numerical score summarizing the severity of clinical pain and accompanying levels of anxiety and depression; each of these dimensions of pain is rated on a 0-to-10 scale of intensity, the axes forming a three-dimensional system of coordinates. Black and Chapman noted that each aspect of pain formed a distinct clinical entity with an accepted, effective therapy (5). For research purposes, they proposed that an overall pain score could be represented by the vector sum of the dimensions represented on the three axes, seemingly an elegant approach to the problem of summarizing pain on several dimensions. Black and Chapman did not pursue the idea further, although it remains an interesting notion.

The names given to pain scales are sometimes quaint. There is the West Haven–Yale Multidimensional Pain Inventory (WHYMPI), which offers a broad-ranging but brief measure of chronic pain. It contains three sections, the first covering five aspects of the pain, the second describing the reactions of significant others to the patient's pain, and the third section covering the level of pain-induced disability (6). There is the Oucher Index, which is a scale for children based on faces depicting increasingly severe pain (7, 8). A useful review of pain measurement in children was given by McGrath (9).

As with the approach used in the Oswestry scale, the theme of pain-related disability was also covered by the Pain Disability Index developed by Tait et al. This uses 0-to-10 ratings of disability in seven areas of activity (10). A related theme is covered by the Pain and Impairment Relationship Scale (PAIRS). Many chronic pain patients believe they cannot function normally because of their pain; the scale uses items such as "Most people expect too much of me, given my chronic pain" to assess the strength of this belief (11).

In the field of measuring emotional reactions to pain, one scale deserves mention if only for its macabre content. As a measure of pain reactivity, Elton et al. showed subjects a color film portraying increasing levels of insult to a human hand; the reactions were recorded. The afflictions included pinching, pricking, hammering, burning, cutting, and, as a finale, severing the hand (12). In spite of reassurances that said hand belonged to a cadaver and even without

the benefit of the color film, *our* reactivity was plainly visible.

There remain, of course, gaps in the repertoire of pain measures. It will be desirable to see greater application of high-quality pain measurement methods in clinical studies than is now the case: frequently clinical studies rely on four-point verbal pain scales. More cross-validation is desirable among the pain measures, especially exploring the equivalence of verbal, behavioral, and analogue methods. The few studies that have compared the various approaches do not show close equivalence, suggesting an area for further investigation that would be of interest to health measurement theory in general.

REFERENCES

(1) Sriwatanakul K, Kelvie W, Lasagna L, et al. Studies with different types of visual analog scales for measurement of pain. Clin Pharmacol Ther 1983;34:234–239.

(2) Dalton JA, Feuerstein M, Carlson J, et al. Biobehavioral Pain Profile: development and psychometric properties. Pain 1994;57:95–107.

(3) Jerome A, Gross RT. Pain Disability Index: construct and discriminant validity. Arch Phys Med Rehabil 1991;72:920–922.

(4) Manniche C, Asmussen K, Lauritsen B, et al. Low Back Pain Rating Scale: validation of a tool for assessment of low back pain. Pain 1994;57:317–326.

(5) Black RG, Chapman CR. SAD Index for clinical assessment of pain. In: Bonica JJ, Albe-Fessard DG, eds. Advances in pain research and therapy. Vol. 1. New York: Raven Press, 1976:301–305.

(6) Kerns RD, Turk DC, Rudy TE. The West Haven–Yale Multidimensional Pain Inventory (WHYMPI). Pain 1985;23:345–356.

(7) Beyer JE, Knapp TR. Methodological issues in the measurement of children's pain. Child Health Care 1986;14:233–241.

(8) Beyer JE, Aradine CR. Convergent and discriminant validity of a self-report measure of pain intensity for children. Child Health Care 1988;16:274–282.

(9) McGrath PA. An assessment of children's pain: a review of behavioral, physiological and direct scaling techniques. Pain 1987;31:147–176.

(10) Tait RC, Pollard CA, Margolis RB, et al.

The Pain Disability Index: psychometric and validity data. Arch Phys Med Rehabil 1987;68:438–441.

(11) Riley JF, Ahern DK, Follick MJ. Chronic pain and functional impairment: assessing beliefs about their relationship. Arch Phys Med Rehabil 1988;69:579–582.

(12) Elton D, Stanley GV, Burrows GD. A new test of pain reactivity. Percept Motor Skills 1978;47:125–126.

9

General Health Status and Quality of Life

Chapter 3 reviewed measurements of physical functioning and the chapters that followed covered the social and emotional, aspects of health. A growing number of health measurements combine these themes in one instrument, and these form the topic of the present chapter. The measures we review cover at least the physical, emotional, and social dimensions of health; many cover much more.

These are variously termed "general health status measures" or "measures of health-related quality of life." Although the trend has been toward calling these instruments quality of life measures, the term is rarely defined and there is no clear distinction between quality of life measures and methods, such as the Sickness Impact Profile, that were described by their authors as general health measures. It seems idle to dispute whether a given instrument measures health status or quality of life, so we will use the labels interchangeably. This is not to say that we approve of the way that the concept of quality of life has been used, however; there is an urgent need to reach agreement over how quality of life should be defined in medicine. Critics have described how the concept has been misused in the medical literature, often obscuring

progress that had painfully been made previously. Marilyn Bergner commented:

One of the striking differences between the notion of quality of life and that of health status is level of conceptualization. Quality of life as it is used in clinical research is a vague term without conceptual clarity. It is what investigators mean it to be. . . . Conceptual frameworks for health status, on the other hand, have appeared in the literature, have been discussed and debated, and have provided the underpinnings of several measures. (1, ppS149–S150)

There are advantages and disadvantages in considering quality of life as an outcome in clinical medicine and health care, and a brief digression into this topic will introduce some of the measurement issues.

MEASURING QUALITY OF LIFE

Medical interest in the quality of life was stimulated by success in prolonging life and by the realization that this may be a mixed blessing: patients want to live, not merely to survive. The questionable quality of survival of people who in the past could not have been saved has fueled debate over topics such as artificial life support, euthanasia, and the definition of death itself (2, 3). The theme, of course, is not new; Jonathan Swift noted that every man desires to live long, but no man wishes to be old.[1] What is new is the development of formal ways to measure quality of life and their routine application in outcome evaluation. As with measuring happiness, we became intrepid to the point that the idea of measuring so abstract and complex a theme as quality of life no longer seemed presumptuous.

Although comparatively new in health research, social scientists have long discussed quality of life. They distinguish it from the concepts of life satisfaction, morale, happiness, and anomie largely in terms of level of subjectivity (4). In the social sciences, quality of life commonly refers to the adequacy of people's material circumstances and to their feelings about these circumstances. Indicators include personal wealth and possessions, level of safety, level of freedom and opportunity; health forms but one of many components in this broad concept. Life satisfaction generally refers to people's subjective assessment of their circumstances, compared to an external reference standard or to their own aspirations. Morale is more subjective still and refers to the sense of optimism, confidence, sadness, or depression that may result from life satisfaction. Happiness commonly refers to short-term, transient feelings of well-being in response to day-to-day events. These distinctions are not rigid; definitions shift with changing social circumstances. Indeed, as wealth increases, indicators of quality of life have expanded from the material terms of income or possessions to include also more spiritual rewards such as satisfaction, personal development, and participation in the community. With the recognition that wealth does not necessarily create happiness, quality of life indicators focused on people's feelings about their circumstances, and economic indicators covered the objective side. This raises the political question of how to balance needs against people's subjective demands as driving forces in planning social and health programs.

The new, subjective indicators of quality of life bear a strong resemblance to familiar indices of emotional well-being and life satisfaction used with the chronically sick and aged. The benefits of quality of life measures in health research lie first in broadening the scope of outcome measures and second in providing a formal means for the patient's judgment to influence treatment. How, for example, do we judge the balance between the increase in survival and the side effects of treatment such as cancer chemotherapy (5)? Quality of life measurement is valuable in comparing treatments that are equivalent in terms of other indices: lumpectomy versus radiation for stage I and II breast cancers (5), or antihypertensive therapy that may be more troublesome than a symptomless disease (6).

The disadvantages of invoking quality of life measures include apparently deliberate attempts to direct attention away from the limited success of some therapy when measured by more objective indicators. The early trials of bypass graft surgery, for example, showed no mortality benefit compared to medical treatment (7, 8). Nonetheless, patients appeared satisfied with the operation, so it was suggested that the operation be evaluated not in terms of morbidity or mortality but via the "satisfaction it provides the individual" or the patient's "achievement of a satisfactory social situation within the limits of perceived physical capacity" (9, p457). This satisfaction was termed quality of life, for example, by the Coronary Artery Surgery Study that reported in 1983 (10), but it remained ill-defined. Part of the difficulty was that different indicators showed different results: if outcomes were defined in terms of treadmill exercise tests, chest pain, or activity limitations, the surgical group performed better than the medical group; in terms of return to employment or recreational

---

1. Isaac Stern recently expressed a similar sentiment when he said "Everyone should die young. But they should delay it as long as possible."

activity, there was no advantage to surgery (10, 11). As a global concept, "quality of life" had intuitive appeal and it formed a convenient rallying call: no one could dispute the virtue of improving a patient's quality of life. However, leaving it undefined gave investigators freedom to select whichever indicators they wished; quality of life had been invoked as much for political goals as out of a scientific interest in evaluating care.

Espousing the idea of quality of life measures did not show how it should be defined. Because the term is intuitively familiar it appears undeserving of close definition: everyone believes he knows when he is better or worse off. Although this represents the central theme, definitions of "well off" seem more closely to reflect the personal values or academic orientation of the researcher than an objective attempt to define the nature of the concept. As a result, a wide variety of measurements began to be called "quality of life" indicators, including scales that bear a striking resemblance to the functional disability indices described in Chapter 3. In practice there is little distinction between quality of life scales and general health measurements, so we will include both types in the present chapter.

SCOPE OF THE CHAPTER

This chapter reviews health profiles, which describe health status in a set of scores, and health indices which summarize health in a single number. The profiles emphasize the diverse aspects of health or quality of life; proponents of this measurement school hold that the dimensions of health should be kept separate and that measurement is only meaningful *within* each domain. Supporters of the health index school agree that health has several dimensions but argue that real-life decisions demand that we combine the impressions from each dimension into an overall score. Numerical indices of health are generally intended for

economic analyses of program output and for comparing results across different programs. By contrast, profiles reflect a clinical perspective, and many scales were derived from symptom check lists and measures intended to monitor the progress of individual patients. We review 18 general health profiles in the first part of this chapter and three health indexes at the end.

In the first part of the chapter, the scales we review are loosely grouped by their intended application: clinical scales; quality of life scales for cancer patients; measures intended for use in primary care; general evaluative methods; and comprehensive indicators of the well-being of elderly people in the community. The chapter opens with reviews of three clinical scales. The Arthritis Impact Measurement Scales represent a disease-specific instrument; this is followed by the Physical and Mental Impairment-of-Function Evaluation, which is appropriate for patients living in institutions and covers the more severe levels of disability, and the Functional Assessment Inventory, which focuses on a patient's potential for vocational rehabilitation. There follow three reviews of quality of life questionnaires developed for cancer patients: the Functional Living Index—Cancer; the European Quality of Life Questionnaire; and Spitzer's Quality of Life Index, which can also be applied to patients with a wide variety of conditions.

The next group of reviews covers measures designed for use in primary care: the Dartmouth COOP Charts, the Functional Status Questionnaire, and the Duke Health Profile. The next instrument, the Nottingham Health Profile, was also designed for use in primary care settings but has since been more widely used as an evaluative instrument. We review five other evaluation tools: the Sickness Impact Profile, the McMaster Health Index Questionnaire, the Multilevel Assessment Instrument, and the two Medical Outcomes Study short-form surveys: the SF-36 and SF-20.

We then describe three scales that provide comprehensive appraisals of the well-being of elderly people living in the community: the Self-Evaluation of Life Function Scale, the Multidimensional Functional Activities Questionnaire developed by the OARS group and the CARE instruments. In their full versions these require lengthy interviews, but they provide results that show good validity and reliability. In the final part of the chapter we review three health indexes that provide numerical summary scores of health. As financial pressure grows, measures of this type are increasingly finding application in economic analyses of the performance of the health care system. We review the Disability and Distress Scale, the new EuroQol Quality of Life Measure, and the Quality of Well-Being Scale.

Table 9.1 compares the quality of the scales in the chapter. They have in general been more thoroughly tested for reliability and validity than the physical disability scales reviewed in Chapter 3. They represent some of the most successful applications of test development procedures to health measurement and, as can be seen from Table 9.1, are often of high quality.

REFERENCES

(1) Bergner M. Quality of life, health status, and clinical research. Med Care 1989; 27(suppl):S148–S156.

(2) Jones MB. Health status indexes: the trade-off between quantity and quality of life. Socio Econ Plan Sci 1977;11:301–305.

(3) Kottke FJ. Philosophic considerations of quality of life for the disabled. Arch Phys Med Rehabil 1982;63:60–62.

(4) Horley J. Life satisfaction, happiness, and morale: two problems with the use of subjective well-being indicators. Gerontologist 1984;24:124–127.

(5) de Haes JCJM, van Knippenberg FCE. The quality of life of cancer patients: a review of the literature. Soc Sci Med 1985; 20:809–817.

(6) Williams GH. Quality of life and its impact on hypertensive patients. Am J Med 1987;82:98–105.

(7) CASS Principal Investigators and their As-sociates. Coronary Artery Surgery Study (CASS): a randomized trial of coronary artery bypass surgery. Survival data. Circulation 1983;68:939–950.

(8) Veterans Administration Coronary Artery Bypass Surgery Cooperative Study Group. Eleven-year survival in the Veterans Administration randomized trial of coronary bypass surgery for stable angina. N Engl J Med 1984;311:1333–1339.

(9) LaMendola WF, Pellegrini RV. Quality of life and coronary artery bypass surgery patients. Soc Sci Med 1979;13A:457–461.

(10) CASS Principal Investigators and their As-sociates. Coronary Artery Surgery Study (CASS): a randomized trial of coronary artery bypass surgery. Quality of life in patients randomly assigned to treatment groups. Circulation 1983;68:951–960.

(11) Scheidt S. Ischemic heart disease: a patient-specific therapeutic approach with emphasis on quality of life considerations. Am Heart J 1987;114:251–257.

THE ARTHRITIS IMPACT MEASUREMENT SCALES
(Robert F. Meenan, 1980, Revised 1991)

Purpose

The Arthritis Impact Measurement Scales (AIMS) cover physical, social, and emotional well-being and were designed as an indicator of the outcome of care for arthritic patients.

Conceptual Basis

Meenan criticized the measurements traditionally used with arthritic patients for their focus on disease activity and functional abilities to the exclusion of other components identified in the WHO definition of health (1). "The major argument in favor of the new questionnaire-based approaches is that they focus on the components of outcome that are the most relevant to the physician and the patient, both of whom are primarily interested in how the patient feels and how he or she functions" (2, p168). The AIMS were intended to be comprehensive and practical, with an

Table 9.1 Comparison of the Quality of General Health Measurements and Quality of Life Scales*

Measurements	Scale	Number of items	Application	Administered by (time)	Studies using method	Reliability Thoroughness	Reliability Results	Validity Thoroughness	Validity Results
Arthritis Impact Measurement Scale (Meenan, 1980)	Guttman	45	clinical	self	many	++	++	+++	++
Physical and Mental Impairment-of-Function Evaluation (PAMIE) (Gurel, 1972)	ordinal	77	clinical	staff (10–15 min)	few	+	+	+	+
Functional Assessment Inventory (Crewe, 1981)	ordinal	40	clinical	staff	few	+	++	++	++
Functional Living Index—Cancer (Schipper, 1984)	ordinal	22	clinical, research	self (< 10 min)	several	+	+	++	++
EORTC Quality of Life Questionnaire (EORTC, 1993)	ordinal	30	clinical, research	self (12 min)	several	+	+	++	++
Quality of Life Index (Spitzer, 1980)	ordinal	5	clinical	self (2 min)	many	++	++	++	++
COOP Charts for Primary Care Practice (Nelson, 1987)	ordinal	9	clinical	self (< 5 min)	many	++	++	+++	++
Functional Status Questionnaire (Jette, 1986)	ordinal	34	clinical, screening	self (15 min)	several	+	++	++	++
DUKE Health Profile (Parkerson, 1990)	ordinal	17	clinical	self	few	++	++	++	++
McMaster Health Index Questionnaire (Chambers, 1976)	ordinal	59	clinical, survey	self (20 min)	several	++	++	++	+
Sickness Impact Profile (Bergner, 1976)	interval	136	research, survey	self, interviewer (20–30 min)	many	+++	+++	+++	+++
Nottingham Health Profile (Hunt, 1981)	interval	45	clinical, survey	self (10–15 min)	many	++	++	++	++
Short-Form-36 Health Survey (Ware, 1990)	ordinal	36	survey	self (5–10 min)	many	+++	+++	+++	+++

Instrument									
Short-Form-20 Health Survey (Stewart, 1988)	ordinal	20	survey	self (3–4 min)	several	++	++	++	++
Self-Evaluation of Life Function Scale (Linn, 1984)	ordinal	54	clinical	self	few	+	++	++	+
Multilevel Assessment Instrument (Lawton, 1982)	ordinal	147	survey	interviewer (50 min)	few	++	++	++	++
OARS Multidimensional Functional Assessment Questionnaire (OARS, 1975)	ordinal	144	clinical	interviewer (45 min)	many	++	++	++	++
Comprehensive Assessment and Referral Evaluation (Gurland, 1977)	ordinal	329 (CORE-CARE)	clinical	interviewer	many	++	++	+++	++
Disability and Distress Scale (Rosser, 1978)	ratio	2	research	expert (< 1 min)	several	+	++	++	++
EuroQol Quality of Life Scale (EuroQol Group, 1990)	ratio	5	research	self	few	+	++	+	++
Quality of Well-Being Scale (Bush and Kaplan, 1973)	ratio	18	research	interviewer (7 min)	many	++	+++	+++	++

* For an explanation of the categories used, see Chapter 1, pages 6–7.

emphasis on proven reliability and validity (3).

Description

The instrument includes 45 items grouped into nine scales that assess mobility, physical activity (walking, bending, lifting), dexterity, household activity (managing money, medications, housekeeping), social activities, activities of daily living, pain, depression, and anxiety. The dexterity and pain scales were developed by Meenan, and other items were adapted from Katz's Index of ADL, the Rand instruments, and the Quality of Well-Being Scale (1). Items were selected for inclusion on the basis of Guttman analyses and internal consistency correlations (3). For each scale the items are listed in Guttman order so that a patient indicating disability on one question will tend also to indicate disability on the items falling below it in that section. An additional 19 questions, not considered here as an integral part of the AIMS, cover general health, health perceptions, and demographic details. The questions are shown in Exhibit 9.1. (The questionnaire was obtained from Dr. Meenan; note that this is a newer, slightly modified version of that shown in reference 3, p149.) Most of the questions refer to problems during the past month. Phrasing of the responses is shown below the exhibit. The instrument is self-administered and takes about 15 minutes to complete.

In scoring the AIMS, the Guttman characteristics are ignored and each item is scored separately; higher scores indicate greater limitation. No item weights are used. Certain questions use a reversed phrasing, so care must be taken in coding replies to these. To convert section scores to a standard range of 0 to 10, Meenan provided simple standardization formulae for each section (4). He recommended forming a total health score by adding the values for six of the scales: mobility, physical and household activities, dexterity, pain, and depression. These details are provided in a three-page user's guide, which is available from the Boston Arthritis Center (4).

Reliability

The Guttman scale coefficients of scalability and reproducibility exceeded 0.60 and 0.90, respectively, for all but the household activity scale, which had a coefficient of reproducibility of 0.88 (3, Table 2). In a study of 625 arthritics, Guttman reproducibility coefficients for all scales exceeded 0.90 (5, Table 2).

The alpha internal consistencies of all nine scales exceeded 0.60; six exceeded 0.80 (2, Table 2). In another study, alpha coefficients exceeded 0.70 for all scales except physical activity (0.63) and social activity (0.69) (5, Table 2).

Test–retest correlations for the nine scales exceeded 0.80 after a two-week delay; the mean test–retest correlation was 0.87 for 100 patients (1, 2, 5). These results were replicated in several diagnostic groups (5). Test–retest reliability ranged from 0.63 to 0.89 for the scales in three groups of patients with chronic disease (6, p352).

Validity

Correlations between the scales and a number of criterion variables were examined. These included age (on the expectation of a reduction in function with age), the patient's perception of general health and of recent disease activity, and a physician's report of functional activity, joint count, and disease activity (3). Meenan et al. commented:

The performance-oriented scales generally correlated closely with age, and all 9 scales were significantly correlated with the patient's estimates of general health and disease activity. Finally, when the psychological scales are excluded, agreement between the scale scores and the doctor's report was significant in 16 of 21 pairs (76%). (3, p150)

Similar analyses were carried out using the data from the study of 625 arthritics.

Exhibit 9.1   The Arthritis Impact Measurement Scales: Questionnaire Items

Mobility
- 4   Are you in bed or chair for most or all of the day because of your health?
- 3   Do you have to stay indoors most or all of the day because of your health?
- 2   When you travel around your community, does someone have to assist you because of your health?
- 1   Are you able to use public transportation?

Physical activity
- 5   Are you unable to walk unless you are assisted by another person or by a cane, crutches, artificial limbs, or braces?
- 4   Do you have any trouble either walking one block or climbing one flight of stairs because of your health?
- 3   Do you have any trouble either walking several blocks or climbing a few flights of stairs because of your health?
- 2   Do you have trouble bending, lifting, or stooping because of your health?
- 1   Does your health limit the kind of vigorous activities you can do such as running, lifting heavy objects, or participating in strenuous sports?

Dexterity
- 5   Can you easily write with a pen or pencil?
- 4   Can you easily turn a key in a lock?
- 3   Can you easily tie a pair of shoes?
- 2   Can you easily button articles of clothing?
- 1   Can you easily open a jar of food?

Household activity
- 7   If you had a telephone, would you be able to use it?
- 6   If you had to take medicine, could you take all your own medicine?
- 5   Do you handle your own money?
- 4   If you had a kitchen, could you prepare your own meals?
- 3   If you had laundry facilities (washer, dryer, etc.), could you do your own laundry?
- 2   If you had the necessary transportation, could you go shopping for groceries or clothes?
- 1   If you had household tools and appliances (vacuum, mops, etc.), could you do your own housework?

Social activity
- 4   About how often were you on the telephone with close friends or relatives during the past month?
- 3   During the past month, about how often did you get together socially with friends or relatives?
- 2   During the past month, about how often have you had friends or relatives to your home?
- 1   During the past month, how often have you visited with friends or relatives at their homes?

Activities of daily living
- 4   How much help do you need to use the toilet?
- 3   How well are you able to move around?
- 2   How much help do you need in getting dressed?
- 1   When you bathe, either a sponge bath, tub or shower, how much help do you need?

Pain
- 4   During the past month, how long has your morning stiffness usually lasted from the time you wake up?
- 3   During the past month, how often have you had pain in two or more joints at the same time?
- 2   During the past month, how often have you had severe pain from your arthritis?
- 1   During the past month, how would you describe the arthritis pain you usually have?

Depression
- 6   During the past month, how often did you feel that others would be better off if you were dead?
- 5   How often during the past month have you felt so down in the dumps that nothing could cheer you up?
- 4   How much of the time during the past month have you felt downhearted and blue?
- 3   How often during the past month did you feel that nothing turned out for you the way you wanted it to?
- 2   During the past month, how much of the time have you been in low or very low spirits?
- 1   During the past month, how much of the time have you enjoyed the things you do?

Exhibit 9.1   *(Continued)*

Exhibit 9.1   *(Continued)*

Anxiety

6   How often during the past month did you find yourself having difficulty trying to calm down?

5   How much have you been bothered by nervousness, or your "nerves" during the past month?

4   During the past month, how much of the time have you felt tense or "high strung"?

3   How much of the time during the past month were you able to relax without difficulty?

2   How much of the time during the past month have you felt calm and peaceful?

1   How much of the time during the past month did you feel relaxed and free of tension?

Response Phrasing for the AIMS Questions:

The *Mobility, Physical Activity,* and *Dexterity* questions use yes/no responses.

The *Household Activity* questions use a three-point scale: without help, with some help, and completely unable.

The *Social Activity* questions use a six-point scale of frequency: every day, several days a week, about once a week, 2 or 3 times in the past month, once in the past month, and not at all in the past month.

The *Activities of Daily Living* questions use the following responses. Question 1: no help at all, help with reaching some parts of the body, help in bathing more than one part of the body. Question 2: no help at all, only need help tying shoes, need help getting dressed. Question 3: able to get in and out of bed or chairs without the help of another person, need help of another person, and don't get out of bed. Question 4: no help at all, some help in getting to or using the toilet, not able to get to the bathroom at all.

Pain is measured on three different six-point frequency scales. The question describing pain grades it as: very severe, severe, moderate, mild, very mild, or none. The question concerning the frequency of the pain and that about pain in two or more joints use: always, very often, fairly often, sometimes, almost never and never. The response modes for the duration of morning stiffness are: over 4 hours, 2 to 4 hours, 1 to 2 hours, 30 minutes to an hour, less than 30 minutes and do not have morning stiffness.

The 12 *Depression and Anxiety* questions use three response scales. Questions on enjoying things, feeling tense, low spirits, feeling relaxed, feeling downhearted and blue, feeling calm, and relaxing without difficulty use: all of the time, most of the time, a good bit of the time, some of the time, a little of the time, and none of the time. The questions about difficulty trying to calm down, feeling nothing turns out, feeling others would be better off if you were dead and feeling down in the dumps use: always, very often, fairly often, sometimes, almost never and never. The scale for how much you have been bothered by nervousness is: extremely so, very much, quite a bit, some, just a little bit and not bothered at all.

Reproduced from the Arthritis Impact Measurement Scales obtained from Dr. Robert F Meenan. With permission.

For 444 of the patients, the nine scales were correlated with disease activity (*r* between 0.14 and 0.52) and with the American Rheumatism Association (ARA) functional class (*r* between 0.24 and 0.52) (2, Table 4). Scales measuring physical functioning showed higher associations with the disease indicators than did the psychological and social scales. The physical scales of the AIMS correlated 0.91 with equivalent scales in the Health Assessment Questionnaire (HAQ); the pain scales in the two instruments correlated 0.64 in a study of 48 arthritics (5). In a different study the AIMS and HAQ correlated 0.89 (7); a lower correlation of 0.48 was obtained between the short AIMS and the modified HAQ for 106 hip replacement patients. The AIMS correlated 0.76 with the Functional Status Questionnaire in the same study (8, Table 3).

A factor analysis of the nine scales provided three factors: physical function, psychological, and pain (5). These results were subsequently precisely replicated (9). Reflecting the three-component factor structure, the results of a multivariate approach to criterion validation showed stronger associations than did the single-variate analyses reported here. Using multiple regression analyses, the AIMS scores achieved multiple correlation coefficients of 0.61 with disease activity and 0.66 with the ARA functional class index (5, p1050). Multiple correlations with a three-item measure of global health status and a visual analogue measure of arthritis impact were 0.84 and 0.75, respectively (5, p1050). Mason et al.

subsequently reconsidered the three-factor solution, arguing that it was theoretically restrictive. They proposed a five-factor solution that presented scores for lower extremity function (mobility, ADL, and physical activity), upper-extremity function (dexterity), affects (anxiety and depression), pain, and social interaction (10).

Sensitivity of the AIMS to change has been studied by several authors. Changes in the scores were correlated with changes in a rating of health following treatment for 120 patients; correlations fell between 0.24 and 0.67 (1, 5). Kazis et al. studied the responsiveness of the AIMS in a study of injectable gold. Seven of the AIMS scales achieved effect sizes that were small; physical activity gave a moderate effect size; and the pain scale gave a large effect size (11, Table 2). In a second trial, effect sizes for pain and anxiety scores were large; those for physical activity and depression were moderate; and the rest were small (11, Table 3). The AIMS scales provide similar effect sizes for rheumatoid and osteoarthritis; again, the pain scale showed the largest effect of treatment in two clinical trials (12). The AIMS total score showed a more significant change in patients following hip-replacement surgery than did the McMaster Health Index Questionnaire (13, Table IV). In a more comprehensive comparison of five scales by Liang et al., the pain, mobility, and overall scores of the AIMS were clearly superior in terms of effect size to those of the SIP, the Quality of Well-Being Scale, the Health Assessment Questionnaire, and the Functional Status Index (14, Table 2). For the global and mobility scores the sample size required by the AIMS to demonstrate a signficant difference would be less than half that required for most of the other measures (14, Table 3).

Alternative Forms

The AIMS has been translated into Spanish (15, 16), Swedish (17), Italian (18), and Canadian French (19). A Dutch version showed internal consistency alphas in excess of 0.80 for six scales and between 0.6 and 0.7 for the remainder (20, Table II). Validity correlations with an independent assessment of functional status ranged from 0.7 to 0.8 for the physical functioning scales (20, Table IV).

An abbreviated version of the AIMS includes 18 items divided into nine scales. The two items with the highest internal consistency and correlation with the total AIMS score were selected from the original AIMS scales. The instrument takes six to eight minutes to complete (21). Using the answer codes in our exhibit, the items are as follows:

mobility 2, 4
physical activity 3, 4
dexterity 2, 3
household activity 1, 4
social activity 1, 3
ADL 1, 2
pain 1, 2
depression 2, 4
anxiety 1, 2 (21, Table 1).

Alpha reliability was only slightly lower than that of the full AIMS, and test–retest reliability was virtually identical (21, Table 2). Likewise, concurrent validity coefficients were very similar for long and short forms (Table 3). In a study of hip patients, the abbreviated version of the AIMS proved more sensitive to change than did the SIP, SF-36, or Functional Status Questionnaire (22, Table 4).

A revised version, called AIMS2, was proposed in 1991 as a more comprehensive and sensitive instrument (23). This contains 57 questions, plus a further 44 that cover satisfaction with health, the impact of arthritis on function, and the patient's priorities for improvement. The 57 core items were derived from the original AIMS, but all were reworded. The nine topic areas of the AIMS were renamed and sections were added on arm function, social support, and work. The answer format was altered to make responses more standard across questions. The questionnaire and a seven-page user's guide are available from Dr. Mason (see Address section). A French version of the AIMS2 has been tested for validity and reliability (24).

The AIMS has been used with children (average age, 9.3 years) with mixed success. The pain scale appeared the most reliable; limited variability on the mobility and ADL scales suggested that they may require modification for use with children (25, p823).

Commentary

The AIMS is one of the most widely used outcome measures in arthritis research. It is well documented and clearly described, and there is strong evidence for its reliability and validity. The use of Guttman scaling in selecting items is appropriate for the questions covering physical disability, and the scaling results obtained for the AIMS appear to be superior to those obtained for other instruments using Guttman scaling, such as the OECD questionnaire. While the AIMS is intended mainly for research, Kazis et al. described a clinical report format for the AIMS that summarized patient profiles on one page; this may make the instrument suitable for routine clinical use (26). The AIMS deserves serious consideration as an outcome indicator for use with arthritic patients.

Address

John H. Mason, PhD, Research and Evaluation Support Core Unit, Boston University Arthritis Center, 80 East Concord Street, Boston, Massachusetts, USA 02118-2394

REFERENCES

(1) Meenan RF. The AIMS approach to health status measurement: conceptual background and measurement properties. J Rheumatol 1982;9:785-788.

(2) Meenan RF. New approaches to outcome assessment: the AIMS questionnaire for arthritis. Adv Int Med 1986;31:167-185.

(3) Meenan RF, Gertman PM, Mason JH. Measuring health status in arthritis: the Arthritis Impact Measurement Scales. Arthritis Rheum 1980;23:146-152.

(4) Boston University Multipurpose Arthritis Center. AIMS user's guide. Boston: Boston University. (Manuscript, nd).

(5) Meenan RF, Gertman PM, Mason JH, et al. The Arthritis Impact Measurement Scales: further investigations of a health status measure. Arthritis Rheum 1982;25:1048-1053.

(6) Burckhardt CS, Woods SL, Schultz AA, et al. Quality of life of adults with chronic illness: a psychometric study. Res Nurs Health 1989;12:347-354.

(7) Hakala M, Nieminen P, Manelius J. Joint impairment is strongly correlated with disability measured by self-report questionnaires. Functional status assessment of individuals with rheumatoid arthritis in a population based series. J Rheumatol 1994; 21:64-69.

(8) Sherbourne CD, Stewart AL, Wells KB. Role functioning measures. In: Stewart AL, Ware JE Jr, eds. Measuring functioning and well-being: the Medical Outcomes Study approach. Durham, North Carolina: Duke University Press, 1992:205-219.

(9) Brown JH, Kazis LE, Spitz PW, et al. The dimensions of health outcomes: a cross-validated examination of health status measurement. Am J Public Health 1984; 74:159-161.

(10) Mason JH, Anderson JJ, Meenan RF. A model of health status for rheumatoid arthritis: a factor analysis of the Arthritis Impact Measurement Scales. Arthritis Rheum 1988;31:714-720.

(11) Kazis LE, Anderson JJ, Meenan RF. Effect sizes for interpreting changes in health status. Med Care 1989;27(suppl):S178-S189.

(12) Anderson JJ, Firschein HE, Meenan RF. Sensitivity of a health status measure to short-term clinical changes in arthritis. Arthritis Rheum 1989;32:844-850.

(13) O'Boyle CA, McGee H, Hickey A, et al. Individual quality of life in patients undergoing hip replacement. Lancet 1992; 339:1088-1091.

(14) Liang MH, Fossel AH, Larson MG. Comparisons of five health status instruments for orthopedic evaluation. Med Care 1990;28:632-642.

(15) Hendricson WD, Russell IJ, Prihoda TJ, et al. Development and initial validation of a dual-language English-Spanish format for the Arthritis Impact Measurement Scales. Arthritis Rheum 1989;32:1153-1159.

(16) Cardiel MH, Abello-Banfi M, Ruiz-Mercado R, et al. How to measure health status in rheumatoid arthritis in non-English speaking patients: validation of a Spanish version of the Health Assessment Questionnaire Disability Index (Spanish HAQ-DI). Clin Exp Rheumatol 1993; 11:117-121.

(17) Archenholtz B, Bjelle A. Reliability and

validity of a Swedish version of the Arthritis Impact Measurement Scales. Scand J Rheumatol 1990;20:219.

(18) Cavalieri F, Salaffi F, Ferracioli GF. Relationship between physical impairment, psychosocial variables and pain in rheumatoid disability. An analysis of their relative impact. Clin Exp Rheumatol 1991;9:47–50.

(19) Sampalis JS, Pouchot J, Beaudet F, et al. Arthritis Impact Measurement Scales: reliability of a French version and validity in adult Still's disease. J Rheumatol 1990; 17:1657–1661.

(20) Taal E, Jacobs JW, Seydel ER, et al. Evaluation of the Dutch Arthritis Impact Measurement Scales (Dutch-AIMS) in patients with rheumatoid arthritis. Br J Rheumatol 1989;28:487–491.

(21) Wallston KA, Brown GK, Stein MJ, Dobbins CJ. Comparing the short and long versions of the Arthritis Impact Measurement Scales. J Rheumatol 1989;16:1105–1109.

(22) Katz JN, Larson MG, Phillips CB, et al. Comparative measurement sensitivity of short and longer health status instruments. Med Care 1992;30:917–925.

(23) Meenan RF, Mason JH, Anderson JJ, et al. AIMS2: the content and properties of a revised and expanded Arthritis Impact Measurement Scales health status questionnaire. Arthritis Rheum 1992;35:1–10.

(24) Poiraudeau S, Dougados M, Ait-Hadad H, et al. Evaluation of a quality of life scale (AIMS2) in rheumatology. Rev Rhumat Maladies Osteoarticulaires 1993;60:561–567.

(25) Coulton CJ, Zborowsky E, Lipton J, et al. Assessment of the reliability and validity of the Arthritis Impact Measurement Scales for children with juvenile arthritis. Arthritis Rheum 1987;30:819–824.

(26) Kazis LE, Anderson JJ, Meenan RF. Health status information in clinical practice: the development and testing of patient profile reports. J Rheumatol 1988;15:338–344.

THE PHYSICAL AND MENTAL IMPAIRMENT-OF-FUNCTION EVALUATION
(Lee Gurel, 1972)

Purpose

The Physical and Mental Impairment-of-Function Evaluation (PAMIE) is a clinical rating scale that records physical, psycho-logical, and social disability in the chronically ill, institutionalized elderly (1).

Conceptual Basis

The PAMIE was based on two previous instruments, the Self-Care Inventory, an ADL rating scale used in Veterans Administration hospitals with severely disabled geriatric patients, and its refinement, the 43-item Patient Evaluation Scale, which assessed the potential for hospital discharge (1). Factor analyses of the latter scale guided the content of the PAMIE, which was intended to cover 12 topics. Subsequent empirical testing of the PAMIE indicated that scores are best presented for ten factors, rather than the 12 hypothesized (1).

Description

The PAMIE is a rating scale completed by a caregiver or clinician familiar with the patient (1). The 77 items are mainly concerned with observable behaviors during the preceding week; all but the first three use a yes/no answer format. Exhibit 9.2 shows a slightly revised version of the PAMIE from that shown in reference 1, Table 1. The instrument takes ten to 15 minutes to complete.

The scoring system for the first three questions is shown in the exhibit; for the remaining questions, the Roman numeral indicates the scale on which it is counted, and its position shows the response that receives one point. Empirical analyses did not confirm the existence of separate factors for irritability and cooperation, and so scores may be provided for the following ten factors (2, p236):

I.   Self-care
II.   Belligerence, irritability
III.   Mental confusion
IV.   Anxiety, depression
V.   Bedfast, moribund
VI.   Behavioral deterioration
VII.   Paranoia, suspicion
VIII.   Sensory and motor function
IX.   Withdrawn, apathetic
X.   Ambulation

Exhibit 9.2   The Physical and Mental Impairment-of-Function Evaluation

On the basis of your knowledge of the patient at the present time will you please rate the following items. Answer items 1, 2 and 3 on this page by circling the number beside the most correct statement. For all other items check either Yes or No. Please do not leave any item unanswered.

1. Which of the following *best* fits the patient? (Circle one)
   - 5 Has no problem in walking
   - 4 Slight difficulty in walking, but manages; may use cane
   - 3 Great difficulty in walking, but manages; may use crutches or stroller
   - 2 Uses wheelchair to get around by himself
   - 1 Uses wheelchair pushed by others
   - 0 Doesn't get around much; mostly or completely bedfast, or restricted to chair

(Factor X)

2. As far as you know, has the patient had one or more strokes (CVA)? (Circle one)
   - 0 No stroke
   - 1 Mild stroke(s)
   - 2 Serious stroke(s)

(Factor VIII)

3. Which of the following *best* fits the patient? (Circle one)
   - 4 In bed all or almost all day
   - 3 More of the waking day in bed than out of bed
   - 2 About half the waking day in bed, about half out of bed
   - 1 More of the waking day out of bed than in bed
   - 0 Out of bed all or almost all day

(Factor V)

	Yes	No	(Check either Yes or No)
4.	___	___	Eats a regular diet
5.	_V_	___	Is given bed baths
6.	_II_	___	Gives sarcastic answers
7.	___	_I_	Takes a bath/shower without help or supervision
8.	_VI_	___	Leaves his clothes unbuttoned
9.	_VI_	___	Is messy in eating
10.	_II_	___	Is irritable and grouchy
11.	_IX_	___	Keeps to himself
12.	_VII_	___	Says he's not getting good care and treatment
13.	_II_	___	Resists when asked to do things
14.	_IV_	___	Seems unhappy
15.	_III_	___	Doesn't make much sense when he talks to you
16.	_II_	___	Acts as though he has a chip on his shoulder
17.	_V_	___	Is IV or tube fed once a week or more
18.	_VIII_	___	Has one or both hands/arms missing or paralyzed
19.	___	_II_	Is cooperative
20.	_V_	___	Is toileted in bed by catheter and/or enema
21.	___	___	Is deaf or practically deaf, even with hearing aid
22.	_IX_	___	Ignores what goes on around him
23.	___	_V_	Knows who he is and where he is
24.	_II_	___	Gives the staff a "hard time"
25.	_VII_	___	Blames other people for his difficulties
26.	_VII_	___	Says, without good reason, that he's being mistreated or getting a raw deal
27.	_II_	___	Gripes and complains a lot
28.	_VII_	___	Says other people dislike him, or even hate him

392

29. ___	___	Says he has special or superior abilities
30. ___	___	Has hit someone or been in a fight in the last six months
31. ___	_I_	Eats without being closely supervised or encouraged
32. _IV_	___	Says he's blue and depressed
33. _IX_	___	Isn't interested in much of anything
34. _III_	___	Has taken his clothes off at the wrong time or place during the last six months
35. ___	___	Makes sexually suggestive remarks or gestures
36. _II_	___	Objects or gives you an argument before doing what he's told
37. _VII_	___	Is distrustful and suspicious
38. ___	_VI_	Looks especially neat and clean
39. _IV_	___	Seems unusually restless
40. _II_	___	Says he's going to hit people
41. _III_	___	Receives almost constant safety supervision (for careless smoking, objects in mouth, self-injury, pulling catheter, etc.)
42. _VI_	___	Looks sloppy
43. _III_	___	Keeps wandering off the subject when you talk with him
44. _VI_	___	Is noisy; talks very loudly
45. ___	_I_	Does things like brush teeth, comb hair, and clean nails without help or urging
46. ___	___	Has shown up drunk or brought a bottle on the ward
47. _IV_	___	Cries for no obvious reason
48. ___	___	Says he would like to leave the hospital
49. _I_	___	Wets or soils once a week or more
50. _III_	___	Has trouble remembering things
51. _VIII_	___	Has one or both feet/legs missing or paralyzed
52. _X_	___	Walks flight of steps without help
53. ___	_V_	When needed, takes medication by mouth
54. _IV_	___	Is easily upset when little things go wrong
55. ___	_I_	Uses the toilet without help or supervision
56. ___	_V_	Conforms to hospital routine and treatment program
57. _VIII_	___	Has much difficulty in speaking
58. _III_	___	Sometimes talks out loud to himself
59. ___	_IX_	Chats with other patients
60. _I_	___	Is shaved by someone else
61. _II_	___	Seems to resent it when asked to do things
62 ___	_I_	Dresses without any help or supervision
63. _II_	___	Is often demanding
64. _IX_	___	When left alone, sits and does nothing
65. _VII_	___	Says others are jealous of him
66. _III_	___	Is confused
67. ___	___	Is blind or practically blind, even with glasses
68. ___	_I_	Decides things for himself, like what to wear, items from canteen (or canteen cart), etc.
69. _II_	___	Swears; uses vulgar or obscene words
70. _III_	___	When you try to get his attention, acts as though lost in a dream world
71. _IV_	___	Looks worried and sad
72. _III_	___	Most people would think him a mental patient

Exhibit 9.2 *(Contunued)*

393

Exhibit 9.2   *(Continued)*

	Yes	No	(Check either Yes or No)
73.	___	_I_	Shaves without any help or supervision, other than being given supplies
74.	_II_	___	Yells at people when he's angry or upset
75.	_I_	___	Is dressed or has his clothes changed by someone
76.	_X_	___	Gets own tray and takes it to eating place
77.	_III_	___	Is watched closely so he doesn't wander

Reproduced from the Physical and Mental Impairment-of-Function Evaluation form obtained from Dr. Lee Gurel. With permission.

Where no numeral is given, the question did not load on a factor in the analyses. Although conceptually distinct, these factors may commonly be found together in the same patient, and so are not independent of one another. Factor scores may be added to give three more general scores representing physical infirmity (factors I, V, VIII, X), psychological deterioration (factors III, VI, IX), and psychological agitation (factors II, IV, VII) (1). Weighted and unweighted factor scores provided essentially identical results, so the unweighted scores are generally used.

Reliability

Alpha internal consistency coefficients for the factor scores ranged from 0.67 to 0.91 (1, Table 2).

Validity

The PAMIE scale was tested on 845 male veterans in nursing homes. Their mean age was 66 years; 47% were general medical and surgical patients, while the remainder had predominantly psychiatric problems, often accompanied by additional medical complaints (1). The factor structure of the PAMIE scale was examined, and nine factors were derived. However, Gurel et al. chose to separate questions on ambulation from the self-care factor, forming the tenth factor that is scored (1). To assess the stability of the factor solution, the analysis was repeated on medical/surgical and psychiatric patients separately, with considerable agreement between them, as indicated by a Harman's coefficient of congruence of

0.86 (1, p85). Several of the factors were substantially correlated, and a second-order factor analysis provided three factors, which the authors named "physical infirmity" (including ambulation, sensory and motor functions, bedfastness), psychological deterioration (including mental confusion, withdrawal/apathy, deterioration in behavior and appearance), and psychological agitation (including paranoia and suspicion, irritability and belligerence, anxiety/depression) (1).

The sample was grouped into those scoring high or low on each of 19 measures reflecting diagnostic and severity ratings. All of the PAMIE scores discriminated between contrasting subgroups in at least three cases. Scores reflecting physical abilities (especially bedfastness, self-care, ambulation) provided significant discriminations between almost all of the criterion dichotomies (1).

Commentary

The PAMIE is a relatively old scale that has not been widely used, but it has the advantage of an identifiable internal structure, broad scope, and relevance for the institutionalized elderly—a group for whom often only ADL questions are used.

REFERENCES

(1) Gurel L, Linn MW, Linn BS. Physical and Mental Impairment-of-Function Evaluation in the aged: the PAMIE scale. J Gerontol 1972;27:83–90.
(2) Goga JA, Hambacher WO. Psychologic and

behavioral assessment of geriatric patients: a review. J Am Geriatr Soc 1977;25:232–237.

THE FUNCTIONAL ASSESSMENT INVENTORY
(Nancy M. Crewe and Gary T. Athelstan, 1981, Revised 1984)

Purpose

The Functional Assessment Inventory (FAI) was developed for clinical use to describe a client's potential for vocational rehabilitation. It summarizes functional limitations and the personal and environmental resources that a client can use to help cope with problems (1). It was intended to be applicable to all types of disability.

Conceptual Basis

The FAI is the first component of a two-part Functional Assessment System. The second part is a goal attainment scaling instrument called the Rehabilitation Goals Identification Form that measures treatment outcomes (1).

The FAI identifies a person's strengths and limitations (whether modifiable or not) that predict ability to return to work, and which should be taken into account in developing a vocational rehabilitation plan. "Pinpointing the obstacles to rehabilitation can be helpful in determining what services are needed even if no attempt will be made to directly modify the limitations" (1, p304). Crewe and Turner noted that existing physical assessment methods such as the Barthel or PULSES scales are not broad enough to assess the potential for vocational rehabilitation: "The vocational counselor . . . requires general information about capacities in a wide variety of physical, emotional, intellectual and social areas that may be relevant to work." (2, p1)

Description

The Functional Assessment Inventory is a rating scale of 30 items describing functional limitations and a ten-item check list of assets or unusual strengths. The strength items are rated as present or absent and are meant to accommodate the instances when a particular asset may compensate for a patient's limitations: considering a patient's strengths may improve the prediction of success in vocational rehabilitation. The functional limitations questions are rated on four-point scales representing current levels of impairment (with aids when used): none, mild, moderate, and severe. The FAI identifies problems that may improve following rehabilitation. Space does not permit showing the complete inventory; the item topics are shown in Exhibit 9.3. Note that the exhibit refers to a revised version, which differs from that published by Crewe and Athelstan (1, p301), two items having been substituted and the order of the items changed. Printed copies of the FAI, an instruction sheet, and an interviewer manual are available (see Address section). Full definitions of each level are given in the questionnaire and the accompanying instruction sheet. As an example, item 25 reads as follows:

25. Skills (See instructions)

   0. No significant impairment.
   1. No available skills that are job-specific. However, possesses general skills (i.e., educational or interpersonal) that could be used in a number of jobs.
   2. Has few general skills. Job-specific skills are largely unusable due to disability or other factors.
   3. Has no job-specific skills and has very few general or personal skills transferable to a job situation.

The instruction sheet adds:

This item refers to skills which the individual possesses after onset of disability.

The Functional Assessment Inventory is completed by a rehabilitation counselor using information available from interviews, observations of the patient, and material drawn from medical records to rate the patient. The ratings concern observable behavior; problems that can only be inferred (e.g., pain, low self-esteem) are excluded

Exhibit 9.3   The Functional Assessment Inventory: Items

Cognition
    1. Learning ability
    2. Ability to read and write
    3. Memory
    4. Spatial and form perception
Vision
    5. Vision
Communication
    6. Hearing
    7. Speech
    8. Language functioning
Motor function
    9. Upper extremity function
    10. Hand function
    11. Motor speed
Physical condition
    12. Mobility
    13. Capacity for exertion
    14. Endurance
    15. Loss of time from work
    16. Stability of condition
Vocational qualifications
    17. Work history
    18. Acceptability to employers
    19. Personal attractiveness
    20. Skills
    21. Economic disincentives

    22. Access to job opportunities
    23. Need for specialized placement or
        accommodations
Adaptive behavior
    24. Work habits
    25. Social support system
    26. Accurate perception of capabilities
        & limitations
    27. Effective interaction with employ-
        ers and co-workers
    28. Judgment
    29. Congruence of behavior with reha-
        bilitation goals
    30. Initiative and problem-solving
        ability
The strength items include exceptional assets in the
following areas:
    31. Physical appearance
    32. Personality
    33. Intelligent or has verbal fluency
    34. Vocational skill in demand
    35. Suitable educational qualifications
    36. Supportive family
    37. Financial resources
    38. Vocational motivation
    39. Job available with employer
    40. Initiative and problem-solving
        ability

Adapted from the Functional Assessment Inventory obtained from Dr. Nancy M Crewe. Copyright University of Minnesota. With permission.

(2). The FAI takes five minutes to complete. A total, unweighted functional limitation score is provided by adding the raw scores for each item. Alternatively, scores may be provided for the seven sections indicated in Exhibit 9.3.

The original version of the FAI (as shown in reference 1) was field tested in three studies, first on 351 physically or mentally disabled patients who were assessed by one of 30 vocational rehabilitation counselors (1). Later it was tested on 1,716 vocational rehabilitation patients, and subsequently on 1,488 patients representing six types of disability: visual, hearing, orthopedic, mental illness, mental retardation, and addiction (2).

Reliability

Alpha internal consistency coefficients were calculated for five subscales of the ques-

tionnaire for 351 patients; the resulting values ranged from 0.70 to 0.85 (1). To assess inter-rater reliability, a series of 51 interviews was observed and rated by pairs of psychologists. Seventy-five percent of the ratings made by the pairs of observers were identical; only 3% of all ratings differed by more than one point on the four-point scales (1, 2).

Validity

The replies of the 351 patients were factor analyzed, providing eight factors that agree quite closely with the item placements shown in the exhibit (1, Table 4). The factor structure held relatively constant when responses from subgroups of the 351 patients with different types of disability were analyzed separately, and analyses of other samples produced similar results (2).

Concurrent validity was assessed by

comparing the FAI limitation and assets scores with judgments made by rehabilitation counselors concerning employability and severity of disability. (Note that these do not represent independent ratings from the FAI responses, as they were recorded by the same rater.) For the 351 patients the correlations with the FAI limitation score were -0.61 for employability and 0.60 for severity of disability (1, p303). For the sample of 1,716 cases the equivalent correlations were -0.57 and 0.55 (3). As might be expected, the correlation between the FAI strength scores and the counselor rating of employability (0.53) was higher than that with disability (-0.21) (1, p303). In a multiple regression analysis, the total functional limitation score plus the total strength score gave a multiple correlation coefficient of 0.70 ($R^2 = 0.49$) with the employability rating. The R^2 value for predicting severity of disability was 0.41 (1, p304).

The third sample of 1,488 patients was divided into those who were admitted for rehabilitation services, those excluded as being too severely disabled, and those excluded as having no impairment. Analyses of variance showed that all FAI scores except for vision and communication distinguished significantly between these groups (2). Strong and logical contrasts were also obtained between different diagnostic groups (2).

Alternative Forms

A self-administered version called the Personal Capabilities Questionnaire has been proposed. This provides the counselor with information on how the client perceives her own limitations.

Commentary

Note that the Functional Assessment Inventory developed by Crewe and Athelstan is completely distinct from the instrument with the same name developed by Pfeiffer as a variant of the OARS Multidimensional Functional Activities Questionnaire. Unfortunately, the two instruments were developed at the same time and were published in different journals, which prevented the duplication of names from being detected.

The Crewe and Athelstan FAI includes clear documentation and instructions. It is innovative in incorporating both limitations and assets, a welcome and unusual approach in assessing disability that would seem to have considerable potential benefit. Like Rosser's Disability and Distress Scale, the FAI can be completed from existing information, so the patient does not necessarily have to be present.

The validity and reliability evidence is promising and uses large samples of patients. Because the FAI is intended to assess the potential for vocational rehabilitation, the results of predictive validity testing are of particular importance, although the preliminary evidence for predictive validity is not strong. Crewe and Turner reported results from 255 of the 351 patients: the data suggest that only about one-half of the FAI items correlated with rehabilitation outcome scores, and the total FAI score did not significantly predict outcome (2). Nonetheless, the FAI seems worth considering as a clinical rating of rehabilitation potential on the basis of the quality of its documentation and its validity and reliability results.

Address

Manual and scoring information: Materials Development Center of the Stout Vocational Rehabilitation Institute, University of Wisconsin—Stout, Menomonie, Wisconsin, USA 54751

REFERENCES

(1) Crewe NM, Athelstan GT. Functional assessment in vocational rehabilitation: a systematic approach to diagnosis and goal setting. Arch Phys Med Rehabil 1981; 62:299–305.
(2) Crewe NM, Turner RR. A functional assessment system for vocational rehabilitation. In: Halpern AS, Fuhrer MJ, eds. Functional assessment in rehabilitation. Baltimore, Maryland: Paul H Brookes, 1984:223–238.

(3) Crewe NM, Athelstan GT, Meadows GK. Vocational diagnosis through assessment of functional limitations. Arch Phys Med Rehabil 1975;56:513–516.

THE FUNCTIONAL LIVING INDEX—CANCER
(H. Schipper, 1984)

Purpose

Schipper et al. developed the Functional Living Index—Cancer (FLIC) to determine the response of cancer patients to their illness and treatment, and they proposed it as an adjunct to clinical assessments of progress and toxicity in clinical trials (1, 2).

Conceptual Basis

Schipper argued for the relevance of quality of life assessments in the absence of a prospect for cure. Palliation implies the preservation of quality of life, but the hospice movement has focused on pain, which forms only one part of the quality of life concept (2, p1120). Schipper notes:

Clinical trials analysts measure tumor size, disappearance, reappearance, and survival. Patients measure quality of life. What is important to the scientist, the very numbers by which he judges the success of his therapy and plans the next steps, may not be relevant to patients. . . . patients frequently prefer function-preserving treatments to more radical curative attempts, even at the expense of survival duration. (2, pp1116–1117)

Schipper identified four components of quality of life: physical/occupational function, psychological state, sociability, and somatic discomfort (2, p1117). These form the basis of the FLIC.

Description

The items in the FLIC were selected from previous instruments by a panel of patients and health professionals in a series of stages (1, p473). The final 22 items are shown in Exhibit 9.4.

The FLIC is intended for inpatients and outpatients with diagnosed malignant cancer. It can be self-administered in less than ten minutes. The questions refer to the past two to four weeks. The response scales are visual analogue scales divided into six categories; patients are instructed to mark the line at the point that best reflects their response (1, p474). For scoring, each interval is divided in half and responses are scored to the nearest whole integer. Scores for questions 3, 6, 8, 10, 12, 15, 16, 18, 19, and 22 are reversed so that higher scores indicates better health. Schipper recommends using the total score on the FLIC, rather than the factor scores (1, p482).

Reliability

Morrow et al. reported alpha internal consistency figures for factor scores they derived; these ranged from 0.64 to 0.87 (3, p293).

Validity

Schipper reported factor analyses from four samples, using slightly different versions of the questionnaire. Four factors were consistently identified, three of which corresponded to the components postulated: physical well-being, emotional state, and sociability. The final factor reflected hardship and disruption due to cancer. A five factor solution was reported by Morrow et al., including physical, emotional, and social functioning; current well-being; and a factor including the pain and nausea symptoms (3, Table 2).

A preliminary version of the questionnaire discriminated significantly between patients in hospital, on active treatment, on adjuvant therapy, off treatment, and being followed up (1, p475). Average scores fell significantly with the extent of the disease. The FLIC has been shown sensitive to the side effects of chemotherapy (4).

The overall scores on the FLIC were correlated with other health measurements for two samples (1, Table 6). Correlations with the Beck Depression Inventory and with the General Health Questionnaire ranged between 0.72 and 0.77; correlations

Exhibit 9.4 The Functional Living Index—Cancer

Please indicate with __/__ your rating.

1. How well do you appear today?

| | | | | | | |
|1|2|3|4|5|6|7|

Extremely   Extremely
Poor   Well

2. Rate your confidence in your prescribed course of treatment.

| | | | | | | |
|1|2|3|4|5|6|7|

No   Very
Confidence   Confident

3. How much of your pain or discomfort over the past 2 weeks was related to your cancer?

| | | | | | | |
|1|2|3|4|5|6|7|

None   All

4. Rate how willing you were to see and spend time with friends, in the past 2 weeks.

| | | | | | | |
|1|2|3|4|5|6|7|

Unwilling   Very
                                              Willing

5. Rate the degree to which you are frightened of the future.

| | | | | | | |
|1|2|3|4|5|6|7|

Constantly   Not
Terrified   Afraid

6. How much nausea have you had in the past 2 weeks?

| | | | | | | |
|1|2|3|4|5|6|7|

None   A Great Deal

7. Rate how willing you were to see and spend time with those closest to you, in the past 2 weeks.

| | | | | | | |
|1|2|3|4|5|6|7|

Unwilling   Very willing

8. How much of your usual household tasks are you able to complete?

| | | | | | | |
|1|2|3|4|5|6|7|

All   None

9. Rate the degree to which your cancer has imposed a hardship on you (personally) in the past 2 weeks.

| | | | | | | |
|1|2|3|4|5|6|7|

Tremendous   No
Hardship   Hardship

10. How much is pain or discomfort interfering with your daily activities?

| | | | | | | |
|1|2|3|4|5|6|7|

Not At All   A Great Deal

11. Rate in your opinion, how disruptive your cancer has been to those closest to you in the past 2 weeks.

| | | | | | | |
|1|2|3|4|5|6|7|

Totally   No
Disruptive   Disruption

12. How uncomfortable do you feel today?

| | | | | | | |
|1|2|3|4|5|6|7|

Not At All   Very
                                    Uncomfortable

13. Rate your satisfaction with your work and your jobs around the house in the past month.

| | | | | | | |
|1|2|3|4|5|6|7|

Very   Very
Dissatisfied   Satisfied

14. Rate how often you feel discouraged about your life.

| | | | | | | |
|1|2|3|4|5|6|7|

Always   Never

15. Rate the degree to which your cancer has imposed a hardship on those closest to you in the past 2 weeks.

| | | | | | | |
|1|2|3|4|5|6|7|

No   Tremendous
Hardship   Hardship

16. Do you feel well enough to make a meal or do minor household repairs today?

| | | | | | | |
|1|2|3|4|5|6|7|

Very Able   Not Able

Exhibit 9.4 *(Continued)*

399

Exhibit 9.4   *(Continued)*

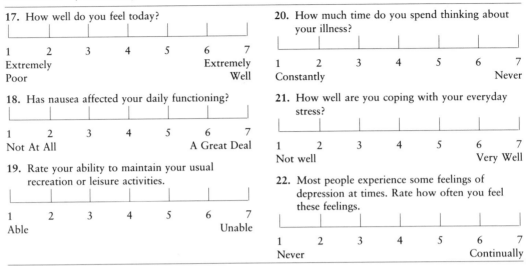

17. How well do you feel today?

| 1 | 2 | 3 | 4 | 5 | 6 | 7 |
Extremely Poor ... Extremely Well

18. Has nausea affected your daily functioning?

| 1 | 2 | 3 | 4 | 5 | 6 | 7 |
Not At All ... A Great Deal

19. Rate your ability to maintain your usual recreation or leisure activities.

| 1 | 2 | 3 | 4 | 5 | 6 | 7 |
Able ... Unable

20. How much time do you spend thinking about your illness?

| 1 | 2 | 3 | 4 | 5 | 6 | 7 |
Constantly ... Never

21. How well are you coping with your everyday stress?

| 1 | 2 | 3 | 4 | 5 | 6 | 7 |
Not well ... Very Well

22. Most people experience some feelings of depression at times. Rate how often you feel these feelings.

| 1 | 2 | 3 | 4 | 5 | 6 | 7 |
Never ... Continually

Reproduced from Schipper H, Levitt M. Measuring quality of life: risks and benefits. Cancer Treat Rep 1985;69:1121. With permission.

with the Karnofsky Scale were 0.62 and 0.69 in the two samples; correlations with the Spielberger anxiety scales ranged from 0.55 to 0.60; and correlations with the McGill Pain Questionnaire were 0.55 and 0.59. Correlations with the Katz Index of ADL were lower: 0.17 and 0.31 in the two samples. Ganz et al. found a correlation of only 0.33 between the FLIC total score and the Karnofsky Scale (5, Figure 3).

Schipper and Levitt reported correlations between the factor scores and criterion measures in two studies. Correlations of the physical factor score and the Katz Index of ADL were 0.21 and 0.23; correlations with the McGill Pain Questionnaire scores were 0.56 and 0.66; correlations with the Karnofsky score were 0.76 and 0.55 (2, Table 1). As expected, the FLIC physical score correlated more highly with the somatic symptoms and social dysfunction scores from the General Health Questionnaire than did the FLIC emotional factor, whereas the emotional factor results correlated more highly than the physical with the anxiety and depression scores. Curiously, however, the physical score correlated more highly (0.57 to 0.64) with the Beck Depression Inventory than did the emotional factor scores (0.52 to 0.53) (2, Table 1). Factors 3 and 4 correlated "only weakly with the validation tests" (1, p478).

Commentary

In the mid-1980s the FLIC caught the attention of cancer researchers searching for a quality of life instrument and was frequently mentioned in the literature. While the coverage of the scale is broad and care was taken in its initial development, the FLIC has seen only limited use.

There may be several reasons for this. Since its initial testing, the scale has received little further development; we still lack information on reliability. The validity findings are varied; Schipper reported higher validity than Ganz, for example. Several of the validity results are based on earlier versions of the scale. The use of a single overall score has been criticized as too coarse to be of optimal clinical value (6, p187). The interpretation of some questions is unclear. For example, in the light of mental imagery in cancer therapy, what is the correct answer to "How much time do you spend thinking about your illness?" The emphasis on function in the title of the scale also does not seem to accurately represent its content. Ganz et al. found that patients with more severe disease experienced difficulty in completing the form themselves and that few patients treated the response scale as a visual analogue scale, instead circling one of the numbers (5). Ganz et al. concluded that "The FLIC should be evaluated more extensively in the clinical trial setting to assess its utility in accurately assessing QOL" (5, p855). More recent scales, such as the European EORTC Quality of Life Questionnaire, may come to replace it.

REFERENCES

(1) Schipper H, Clinch J, McMurray A, et al. Measuring the quality of life of cancer patients: the Functional Living Index—Cancer: development and validation. J Clin Oncol 1984;2:472–483.

(2) Schipper H, Levitt M. Measuring quality of life: risks and benefits. Cancer Treat Rep 1985;69:1115–1123.

(3) Morrow GR, Lindke J, Black P. Measurement of quality of life in patients: psychometric analyses of the Functional Living Index—Cancer (FLIC). Qual Life Res 1992;1:287–296.

(4) Lindley CM, Hirsch JD, O'Neill CV, et al. Quality of life consequences of chemotherapy-induced emesis. Qual Life Res 1992;1:331–340.

(5) Ganz PA, Haskell CM, Figlin RA, et al. Estimating the quality of life in a clinical trial of patients with metastatic lung cancer using the Karnofsky performance status and the Functional Living Index—Cancer. Cancer 1988;61:849–856.

(6) Aaronson NK, Ahmedzai S, Bullinger M, et al. The EORTC core quality-of-life questionnaire: interim results of an international field study. In: Osoba D, ed. Effect of cancer on quality of life. Boca Raton, Florida: CRC Press, 1991:185–203.

THE EORTC QUALITY OF LIFE QUESTIONNAIRE
(European Organization for Research and Treatment of Cancer [EORTC], 1993)

Purpose

The Quality of Life Questionnaire (QLQ) is a modular system for evaluating the quality of life of cancer patients participating in international clinical trials. The system includes the core module described here and diagnosis-specific additional questionnaires.

Conceptual Basis

The European Organization for Research and Treatment of Cancer (EORTC) created a study group on quality of life in 1980. This brought together clinicians and behavioral scientists to advise on the design of clinical trials and to achieve consensus on how to define and measure quality of life (1). In 1986 the study group initiated a program to develop an outcome measurement system for cancer trials; the QLQ was developed by a consortium representing 13 countries.

The design requirements specified that the QLQ be relevant to cancer patients, cross-culturally applicable, and sensitive to change following treatment. To capture the advantages of generic and disease-specific instruments, the measurement system includes a generic core questionnaire (the QLQ-C30 described here), to which disease- and treatment-specific modules can be added. The core component contains questions applicable to all cancer patients while the additional modules address questions of relevance in a given clinical trial; tumor-specific forms covering breast, lung, colorectal, head and neck cancer have been developed to supplement the core instrument. Reports from the EORTC group discuss the design of quality of life instruments (2) and give conceptual justification for the dimensions covered (3); guidelines for the development of disease-specific modules have been published (4).

Description

A first-generation core questionnaire contained 36 items (1); following reliability and validity testing on patients from 15 countries this was revised to produce the 30-item version shown here. The QLQ-C30 includes nine multi-item scales: five cover function, three cover symptoms, and one provides an overall judgment of health status and quality of life (5). Additional items cover common physical problems of cancer and its treatment (5). The core questionnaire is shown in Exhibit 9.5. The subscales and items comprising each are as follows: physical function, items 1–5; role function, items 6, 7; cognitive function, items 20, 25; emotional function, items 21–24; social function, items 26, 27. The symptom scales include fatigue (items 10, 12, 18), nausea and vomiting (items 14, 15) and pain (items 9, 19). The global quality of life subscale includes items 29 and 30. The single items cover dyspnea (item 8), sleep disturbance (item 11), appetite loss (item 13), constipation (item 16), diarrhea (item 17), and the financial impact of cancer (item 28). It should be noted, however, that the QLQ is still under development and that recent studies have proposed altering some of the content of the subscales (6).

The questionnaire can be self- or interviewer-administered in eleven to twelve minutes (5, p368); a minority of patients require assistance to complete it (1, p191). Separate profile scores are calculated for the nine scales and for the individual items; the raw scores for items are added, then divided by the number of items in the scale, and then linearly transformed to a 0–to–100 scale, with a higher score representing a higher level of function. The transformation for each scale takes the form of

$$100 - [(\text{Scale score} -1) \times 100 /\\ (\text{Response scale range} -1)]$$

Aaronson et al. do not propose adding these to form an overall score, arguing that a profile more accurately reflects the multidimensional character of quality of life (5, p373).

The QLQ-C30 is a copyrighted instrument, with all rights reserved. Permission is required from the EORTC for its use.

Reliability

Multitrait analyses confirmed that the items fall on the nine hypothesized scales.

Mean item-scale correlations were 0.53 and 0.59 in two administrations of the questionnaire (5, p368). Alpha internal consistency coefficients for the nine scales fell in the range 0.52 (role functioning) to 0.89 (global QoL) (5, Table 3). Coefficients were similar across cultural groups with the exception of the nausea subscale. A similar range of alpha coefficients was reported for the 36-item version from a Swedish study ($\alpha = 0.61$ to 0.89) (7, Table 2).

Modifications have been proposed to the composition of certain subscales; Ringdal and Ringdal presented alpha values for the original and the modified scales ranging from 0.55 to 0.86. Eight of the 14 coefficients exceeded 0.80 (6, Table 3).

Validity

In the original validation study, correlations among the subscales appear moderate; those between the physical function, role function, and fatigue scales were the highest, ranging from 0.54 to 0.63 (5, p369). A factor analysis of the subscales identified a strong physical factor and a weaker psychological factor, which correlated 0.47 with each other (6, p137).

Comparisons of QLQ-C30 scores between diagnostic groups and by factors such as extent of weight loss, performance scores, and toxicity ratings demonstrated that many, but not all, of the subscales showed significant variations (5, Figures 1, 2). Responsiveness to change was evaluated by grouping 262 lung cancer patients into those who improved, those who deteriorated, and those whose condition did not change during treatment on the basis of the Eastern Cooperative Oncology Group performance status scale. The QLQ-C30 physical, role, fatigue, and nausea scales showed significant contrasts between these groupings (5, Table 5).

Multitrait validation has been applied to the original 36-item version and to the C30. In 96% of comparisons the convergent coefficients exceeded the discriminant; errors occurred with the role functioning scale (8, p385).

Exhibit 9.5   The EORTC Quality of Life Questionnaire (QLQ-C30)

We are interested in some things about you and your health. Please answer all of the questions yourself by circling the number that best applies to you. There are no "right" or "wrong" answers. The information that you provide will remain strictly confidential.

	No	Yes
1. Do you have any trouble doing strenuous activities, like carrying a heavy shopping bag or a suitcase?	1	2
2. Do you have any trouble taking a *long* walk?	1	2
3. Do you have any trouble taking a *short* walk outside of the house?	1	2
4. Do you have to stay in bed or a chair for most of the day?	1	2
5. Do you need help with eating, dressing, washing yourself, or using the toilet?	1	2
6. Are you limited in any way in doing either your work or doing household jobs?	1	2
7. Are you completely unable to work at a job or to do household jobs?	1	2

During the past week:	Not at All	A Little	Quite a Bit	Very Much
8. Were you short of breath?	1	2	3	4
9. Have you had pain?	1	2	3	4
10. Did you need to rest?	1	2	3	4
11. Have you had trouble sleeping?	1	2	3	4
12. Have you felt weak?	1	2	3	4
13. Have you lacked appetite?	1	2	3	4
14. Have you felt nauseated?	1	2	3	4
15. Have you vomited?	1	2	3	4
16. Have you been constipated?	1	2	3	4
17. Have you had diarrhea?	1	2	3	4
18. Were you tired?	1	2	3	4
19. Did pain interfere with your daily activities?	1	2	3	4
20. Have you had difficulty in concentrating on things, like reading a newspaper or watching television?	1	2	3	4
21. Did you feel tense?	1	2	3	4
22. Did you worry?	1	2	3	4
23. Did you feel irritable?	1	2	3	4
24. Did you feel depressed?	1	2	3	4
25. Have you had difficulty remembering things?	1	2	3	4
26. Has your physical condition or medical treatment interfered with your *family* life?	1	2	3	4
27. Has your physical condition or medical treatment interfered with your *social* activities?	1	2	3	4
28. Has your physical condition or medical treatment caused you financial difficulties?	1	2	3	4

For the following questions please circle the number between 1 and 7 that best applies to you

29. How would you rate your overall *physical condition* during the past week?

1	2	3	4	5	6	7
Very poor						Excellent

30. How would you rate your overall *quality of life* during the past week?

1	2	3	4	5	6	7
Very poor						Excellent

Reproduced from Aaronson NK, Ahmedzai S, Bergman B, et al. The European Organization for Research and Treatment of Cancer QLQ-C30: a quality-of-life instrument for use in international clinical trials in oncology. J Natl Cancer Inst 1993;85:373–374. With permission.

Correlations with other scales have been reported in several studies. The emotional function score correlated 0.71 with scores on the Hospital Anxiety and Depression Scale, from which the QLQ emotional items were drawn (6, p135). Spearman correlations of the subscales with equivalent scores from the Sickness Impact Profile included 0.73 for the physical scale, 0.58 for the cognitive and the fatigue scales, 0.55 for the role scale, and 0.48 for the emotional and the social scales (9, Table 3). Spearman correlations with subscales of the Cancer Rehabilitation Evaluation System (CARES) were similar, including 0.71 for the physical scales, 0.56 for the emotional scales, 0.46 for the social scale, and 0.69 for the pain scale (9, Table 4). The QLQ psychological score correlated 0.61 with the General Health Questionnaire overall score (9, Table 5). Finally, the pain subscale correlated 0.57 and 0.53 with the sensory and present pain scores from the McGill Pain Questionnaire (9, Table 6).

Alternative Forms

Although the original questionnaire was developed in English, this was done with the direct input of people from a range of countries. The QLQ-C30 was field tested simultaneously in 13 countries, including most of the Western European countries, Canada, Australia, and Japan. Validity and reliability information is available for several languages, mainly for the earlier, 36-item version (8, p386).

Commentary

The scope of the QLQ-C30 is broad, and its design reflects a sensible plan for blending generic with disease-specific questions. The items are clearly phrased and would appear to be relevant to patients beyond those with cancer. An advantage is the careful attention to cross-cultural applicability. This should be especially relevant for the growing number of international clinical trials.

The instrument is still in the early stages of field testing, but the early results appear strong. Correlations with other, established scales are high and follow a logical pattern. The QLQ-C30 appears able to detect change, and the reliability scores are moderate to high (as might be expected in a broad-ranging but brief instrument). However, Aaronson et al. commented on the need to modify the role functioning scale, so the version shown here is likely to be revised (5, p372). With the EORTC's strong collaborative network of researchers, it is likely that we will see more testing of this promising instrument.

Address

The European Organization for Research and Treatment of Cancer, Avenue E. Mounier 83, Bte 11, 1200 Brussels, Belgium

Neil K. Aaronson, PhD, Head, Division of Psychosocial Research and Epidemiology, The Netherlands Cancer Institute, Plesmanlaan 121, 1066 CX Amsterdam, The Netherlands

REFERENCES

(1) Aaronson NK, Ahmedzai S, Bullinger M, et al. The EORTC core quality-of-life questionnaire: interim results of an international field study. In: Osoba D, ed. Effect of cancer on quality of life. Boca Raton, Florida: CRC Press, 1991:185–203.

(2) Aaronson NK. Quantitative issues in health-related quality of life assessment. Health Policy 1988;10:217–230.

(3) Aaronson NK, Bullinger M, Ahmedzai S. A modular approach to quality-of-life assessment in cancer clinical trials. Recent Results Cancer Res 1988;111:231–249.

(4) Sprangers MAG, Cull A, Bjordal K, et al. The European Organization for Research and Treatment of Cancer approach to quality of life assessment: guidelines for developing questionnaire modules. Qual Life Res 1993;2:287–295.

(5) Aaronson NK, Ahmedzai S, Bergman B, et al. The European Organization for Research and Treatment of Cancer QLQ-C30: a quality-of-life instrument for use in international clinical trials in oncology. J Natl Cancer Inst 1993;85:365–376.

(6) Ringdal GI, Ringdal K. Testing the EORTC Quality of Life Questionnaire on cancer

patients with heterogeneous diagnoses. Qual Life Res 1993;2:129–140.

(7) Sigurdardóttir V, Bolund C, Brandberg Y, et al. The impact of generalized malignant melanoma on quality of life evaluated by the EORTC questionnaire technique. Qual Life Res 1993;2:193–203.

(8) Anderson RT, Aaronson NK, Wilkin D. Critical review of the international assessments of health-related quality of life. Qual Life Res 1993;2:369–395.

(9) Niezgoda HE, Pater JL. A validation study of the domains of the core EORTC Quality of Life Questionnaire. Qual Life Res 1993;2:319–325.

THE QUALITY OF LIFE INDEX
(W.O. Spitzer, 1980)

Purpose

The Quality of Life Index (QL Index) measures the general well-being of patients terminally ill with cancer or other chronic diseases. It was intended as a brief instrument for evaluating the effects of treatment and programs such as palliative care, but it has subsequently been used more broadly.

Conceptual Basis

Spitzer's index is one of the earliest scales to be designated a "quality of life" measurement. It sought to extend outcome assessment beyond morbidity and mortality by providing a simple and quantified scale that might become the equivalent of the neonatal Apgar score (1). The theme of quality of life was seen as pertinent for patients with terminal illness, for whom extending the length of life is not feasible and for whom, therefore, the prime objective of treatment is to maintain quality of life.

Spitzer saw several dimensions to quality of life, including a positive mood state, supportive relationships, and the absence of physical or psychological distress (2). Hence a measurement of quality of life should consider physical, social, and emotional function, attitudes to illness, the adequacy of family interactions, and the cost of illness to the individual (3).

Description

Potential themes for inclusion in the QL Index were selected empirically from an opinion survey among chronic disease patients, their relatives, health professionals, and well people concerning the factors that enhance or detract from the quality of life (4, p37). Fourteen themes were identified, including absence of symptoms, mental alertness, and financial independence. Questions measuring these were incorporated in draft versions of the QL Index. Pilot testing led to the selection of the five themes in the eventual index: activity level (including occupation), activities of daily living, feelings of healthiness, quality of social support, and psychological outlook (3). The resulting scale takes about two minutes to complete and is administered by a physician or other health professional. This version is shown in Exhibit 9.6, and a self-administered version is shown in Exhibit 9.7. Scores of 0, 1, or 2 for each category reflect increasing well-being and may be summed to give a total score ranging from 0 to 10. In the interests of simplicity, differential weights for the categories are not used.

Along with the QL Index, Spitzer developed a QL Uniscale. This is a visual analogue scale ranging from "lowest quality" to "highest quality"; it may be included in the interviewer and self-administered versions.

Reliability

Spearman rho correlations among the five items ranged from 0.21 to 0.71; three coefficients were 0.5 or above (3, Table 1; 4, Table 4). Internal consistency was assessed on 91 patients in an Australian study, giving an alpha of 0.77 (3, p594). Alpha was also calculated for a sample of 261 patients in Canada, giving a value of 0.78, and of 0.85 for a subset of patients with cancer (2). Other estimates of internal consistency include $\alpha = 0.66$ (5), 0.77, and 0.80 (6). Item-total corrrelations ranged from 0.49 (activity) to 0.86 (outlook) (7, Table 2).

Exhibit 9.6 The Quality of Life Index: Clinician Rating Version

Score each heading 2, 1 or 0 according to your most recent assessment of the patient.

Activity

During the last week, the patient

- has been working or studying full-time or nearly so, in usual occupation; or managing own household; or participating in unpaid or voluntary activities, whether retired or not   2
- has been working or studying in usual occupation or managing own household or participating in unpaid or voluntary activities; but requiring major assistance or a significant reduction in hours worked or a sheltered situation or was on sick leave   1
- has not been working or studying in any capacity and not managing own household   0

☐

Daily living

During the last week, the patient

- has been self-reliant in eating, washing, toileting and dressing; using public transport or driving own car   2
- has been requiring assistance (another person or special equipment) for daily activities and transport but performing light tasks   1
- has not been managing personal care nor light tasks and/or not leaving own home or institution at all   0

☐

Health

During the last week, the patient

- has been appearing to feel well or reporting feeling "great" most of the time   2
- has been lacking energy or not feeling entirely "up to par" more than just occasionally   1
- has been feeling very ill or "lousy," seeming weak and washed out most of the time or was unconscious   0

☐

Support

During the last week

- the patient has been having good relationships with others and receiving strong support from at least one family member and/or friend   2
- support received or perceived has been limited from family and friends and/or by the patient's condition   1
- support from family and friends occurred infrequently or only when absolutely necessary or patient was unconscious   0

☐

Outlook

During the past week the patient

- has usually been appearing calm and positive in outlook, accepting and in control of personal circumstances, including surroundings   2
- has sometimes been troubled because not fully in control of personal circumstances or has been having periods of obvious anxiety or depression   1
- has been seriously confused or very frightened or consistently anxious and depressed or unconscious   0

☐

QL-Index total   ☐☐

☐

How confident are you that your scoring of the preceding dimensions is accurate? Please ring [circle] the appropriate category.

Absolutely confident	Very confident	Quite confident	Not very confident	Very doubtful	Not at all confident
1	2	3	4	5	6

Reproduced from Spitzer WO, Dobson AJ, Hall J, Chesterman E, Levi J, Shepherd R, Battista RN, Catchlove BR. Measuring the quality of life of cancer patients: a concise QL-Index for use by physicians. J Chronic Dis 1981;34:591, Figure 2, Pergamon Press Ltd.

Exhibit 9.7 The Quality of Life Index: Self-Assessment

Each of the next five headings has three choices. Under each heading put a circle around the number that best describes your quality of life during the last week.

Activity—*What is your "main" activity?*

1. I work full-time (or nearly so) in my usual occupation or study full-time (or nearly so) or manage my own household or take part in as much unpaid or voluntary activity as I wish, whether retired or not.

2. I work or study in my usual occupation or manage my own household or participate in unpaid or voluntary activities; but I need a lot of help to do so or I work greatly reduced hours.

3. I do not work in any capacity nor do I study nor do I manage my own household.

Daily living—*Ability to look after yourself.*

1. I am able to eat, wash, go to the toilet and dress without assistance. I drive a car or use public transport without assistance.

2. I can travel and perform daily activities only with assistance (another person or special equipment) but can perform light tasks.

3. I am confined to my home or an institution and cannot manage personal care or light tasks at all.

Health—*What is your state of health?*

1. I feel well most of the time.

2. I lack energy or only feel "up to par" some of the time.

3. I feel very ill or "lousy" most of the time.

Support—*What support do you receive from others?*

1. I have good relationships with others and receive strong support from *at least one* family member and/or friend.

2. The support I receive from family and friends is limited.

3. The support I receive from family and friends occurs infrequently or only when absolutely necessary.

Outlook—*How do you feel about your life?*

1. I am basically a calm person. I generally look forward to things and am able to make my own decisions about my life and surroundings.

2. I am sometimes troubled and there are times when I do not feel fully in control of my personal life. I am anxious and depressed at times.

3. I feel frightened and completely confused about things in general.

Adapted from an original provided by Dr. Spitzer. With permission.

Inter-rater reliability was studied by comparing pairs of ratings made by different physicians; Spearman correlations for various samples ranged from 0.74 to 0.84 (3; 4, Table 5). When five raters judged each patient, they agreed completely on only 45% of ratings (coefficient of concordance = 0.54) (8). Several studies have compared the self-report and physician rating versions of the QL Index. For 161 Australian patients the Spearman correlation was 0.61; for 51 Canadian patients it was 0.69 (3, p595). Other studies obtained correlations of 0.45 (2) and 0.72 (9) and a Kendall correlation of 0.72 (9, Table 1). Pearson correlations between self-report and ratings of relatives was 0.63 for 261 Canadian patients (2).

Stability was assessed by having patients rate themselves daily for five days; their scores agreed completely 80% of the time and fell within one point 95% of the time (8). The QL Index was administered twice to breast cancer patients who, in the judgment of a nurse, had not changed physical or emotional functioning over a two-week period. The QL Index (like a second scale, the Breast Cancer Questionnaire) showed a significant decline, suggesting either that the nurse's rating missed a deterioration or that there is measurement error in the scales (10).

Validity

The content validity of the QL Index was checked by asking patients, well people, physicians, and researchers to judge its scope and design (2).

Ten items from the initial item pool that were not used in the QL Index were formed into a more extensive quality of life scale. This instrument was administered with the QL Index to 476 patients and well people in Australia. The correlations between the QL Index and the comprehensive scale were highest for samples of cancer patients (ρ = 0.61 to 0.71), intermediate for other chronically sick patients, and low (ρ = 0.29 to 0.49) for well people (3, Table 2). Replication of these analyses in a Canadian study yielded correlations between 0.66 and 0.84 for cancer patients (2, Table 4). Correlations between the QL Index and the Uniscale were higher for cancer patients (0.49 to 0.61) than for well people (0.17 to 0.39).

Spitzer et al. reported mean scores for healthy people and various patient groups, showing that the index discriminates between healthy people and various categories of patients (3). Scores on the QL Index have shown a decline with age in several studies (see 1, p175). In a study of congestive heart failure, the QL Index showed greater ability to discriminate between experimental and control groups than the Sickness Impact Profile or the Quality of Well-Being Scale (11).

The QL Index has been compared to the Karnofsky Performance Status Scale in several studies with variable results: correlations of 0.72 (12), 0.41, and 0.83 (5). A study of 45 elderly patients reported moderate correlations with three ADL scales: 0.52 with the Barthel Index, 0.45 with the Functional Independence Measure, and 0.48 with Katz's Index of ADL (13, Table 2). Index scores correlated 0.42

with a Breast Cancer Questionnaire (10). A Kendall rank correlation of 0.53 was reported between the Index scores and a visual analogue scale (similar to the QL Uniscale). While this does not seem high enough to indicate that the QL Index could be replaced by the simpler scale, it is not very much lower than the typical correlation between self-administered and interview versions of the QL Index of about 0.70. The social support item correlated 0.72 with Wortman's social support scale (7, Table 5). The outlook item correlated −0.68 with the Hamilton Rating Scale for Depression and −0.63 with the Brief Symptom Inventory anxiety scale (7, Table 7).

Alternative Forms

Morris et al. replaced the activity item by one on mobility, arguing that the activity item was inappropriate for terminally ill patients; they also reworded items for verbal presentation (14). These changes seem to offer little advantage in terms of power or efficiency of the QL Index, however (1, p173).

The QL Index has been translated into French (2), German (12), and Italian (15, p388).

Reference Standards

Representative scores from well and ill respondents are given by Spitzer. Mean scores for two samples of healthy people were 8.8 and 9.2; means for those with chronic disease were 7.3, and for seriously ill patients the mean was 3.3 (3, Table 3).

Commentary

The emphasis in the QL Index is on practicality; it is brief and easy to administer in a clinical setting and yet broad in scope: "The QL Index, like the Apgar score, should be thought of as a composite of dissimilar items" (1, p181). It has proved acceptable to clinicians and has been widely cited in the literature. The development of the QL Index was carefully undertaken, involving extensive consultation with patients and clinicians; the approach has served as a model for subsequent investigators (1). The QL Index has been used in Australia, Britain, Canada, Germany, and the United States. Reliability and validity results are good; the pattern of validity results suggests that the instrument achieves its aims.

A brief scale that is also broad in scope may be expected to sacrifice some psychometric properties, but the internal consistency alphas of 0.77 and above are reasonably high. The finding that agreement between patient and physician ratings is modest (in the range of 0.6 to 0.7) may not indicate a failure of reliability so much as remind us that the perspectives differ and that both types of rating are needed. The modest agreement also indicates that the scale must be consistently completed by one type of respondent in a before and after evaluative design. Suissa et al. identified systematic variations in QL Index scores by age, sex, and disease categories, suggesting that these confounding variables should be controlled in research studies (2). It should also be recognized that the QL Index may be less sensitive to short-term changes than some other, disease-specific instruments. Its reliance on physical functioning and on observer assessments may be at the expense of sensitivity to the impact of cancer on the patient's social activities or emotional status (15, p389). The instrument is more suited to global assessments of seriously sick patients over the long term than to detailed evaluation of short-term outcomes (1, p182). The instrument is not suitable for healthy respondents, for whom survey measures such as the SF-36 would be more appropriate (3).

REFERENCES

(1) Wood-Dauphinee S, Williams JI. The Spitzer Quality-of-Life Index: its performance as a measure. In: Osoba D, ed. Effect of cancer on quality of life. Boca Raton, Florida: CRC Press, 1991:169–184.

(2) Suissa S, Shenker SC, Spitzer WO. Measuring the quality of life of cancer and chronically ill patients: cross-validation studies of the Quality of Life Index. Montreal, Quebec: Department of Clinical Epidemiology, McGill University, 1984. (Manuscript.)

(3) Spitzer WO, Dobson AJ, Hall J, et al. Measuring the quality of life of cancer patients: a concise QL-Index for use by physicians. J Chronic Dis 1981;34:585–597.

(4) Spitzer WO. Quality of life. In: Burley D, Inman WHW, eds. Therapeutic risk: perception, measurement, management. New York: John Wiley & Sons, 1988: 35–46.

(5) Mor V. Cancer patients' quality of life over the disease course: lessons from the real world. J Chronic Dis 1987;40:535–544.

(6) Mor V, Stalker MZ, Gralla R, et al. Day hospital as an alternative to inpatient care for cancer patients: a random assignment trial. J Clin Epidemiol 1988;41:771.

(7) Williams JBW, Rabkin JG. The concurrent validity of items in the Quality-of-Life Index in a cohort of HIV-positive and HIV-negative gay men. Controlled Clin Trials 1991;12(suppl):129S-141S.

(8) Slevin ML, Plant H, Lynch D, et al. Who should measure quality of life, the doctor or the patient? Br J Cancer 1988;57:109–112.

(9) Gough IR, Furnival CM, Schilder L, et al. Assessment of the quality of life of patients with advanced cancer. Eur J Cancer Clin Oncol 1983;19:1161–1165.

(10) Levine MN, Guyatt GH, Gent M, et al. Quality of life in stage II breast cancer: an instrument for clinical trials. J Clin Oncol 1988;6:1798–1810.

(11) Tandon PK, Stander H, Schwarz RP Jr. Analysis of quality of life data from a randomized, placebo-controlled heart-failure trial. J Clin Epidemiol 1989;42:955–962.

(12) Köster R, Gebbensleben B, Stützer H, et al. Quality of life in gastric cancer. Karnofsky's scale and Spitzer's index in comparison at the time of surgery in a cohort of 1081 patients. Scand J Gastroenterol 1987;22(suppl 133):102–106.

(13) Rockwood K, Stolee P, Fox RA. Use of goal attainment scaling in measuring clinically important change in the frail elderly. J Clin Epidemiol 1993;46:1113–1118.

(14) Morris JN, Suissa S, Sherwood S, et al. Last days: a study of the quality of life of terminally ill cancer patients. J Chronic Dis 1986;39:47–62.

(15) Anderson RT, Aaronson NK, Wilkin D. Critical review of the international assessments of health-related quality of life. Qual Life Res 1993;2:369–395.

THE COOP CHARTS FOR PRIMARY CARE PRACTICE
(Eugene C. Nelson, 1987)

Purpose

The COOP Charts provide a rapid way to assess the health and functioning of patients in primary care (1–3). They are intended for use in routine clinical practice, rather than as research instruments.

Conceptual Basis

The Dartmouth Primary Care Cooperative Information Project (or COOP) in New Hampshire was established to create a practical system for measuring health status in physicians' offices. Nelson et al. argued that, beyond safeguarding biological function, care should be concerned with improving patients' physical, mental, and role function. The functioning of the person as a whole is more important than that of separate organ systems, so indicators of organ system function are not sufficient as indicators of health (3, 4). Several design requirements were made of the COOP Charts: they had to be reliable, valid, acceptable in routine practice, applicable to a wide range of diagnoses, easily interpretable—and they had to provide clinically useful information (1; 5, pp97–98).

The COOP information model contains five stages: screening, assessment, diagnosis, treatment, and monitoring, of which the charts form the screening stage (1, p61).

Used correctly, the Charts allow practitioners to screen patients quickly and efficiently and to highlight those individuals who might benefit from a more comprehensive inquiry of functioning and health-related quality of life. The screening instrument should be used periodically to monitor the progression of chronic disease of a patient and to diagnose the onset of new disease. (6, p152)

Wasson et al. illustrate how the screening information is used in routine clinical practice (7). Time constraints in practice demand an instrument that is quick to complete and to score, that can be applied to a wide range of problems and diagnoses, and that can provide clinically useful informa-

tion. With this in mind, the instrument was designed in the form of charts, similar in concept to the familiar Snellen Charts used to measure visual acuity.

Description

Originally three charts covered physical, emotional, and role function (1). Successful pretesting led to an expansion of the method to produce nine charts, each with a single question about health during the past month. They are shown in Exhibit 9.8. Three charts cover function (physical fitness, daily and social activities), three cover health perceptions (quality of life, overall health, and change in health), two cover symptoms and feelings (pain, emotional status), and one (social support) is seen as a factor influencing health. Each chart includes a descriptive title, a question relating to the past four weeks, and a five-point answer scale illustrated by simple pictures; a score of 5 represents the most severe limitations. A randomized trial that compared the charts with and without the pictures showed no difference in mean scores between the two versions (8).

Nelson et al. originally recommended that the charts be administered by trained office staff (2, p1121) but they can also be completed by the patient in the waiting room in less than five minutes (2, p1119; 5). Administration by staff is typically done at the beginning of the office visit while routine data are being collected (1). The diagrams can be displayed on the wall, or the patient may be handed copies. The answer sheet is stored in the patient's medical record. The nine charts are considered as separate dimensions of functioning, and an overall score is not calculated.

Nelson initially tested the charts on 117 patients (1), demonstrating their feasibility and acceptability and collecting preliminary data on validity and reliability. The charts were revised and subsequently tested in a series of studies (2; 5, Table 8.2). The largest included 2,349 patients participating in the Rand Medical Outcomes Study (MOS), in which the COOP Charts were included.

Exhibit 9.8 The Dartmouth COOP Charts

PHYSICAL FITNESS

During the past 4 weeks . . .
   What was the hardest physical activity
   you could do for at least 2 minutes ?

Very heavy, (for example)
•Run, fast pace
•Carry a heavy load
   upstairs or uphill
   (25 lbs/10 kgs)
		1

Heavy, (for example) •Jog, slow pace •Climb stairs or a hill moderate pace		2

Moderate, (for example)
•Walk, medium pace
•Carry a heavy load
   level ground
   (25 lbs/10 kgs)
		3

Light, (for example)
•Walk, medium pace
•Carry light load
   on level ground
   (10 lbs/5kgs)
		4

Very light, (for example) •Walk, slow pace •Wash dishes		5

FEELINGS

During the past 4 weeks . . .
   How much have you been bothered by
   emotional problems such as feeling anxious,
   depressed, irritable or downhearted and blue ?

Not at all		1
Slightly		2
Moderately		3
Quite a bit		4
Extremely		5

DAILY ACTIVITIES

During the past 4 weeks . . .
   How much difficulty have you had doing your usual
   activities or task, both inside and outside the house
   because of your physical and emotional health ?

No difficulty at all		1
A little bit of difficulty		2
Some difficulty		3
Much difficulty		4
Could not do		5

SOCIAL ACTIVITIES

During the past 4 weeks . . .
   Has your physical and emotional health limited
   your social activities with family, friends,
   neighbors or groups ?

Not at all		1
Slightly		2
Moderately		3
Quite a bit		4
Extremely		5

Exhibit 9.8   (Continued)

Exhibit 9.8 *(Continued)*

PAIN

During the past 4 weeks . . .
    How much bodily pain have you
    generally had ?

No pain		1
Very mild pain		2
Mild pain		3
Moderate pain		4
Severe pain		5

CHANGE IN HEALTH

How would you rate your overall health
now compared to 4 weeks ago ?

Much better	▲▲	++	1
A little better	▲	+	2
About the same	◄►	=	3
A little worse	▼	—	4
Much worse	▼▼	— —	5

OVERALL HEALTH

During the past 4 weeks . . .
    How would you rate your health in general ?

Excellent		1
Very good		2
Good		3
Fair		4
Poor		5

SOCIAL SUPPORT

During the past 4 weeks . . .
    Was someone available to help you if you
    needed and wanted help? For example if you
— felt very nervous, lonely, or blue
— got sick and had to stay in bed
— needed someone to talk to
— needed help with daily chores
— needed help just taking care of yourself

Yes, as much as I wanted		1
Yes, quite a bit		2
Yes, some		3
Yes, a little		4
No, not at all		5

412

QUALITY OF LIFE

How have things been going for you during the past 4 weeks?

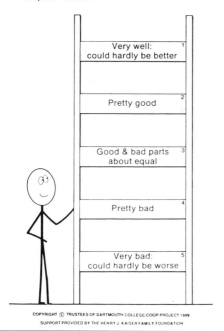

Very well: could hardly be better   1

Pretty good   2

Good & bad parts about equal   3

Pretty bad   4

Very bad: could hardly be worse   5

Adapted from an original provided by Dr. E Nelson. With permission.

Reliability

Inter-rater agreement between tests administered by a physician and a nurse measured by the intraclass correlation averaged 0.77 across the charts; the range was 0.50 to 0.98 (2, Table 1); eight of the nine correlation coefficients were 0.76 or above (four had kappa coefficients above 0.65) (5, Table 8.5).

Nelson et al. have reported reliability from four samples (5, Table 8.5). One-hour retest reliability averaged $r = 0.93$ for the nine charts, with a range of 0.78 to 0.98 (N = 53); in a different sample of 51 outpatients, reliability averaged 0.88 (range 0.73 to 0.98) (2, Table 1). Retest reliability at two weeks was lower, averaging 0.67 (range 0.42 to 0.88) (2, Table 1). Reliability at one week ranged from 0.67 (physical condition) to 0.82 (daily work) for the Dutch version of the charts (9, Table 9.1).

McHorney et al. compared the reliability of the individual chart ratings and the global ratings from the MOS instrument (10). The two instruments had the same number of scale levels but only the COOP instrument had illustrations. The MOS ratings showed markedly higher reliabilities: for example, 0.57 compared to 0.37 for physical functioning and 0.65 compared to 0.54 for emotional functioning (10, Table 2). The intercorrelations among scores for the nine charts averaged 0.37 (range 0.06 to 0.68) (11, p176).

Validity

The validity of the COOP Charts has been tested in numerous studies, often with large samples. Nelson evaluated acceptability of the charts by interviewing office staff and patients in ten practices that had been using them. Interviews with 225 patients indicated that 97% understood the charts, 89% enjoyed them, 93% liked the pictures, and 74% rated the charts as useful (6, Table 10.3). Physicians reported that in one-quarter of cases the charts provided them with new information and that in 40% of these, the information led to a change in management (5, p117). For 13% of patients doctors reported that the charts had a positive effect on communication but for 2% they had a negative effect (2, p1120).

Nelson et al. compared the chart scores to a range of criterion variables in a study of 784 patients as part of the MOS. Convergent coefficients fell in the range 0.40 to 0.50 for most charts (5, Table 8.6). The correlations between chart scores and numbers of symptoms ranged from 0.25 (for "health change") to 0.51 ("overall health") (2, p1117). McHorney et al. evaluated the ability of each COOP Chart to discriminate between medical patients with minor and serious complaints and psychiatric patients; they also compared this discrimination with that of MOS global indicators (10, Tables 3–8). The COOP Charts all proved capable of discriminating between categories of patient; in general they performed less well than the equivalent MOS indicators for medical patients, but better for psychiatric patients. Nelson et al. also compared the discriminal ability of the charts and MOS scores. Interestingly, they found the two methods similar for physical illness, and the charts superior for emotional symptoms (5, pp111, 116).

The COOP Charts have been compared to various short forms of the Medical Outcomes Study measures, including the Short-Form-20 survey (SF-20) (2, 10, 12, 13). Nelson et al. compared the three original COOP physical, emotional, and role function charts to equivalent scales from the 28-item short-form MOS instrument (1). Convergent validity correlations (those between scales purporting to measure the same theme) were 0.71 (for physical functioning) and 0.74 (emotional) and 0.40 (daily activities) (1, Table 2; 1, Table 2); equivalent figures from a study testing the revised version of the COOP Charts were 0.59, 0.69, and 0.60 (2, Table 2). The average convergent correlations in two samples were 0.62 and 0.46 (2, Table 1). As expected, these exceeded correlations between scales measuring different attributes; the average divergent correlations were 0.39 and 0.32 (2, p1117). Convergent validity coefficients in the range 0.48 to 0.78 were reported from three samples (total sample size of over 1,000) (5, Table 8.8). Two multitrait-multimethod analyses showed an average convergent coefficient of 0.60, and an average divergent correlation of 0.16 (5, p111). In a comparison with the Nottingham Health Profile, the COOP Charts proved more sensitive to minor deviations from complete well-being (14). Four of the COOP Charts were compared to the Nottingham scales in a Dutch study; convergent correlation coefficients fell in the range 0.35 to 0.58 (9, Table 9.2).

The correlations between the emotional condition chart and the General Health Questionnaire (GHQ) was 0.60 in a Dutch study. The correlation between the GHQ and the daily work section was 0.61, suggesting that the daily work chart reflects emotional difficulties as much as physical (9, Table 9.2).

Regression analyses compared the sensitivity of the COOP Charts and SF-20 scales in reflecting the impact of selected chronic conditions on functioning. The variance explained by the physical function scale was slightly superior for the COOP Chart, whereas for the emotional, role, and overall scales, the SF-20 scales were better (markedly so for the emotional questions: $R^2 = 0.29$ for the COOP Charts versus 0.52 for the Rand questions) (2, Table 3). Correlations with number of symptoms ranged from 0.27 (social support) to 0.51 (overall health) for 231 elderly people (5, Table 8.7).

Siu et al. compared the convergent and divergent validity of *change* scores on the COOP and SF-20. The average convergent validity correlation was 0.37, and the average divergent correlation was 0.18 (12, p1096). Moderate to strong convergent correlations were observed only for pain, social, and mental scores; convergent validity between change on the physical function measures was only 0.05 (12, p1096). The COOP function score failed to detect changes in physical function as measured by performance based measures of gait and balance or the 50-foot walk time (12, Table 5). Siu et al. commented that while cross-sectional studies have supported the convergent and discriminant validity of the SF-20 and COOP instruments, the results may not hold for changes in functional status (12, p1100).

A study of elderly patients compared the validity of COOP and SF-20 scores in predicting future health status; both provided significant and almost identical predictors of nursing home placement and hospitalization (13). Wasson et al. noted that the predictive value of a good emotional health score on the COOP Charts lies somewhere between 96% and 99%: the emotional chart is adequate to rule out psychiatric illness (7, pMS46).

Alternative Forms

In 1988 the World Organization of National Colleges, Academies, and Academic Associations of General Practitioners and

Family Physicians (WONCA) adopted the COOP Charts as the basis of their international system for measuring functional status (15, 16). The WONCA group modified the charts in several ways, changing the titles and wording of the questions, omitting the quality of life and social support charts, and changing the physical chart to cover walking only (16; 17; 18, p383). Four-week test–retest reliability correlations for this version ranged from 0.42 to 0.62. Some validity results have also been published (18, p384).

The COOP Charts have been used in the Netherlands (9), Japan (19), and Hong Kong with positive results (20). Along with the translation, the illustrations are usually altered, occasionally offering intriguing cross-cultural insights. The Dutch version, for example, depicts strenuous physical activity by a woman positively rushing up stairs two steps at a time (9, p134); the original COOP man climbs more steadily, one step at a time. The WONCA version is also available in Danish, Finnish, Norwegian, Spanish, German, Hebrew, and Urdu (17).

The COOP Chart approach has been adapted for adolescents; six charts cover physical fitness, feelings, school work, social support, family communications, and health habits. The charts appear acceptable to adolescents and they correlate well with questionnaire measures (21).

Commentary

The COOP Charts offer an imaginative and innovative approach to routine measurement in clinical practice. They are quick and easy to use; they are acceptable to patients; and they are judged clinically useful by physicians (1). The visual metaphors are attractive and may speed up administration; they may also help to overcome language barriers in cross-cultural applications, where patients are marginally literate, or with patients unfamiliar with thinking in abstract concepts (22). Methodologically, the charts represent one side in the debate over how brief a measure can

be and still achieve the precision required in clinical practice and research (10). An impressive amount of data have been collected attesting to the validity and reliability of the charts; the Dartmouth COOP project team has been a solid force in overseeing this. The comparison between the charts and the MOS instruments has in part been fueled by a desire to guide the balance between brevity and accuracy of measurement. The results thus far seem to suggest that the single-item measures in the charts can provide quite good indications of present state but are too coarse to detect minor changes in function over time. The reliability and validity studies have been undertaken in several testing sites and offer a more extensive and varied testing protocol than applied in most reliability and validity studies. The low reliability results compared to the MOS global ratings gives cause for concern (10).

The illustrations in the COOP Charts have raised considerable interest, as have the smiling faces scales reviewed in Chapter 5. The approach appears attractive to respondents, although the consistency of interpreting illustrations by different cultural groups is a point of concern. Furthermore, pictures are usually more specific than a verbal description, and so may focus attention on a narrow interpretation of the question (22). McHorney et al. concluded that the illustrations appeared to improve the charts' sensitivity to psychological distress, but not to physical impairment. They commented: "Similarly, the use of a smiling face for no pain and a sad face with drooping shoulders for severe pain appears to have increased the sensitivity of the pain chart to emotional distress at the expense of its sensitivity to physical health." (10, pMS263)

Although brief, the charts agree surprisingly well with the lengthier MOS scales. The charts offer a brief screen that is accurate enough to give a global impression of a patient's well-being, but may miss changes in condition over time. The ratings of physical function and of pain may include a strong measure of psychological reaction to any physical problems present.

REFERENCES

(1) Nelson EC, Wasson J, Kirk J, et al. Assessment of function in routine clinical practice: description of the COOP Chart method and preliminary findings. J Chronic Dis 1987;40(suppl 1):55S-63S.

(2) Nelson EC, Landgraf JM, Hays RD, et al. The functional status of patients. How can it be measured in physicians' offices? Med Care 1990;28:1111-1126.

(3) Nelson EC, Landgraf JM, Hays RD, et al. Dartmouth COOP proposal to develop and demonstrate a system to assess functional health status in physicians' offices. Final report to Henry J. Kaiser Family Foundation. Hanover, New Hampshire: Department of Community and Family Medicine, Dartmouth Medical School, 1987.

(4) Greenfield S, Nelson EC. Recent developments and future issues in the use of health status assessment measures in clinical settings. Med Care 1992;30(suppl):MS23-MS41.

(5) Nelson EC, Landgraf JM, Hays RD, et al. The COOP Function Charts: a system to measure patient function in physicians' offices. In: Lipkin M, ed. Functional status measurement in primary care. New York: Springer-Verlag, 1990:97-131.

(6) Landgraf JM, Nelson EC, Hays RD, et al. Assessing function: does it really make a difference? A preliminary evaluation of the acceptability and utility of the COOP Function Charts. In: Lipkin M, ed. Functional status measurement in primary care. New York: Springer-Verlag, 1990:150-161.

(7) Wasson J, Keller A, Rubenstein L, et al. Benefits and obstacles of health status assessment in ambulatory settings: the clinician's point of view. Med Care 1992;30(suppl):MS42-MS49.

(8) Larson CO, Hays RD, Nelson EC. Do the pictures influence scores on the Dartmouth COOP Charts? Qual Life Res 1992;1:247-249.

(9) Meyboom-de Jong B, Smith RJA. Studies with the Dartmouth COOP Charts in general practice: comparison with the Nottingham Health Profile and the General Health Questionnaire. In: Lipkin M, ed. Functional status measurement in primary care. New York: Springer-Verlag, 1990:132-149.

(10) McHorney CA, Ware JE Jr, Rogers W, et al. The validity and relative precision of MOS short- and long-form health status scales and Dartmouth COOP charts. Med Care 1992;30(suppl):MS253-MS265.

(11) Westbury RC. Use of the Dartmouth COOP Charts in a Calgary practice. In: Lipkin M, ed. Functional status measurement in primary care. New York: Springer-Verlag, 1990:166-180.

(12) Siu AL, Ouslander JG, Osterweil D, et al. Change in self-reported functioning in older persons entering a residential care facility. J Clin Epidemiol 1993;46:1093-1101.

(13) Siu AL, Reuben DB, Ouslander JG, et al. Using multidimensional health measures in older persons to identify risk of hospitalization and skilled nursing placement. Qual Life Res 1993;2:253-261.

(14) Coates AK, Wilkin D. Comparing the Nottingham Health Profile with the Dartmouth COOP Charts. In: Scholten JHG, ed. Functional status assessment in family practice. Lelystad, Netherlands: Meditekst, 1992:81-86.

(15) Landgraf JM, Nelson EC. Dartmouth COOP primary care network. Summary of the WONCA/COOP international health assessment field trial. Aust Fam Phys 1992;21:255-269.

(16) Froom J. Preface: WONCA committee on international classification. Statement on functional status assessment Calgary, October 1988. In: Lipkin M, ed. Functional status measurement in primary care. New York: Springer-Verlag, 1990:xiii-xvii.

(17) Scholten JHG, van Weel C. Manual for the use of the Dartmouth COOP functional health assessment charts/WONCA in measuring functional status in family practice. In: Scholten JHG, ed. Functional status assessment in family practice. Lelystad, Netherlands: Meditekst, 1992:17-50.

(18) Anderson RT, Aaronson NK, Wilkin D. Critical review of the international assessments of health-related quality of life. Qual Life Res 1993;2:369-395.

(19) Shigemoto H. A trial of the Dartmouth COOP Charts in Japan. In: Lipkin M, ed. Functional status measurement in primary care. New York: Springer-Verlag, 1990:181-187.

(20) Lam CL, van Weel C, Lauder IJ. Can the Dartmouth COOP/WONCA charts be used to assess the functional status of Chinese patients? Fam Pract 1994;11:85-94.

(21) Wasson JH, Kairys SW, Nelson EC, et al. A short survey for assessing health and social problems of adolescents. J Fam Pract 1994;38:489-494.

(22) Palmer RH. Commentary: assessment of function in routine clinical practice. J Chronic Dis 1987;40(suppl 1):65S-69S.

THE FUNCTIONAL STATUS QUESTIONNAIRE
(Alan M. Jette, 1986)

Purpose

The Functional Status Questionnaire (FSQ) is a brief, self-administered questionnaire that assesses physical, psychological, and social role functioning in ambulatory patients. It was designed as a clinical tool to screen for disability and to monitor changes in function among people attending primary care practices (1, 2).

Conceptual Basis

Following the WHO, Jette defined functional disability in terms of departure from normal performance. Three common purposes of monitoring functional disability include describing a patient's status, assessing need for treatment, and monitoring progress. An assessment instrument has to be more detailed than a descriptive one and a monitoring instrument, in addition, has to be sensitive to change (2, p1854).

Description

The FSQ was adapted from existing scales by researchers at the Beth Israel Hospital in Boston and at UCLA in California. It covers physical function (three ADL and six IADL items), psychological function (five items), work performance (six items), social activity (three items) and quality of social interaction (five items). Four-, five-, and six-point ratings are used, referring to health in the past month. Six additional questions cover sick days, interpersonal relationships, and feelings about health. The questionnaire takes about 15 minutes to complete (2, p1855).

The 34 items are scored by computer to provide six summary scale scores and six single-item scores (see Exhibit 9.9). The scale scores are standardized to a 0-to-100 range, with high scores indicating better function. The computer prints a one-page summary report of responses, indicating areas that are of potential clinical concern based on cutting points determined by a panel of experienced clinicians (1, 2). An illustration of routine clinical use of the FSQ is given by Rubenstein et al. (3).

Reliability

Based on the responses of 1,153 ambulatory primary care patients, the internal consistencies of the six scale scores ranged from 0.64 to 0.82 (2, Table 1). In a different study, Jette obtained an alpha internal consistency coefficient of 0.87 for an emotional function scale that combines the five psychological function questions with the five quality of interaction questions (4, Table 2). A Swedish study obtained an alpha coefficient of 0.77 for the basic ADL, of 0.87 for the instrumental ADL score, of 0.88 for the mental functioning score, of 0.75 for social activities, and of 0.79 for quality of interaction (5, Table V).

Validity

As an indicator of the acceptability of the FSQ to physicians, a randomized trial compared patient management by physicians who received, or did not receive, FSQ profiles of the patients they were seeing. Forty-three percent of physicians reported that the FSQ information led them to alter their therapy; 97% reported that the information was useful (3, Table 4). There were, however, no significant differences in health outcomes between the experimental and control groups.

Jette reported the correlations among the six scales but did not present a factor analysis. The correlations ranged from 0.14 to 0.75 and showed intercorrelations exceeding 0.62 among the three scales requiring physical ability: basic ADL, instrumental ADL (IADL), and social activity (2, Table 2). Very similar correlations were reported from a Swedish study (5, Table VI).

Jette et al. present construct validity cor-

Exhibit 9.9 The Functional Status Questionnaire

Note: An asterisk indicates items for which scores are reversed.

Category	Item

Physical function: During the past month have you had difficulty:

Basic activities of daily living (ADL)

Taking care of yourself, that is, eating, dressing or bathing?
Moving in and out of a bed or chair?
Walking indoors, such as around your home?

Intermediate ADL

Walking several blocks?
Walking one block or climbing one flight of stairs?
Doing work around the house such as cleaning, light yard work, home maintenance?
Doing errands, such as grocery shopping?
Driving a car or using public transportation?
Doing vigorous activities such as running, lifting heavy objects or participating in strenuous sports?

Responses: usually did with no difficulty (4), some difficulty (3), much difficulty (2), usually did not do because of health (1), usually did not do for other reasons (0).

Psychological function: During the past month:

Mental health

Have you been a very nervous person?
Have you felt calm and peaceful?*
Have you felt downhearted and blue?
Were you a happy person?*
Did you feel so down in the dumps
  that nothing could cheer you up?

Responses: all of the time (1), most of the time (2), a good bit of the time (3), some of the time (4), a little of the time (5), none of the time (6).

Social/role function: During the past month have you:

Work performance (for those employed, during the preceding month)

Done as much work as others in similar jobs?*
Worked for short periods of time or taken frequent rests because of your health?
Worked your regular number of hours?*
Done your job as carefully and accurately as others with similar jobs?*
Worked at your usual job, but with some changes because of your health?
Feared losing your job because of your health?

Responses: all of the time (1), most of the time (2), some of the time (3), none of the time (4).

Social activity

Had difficulty visiting with relatives or friends?
Had difficulty participating in community activities, such as religious services, social activities, or volunteer work?
Had difficulty taking care of other people such as family members?

Responses: Usually did with no difficulty (4), some difficulty (3), much difficulty (2), usually did not do because of health (1), usually did not do for other reasons (0).

Quality of interaction

Isolated yourself from people around you?
Acted affectionate toward others?*
Acted irritable toward those around you?
Made unreasonable demands on your family and friends?
Gotten along well with other people?*

Responses: all of the time (1), most of the time (2), a good bit of the time (3), some of the time (4), a little of the time (5), none of the time (6).

418

Single item questions:

Which of the following statements best describes your work situation during the past month?
Responses: working full-time; working part-time; unemployed; looking for work; unemployed because of my health; retired because of my health; retired for some other reason.

During the past month, how many days did illness or injury keep you in bed all or most of the day?
Response: 0–31 days.

During the past month, how many days did you cut down on the things you usually do for one-half day or more because of your own illness or injury? *Response:* 0–31 days.

During the past month, how satisfied were you with your sexual relationships? *Responses:* very satisfied; satisfied; not sure; dissatisfied; very dissatisfied; did not have any sexual relationships.

How do you feel about your own health? *Responses:* very satisfied; satisfied; not sure; dissatisfied; very dissatisfied.

During the past month, about how often did you get together with friends or relatives, such as going out together, visiting in each other's homes, or talking on the telephone? *Responses:* every day; several times a week; about once a week; two or three times a month; about once a month; not at all.

Reproduced from Jette AM, Davies AR, Cleary PD, et al. The Functional Status Questionnaire: reliability and validity when used in primary care. J Gen Intern Med 1986;1:144. With permission.

relations for the FSQ scale scores and criterion variables (1, Table 4). Illustrative results include: the ADL scale of the FSQ correlated −0.33 with restricted activity days and −0.44 with limitations in work role. Equivalent correlations for the IADL scale were −0.36 and −0.61. The mental health scale correlated 0.45 with satisfaction with health; quality of interaction correlated 0.26 with number of social contacts. Equivalent correlations were reported from the Swedish study: the number of restricted activity days correlated −0.42 with the ADL score and −0.44 with the IADL score; the frequency of social contacts correlated 0.29 with the FSQ quality of interaction scale and 0.35 with the social activities score (5, Table VI). Correlations of the FSQ scores with the Current Health Perceptions scale of the SF-20 ranged from 0.30 to 0.46 (6, p667). A correlation of 0.82 was obtained between the global dimension and the SIP, and of 0.83 with the SF-36 in a study of 106 hip replacement patients (7, Table 3). The FSQ physical scores correlated 0.76 with the modified Health Assessment Questionnaire.

The predictive validity of the FSQ has been tested in several studies. FSQ ADL and IADL scores proved better able to predict outcomes of valvuloplasty and recur-

rences in patients with aortic stenosis than the New York Heart Association classification (8). In a four-year prospective study of risk factors for mortality, the IADL and quality of interaction scores were independently associated with mortality after controlling for age, race, marital status, and other variables (6).

Sensitivity to change was tested for 106 hip replacement patients and compared to that of the SIP, SF-36, and shortened Arthritis Impact Measurement Scales. The FSQ overall score ranked second in sensitivity to change (7, Table 4).

Alternative Forms

Results of using a Swedish version of the FSQ have been described above (5).

Commentary

This measure was designed as a screen for disability in primary care settings, among ambulatory adults of all ages, and it was designed to be scored and summarized using the doctor's office computer. The aim of giving a routine and systematic review of functional status for ambulatory patients is similar to that of the COOP Charts, and practical testing of the FSQ along the lines used with the COOP Charts is beginning to be reported (3). The main difference in the two instruments lies in their length: the Charts provide only summary ratings in each area, compared to FSQ's more conventional, psychometric approach of summing responses to several questions to form response scales. In addition to its use by physicians, Jette notes that the FSQ could be adapted for clinical use by physical therapists (2).

As a new scale, further testing is required. Jette notes that, partly because of the brevity of the scales, reliability is not sufficient to make comparisons between individual patients. The FSQ may, however, prove adequate to study the same patient across time and to compare groups of patients. Further validity testing is desirable, and the practical aspects of using it routinely in medical practice (perhaps using computer instead of paper and pencil) remain to be tested. The method should also be used in other centers before it can be fully recommended.

Address

Scoring software is available from Michael McCoy, MD, Department of Medicine, UCLA, Los Angeles, California, USA 90024

REFERENCES

(1) Jette AM, Davies AR, Cleary PD, et al. The Functional Status Questionnaire: reliability and validity when used in primary care. J Gen Intern Med 1986;1:143–149.

(2) Jette AM, Cleary PD. Functional disability assessment. Phys Ther 1987;67:1854–1859.

(3) Rubenstein LV, Calkins DR, Young RT, et al. Improving patient function: a randomized trial of functional disability screening. Ann Intern Med 1989;111:836–842.

(4) Jette AM, Harris BA, Cleary PD, et al. Functional recovery after hip fracture. Arch Phys Med Rehabil 1987;68:735–740.

(5) Einarsson G, Grimby G. Disability and handicap in late poliomyelitis. Scand J Rehabil Med 1990;22:1–9.

(6) Reuben DB, Rubenstein LV, Hirsch SH, et al. Value of functional status as a predictor of mortality: results of a prospective study. Am J Med 1992;93:663–669.

(7) Katz JN, Larson MG, Phillips CB, et al. Comparative measurement sensitivity of short and longer health status instruments. Med Care 1992;30:917–925.

(8) Tedesco C, Manning S, Lindsay R, et al. Functional assessment of elderly patients after percutaneous aortic balloon valvuloplasty: New York Heart Association classification versus Functional Status Questionnaire. Heart Lung 1990;19:118–125.

THE DUKE HEALTH PROFILE
(George R. Parkerson, 1990)

Purpose

The Duke Health Profile (DUKE) is intended as a brief and practical measure to evaluate patient health status in primary care settings.

Conceptual Basis

The DUKE was derived from the Duke–UNC Health Profile (DUHP), a 63-item measure designed to measure outcomes in primary care settings (1). Limitations in the DUHP stimulated the development of the abbreviated version. The limitations included grouping all symptoms together rather than distributing them among physical and mental scales, reliance on self-esteem as the sole indicator of emotional health, and measuring social function in terms of social role performance only (2, p1057).

The abbreviated DUKE instrument extends the WHO triad of physical, mental, and social by adding self-esteem and self-perceived health; positive and negative aspects of health are covered separately.

Description

The DUKE is a 17-item generic health status profile from which six health measures and five dysfunction measures are generated. The health measures cover physical, mental, social, general, and perceived health, and self-esteem, as shown in Exhibit 9.10. The dysfunction scores cover anxiety, depression, pain, and disability. An anxiety-depression scale combines items from the anxiety and depression subscales. The

Exhibit 9.10 The Duke Health Profile, Showing the Raw Scores for Each Response

Note: The scores shown are used in calculating the seven health measures. In calculating the four negative measures, the scoring for items 2, 4, 5, 7, 10–14 and 17 is reversed (see text). The scores are omitted from the version completed by the respondent.

Instructions:

Here are a number of questions about your health and feelings. Please read each question carefully and check (√) your best answer. You should answer the questions in your own way. There are no right or wrong answers.

	Yes, describes me exactly	Somewhat describes me	No, doesn't describe me at all
1. I like who I am	2	1	0
2. I am not an easy person to get along with	0	1	2
3. I am basically a healthy person	2	1	0
4. I give up too easily	0	1	2
5. I have difficulty concentrating	0	1	2
6. I am happy with my family relationships	2	1	0
7. I am comfortable being around people	2	1	0

Today would you have any physical trouble or difficulty:	None	Some	A Lot
8. Walking up a flight of stairs	2	1	0
9. Running the length of a football field	2	1	0

During the *past week:*

How much trouble have you had with:	None	Some	A Lot
10. Sleeping	2	1	0
11. Hurting or aching in any part of your body	2	1	0
12. Getting tired easily	2	1	0
13. Feeling depressed or sad	2	1	0
14. Nervousness	2	1	0

During the *past week:*

How often did you:	None	Some	A Lot
15. Socialize with other people (talk or visit with friends or relatives)	0	1	2
16. Take part in social, religious, or recreation activities (meetings, church, movies, sports, parties)	0	1	2

During the *past week:*

How often did you:	None	1–4 Days	5–7 Days
17. Stay in your home, a nursing home, or hospital because of sickness, injury, or other health problem	2	1	0

Adapted from Parkerson GR, Broadhead WE, Tse C-KJ. The Duke Health Profile: a 17–item measure of health and dysfunction. Med Care 1990;28:1070. With permission.

questionnaire is self-completed; the time frame refers to the present or the past week (2, p1062).

The raw scores for each response are indicated in Exhibit 9.10. Scores for each measure are calculated by summing the raw scores for the items on that measure, dividing by the maximum raw score, and then multiplying by 100. The resulting scores run from 0 to 100, with high scores for health measures indicating good health and high scores for the dysfunction measures indicating poor health. The items to be added on each measure, and the scaling factors for the six health measures, are as follows:

Physical health: items 8 to 12 ($\div$ 10 $\times$ 100)

Mental health: items 1, 4, 5, 13, 14 ($\div$ 10 $\times$ 100)

Social health: items 2, 6, 7, 15, 16 ($\div$ 10 $\times$ 100)

General health: (add above three scores and divide by 3)

Perceived health: item 3 ($\div$ 2 $\times$ 100)

Self-esteem: items 1, 2, 4, 6, 7 ($\div$ 10 $\times$ 100).

In scoring the five negative measures, the raw scores for each item listed below are first subtracted from 2 to reverse the direction of each raw score.

Anxiety: items 2, 5, 7, 10, 12, 14 ($\div$ 12 $\times$ 100)

Depression: items 4, 5, 10, 12, 13 ($\div$ 10 $\times$ 100)

Pain: item 11 ($\div$ 2 $\times$ 100)

Disability: item 17 ($\div$ 2 $\times$ 100)

Anxiety-Depression: items 4, 5, 7, 10, 12, 13, 14 ($\div$ 14 $\times$ 100).

Note that several items are counted on one (or more than one) of the health measures; then the score is reversed and the item is included on one of the dysfunction measures as well. If one or more responses is missing, scores cannot be calculated for any scale that involves that item (2).

Reliability

Parkerson et al. reported correlations between each item and the remainder of the multi-item scales; these were relatively low, ranging from 0.37 to 0.45 for the physical health items, from 0.38 to 0.45 for the mental health items, and from 0.26 to 0.35 for the social health items (2, p1062). Alpha coefficients for the eight multi-item

measures ranged from 0.55 to 0.78; test–retest coefficients for the eleven measures ranged from 0.30 to 0.78 and exceeded 0.5 for all except pain and disability (2, Table 2). Alpha reliability results in a study of 314 ambulatory patients ranged from 0.49 to 0.70 for the scale scores, while test–retest coefficients ranged from 0.41 to 0.72 (3, Table 1).

An intraclass coefficient of 0.59 for the general health dimension was obtained for 49 musculoskeletal patients; this figure was lower than that found using the SF-36, Sickness Impact Profile, or Nottingham Health Profile (4). In a sample of healthy people, the alpha coefficient was 0.38 for the physical health scale (compared to 0.58 for the equivalent scale in the MOS Short-Form-20 instrument); the alpha coefficient for the mental health score was 0.47, compared to 0.82 for the SF-20 scale (5, p681).

Validity

The correlations between selected DUKE scales and the equivalent scales from the DUHP instrument they were derived from were 0.72 (physical health), 0.70 (mental health), and 0.61 (social); the correlation of the overall scores was 0.86 (2, p1063).

Parkerson et al. compared the DUKE and the Short-Form-20 survey in a sample of healthy students (5). A multitrait-multimethod analysis lent support to the disability, pain, mental, and perceived health dimensions in which the convergent correlations clearly exceeded the divergent (5, Table 3). Support for the physical and social health dimensions was less clear; physical health correlated most strongly with the SF-20 pain score, and only 0.18 with the SF-20 physical function score. Likewise, social functioning correlated only 0.07 with the equivalent SF-20 score (5, Table 3). Parkerson et al. discussed the contrasting content of the DUKE and SF-20 scales (5, p682). A comparison of the DUKE and Sickness Impact Profile (SIP) showed an overall correlation of −0.70. Correlations between individual scales were: −0.63 for the physical health scales,

−0.48 for mental health, −0.41 for social, and +0.36 for disability. It was notable that there was comparatively little contrast between convergent and discriminant coefficients for the physical health measure, which correlated relatively highly with most of the SIP scales (2, Table 3). Scores on the self-esteem measure correlated 0.80 with scores on the Tennessee Self-Concept Scale; correlations with the other DUKE health measures (except physical) fell between 0.60 and 0.64 (2, Table 4). The Zung depression scale showed a correlation of −0.70 with the DUKE mental health score, −0.58 with self-esteem, and +0.63 with both the anxiety and depression scores (2, p1065).

In terms of group differences, DUKE scores showed some significant differences between primary care patients consulting for physical, mental, or health maintenance reasons (2, Table 5). Highly significant differences were found in DUKE scores between patients judged as having high and low disability (3, Table 2). DUKE scores also predicted ambulatory care utilization in an 18-month follow-up study (6, Table 1).

An effect size of 0.34 was identified in a study of musculoskeletal patients, smaller than that obtained for other leading health measures (4).

Alternative Forms

Translations into nine languages are included in the user's guide for the DUKE (7, Appendix D). The user's guide is available from Dr. Parkerson.

Reference Standards

Norms by age and sex are shown in the user's guide (7, Appendix B). These are based on 1,916 primary care patients and on 3,521 health insurance policyholders.

Commentary

The DUKE scale derives from the established Duke-UNC Health Profile and reacts to the need for a brief and practical measure for primary care settings. The DUKE has been shown acceptable to patients, being quicker and easier to complete than the SF-20 (8). It is longer and more broadranging than the COOP Charts, but briefer than the SF-36 or Nottingham Health Profile. Correlations with much longer scales are moderate to high. The main distinctive feature of the DUKE is its inclusion of selfesteem. The early evidence for reliability and validity suggests that the emotional components are sound but that the physical health scale is not comparable with that in other measures.

The DUKE offers a broad-ranging instrument with a number of subscores. However, five of these share items with other scales and so cannot be seen as independent measures (an issue that also occurs with the McMaster Health Index Questionnaire). Nor are all the scales homogeneous: the physical scale, for example, includes two ADL items, one on sleep, one on tiredness, and one on pain. Because the component scales lack specificity, it is not surprising that some of the convergent validity correlations are similar in strength to the divergent ones, and the low alpha coefficients are to be expected.

For use as a general outcome measure in primary care settings, the DUKE is worthy of consideration, although precise interpretation of some of the subscores may be uncertain.

Address

Dr. G.R. Parkerson, Department of Family and Community Medicine, Box 3886, Duke University Medical Center, Durham, North Carolina, USA 27710

REFERENCES

(1) Parkerson GR Jr, Gehlbach SH, Wagner EH, et al. The Duke-UNC Health Profile: an adult health status instrument for primary care. Med Care 1981;19:806–828.
(2) Parkerson GR Jr, Broadhead WE, Tse C-KJ. The Duke Health Profile: a 17-item measure of health and dysfunction. Med Care 1990; 28: 1056–1072.

(3) Parkerson GR Jr, Broadhead WE, Tse C-J. Quality of life and functional health of primary care patients. J Clin Epidemiol 1992; 45: 1303–1313

(4) Beaton DE, Bombardier C, Hogg-Johnson S. Choose your tool: a comparison of the psychometric properties of five generic health status instruments in workers with soft tissue injuries. Qual Life Res 1994; 3:50–56.

(5) Parkerson GR Jr, Broadhead WE, Tse C-KJ. comparison of the Duke Health Profile and the MOS Short-Form in healthy young adults. Med Care 1991;29:679–683.

(6) Parkerson GR Jr, Broadhead WE, Tse C-KJ. Health status and severity of illness as predictors of outcomes in primary care. Med Care 1995;33:53–66.

(7) Parkerson GR Jr. User's guide for the Duke Health Profile (DUKE). Durham, North Carolina: Duke University Medical Center, 1994.

(8) Chen AL-T, Broadhead WE, Doe EA, Broyles WK. Patient acceptance of two health status measures: the Medical Outcomes Study Short-Form General Health Survey and the Duke Health Profile. Fam Med 1993;25:536–539.

THE McMASTER HEALTH INDEX QUESTIONNAIRE
(Larry W. Chambers, 1976, revised 1984)

Purpose

The McMaster Health Index Questionnaire (MHIQ) provides a profile of scores describing physical, emotional, and social function. The MHIQ is intended for use in health services evaluation and in clinical research, principally with outpatients and those living in the community.

Conceptual Basis

The WHO definition of health was used to guide the content, which covers physical, social, and mental well-being (1).

Description

Items were drawn from a range of existing scales, including those of Bennett and Garrad, and the Katz Index of ADL (reviewed in Chapter 3). An early version of the MHIQ contained 150 items (2, 3); this was abbreviated to the present 59-item version in the early 1980s (4). The 59 items were selected on the basis of agreement with family physician ratings of physical, mental, and social health, and of their sensitivity to change (1). Equal numbers of items cover physical, emotional, and social function. The physical items cover physical activities, mobility, self-care, and communication. The social function items cover general well-being, role performance, family participation, and relations with friends. The items on emotional function cover feelings of self-esteem, feelings toward personal relationships, thoughts of the future, and life events (5). The time reference for most items is the present, and most record performance rather than capacity. The questionnaire can be used in self-completed mode (20 minutes) or via personal or telephone interviews. A comparison of these three modes showed that physical function scores did not differ, nor did the size of change scores (6, p474). However, for the emotional and social scores self-completion gave slightly lower scores than telephone administration (6, Table 1).

Each item is scored by awarding one point to good function, and scores are added to provide the three scale scores. The responses that are scored are shown in Exhibit 9.11, which also indicates to which scale each item belongs. Note that for items 8 and 9 a point is awarded only if both of the "never" responses in either column are checked. Note, also, that the answer categories for question 35 are incorrect in some published versions of the MHIQ (1, 4). The items in question 42 are scored for both social and emotional scales. Questions not answered are scored to indicate poor function. The raw scores are standardized to a 0 (extremely poor function)-to-1 (extremely good function) scale; this involves dividing the raw score by 19 for the physical scale and by 25 for the other two scales. A weighted scoring system has been described for chronic respiratory disease patients (5); this correlated 0.98 with the unweighted score (1, Figure 6.7).

Exhibit 9.11 The McMaster Health Index Questionnaire

Note: We have indicated the responses that are scored by letters following one of the response options for each question. These letters are omitted from the version given to the respondent. The responses marked "P" count one point to the physical score. In questions 8 and 9, *both* responses marked "p" must be checked to count one point. Responses marked "E" count one point to the emotional score; for questions 10–27, *either* of two responses in each question earns one point. Responses marked "S" count one point to the social function score. For question 34 there are several alternative answers; a maximum of one point can be awarded for this question.

SECTION A: The questions in the first section ask about your health and whether you are able to do certain things.

1. Today, are you physically able to run a short distance, say 300 feet, if you are in a hurry? (This is about the length of a football field or soccer pitch.)
   1 NO
   2 YES   P

2. Today, do you (or would you) have any physical difficulty at all with

		Difficulty	No Difficulty
a.	walking as far as a mile?	1	2 P
b.	climbing up 2 flights of stairs?	1	2 P
c.	standing up from and/or sitting down in a chair?	1	2 P
d.	feeding yourself?	1	2 P
e.	undressing?	1	2 P
f.	washing (face and hands), shaving (men), and/or combing hair?	1	2 P
g.	shopping?	1	2 P
h.	cooking?	1	2 P
i.	dusting and/or light housework?	1	2 P
j.	cleaning floors?	1	2 P

3. Today, are you physically able to take part in any sports (hockey, swimming, bowling, golf, and so forth) or exercise regularly?
   1 NO
   2 YES   P

4. At present, are you physically able to walk out-of-doors by yourself when the weather is good?

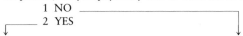
          1 NO
          2 YES

   a. What is the farthest you can walk by yourself?
      1 ONE MILE OR MORE   P
      2 LESS THAN 1 MILE BUT MORE THAN 30 FEET (ABOUT THE SIDE OF A HOUSE)
      3 LESS THAN 30 FEET
   b. Are you able to walk by yourself?
      4 BETWEEN ROOMS
      5 ONLY WITHIN A ROOM
      6 CAN'T WALK AT ALL

5. Today, do you (or would you) have any physical difficulty at all travelling by bus whenever necessary? (Circle your answer)
   1 NO   P
   2 YES

6. Today, do you have any physical difficulty at all travelling by car whenever necessary?
   1 NO   P
   2 YES

7. Do you have any physical difficulty at all driving a car by yourself?

   1 NO (or do not have a licence) P   ⟶   │ Go to Q. 8 │

   2 YES a. Is this because of a physical disability?
      1 NO
      2 YES

Exhibit 9.11   *(Continued)*

Exhibit 9.11 *(Continued)*

8. Do you wear glasses?
       1 NO ⎯⎯⎯⎯⎯⎯⎯⎯⎯⎯⎯⎯⎯⎯⎯⎯⎯⎯⎯⎯⎯
       2 YES ⎯⎯⎯⎯⎯⎯⎯⎯⎯⎯⎯⎯⎯⎯⎯⎯

a. Do you have any trouble seeing ordinary newsprint when you wear your glasses?
   1 NEVER p
   2 SOMETIMES
   3 ALWAYS

b. Do you have a headache after watching television or reading when you wear your glasses?

   1 NEVER p

   2 SOMETIMES   ⎫   Go to Q. 9

   3 ALWAYS

c. Do you have any trouble seeing ordinary newsprint?
   1 NEVER p
   2 SOMETIMES
   3 ALWAYS

d. Do you have a headache after watching television or reading?

   1 NEVER p

   2 SOMETIMES   ⎫   Go to Q. 9

   3 ALWAYS

9. Do you wear a hearing aid?
       1 NO ⎯⎯⎯⎯⎯⎯⎯⎯⎯⎯⎯⎯⎯⎯⎯⎯⎯⎯⎯⎯⎯
       2 YES ⎯⎯⎯⎯⎯⎯⎯⎯⎯⎯⎯⎯⎯⎯⎯⎯

a. Do you have trouble hearing in a normal conversation with several other persons when you wear your hearing aid?
   1 NEVER p
   2 SOMETIMES
   3 ALWAYS

b. Do you have trouble hearing the radio or television when you wear your hearing aid?
   1 NEVER p
   2 SOMETIMES
   3 ALWAYS

c. Do you have trouble hearing in a normal conversation with several other persons?
   1 NEVER p
   2 SOMETIMES
   3 ALWAYS

d. Do you have trouble hearing the radio or television?
   1 NEVER p
   2 SOMETIMES
   3 ALWAYS

SECTION B: Often people's health affects the way they feel about life. For these next questions, please circle the choice that is closest to the way you feel about each statement.
    If you STRONGLY AGREE, circle 1
    If you AGREE, circle 2
    If you are NEUTRAL, circle 3
    If you DISAGREE, circle 4
    If you STRONGLY DISAGREE, circle 5

	STRONGLY AGREE				STRONGLY DISAGREE	
10. I sometimes feel that my life is not very useful.	1	2	3	4	5	E
11. Everyone should have someone in his life whose happiness means as much to him as his own.	1	2	3	4	5	E
12. I am a useful person to have around.	1	2	3	4	5	E
13. I am inclined to feel that I'm a failure.	1	2	3	4	5	E
14. Many people are unhappy because they do not know what they want out of life.	1	2	3	4	5	E
15. In a society where almost everyone is out for himself, people soon come to distrust each other.	1	2	3	4	5	E
16. I am a quick thinker.	1	2	3	4	5	E

17. Some people feel that they run their lives pretty much the way they want to and this is the case with me.   <u>1</u>   <u>2</u>   3   4   5   E

18. There are many people who don't know what to do with their lives.   1   2   3   <u>4</u>   <u>5</u>   E

19. Most people don't realize how much their lives are controlled by plots hatched in secret by others.   1   2   3   <u>4</u>   <u>5</u>   E

20. People feel affectionate toward me.   <u>1</u>   <u>2</u>   3   4   5   E

21. I would say I nearly always finish things once I start them.   <u>1</u>   <u>2</u>   3   4   5   E

22. When I make plans ahead, I usually get to carry out things the way I expected.   <u>1</u>   <u>2</u>   3   4   5   E

23. I think most married people lead trapped (frustrated or miserable) lives.   1   2   3   <u>4</u>   <u>5</u>   E

24. It's hardly fair to bring children into the world the way things look for the future.   1   2   3   <u>4</u>   <u>5</u>   E

25. Some people feel as if other people push them around a good bit, and I feel this way too.   1   2   3   <u>4</u>   <u>5</u>   E

26. I am usually alert.   <u>1</u>   <u>2</u>   3   4   5   E

27. Nowadays a person has to live pretty much for today and let tomorrow take care of itself.   1   2   3   <u>4</u>   <u>5</u>   E

SECTION C: This section contains some questions on general health and on your social activities.

28. How would you say your health is today? Would you say your health is (Circle your answer)
     1 VERY GOOD
     2 PRETTY GOOD   } S
     3 NOT TOO GOOD

29. Taking all things together, how would you say things are today? Would you say you are
     1 VERY HAPPY
     2 PRETTY HAPPY   } S
     3 NOT TOO HAPPY

30. In general, how satisfying do you find the way you're spending your life today? Would you call it
     1 COMPLETELY SATISFYING
     2 PRETTY SATISFYING   } S
     3 NOT VERY SATISFYING

31. How would you say your *physical* functioning is today? (By this we mean the ability to move around, see, hear, and talk.)
     1 GOOD
     2 GOOD TO FAIR   } P
     3 FAIR
     4 FAIR TO POOR
     5 POOR

32. How would you say your *social* function is today? (By this we mean your ability to work, to have friends, and to get along with your family.)
     1 GOOD
     2 GOOD TO FAIR   } S
     3 FAIR
     4 FAIR TO POOR
     5 POOR

33. How would you say your *emotional* functioning is today? (By this we mean your ability to remain in good spirits most of the time and to be usually happy and satisfied with your life.) (Circle your answer)
     1 GOOD
     2 GOOD TO FAIR   } E

Exhibit 9.11 *(Continued)*

Exhibit 9.11 *(Continued)*

3 FAIR
4 FAIR TO POOR
5 POOR

34. Are you presently working on a job for wages, either full- or part-time?

1 YES ⟶ | GO TO Q.35 | S

2 NO . . a. Are you presently
1 ON VACATION   S
2 ON SICK LEAVE
3 RETIRED
4 A STUDENT   S
5 A HOUSEWIFE   S
6 OTHER (please specify):
_____

35. How much time, in a one-week period, do you usually spend watching television?
1 NONE
2 LESS THAN THREE HOURS A WEEK   S
3 LESS THAN TWO HOURS A DAY
4 TWO OR MORE HOURS A DAY

36. Which of the following describe your usual social and recreational activities?
a. going to church?
1 NO
2 YES   S
b. going to a relative's home?
1 NO
2 YES   S
c. any other activities? (please specify)
_____ S (yes)

37. Has anyone visited you in the last week? (Circle your answer)
a. a relative?
1 NO
2 YES   S
b. a friend?
1 NO
2 YES   S
c. a religious group member?
1 NO
2 YES   S
d. a social agency representative?
1 NO   S
2 YES

38. Do you have a telephone?

1 NO ⟶ | GO TO Q. 41 |

2 YES   S

39. Have you used your telephone in the last week to call
a. a friend?
1 NO
2 YES   S
b. a religious group member?
1 NO
2 YES   S
c. a social agency representative?
1 NO   S
2 YES

40. Have you been called in the last week by a social agency representative?
    1 NO S
    2 YES

41. How long has it been since you last had a holiday?
    (Write in number "0" if presently on holidays.)
    _____ MONTHS *or* _____ YEARS S (≤ 12 months)

42. *During the last year,* have any of the following things happened to you?
    a. separation from your spouse?
       1 NO S,E
       2 YES
    b. divorce?
       1 NO S,E
       2 YES
    c. going on welfare during the last year?
       1 NO S,E
       2 YES
    d. trouble getting along with friends/relatives during the last year?
       1 NO S,E
       2 YES
    e. retired from work during the last year?
       1 NO S,E
       2 YES
    f. some other problem or change in your life? (please specify)

    _____

    _____

    _____ S, E (if no problems listed)

Adapted from an original provided by Dr. L Chambers. With permission.

Reliability

Intraclass one–week test–retest reliability coefficients were 0.53 for the physical function scores, 0.70 for the emotional, and 0.48 for the social scores for 30 physiotherapy patients (1, p134). For 40 psychiatry patients, test–retest reliability was 0.95 for the physical scores, 0.77 for the emotional, and 0.66 for social function scores. Fortin and Kérouac report inter-rater agreement for the physical section of the original version of the MHIQ, to which they made "extensive changes" (7, p129). Kendall's coefficient of concordance between four raters was 0.71 (7, Table 6). [Note that a figure of 0.80, representing agreement between only two of these raters, is quoted in some reviews of the MHIQ (1, p134; 4, p162).]

Internal consistency was assessed using the Kuder-Richardson formula, giving values of 0.76 for the physical scale, 0.67 for the emotional, and 0.51 for the social scale for 40 rheumatoid arthritics (5, p781).

Validity

Chambers et al. have compared scores from contrasting groups of patients. As hypothesized, physiotherapy patients scored significantly lower (i.e., worse functioning) than psychiatric patients on the physical scale; the reverse held for the emotional and social scales (1, Figure 6.2). Family practice patients showed less physical disability than did respiratory or physiotherapy patients, but more emotional distress (1, Figures 6.3, 6.5).

Physical function scores were compared to ratings made by occupational therapists for 40 patients; the R^2 was 0.26 ($r = 0.51$) (1, Figure 6.1). For 40 patients with rheumatoid arthritis, MHIQ physical function scores were compared to clinical assessments, and they showed an association with morning stiffness, with the Ritchie Articular Index, and with age (no statistical measure of association was provided) (5, Table 1). The social and emotional function scores showed no association with these variables. Physical scores also correlated with a rating of disease severity for 246 patients with multiple sclerosis ($\rho = -0.70$) (8, p307). The emotional function scores correlated 0.31 and 0.51 with Bradburn's Affect Balance Scale on two occasions (6, p476).

A randomized trial with physiotherapy patients examined the sensitivity of the MHIQ to detecting change with treatment. The main effect of change over time was significant for the physical function scores, which also identified different amounts of improvement in different patients (6, p474). The power of the MHIQ (its ability to detect differences of half a standard deviation) was greater than 0.9 for all three modes of administration (6, p474). Compared with the McMaster-Toronto Arthritis and Rheumatism (MACTAR) questionnaire, the MHIQ showed less sensitivity to change in rheumatoid arthritis patients (9). The MHIQ showed a significant change in patients following hip replacement surgery but a less marked change than that identified by the Arthritis Impact Measurement Scales (10, Table IV).

Alternative Forms

A Canadian French translation is available (7, p129).

Commentary

Two of the distinguishing features of the MHIQ are its wide range of coverage (including disability and handicap and topics such as life events that are not included in other scales) and the even balance between physical, emotional, and social coverage. As it only provides three scores, however, variations in the components of the questionnaire may not be reflected in the final scores. The MHIQ has mainly been used in studies at McMaster University in Canada.

The questionnaire has undergone a protracted development phase; Chambers noted that he was reporting "major findings with the instrument some 22 years after it was initially conceived" (1, p132). This has compromised the consistency of

the validity and reliability testing in that several of the trials of the MHIQ used the initial version, so results cannot be directly applied to the revised form. Some results are in unpublished documents; other studies used parts of the questionnaire only (8), or modified it (7), and some reports provide descriptive, rather than quantitative, evidence for validity (1, Figures 6.2–6.5; 5). Fuller information on validity is needed, including comparisons with other, more recent scales as well as additional validation of the emotional and social scales.

The inclusion of the same items on both social and emotional scales is unusual, although appears in even more extreme form in the DUKE instrument. Being counted twice, they carry more weight than other items, although this approach may represent an honest recognition of the difficulty of operationally separating different dimensions of health. While this instrument has some attractive design features, the lack of reliability and validity data means that users will be likely to find an alternative scale that has undergone more extensive testing.

REFERENCES

(1) Chambers LW. The McMaster Health Index Questionnaire: an update. In: Walker SR, Rosser RM, eds. Quality of life assessment: key issues in the 1990s. Dordrecht, Netherlands: Kluwer Academic Publishers, 1993:131–149.

(2) Chambers LW, Sackett DL, Goldsmith CH. Development and application of an index of social function. Health Serv Res 1976;11:430–441.

(3) Sackett DL, Chambers LW, MacPherson AS, et al. The development and application of indices of health: general methods and a summary of results. Am J Public Health 1977;67:423–428.

(4) Chambers LW. The McMaster Health Index Questionnaire. In: Wenger NK, Mattson ME, Furberg CD, Elinson J, eds. Assessment of quality of life in clinical trials of cardiovascular therapies. New York: Le Jacq, 1984:160–164.

(5) Chambers LW, MacDonald LA, Tugwell P, et al. The McMaster Health Index Ques-

tionnaire as a measure of quality of life for patients with rheumatoid disease. J Rheumatol 1982;9:780–784.

(6) Chambers LW, Haight M, Norman G, et al. Sensitivity to change and the effect of mode of administration on health status measurement. Med Care 1987;25:470–479.

(7) Fortin F, Kérouac S. Validation of questionnaires on physical function. Nurs Res 1977;26:128–135.

(8) Harper AC, Harper DA, Chambers LW, et al. An epidemiological description of physical, social and psychological problems in multiple sclerosis. J Chronic Dis 1986;39:305–310.

(9) Tugwell P, Bombardier C, Buchanan WW, et al. The MACTAR Patient Preference Disability Questionnaire: an individualized functional priority approach for assessing improvement in physical disability in clinical trials in rheumatoid arthritis. J Rheumatol 1987;14:446–451.

(10) O'Boyle CA, McGee H, Hickey A, et al. Individual quality of life in patients undergoing hip replacement. Lancet 1992; 339:1088–1091.

THE SICKNESS IMPACT PROFILE
(Marilyn Bergner, 1976, Revised 1981)

Purpose

The Sickness Impact Profile (SIP) indicates the changes in a person's behavior due to sickness (1). It is broadly applicable and was intended for use in measuring the outcomes of care, in health surveys, in program planning and policy formation, and in monitoring patient progress (2).

Conceptual Basis

The conceptual development originated from the observation that the ultimate aim of most health care is to reduce sickness or modify its effect on everyday activities (3). "Sickness" denotes the individual's own experience of illness, perceived through its effect on daily activities, feelings, and attitudes. In this sense, sickness differs from disease, which denotes a professional definition of illness based on clinical observations (4).

The SIP measures health status by assessing the way sickness changes daily activities and behavior. Its concentration on behavior holds several advantages over recording feelings or clinical reports. Behaviors are observable and so accessible to external validation; feelings are variable and can be hard to measure. Clinical assessments are limited to patients under care and may require medical interpretation of symptoms. Behavioral reports, by contrast, can be verified by observation and they can be obtained whether or not a patient is receiving care; they may also be less subject to cultural bias than reports of feelings (1).

The items in the SIP all concentrate on changes in performance rather than capacity (3). The behaviors included in the profile are considered significant from the individual, social, and health care points of view. They are held to represent universal patterns of limitations that may be affected by sickness or disease, regardless of the specific conditions, treatment, individual characteristics, or prognosis concerned (1).

Description

Work on the SIP began in 1972; statements describing changes in behavior attributable to sickness were compiled from professionals, from interviews with healthy and ill lay persons, and from a literature review. Following a succession of field trials (total sample = 1,108), the prototype, containing 312 statements grouped into 14 categories of activities, was refined to a final version with 136 statements in 12 categories. The SIP is composed of statements such as, "I have difficulty reasoning and solving problems" and "I do not walk at all," each of which describes a change in behavior and specifies the extent of limitation. The full instrument is too long to reproduce here; a copy is included in the appendix to the book by Wenger et al. on quality of life assessment (5, pp334–341). Exhibit 9.12 indicates the scope of the SIP and illustrates the types of items used.

Respondents check only the items that describe them on a given day and are related to their health, although the actual

Exhibit 9.12 The Sickness Impact Profile: Categories and Selected Items

Dimension	Category	Items describing behavior related to	Selected items
Independent categories	SR	Sleep and Rest	I sit during much of the day I sleep or nap during the day
	E	Eating	I am eating no food at all, nutrition is taken through tubes or intravenous fluids I am eating special or different food
	W	Work	I am not working at all I often act irritable toward my work associates
	HM	Home management	I am not doing any of the maintenance or repair work around the house that I usually do I am not doing heavy work around the house
	RP	Recreation and pastimes	I am going out for entertainment less I am not doing any of my usual physical recreation or activities
Physical	A	Ambulation	I walk shorter distances or stop to rest often I do not walk at all
	M	Mobility	I stay within one room I stay away from home only for brief periods of time
	BCM	Body care and movement	I do not bathe myself at all, but am bathed by someone else I am very clumsy in body movements
Psychosocial	SI	Social interaction	I am doing fewer social activities with groups of people I isolate myself as much as I can from the rest of the family
	AB	Alertness behavior	I have difficulty reasoning and solving problems, for example, making decisions, learning new things I sometimes behave as if I were confused or disoriented in place or time, for example, where I am, who is around, directions, what day it is
	EB	Emotional behavior	I laugh or cry suddenly I act irritable and impatient with myself, for example, talk badly about myself, swear at myself, blame myself for things that happen
	C	Communication	I am having trouble writing or typing I do not speak clearly when I am under stress

Reproduced from Bergner M, Bobbitt RA, Carter WB, Gilson BS. The Sickness Impact Profile: development and final revision of a health status measure. Med Care 1981;19:789, Table 1. With permission.

medical condition is not an issue (1). Item weights indicate the relative severity of limitation implied by each statement. The weights were derived from equal-appearing interval scaling procedures involving more than 100 judges (6, 7).

The scaling permits the calculation of an SIP percent score which is the sum of the scale values of items checked divided by the sum of the scale values for all items multiplied by 100. This SIP percent score may be calculated for the entire SIP (the SIP overall score) as well as for each of the categories. (8, p58)

The 12 categories may be scored separately, or (as shown in the exhibit) two dimension scores may be formed: ambulation, mobility, and body care and movement can be summed to form a physical score, and social interaction, alertness, emotional behavior, and communication can form a psychosocial dimension score (6). The remaining five categories are scored separately.

The profile can be administered by an interviewer in 20 to 30 minutes, or it can be self-administered. It takes five to 10 minutes to score the SIP (9, p1004). User's and trainer's manuals are available (3). Self-report has been compared to proxy report (typically by the caregivers of elderly respondents), often showing considerable differences. Rothman et al. found significant differences between self- and proxy ratings for both physical and psychosocial scores, with proxies rating patients as more impaired (10, p119). DeBruin et al. concluded that the two sources of information cannot be regarded as interchangeable (9, p1009).

Reliability

In a comprehensive discussion of reliability, Pollard et al. reported the results of various tests of the 235-item and 146-item versions of the SIP (11, 12) while reliability results for the final 136-item version were reported by Bergner et al. (6). Test–retest reliability in these various trials was consistently high

(0.88 to 0.92) for the overall scores. Reliability was higher for the interviewer-administered (0.97) than for the self-administered version (0.87). Reproducibility of the individual items averaged 0.50, while for the 12 category scores it was 0.82 (6, pp793, 796). The reliability of overall scores did not vary by type or level of sickness; the short form was as reliable as the long form (6, 11, 12). Deyo et al. applied the SIP in a study of 79 arthritics (mean age, 57 years). Test–retest reliability (Spearman correlation) was 0.91 for 23 patients ($\kappa = 0.87$) (13, Table 6). Lower intraclass correlation values, of 0.61 for the overall score and ranging from 0.30 to 0.93 for the dimension scores, were reported for Spanish- and English-speaking samples (14, Table 1). DeBruin et al. summarize results from several studies: test–retest reliability for the overall SIP score ranges from 0.75 to 0.92; reliabilities for dimension scores range from 0.79 to 0.91; and category score reliabilities range from 0.50 to 0.95 (9, Table 2).

Internal consistency has been widely examined for the American version, and also for many of the translated versions of the SIP. Alpha coefficients for the overall score were 0.97 for the 235-item version and 0.94 for the final 136-item version, although a mailed, self-administered version had a lower alpha of 0.81 (6, p793). In a nursing-home study, the alpha for the overall score was 0.95, while section score alphas ranged from 0.59 to 0.93 (15, Table 7). An intraclass correlation of 0.92 was reported on a sample of musculoskeletal patients (16). Alpha values for the category scores ranged from 0.60 to 0.84 in another nursing home sample (17, Table 1). The summary by DeBruin et al. cites alpha coefficients ranging from 0.91 to 0.95 for the overall score, from 0.84 to 0.93 for dimension scores, and from 0.60 to 0.90 for category scores (9, Table 2).

Inter-rater reliabilities of $r = 0.92$ and $\kappa = 0.87$ have been reported for the overall score (9, Table 2).

Validity

Early validation studies compared the SIP with other subjective ratings and with clinical assessments. The SIP scores correlated 0.69 with a self-assessment of functional limitation; 0.63 with a self-assessment of sickness; 0.50 with a clinician's assessment of limitation; and 0.40 with a clinician's assessment of sickness (6, Table 4). Responses to the SIP were compared to clinical indicators for patients in diagnostic groups in which clinical tests could be expected to reflect patient functioning to varying extents. For 15 hip replacement patients, for example, the overall SIP score correlated 0.81 with an index of physical functioning. A similar comparison for 15 patients with rheumatoid arthritis yielded a correlation of 0.66. For hyperthyroid patients the overall SIP score correlated 0.41 with thyroid function measurements (6, Table 8). Read et al. compared SIP scores with indicators of overall health; correlations were 0.53 with the number of self-reported symptoms, 0.57 with a mental health scale, 0.63 with time achieved on treadmill, and 0.34 with forced expiratory capacity (18, pS15). Deyo et al. reported correlations between SIP physical and psychosocial scores and several indicators of disease severity for 79 arthritic patients (13). The results are shown in Table 9.2. Correlations with the American Rheuma-

tism Association's four-point functional rating were 0.36 for the SIP physical dimension and 0.02 for the psychosocial dimension (13, Table 3). Correlations with neurological tests in a sample of head-injured patients were modest, falling in the range of 0.25 to 0.40; this was explained in terms of the narrow focus of the neurological tests, compared to the broad scope of the SIP (19, p54). DeBruin et al. found correlations with self-assessed health status falling mainly in the range of 0.55 to 0.65; correlations with clinicians' ratings were lower, typically in the range 0.45 to 0.55 (9, Table 3).

The SIP has been compared to most of the leading health indices; DeBruin et al. show correlations of the SIP overall score with 13 other health measures, almost all exceeding 0.50 (9, Table 3). The rank correlation between SIP overall scores and Katz's Index of Activities of Daily Living (ADL) was 0.46 for 73 rehabilitation patients (8, p65) and 0.42 in a nursing-home sample (15, Table 6). The low correlations presumably reflect the broader scope of the SIP overall score; other studies show clearly that the association increases as successively narrower samples of SIP items are compared with the ADL scale. Thus the ADL scale correlated 0.64 with a combined score for the five SIP categories that include ADL behaviors (8, p65). A higher correlation of 0.74 was obtained between the SIP

Table 9.2 Correlations Between SIP Scores and Criterion Variables

	SIP		
	Overall score	Physical dimension	Psychosocial dimension
Duration of rheumatoid arthritis	0.26*	0.36†	0.03
Morning stiffness	0.23*	0.15	0.32†
Hematocrit	—0.29*	—0.26*	—0.12
Sedimentation rate (ESR)	0.36*	0.44†	0.11
Anatomic stage	0.17	0.31†	—0.01
Evidence of mental health problems	0.11	—0.03	0.27†

*p<0.05
†p<0.01
Adapted from Deyo RA, Inui TS, Leininger JD, Overman SS. Measuring functional outcomes in chronic disease: a comparison of traditional scales and self-administered health status questionnaire in patients with rheumatoid arthritis, Med Care 1983;21:187, Table 2

physical dimension alone and the ADL in a nursing–home study; the equivalent correlation with the Barthel Index was also 0.74 (17, pS162). An even higher correlation of 0.88 was found between the ADL score and a score based on the 14 SIP items most closely matching the content of the ADL scale; the equivalent correlation with the Barthel Index was 0.90 (17, pS163). This consistent pattern of correlations illustrates the contrast between a specific scale (here, the function-specific ADL scale) and a generic scale like the SIP.

SIP scores correlated 0.55 with the National Health Interview Survey questions on activity limitation (6, p795). The overall scores of the SIP and the Arthritis Impact Measurement Scales (AIMS) correlated 0.83; their physical scales correlated 0.86; and their psychosocial scales correlated 0.65 (14, p964). A correlation of 0.73 with the abbreviated AIMS was reported (20, Table 3). The SIP psychosocial subscale correlated 0.72 with the Carroll Rating Scale for Depression; the correlation between the physical scale and the Carroll was 0.44 (21, p793). A correlation of 0.54 between the SIP overall score and the Geriatric Depression Scale has been reported (15, Table 6). Correlations with the Katz Adjustment Scale were 0.45 for the overall score and 0.57 for the withdrawal subscale (22, Table 5). Anderson et al. comment that "Perhaps reflecting its behavioral content, the SIP psychosocial component has demonstrated only moderate correlations (r = 0.40 to 0.60) with traditional depression and anxiety measures" (23, p375). A factor analysis of the SIP identified two main factors, distinguishing the physical and psychosocial subscales (21). Several other studies have reported factor analyses of the SIP combined with other measures; very few report on the SIP alone (9, p1007).

The ability of the SIP to reflect change has been reported in various studies. An effect size of 0.52 was reported for musculoskeletal patients, somewhat lower than that of the SF-36 or the Nottingham Health Profile (16). Deyo and Inui compared changes in SIP scores over time with clinicians' ratings of change in the status of arthritic patients. The SIP showed only a 50% sensitivity to clinically estimated improvement and a 43% sensitivity in detecting clinical deterioration (24, Table 4). Sensitivity to change for hip replacement patients was compared to that of other measures; the SIP overall score proved less sensitive to change than that of the SF-36, the AIMS, and the Functional Status Questionnaire (20, Table 4). The SIP proved no better than a seven-point patient self-rating scale in reflecting clinically judged changes, and both showed similar correlations with physical signs such as hematocrit, erythrocyte sedimentation rate (ESR), and grip strength (24, Table 5). A similar caution was raised by MacKenzie et al., who found that the SIP was comparatively insensitive to change (as judged by asking patients directly about their change in health status) (25). It identified deterioration more reliably than improvement, and variance in patients who apparently remained stable was large (25, p436). For patients with low back pain, briefer, disease-specific scales were found to be more responsive to change than the complete SIP (26). DeBruin et al. concluded, "a definite conclusion about the responsiveness of the SIP cannot yet be drawn. . . . Findings suggest that the instrument is not sensitive to small, daily changes in a patient's situation, but changes occurring over a longer period of time seem to be mirrored in SIP scores" (9, p1011). A somewhat different conclusion can be drawn from Liang's comparison of five health measures: the effect size for the SIP was second only to that of the AIMS for mobility and overall scores, and the SIP was also second on the social score, this time to the Health Assessment Questionnaire (27, Tables 2, 3).

Alternative Forms

The SIP was adapted for use in England and renamed the Functional Limitations Profile (FLP). Linguistic changes were made and scale weights were recalculated, although these agreed closely with the original weights for the United States (28). The FLP is the version normally used in British studies. In a study of 105 arthritics, the FLP overall score correlated -0.66 with grip strength, 0.62 with the Ritchie index, 0.29 with ESR, and 0.49 with a rating of morning stiffness (29, Table 2). Sensitivity to improvement in disease state over 15 months was a modest 55% (specificity 56%), while sensitivity to deterioration was 73% (specificity 69%). These results for the FLP compared closely with those obtained for the Health Assessment Questionnaire.

The SIP has been translated into Dutch (30, 31), Spanish (14, 32–35), French (36), Swedish (37), and several other European languages (9, 23).

Abbreviations of the SIP have been proposed. A 64-item version was designed for patients with rheumatoid arthritis (38). A 66-item version was developed for use in nursing homes; this correlated 0.98 with the complete SIP (15). Roland et al. selected 24 items from the FLP that seemed most appropriate for back pain (39). This disease-specific abbreviation may be more responsive to change in low back pain patients than the complete SIP (26).

Reflecting the 1980s debate over disease-specific versus generic instruments, Temkin and others proposed a version of the SIP for patients with head injuries. The modified form added items relevant to head injury, deleted items not relevant to individual respondents (e.g., items on work for those not working), and altered the relative weighting between sections (19, 22). While the modifications did improve the discrimination ability of the SIP, Temkin concluded that the advantages were not "sufficiently large or consistent to provide a practical advantage over the SIP. . . Until other factors, such as emotional status and response style, are better controlled, little benefit is likely to be obtained from creating disease-specific psychosocial measures" (22, pS44).

Slight modifications to the SIP instruc-

tions were proposed for use with elderly nursing-home patients (17). These included abbreviation, adding examples, and interpreting the theme of impairments being "due to your health" for people with chronic conditions. The SIP items were changed from statements into questions by Johnson et al. to facilitate administration in an interview (40).

Commentary

The Sickness Impact Profile was developed with exemplary care and thoroughness, and with the death of Marilyn Bergner at the end of 1992, the health measurement field lost one of its most highly respected leaders. The quality of the SIP is tacitly acknowledged in that it frequently serves as the gold standard against which other scales are evaluated. An illustration of the many types of study in which the SIP has been used is given by DeBruin et al. (9, Table 1).

The SIP illustrates the philosophy of the generic instrument: it seeks to be applicable in any country, to all age groups, and to any medical condition. It appears to achieve this objective. For example, the study that modified the SIP for patients with head injuries found that the revised version performed little better than the generic SIP; the authors concluded that the standard version should be used (19). Nonetheless, this broad applicability may come at a cost. The SIP is long, and although it can be used successfully in general practice settings (30), there are pressures to design abbreviated versions. Some of these appear to perform equally well, especially in measuring change, where length is not an advantage.

The reliability results for the SIP are good, and it appears valid as a discriminative method, particularly in group analyses. Correlations with various clinical assessments are moderate to good, falling in the range 0.40 to 0.65; correlations with self-ratings are higher and follow a very logical pattern in which correlations between narrow (e.g., function-specific) scales and the

SIP overall are modest, but successively narrower selections of SIP items correlate increasingly highly with the specific scale. The evidence gives strong support for the concurrent validity of the SIP. Its use as an evaluative index for use in detecting changes, however, appears less certain. The emphasis on behaviors may limit sensitivity to change and section scores should be used rather than the overall score, for diluted among 136 items, a change in one area is unlikely to be reflected in changes in the overall score.

The SIP is very well established, has been extensively used and is appropriate where a comprehensive assessment is required, and can be applied to populations with a wide range of levels of sickness.

REFERENCES

(1) Bergner M, Bobbitt RA, Kressel S, et al. The Sickness Impact Profile: conceptual formulation and methodology for the development of a health status measure. Int J Health Serv 1976;6:393–415.

(2) The Sickness Impact Profile: a brief summary of its purpose, uses and administration. Seattle, Washington: University of Washington, Department of Health Services, 1978.

(3) Gilson BS, Bergner M, Bobbitt RA, et al. The Sickness Impact Profile: final development and testing, 1975–1978. Seattle, Washington: University of Washington, Department of Health Services, 1979.

(4) Gilson BS, Gilson JS, Bergner M, et al. The Sickness Impact Profile: development of an outcome measure of health care. Am J Public Health 1975;65:1304–1310.

(5) Bergner M. The Sickness Impact Profile (SIP). In: Wenger NK, Mattson ME, Furberg CD, Elinson J, eds. Assessment of quality of life in clinical trials of cardiovascular therapies. New York: LeJacq, 1984:152–159.

(6) Bergner M, Bobbitt RA, Carter WB, et al. The Sickness Impact Profile: development and final revision of a health status measure. Med Care 1981;19:787–805.

(7) Carter WB, Bobbitt RA, Bergner M, et al. Validation of an interval scaling: the Sickness Impact Profile. Health Serv Res 1976;11:516–528.

(8) Bergner M, Bobbitt RA, Pollard WE, et al. The Sickness Impact Profile: validation of a health status measure. Med Care 1976;14:57–67.

(9) DeBruin AF, De Witte LP, Stevens F, et al. Sickness Impact Profile: the state of the art of a generic functional status measure. Soc Sci Med 1992;35:1003–1014.

(10) Rothman ML, Hedrick SC, Bulcroft KA, et al. The validity of proxy-generated scores as measures of patient health status. Med Care 1991;29:115–124.

(11) Pollard WE, Bobbitt RA, Bergner M, et al. The Sickness Impact Profile: reliability of a health status measure. Med Care 1976; 14:146–155.

(12) Pollard WE, Bobbitt RA, Bergner M. Examination of variable errors of measurement in a survey-based social indicator. Soc Indicat Res 1978;5:279–301.

(13) Deyo RA, Inui TS, Leininger JD, et al. Measuring functional outcomes in chronic disease: a comparison of traditional scales and a self-administered health status questionnaire in patients with rheumatoid arthritis. Med Care 1983;21:180–192.

(14) Hendricson WD, Russell IJ, Prihoda TJ, et al. An approach to developing a valid Spanish language translation of a health-status questionnaire. Med Care 1989; 27:959–966.

(15) Gerety MB, Cornell JE, Mulrow CD, et al. The Sickness Impact Profile for Nursing Homes (SIP-NH). J Gerontol 1994; 49:M2–M8.

(16) Beaton DE, Bombardier C, Hogg-Johnson S. Choose your tool: a comparison of the psychometric properties of five generic health status instruments in workers with soft tissue injuries. Qual Life Res 1994; 3:50–56.

(17) Rothman ML, Hedrick S, Inui T. The Sickness Impact Profile as a measure of the health status of noncognitively impaired nursing home residents. Med Care 1989; 27(suppl):S157–S167.

(18) Read JL, Quinn RJ, Hoefer MA. Measuring overall health: an evaluation of three important approaches. J Chronic Dis 1987;40(suppl 1):S7–S21.

(19) Temkin N, McLean A Jr, Dikmen S, et al. Development and evaluation of modifications to the Sickness Impact Profile for head injury. J Clin Epidemiol 1988;41:47–57.

(20) Katz JN, Larson MG, Phillips CB, et al. Comparative measurement sensitivity of short and longer health status instruments. Med Care 1992;30:917–925.

(21) Brooks WB, Jordan JS, Divine GW, et al. The impact of psychologic factors on measurement of functional status: assess-

ment of the Sickness Impact Profile. Med Care 1990;28:793–804.

(22) Temkin NR, Dikmen S, Machamer J, et al. General versus disease-specific measures: further work on the Sickness Impact Profile for head injury. Med Care 1989;27(suppl):S44–S53.

(23) Anderson RT, Aaronson NK, Wilkin D. Critical review of the international assessments of health-related quality of life. Qual Life Res 1993;2:369–395.

(24) Deyo RA, Inui TS. Toward clinical applications of health status measures: sensitivity of scales to clinically important changes. Health Serv Res 1984;19:275–289.

(25) MacKenzie CR, Charlson ME, DiGioia D, et al. Can the Sickness Impact Profile measure change? An example of scale assessment. J Chronic Dis 1986;39:429–438.

(26) Deyo RA, Centor RM. Assessing the responsiveness of functional scales to clinical change: an analogy to diagnostic test performance. J Chronic Dis 1986;39:897–906.

(27) Liang MH, Fossel AH, Larson MG. Comparisons of five health status instruments for orthopedic evaluation. Med Care 1990;28:632–642.

(28) Patrick DL, Sittampalam Y, Somerville SM, et al. A cross-cultural comparison of health status values. Am J Public Health 1985;75:1402–1407.

(29) Fitzpatrick R, Newman S, Lamb R, et al. A comparison of measures of health status in rheumatoid arthritis. Br J Rheumatol 1989;28:201–206.

(30) Jacobs HM, Luttik A, Touw-Otten FWMM, et al. Measuring impact of sickness in patients with nonspecific abdominal complaints in a Dutch family practice setting. Med Care 1992;30:244–251.

(31) Jacobs HM, Luttik A, Touw-Otten FW, et al. The Sickness Impact Profile (SIP): results of an evaluation study of the Dutch version. Nederlands Tijdschr Geneeskd 1990; 134:1950–1954.

(32) Esteva M, Gonzalez N, Ruiz M. Reliability and validity of a Spanish version of the Sickness Impact Profile. Arthritis Rheum 1992;35(suppl):S219.

(33) Gilson BS, Erickson D, Chavez CT, et al. A Chicano version of the Sickness Impact Profile. Cult Med Psychiatry 1980;4:137–150.

(34) Deyo RA. Pitfalls in measuring the health status of Mexican Americans: comparative validity of the English and Spanish Sickness Impact Profile. Am J Public Health 1984;74:569–573.

(35) Badia X, Alonso J. Reliability of the Span-ish version of the Sickness Impact Profile. Qual Life Res 1994;3:65.

(36) Chwalow AJ, Lurie A, Bean K. A French version of the Sickness Impact Profile (SIP): stages in the cross cultural validation of a generic quality of life scale. Fundam Clin Pharmacol 1992;6:319–326.

(37) Sullivan M, Ahlmen M, Archenholtz B. Measuring health in rheumatic disorders by means of a Swedish version of the Sickness Impact Profile: results from a population study. Scand J Rheumatol 1986;15:193–200.

(38) Sullivan M, Ahlmen M, Bjelle A, et al. Health status assessment in rheumatoid arthritis. II. Evaluation of a modified Shorter Sickness Impact Profile. J Rheumatol 1993;20:1500–1507.

(39) Roland M, Morris R. A study of the natural history of back pain. Part I: Development of a reliable and sensitive measure of disability in low-back pain. Spine 1983; 8:141–144.

(40) Johnson J, King K, Murray R. Measuring the impact of sickness on functions of radiation therapy patients. Oncol Nurs Forum 1983;10:36–39.

THE NOTTINGHAM HEALTH PROFILE
(Sonja Hunt, 1981)

Purpose

The Nottingham Health Profile (NHP) was designed to give a brief indication of perceived physical, social, and emotional health problems (1). Originally intended for use in primary medical care settings, the NHP has also been used to assess demand for care in population health surveys and has been used in clinical trials (2).

Conceptual Basis

The design and content of the NHP was influenced by the Sickness Impact Profile. One difference, however, is that the NHP asks about feelings and emotional states directly, rather than via changes in behavior. The emphasis is on the respondent's subjective assessment of her health status: this is seen as the major factor predicting use of medical services and satisfaction with outcomes (3). The questions reflect the WHO definition of disability and the profile may be viewed as an indicator of perceived distress.

Description

The pool of items used in constructing the NHP was formed through surveys of 768 patients with acute and chronic ailments, supplemented by items drawn from other health indices such as the Sickness Impact Profile. Each item refers to

departures from "normal" functioning because, in the field of health especially, it is easier to obtain, record, and provide some measure of departures from the norm than it is to specify the norm itself. Respondents were asked to answer "Yes" or "No" according to whether or not they feel the item applies to them "in general" (4, p282).

The original version of the NHP (called the Nottingham Health Index) contained 33 items; it was tested on rehabilitation patients (5) and surgical patients undergoing hip replacements (2). The revised Nottingham Health Profile is similar in content and was constructed from the same pool of items. Part I of the NHP contains 38 items grouped into six sections: physical abilities (in Exhibit 9.13 designated PA, with 8 items), pain (P = 8 items), sleep (S = 5), social isolation (SI = 5), emotional reactions (ER = 9), and energy level (EL = 3 items) (6). Part II provides a brief indicator of handicap, and contains seven items that record the effect of health problems on occupation, jobs around the house, personal relationships, social life, sex life, hobbies and holidays (7). Part II is optional as some items (e.g., work, sex life) may not be applicable (8, p5). Yes/no responses are used throughout. The NHP is self-administered and takes approximately ten to 15 minutes to complete. Exhibit 9.13 shows the items, the section to which each pertains, and the scale weights. Note that the version shown represents the definitive version (S. McKenna, personal communication, 1995); the instructions and two items have been slightly modified from the version presented in our first edition.

Hunt recommends that section scores in Part I be presented as a profile. The items were scaled for severity using a paired comparisons technique involving 1,200 outpatient interviews (7, 9). The weights are transformed to yield scores from 0 (no problems) to 100 (all items checked) for each scale. A simpler scoring system is often used which counts the number of affirmative responses in each section. Weighted and unweighted scores correlate highly, raising the question of the usefulness of the weights; Jenkinson calculated correlations between weighted and unweighted section scores on three samples of respondents and found that none of the 18 correlations fell below 0.98 (10, p1415). Although not recommended by the developers of the NHP, some users present results as an overall score, and O'Brien et al. suggest three options for this which all provide a 0-to-1 (poor-to-good health) overall score (11). First, the proportion of the 38 items to which an affirmative response is given is subtracted from 1. Second, the item weights for items answered affirmatively are added, and this total is divided by 600 (the sum of all item weights); the result is subtracted from 1. Third, because there are different numbers of statements in the dimensions, a weight can be used to give each section the same contribution to the overall score. In this method, weights for items answered affirmatively are summed within each section, and the section scores are multiplied by one-sixth the number of items in that section; the resulting section scores are added and this sum subtracted from 1 (11, ppS152–S153). These three scores provided virtually identical results (11, pS148).

Part II of the NHP is scored by summing the number of positive responses; no item weights are used.

Reliability

For the original version, correlations of items with section scores were examined in two studies (2, 5).

The four-week test–retest reliability of

Exhibit 9.13   The Nottingham Health Profile, Showing the Sections on Which Each Item Is Scored and the Weights for Positive Responses

Note: EL = energy level, P = pain, ER = emotional reactions, S = sleep, SI = social isolation, PA = physical abilities. The columns headed Section and Weight are not included in the version used by the repondent.

Part I

Listed below are some problems people might have in their daily lives.

Read the list carefully and put a tick in the box ☐ under *Yes* for any problem that applies to you *at the moment*. Tick the box under *No* for any problem that does not apply to you. *Please answer every question.* If you are not sure whether to answer Yes or No, tick whichever answer you think is *most* true at the moment.

	Yes	No	Section	Weight
I'm tired all the time	☐	☐	EL	39.20
I have pain at night	☐	☐	P	12.91
Things are getting me down	☐	☐	ER	10.47
	Yes	No		
I have unbear able pain	☐	☐	P	19.74
I take tablets to help me sleep	☐	☐	S	22.37
I've forgotten what it's like to enjoy myself	☐	☐	ER	9.31
	Yes	No		
I'm feeling on edge	☐	☐	ER	7.22
I find it painful to change position	☐	☐	P	9.99
I feel lonely	☐	☐	SI	22.01
	Yes	No		
I can only walk about indoors	☐	☐	PA	11.54
I find it hard to bend	☐	☐	PA	10.57
Everything is an effort	☐	☐	EL	36.80
	Yes	No		
I'm waking up in the early hours of the morning	☐	☐	S	12.57
I'm unable to walk at all	☐	☐	PA	21.30
I'm finding it hard to make contact with people	☐	☐	SI	19.36

Remember if you are not sure whether to answer "Yes" or "No" to a problem, tick whichever answer you think *more true at the moment.*

	Yes	No	Section	Weight
The days seem to drag	☐	☐	ER	7.08
I have trouble getting up and down stairs and steps	☐	☐	PA	10.79
I find it hard to reach for things	☐	☐	PA	9.30
	Yes	No		
I'm in pain when I walk	☐	☐	P	11.22
I lose my temper easily these days	☐	☐	ER	9.76
I feel there is nobody I am close to	☐	☐	SI	20.13
	Yes	No		
I lie awake for most of the night	☐	☐	S	27.26
I feel as if I'm losing control	☐	☐	ER	13.99
I'm in pain when I'm standing	☐	☐	P	8.96

	Yes	No		
I find it hard to dress myself	☐	☐	PA	12.61
I soon run out of energy	☐	☐	EL	24.00
I find it hard to stand for long (e.g., at the kitchen sink, waiting for a bus)	☐	☐	PA	11.20
	Yes	No		
I'm in constant pain	☐	☐	P	20.86
It takes me a long time to get to sleep	☐	☐	S	16.10
I feel I am a burden to people	☐	☐	SI	22.53
	Yes	No		
Worry is keeping me awake at night	☐	☐	ER	13.95
I feel that life is not worth living	☐	☐	ER	16.21
I sleep badly at night	☐	☐	S	21.70
	Yes	No		
I'm finding it hard to get on with people	☐	☐	SI	15.97
I need help to walk about outside (e.g., a walking aid or someone to support me)	☐	☐	PA	12.69
	Yes	No		
I'm in pain when going up and down stairs or steps	☐	☐	P	5.83
I wake up feeling depressed	☐	☐	ER	12.01
I'm in pain when I'm sitting	☐	☐	P	10.49

Part II

Now we would like you to think about the activities in your life which may be affected by health problems. In the list below, tick *Yes* for each activity in your life which is being affected by your state of health. Tick *No* for each activity which is not being affected, *or which does not apply to you.*

Is your present state of health causing problems with your . . .

	Yes	No
Job or work? (That is, paid employment)	☐	☐
Looking after the home? (Examples: cleaning and cooking, repairs, odd jobs around the home, etc.)	☐	☐
Social life? (Examples: going out, seeing friends, going to the pub, etc.)	☐	☐
Home life? (That is: relationships with other people in your home)	☐	☐
Sex life?	☐	☐
Interests and hobbies? (Examples: sports, arts and crafts, do-it-yourself, etc.)	☐	☐
Holidays? (Examples: summer or winter holidays, weekends away, etc.)	☐	☐

Now please go back to page 1 and make sure that you have answered "Yes" or "No" to every question, in all pages of this questionnaire.

Thank you for your help.

Part I of the revised NHP was reported by Hunt et al. for 58 arthritics and 93 patients with peripheral vascular disease; coefficients for the six sections ranged from 0.75 to 0.88 (1, Table 2; 12). Test–retest reliability for the seven items in Part II ranged from 0.44 to 0.86 in one sample and from 0.55 to 0.89 in the other (1, Table 3).

Spearman correlations among domain scores ranged from 0.32 (sleep and social isolation) to 0.70 (pain and physical mobility) in a sample of cardiac patients; most fell in the range 0.41 to 0.58 (13, Table 4).

Reliability measured by intraclass correlation was 0.95, with an effect size of 0.52 in people with musculoskeletal disorders (14). The high reliability balanced by modest effect size was attributed in part to the fact that many respondents achieved the maximum score.

Validity

In the initial development considerable attention was paid to content validity. Items were based on patients' descriptions of their experience, and formal tests of linguistic clarity were applied in an effort to simplify the item wording.

The NHP has repeatedly been shown to discriminate between different types of patient. The original Nottingham Health Index showed marked differences between arthritic patients before and after hip replacement surgery. Concurrent evidence for differences between the groups was provided by the McGill Pain Questionnaire and a physical assessment made by a physiotherapist (2). The revised NHP also showed clear differences between hip replacement patients and their spouses who served as a comparison group (15). It showed contrasts between rehabilitation patients with physical and mental handicaps (5, Table 5) and between stroke patients and normal controls (16, Table 1). The NHP was tested on four groups of elderly people, ranging from those with chronic illness and physical, social, and emotional disabilities to physically fit people who had recently sought medical care (4). Kruskal-Wallis tests showed significant differences between the groups on all six sections ($p < 0.001$). In a study of cardiac patients, NHP domain scores discriminated significantly between patients in different New York Heart Association (NYHA) classes, and according to Karnofsky scores

(13, Tables 2, 3). Spearman correlations with the NYHA classification ranged from 0.30 (social isolation) to 0.52 (energy level); correlations with the Karnofsky scale were almost identical (13, Table 4). Hunt et al. summarized studies that applied the NHP to nine different patient groups; the results showed clear and clinically plausible contrasts in scores (1).

The correlation between the first version and the McGill Pain Questionnaire was 0.74, with a range from 0.50 for the social activities section to 0.78 for the pain section. The overall score correlated 0.65 with a physiotherapist's rating; correlations for each item ranged from 0.16 to 0.47 (2, Table 3). Equivalent data were collected in the rehabilitation study, correlations being drawn between the questionnaire and a set of ratings made by a physician (5). Kendall correlations for the walking questions ranged from 0.47 to 0.56, while those for dressing and self-care ranged between 0.40 and 0.48; coefficients for body movements ranged from 0.44 to 0.55 (5, Table 4). The emotional questions correlated 0.71 (Spearman rho) with scores on the General Health Questionnaire (GHQ) (16, p167). Using the GHQ as a criterion, the sensitivity of the NHP for detecting depression was examined. The best result was obtained by calculating a summary score for the entire NHP less the physical mobility section; sensitivity was 91% and specificity 82% (16, p167). While the emotional questions alone achieved high sensitivity, specificity was greatly increased by including responses to the other four sections. A separate study found a correlation of 0.76 between the 12-item GHQ scores and the emotional reactions scale of the NHP (8, p49).

A factor analysis of the 33 items in the original version identified eight factors, reflecting pain, mobility, body movement, sleep, anxiety, getting out of the house, loneliness, and depression (2).

There is some indication, acknowledged by Hunt, that the NHP has a floor effect, whereby it does not identify low levels of disability. A comparison with the Dartmouth COOP Charts, for example, showed that the COOP Charts were more sensitive to minor deviations from complete well-being (17). Similarly, in a sample of well people, scores on the SF-36 were less skewed than those on the NHP, such that the SF-36 identified minor levels of discomfort missed by the Nottingham scale (18).

There are some reports of the NHP's sensitivity to change; all six sections showed strong contrasts before and after heart transplant surgery (11, Table 4). Hunt et al. demonstrated no contrast in the status of a group of patients a week before surgery and 6 to 8 weeks after (7, Table VII).

Alternative Forms

The NHP has been translated into most European languages, plus Arabic (19) and Urdu (20). A Danish version showed an overall test–retest reliability of 0.93, with reliabilities for the sections ranging from 0.76 to 0.86 (21). A Spanish version (22) showed an internal consistency of 0.91 (range across sections 0.58 to 0.86) and test–retest reliabilities ranging from 0.69 to 0.85 for the six sections (23). Alpha internal consistency coefficients for a Dutch version ranged from 0.55 (physical mobility) to 0.81 (pain); four of six coefficients exceeded 0.70 (24, Table 9.2).

Translations that have also developed their own weighting schemes include Swedish (25) and French (26). Correlations between the original and the French weights exceeded 0.9 for most sections, although the correlation for pain was only 0.76 and emotional reaction was 0.58 (26). The Swedish version of the NHP has been extensively used, and considerable information is available on its reliability and validity (25, 27–30). Rank correlations of item weights between Swedish and the original weights are in the high 0.80s: valuations of health states seem quite similar in both cultures (31, p373). Test–retest reliability at four weeks was 0.92; internal consis-

tency for the sections ranged from 0.34 (social isolation) to 0.81 (emotional reactions) (31, p373).

Based on their experience in producing so many versions, Hunt and her group have proposed guidelines for the development of culturally equivalent versions of a measurement (19, 32).

Reference Standards

Reference scores for the NHP are available for healthy people (by age group, sex, and social class) and for various categories of patients (1, Table 1; 33; 34).

Commentary

The NHP is one of the more frequently used measures, especially in Europe. It has been applied to a variety of people in medical and nonmedical settings: to miners and firemen in good physical health (35), to elderly people and patients frequently visiting their general practitioner (36), and in a study of social class differences in perceived health (1). The strengths of the method include its simplicity and its broad coverage.

The NHP has, however, encountered spirited criticism. The first issue derives from confusion over the applications for which it is best suited. Early articles describing the scale suggested that it was suitable for use in health surveys, but subsequent use indicated a clear floor effect whereby healthy respondents or those with minor ailments tend to show, perfect scores and hence have no scope for improvement; comparison with other instruments shows that such scores do not necessarily indicate an absence of problems (1, 17). The NHP does not include items indicating positive well-being. Community surveys typically find that around two thirds of the population record no problems on the NHP; the figure was 46% in a British survey (37). Sleep and energy level form the mildest and therefore the most common problems (38); the range of disability covered by each dimension is uneven. Hunt and McKenna subsequently suggested that the NHP should not be used as a survey instrument (39). The floor effect presumably results from its original design as an instrument for people seeking care, deliberately focusing on people with disabilities; only later was the NHP used in healthy populations. A balanced view would hold that the NHP is suitable as a survey tool in populations, such as the elderly, where there are likely to be people with significant disability (8, p3; 40). Kind and Carr-Hill suggest that if the NHP is used as a screen for disability, it is unnecessarily long and contains considerable redundancy (37, p909). Readers should carefully consider alternative scales before using the NHP as a survey instrument in general populations.

Debate also surrounds the scoring. First, there is discussion over the choice between a total score and scores for each section. Hunt et al. argued that an overall score was inappropriate, as the large number of possible routes to an intermediate score would not provide an interpretable picture of a person's disability (1). However, if section scores are to be used, the sections should measure different things. The assignment of items to separate sections has been criticized as arbitrary, and the correlations among items in some categories are lower than those between categories (37, Tables 5, 6). Second, there have been criticisms of the weighting system used (31, p371). One difficulty concerns how to score people whose disabilities limit their roles, making questions on role performance inapplicable. Jenkinson noted that a person who cannot walk will receive a less severe weighted score than one who has difficulty with stairs and can only walk about indoors (10). Another example concerns scores for those who do not work at all, compared to others who are working, but with limitations. The criticism has also been made that items on several of the NHP sections do not show a wide range of scores (10).

Certain of the norms quoted by Hunt et al. do not form smooth trends across the age, sex, or social class groups; either the populations used were not homogeneous, or the samples were simply too small to derive stable estimates. They may need to be smoothed before using them as reference standards.

The NHP continues to be used and tested and holds considerable utility as a clinical instrument. Until the advent of the SF-36 it was one of the most popular instruments in Europe; time will tell how the turf is divided between them.

REFERENCES

(1) Hunt SM, McEwen J, McKenna SP. Measuring health status: a new tool for clinicians and epidemiologists. J R Coll Gen Pract 1985;35:185–188.

(2) McDowell IW, Martini CJM, Waugh W. A method for self-assessment of disability before and after hip replacement operations. Br Med J 1978;2:857–859.

(3) Hunt SM, McKenna SP, McEwen J, et al. The Nottingham Health Profile: subjective health status and medical consultations. Soc Sci Med 1981;15:221–229.

(4) Hunt SM, McKenna SP, McEwen J, et al. A quantitative approach to perceived health status: a validation study. J Epidemiol Community Health 1980;34:281–286.

(5) Martini CJ, McDowell I. Health status: patient and physician judgments. Health Serv Res 1976;11:508–515.

(6) Hunt SM, McEwen J. The development of a subjective health indicator. Sociol Health Illness 1980;2:231–246.

(7) Hunt SM, McEwen J, McKenna SP, et al. Subjective health assessments and the perceived outcome of minor surgery. J Psychosom Res 1984;28:105–114.

(8) Hunt SM, McKenna SP, McEwen J. The Nottingham Health Profile: user's manual. Revised ed. Manchester, England: (Manuscript), 1989.

(9) McKenna SP, Hunt SM, McEwen J. Weighting the seriousness of perceived health problems using Thurstone's method of paired comparisons. Int J Epidemiol 1981;10:93–97.

(10) Jenkinson C. Why are we weighting? A critical examination of the use of item weights in a health status measure. Soc Sci Med 1991;32:1413–1416.

(11) O'Brien BJ, Buxton MJ, Ferguson BA. Measuring the effectiveness of heart transplant programmes: quality of life data and

their relationship to survival analysis. J Chronic Dis 1987;40:S137–S153.

(12) Hunt SM, McKenna SP, Williams J. Reliability of a population survey tool for measuring perceived health problems: a study of patients with osteoarthrosis. J Epidemiol Community Health 1981;35:297–300.

(13) O'Brien BJ, Buxton MJ, Patterson DL. Relationship between functional status and health-related quality-of-life after myocardial infarction. Med Care 1993;31:950–955.

(14) Beaton DE, Bombardier C, Hogg-Johnson S. Choose your tool: a comparison of the psychometric properties of five generic health status instruments in workers with soft tissue injuries. Qual Life Res 1994;3:50–56.

(15) McKenna SP, McEwen J, Hunt SM, et al. Changes in the perceived health of patients recovering from fractures. Public Health 1984;98:97–102.

(16) Ebrahim S, Barer D, Nouri F. Use of the Nottingham Health Profile with patients after a stroke. J Epidemiol Community Health 1986;40:166–169.

(17) Coates AK, Wilkin D. Comparing the Nottingham Health Profile with the Dartmouth COOP Charts. In: Scholten JHG, ed. Functional status assessment in family practice. Lelystad, Netherlands: Meditekst, 1992:81–86.

(18) Brazier JE, Harper R, Jones NMB, et al. Validating the SF-36 Health Survey questionnaire: new outcome measure for primary care. Br Med J 1992;305:160–164.

(19) Hunt SM. Cross-cultural issues in the use of socio-medical indicators. Health Policy 1986;6:149–158.

(20) Ahmad WIU, Kernohan EEM, Baker MR. Cross-cultural use of socio-medical indicators with British Asians. Health Policy 1989;13:95–102.

(21) Thorsen H, McKenna SP, Gottschalck L. The Danish version of the Nottingham Health Profile: its adaptation and reliability. Scand J Prim Health Care 1993; 11:124–129.

(22) Alonso J, Anto JM, Moreno C. Spanish version of the Nottingham Health Profile: translation and preliminary validity. Am J Public Health 1990;80:704–708.

(23) Badia X, Alonso J, Brosa M, Lock P. Reliability of the Spanish version of the Nottingham Health Profile in patients with stable end-stage renal disease. Soc Sci Med 1994;38:153–158.

(24) Meyboom-de Jong B, Smith RJA. Studies with the Dartmouth COOP Charts in general practice: comparison with the Notting-ham Health Profile and the General Health Questionnaire. In: Lipkin M, ed. Functional status measurement in primary care. New York: Springer-Verlag, 1990:132–149.

(25) Hunt SM, Wiklund I. Cross-cultural variation in the weighting of health statements: a comparison of English and Swedish valuations. Health Policy 1987;8:227–235.

(26) Bucquet D, Condon S, Ritchie K. The French version of the Nottingham Health Profile. A comparison of items weights with those of the source version. Soc Sci Med 1990;30:829–835.

(27) Wiklund I, Romanus B, Hunt SM. Self-assessed disability in patients with arthrosis of the hip joint. Reliability of the Swedish version of the Nottingham Health Profile. Int Disabil Stud 1988;10:159–163.

(28) Wiklund I. The Nottingham Health Profile—a measure of health-related quality of life. Scand J Prim Health Care 1990; 8(suppl 1):15–18.

(29) Wiklund I, Welin C. A comparison of different psychosocial questionnaires in patients with myocardial infarction. Scand J Rehabil Med 1992;24:195–202.

(30) Wiklund I, Karlberg J. Evaluation of quality of life in clinical trials. Controlled Clin Trials 1991;12:204S–216S.

(31) Anderson RT, Aaronson NK, Wilkin D. Critical review of the international assessments of health-related quality of life. Qual Life Res 1993;2:369–395.

(32) Hunt SM, Alonso J, Bucquet D, et al. Cross-cultural adaptation of health measures. Health Policy 1991;19:33–44.

(33) Hunt SM, McEwen J, McKenna SP. Perceived health: age and sex comparisons in the community. J Epidemiol Community Health 1984;38:156.

(34) Hunt SM, McKenna SP. The Nottingham Health Profile user's manual, revised. Manchester, England: Galen Research and Consultancy, 1991.

(35) McKenna SP, Hunt SM, McEwen J. Absence from work and perceived health among mine rescue workers. J Soc Occup Med 1981;31:151–157.

(36) McKenna SP, Hunt SM, McEwen J, et al. Looking at health from the consumers' point of view. Occup Health 1980; 32:350–355.

(37) Kind P, Carr-Hill R. The Nottingham Health Profile: a useful tool for epidemiologists? Soc Sci Med 1987;25:905–910.

(38) Kind P, Gudex CM. Measuring health status in the community: a comparison of methods. J Epidemiol Community Health 1994;48:86–91.

(39) Hunt SM, McKenna SP. Validating the SF-36. Br Med J 1992;305:645.

(40) Hunt SM. Nottingham Health Profile. In: Wenger NK, Mattson ME, Furberg CD, Elinson J, eds. Assessment of quality of life in clinical trials of cardiovascular therapies. New York: Le Jacq, 1984:165–169.

THE SHORT-FORM-36 HEALTH SURVEY
(Rand Corporation and John E. Ware, 1990)

Purpose

The 36-item short form of the Medical Outcomes Study questionnaire (SF-36) was designed as a generic indicator of health status for use in population surveys and evaluative studies of health policy. It can also be used in conjunction with disease-specific measures as an outcome measure in clinical practice and research (1).

Conceptual Basis

The SF-36 derived from the work of the Rand Corporation of Santa Monica during the 1970s. Rand's Health Insurance Experiment compared the impact of alternative health insurance systems on health status and utilization (2). The outcome measures developed for the study have been widely used and several are described in this book. They were subsequently refined and used in Rand's Medical Outcomes Study (MOS), which focused more narrowly on care for chronic medical and psychiatric conditions (3, 4). A 20-item shortened form of the MOS instrument was published in 1988 (see the review that follows), and the SF-36 was designed in response to criticisms that the SF-20 was too brief to be sensitive to changes in health status (5). The SF-36 extends the scope of the SF-20 by adding items applicable to retired people and items on vitality, and by distinguishing role changes due to physical from those due to mental problems. Note that the ten physical functioning items in the SF-36 are also contained in the MOS Physical Functioning Measure, which is reviewed in Chapter 3. Fuller details of the origins of the items in the SF-36 are given in the SF-36 manual (6). The development of the SF-36 is now coordinated by The Health Institute, based in Boston (see Address section).

As a generic instrument, the SF-36 was designed to be applicable to a wide range of types and severities of conditions. Generic instruments are useful for monitoring patients with multiple conditions, for comparing the health status of patients with different conditions, and for comparing patients to the general population (3, p912). Ware argued that a generic measure should cover both physical and mental concepts and should measure each concept in several contrasting ways. These include behavioral functioning, perceived well-being, social and role disability, and personal evaluations of health in general (6, p3:2). Measures of behavioral functioning and role limitations include questions on work, self-care, mobility, etc. Perceived well-being is subjective and cannot be completely inferred from behavior; hence the SF-36 includes questions on feeling states. The questions on overall evaluation of health provide a summary indicator and capture the impact of health problems not directly included in the other questions (6, p3:3).

Description

The items in the SF-36 were drawn from the original 245-item MOS questionnaire; nine items from the SF-20 were retained in the SF-36 while a further five were reworded, as were several of the answer categories. Several of the mental health items originated from the General Well-Being Schedule of Dupuy. Ware and Sherbourne give an extended description of the origins of the SF-36 and of its links with the other MOS instruments (1). The SF-36 includes multi-item scales to measure the following eight dimensions (the question numbers refer to those in Exhibit 9.14):

Physical functioning (ten items in question 3)

Role limitations due to physical health problems (four items in question 4)

Bodily pain (questions 7 and 8)

Social functioning (questions 6 and 10)

Exhibit 9.14 The Short-Form-36 Health Survey

Instructions: This survey asks for your views about your health. This information will help keep track of how you feel and how well you are able to do your usual activities.

Answer every question by marking the answer as indicated. If you are unsure about how to answer a question, please give the best answer you can.

---

1. In general, would you say your health is:

(Circle one)

Excellent 1
Very Good 2
Good 3
Fair 4
Poor 5

2. *Compared to one year ago,* how would you rate your health in general *now?*

(Circle one)

Much better now than one year ago 1
Somewhat better now than one year ago 2
About the same now as one year ago 3
Somewhat worse now than one year ago 4
Much worse now than one year ago 5

3. The following items are about activities you might do during a typical day. Does *your health* now limit you in these activities? If so, how much?

(Circle one number on each line)

Activities	Yes, Limited A Lot	Yes, Limited A Little	No, Not Limited At All
a. **Vigorous activities,** such as running, lifting heavy objects, participating in strenuous sports	1	2	3
b. **Moderate activities,** such as moving a table, pushing a vacuum cleaner, bowling, or playing golf	1	2	3
c. Lifting or carrying groceries	1	2	3
d. Climbing **several** flights of stairs	1	2	3
e. Climbing **one** flight of stairs	1	2	3
f. Bending, kneeling, or stooping	1	2	3
g. Walking **more than a mile**	1	2	3
h. Walking **several blocks**	1	2	3
i. Walking **one block**	1	2	3
j. Bathing or dressing yourself	1	2	3

4. During the *past 4 weeks,* have you had any of the following problems with your work or other regular daily activities *as a result of your physical health?*

(Circle one number on each line)

	Yes	No
a. Cut down on the **amount of time** you spent on work or other activities	1	2
b. **Accomplished less** than you would like	1	2

Exhibit 9.14 *(Continued)*

Exhibit 9.14 *(Continued)*

(Circle one number on each line)

	Yes	No
c. Were limited in the **kind** of work or other activities	1	2
d. Had **difficulty** performing the work or other activities (for example, it took extra effort)	1	2

5. During the *past 4 weeks,* have you had any of the following problems with your work or other regular activities *as a result of any emotional problems* (such as feeling depressed or anxious)?

(Circle one number on each line)

	Yes	No
a. Cut down on the **amount of time** you spent on work or other activities	1	2
b. **Accomplished less** than you would like	1	2
c. Didn't do work or other activities as **carefully** as usual	1	2

6. During the *past 4 weeks,* to what extent has your physical health or emotional problems interfered with your normal social activities with family, friends, neighbors, or groups?

(Circle one)

Not at all 1
Slightly 2
Moderately 3
Quite a bit 4
Extremely 5

7. How much *bodily* pain have you had during the *past 4 weeks?*

(Circle one)

None 1
Very mild 2
Mild 3
Moderate 4
Severe 5
Very severe 6

8. During the *past 4 weeks,* how much did *pain* interfere with your normal work (including both work outside the home and housework)?

(Circle one)

Not at all 1
A little bit 2
Moderately 3
Quite a bit 4
Extremely 5

9. These questions are about how you feel and how things have been with you *during the past 4 weeks.* For each question, please give the one answer that comes closest to the way you have been feeling. How much of the time during the *past 4 weeks -*

(Circle one number on each line)

	All of the Time	Most of the Time	A Good Bit of the Time	Some of the Time	A Little of the Time	None of the Time
a. Did you feel full of pep?	1	2	3	4	5	6
b. Have you been a very nervous person?	1	2	3	4	5	6

c. Have you felt so down in the dumps that nothing could cheer you up?	1	2	3	4	5	6
d. Have you felt calm and peaceful?	1	2	3	4	5	6
e. Did you have a lot of energy?	1	2	3	4	5	6
f. Have you felt downhearted and blue?	1	2	3	4	5	6
g. Did you feel worn out?	1	2	3	4	5	6
h. Have you been a happy person?	1	2	3	4	5	6
i. Did you feel tired?	1	2	3	4	5	6

10. During the *past 4 weeks,* how much of the time has your *physical health or emotional problems* interfered with your social activities (like visiting with friends, relatives, etc.)?

(Circle one)

All of the time 1
Most of the time 2
Some of the time 3
A little of the time 4
None of the time 5

11. How TRUE or FALSE is *each* of the following statements for you?

(Circle one number on each line)

	Definitely True	Mostly True	Don't Know	Mostly False	Definitely False
a. I seem to get sick a little easier than other people	1	2	3	4	5
b. I am as healthy as anybody I know	1	2	3	4	5
c. I expect my health to get worse	1	2	3	4	5
d. My health is excellent	1	2	3	4	5

From Ware JE Jr, Snow KK, Kosinski M, Gandek B. SF-36 Health Survey: manual and interpretation guide. Boston, MA: The Health Institute, New England Medical Center, 1993:B1–B5. With permission.

General mental health, covering psychological distress & well-being (five items: questions 9 b, c, d, f, and h)

Role limitations due to emotional problems (questions 5 a, b, and c)

Vitality, energy or fatigue (four items: questions 9 a, e, g, and i)

General health perceptions (five items: questions 1 and 11 a–d)

In addition, question 2 covers change in health status over the past year; this is not counted in scoring the eight dimensions, but is used to estimate change in health from a cross-sectional administration of the SF-36 (6, p9:15). The exhibit shows the Standard Version of the SF-36; note that this is the definitive version and contains minor variations from those published previously. Differences between versions are indicated in the manual (6, Table 3.4).

The SF-36 may be self-administered or used in personal or telephone interviews; machine-readable forms and instruction sheets for each version are available from the Health Institute. McHorney et al. compared mail and telephone survey administration; mail was significantly cheaper, and provided a higher response rate; mail also identified a higher level of disability (7). The questions generally take five to ten minutes to complete; elderly respondents may require up to 15 minutes (8). Self-administration appears acceptable and feasible for most patients, although the optical scan forms may be difficult for people with vision problems (9). Nonresponse rates averaged 3.9% across the 36 items in a large study of people with chronic conditions (10, p46). Detailed administration instructions are contained ti Chapter 4 of the manual.

Scoring. Two slightly different approaches to scoring have been proposed: a simpler one by the Rand group and one developed by The Health Institute that gives different weights to certain responses. The Rand approach recodes the answers of each question into a 0-to-100 score, oriented so that high values represent more favorable states (11, Table 1). Questions with three-category response scales are coded 0, 50, or 100. Five-category responses are coded in steps of 25, again ensuring that higher scores represent better health. Six-point scales (e.g., question 7) are coded in steps of 20. Then, scores for items in the same health dimensions are averaged to create the eight scale scores ranging from 0 to 100. Items not answered are ignored when calculating the scale scores.

The alternative scoring approach is the recommended one and is fully described in Chapter 6 of the manual. Scoring can be automated using software from Response Technologies, Inc., which sells or rents a self-contained system for processing and interpreting the SF-36 forms (see Address section). The unit optically scans the SF-36 form, computes scale scores, and prints a graphical display of results within about five seconds (9). The scoring system orients all items so that a higher score represents

better health. Values for items 1, 7, and 8 are recoded, using weights derived for Likert analyses. For item 1, excellent is scored 5.0, very good = 4.4, good = 3.4, fair = 2.0, and poor = 1.0. For item 7, none = 6.0, very mild = 5.4, mild = 4.2, moderate = 3.1, severe = 2.2, and very severe = 1.0. Scores for item 8 take account of the answers to item 7: if no pain is recorded on either item, then item 8 is scored 6. If item 8 is answered not at all, but item 7 > none, then item 8 is scored 5. For the remaining categories of item 8, a little bit = 4, moderately = 3, quite a bit = 2, and extremely = 1. Next, scores for items on each scale (see above) are added to give scale scores. Finally, these are linearly transformed to a 0-to-100 scale (6, Table 6.11; 10; 12). The formula is

Transformed scale =

$$\frac{(\text{Actual score} - \text{Lowest possible score})}{\text{Possible raw score range}} \times 100$$

A missing value is given for a scale if over half of the items are missing; where fewer items are missing, these are replaced by that respondent's mean scores on the remaining items in the scale (10, p44).

Reliability

McHorney et al. based comprehensive analyses of item response, reliability, and validity on a sample of 3,445 patients with chronic medical or psychiatric conditions drawn from the MOS study (10). Item analyses confirmed the assignment of the items to the eight scales; this was replicated in different patient groups (10, p51).

Alpha internal consistency coefficients for the eight scales have been reported from many studies; Ware et al. list results from 14 (6, Table 7.2). Combining results from these studies, the median alpha reliability for all scales exceeds 0.80, except for the two-item social functioning scale (0.76). Typical results are illustrated in Table 9.3. Slightly lower values were reported by Kurtin et al. (9, Table 5). All scales appear sufficiently reliable for comparing

Table 9.3 Cronbach Alpha Coefficients for SF-36 Scales from Several Studies

Scale	Kantz et al. (16)	McHorney et al. (10)	Brazier et al. (14)	Jenkinson et al. (17)	Manual, Table 8.2 (6)
Physical functioning	0.88	0.93	0.93	0.90	0.93
Role limitations (physical problems)	0.90	0.84	0.96	0.88	0.89
Pain	0.80	0.82	0.85	0.82	0.90
Social functioning	0.77	0.85	0.73	0.76	0.68
Mental health	0.82	0.90	0.95	0.83	0.84
Role limitations (emotional problems)	0.80	0.83	0.96	0.80	0.82
Vitality	0.88	0.87	0.96	0.85	0.86
General health perceptions	0.83	0.78	0.95	—	0.81

groups, and the physical functioning scale appears reliable enough for comparing individuals. The intraclass correlation was 0.85 for patients with musculoskeletal problems (13). Item-total correlations typically lie in the mid-0.70s (6, Table 5.2).

Two-week test–retest correlations exceeded 0.8 for physical function, vitality, and general health perceptions; the lowest coefficient was 0.6 for social function (14, Table II). Assessing agreement, the mean of the differences in scores did not exceed one point on the 100-point scale (14, p162). Test–retest correlations for the scales after a delay of six months ranged between 0.60 and 0.90, except for the pain dimension, with a correlation of 0.43 (15, Table 5).

Validity

The SF-36 manual presents criterion validity information on the scales, comparing scale scores to ability to work, symptoms, utilization of care, and to a range of criteria for the mental health scale (6, Chapter 9). Each comparison suggested significant and consistent associations with the validation criteria. Item 2, on self-reported change, was evaluated in a study that applied a general health rating twice, at an interval of one year (6, Table 9.11). There was substantial agreement, although there were some errors at the ends of the scale: 6.9% of those who said they were much better

had worsened, and 3.4% of those who reported being much worse had improved. McHorney et al. compared SF-36 scale scores for patients with varying levels of medical and psychiatric conditions and with combinations of both. The scales discriminated between types and levels of disease and were also able to distinguish people with a chronic medical condition alone from those who had a medical disorder combined with a psychological one (18, pp255–259; 6, pp9:21–9:23). From these analyses, McHorney et al. provided guidelines for interpreting the eight scales. The physical functioning and mental health scales are relatively pure, being specific to medical or to psychiatric disorders. The two role scales chiefly reflect physical or mental conditions, but not exclusively. By design, the social functioning and vitality scales reflect both physical and mental conditions. The general health perceptions scale appears to be most sensitive to physical health problems. Nerenz et al. compared patient SF-36 ratings with physicians' ratings of the eight dimensions; these fell between 0.39 and 0.64 (15, pMS117). In general, physicians rated patients healthier than did the patients themselves.

Principal components analyses of the MOS data indicated that a general health dimension was common to all eight SF-36 scales, explaining 55% of the variance (18, p254). When a two-component solution was extracted, physical and mental dimensions were identified; the vitality scale loaded on both, and the general health perceptions scale loaded mainly on the physical component (6, Table 9.12; 18, Table 1). Correlations among the eight scales were reported by Nerenz et al. (15, Table 2). These broadly correspond to the groupings found by McHorney, except that the social functioning scale was more closely associated with physical than mental functioning in the Nerenz study.

Correlations with the Sickness Impact Profile (SIP) were 0.78 for 106 hip surgery patients (19, Table 3); in a separate study the correlations were 0.73 for overall functioning, 0.78 for physical function, and 0.67 for social function (N = 25 elderly males) (8, Table 2). A comparison of the SF-36 and the Quality of Well-Being Scale (QWB) for 916 respondents indicated that the SF-36 accounted for 55.7% of the variance in the QWB scores; conversely, the QWB accounted for 63.7% of the variance in SF-36 physical functioning scores, for 33.8% of variance in general health perceptions, and for 49.2% of physical role functioning (20). Correlations of the eight scales of the British version of the SF-36 with the EuroQol Quality of Life Index ranged from 0.48 to 0.60 ($p < 0.01$) (21, p173). In a general population sample, the SF-36 demonstrated less of a ceiling effect than the EuroQol, on which between 64% and 95% of respondents achieved maximum scores on the dimensions of the instrument, compared to 37% to 72% for the various dimensions of the SF-36 (21, p173). Ware et al. present a table listing correlations between the SF-36 and 15 other health measures. Correlations for the mental health scale range from 0.51 to 0.82 with the corresponding scales in other leading measures; equivalent correlations for the physical function scale range from 0.52 to 0.85 (6, Table 9.16). Brazier et al. present a full multitrait–multimethod correlation matrix comparing the SF-36 dimension scores with those of the Nottingham Health Profile. While the correlations

between comparable dimensions in the two instruments exceeded those between noncomparable dimensions, the coefficients were not high (0.52 for the physical scale, 0.55 for pain, 0.67 for mental health, and 0.68 for vitality) (14, Table IV).

The SF-36 appears sensitive to change: an effect size of 0.67 in a study of musculoskeletal patients was higher than that for the Nottingham Health Profile, SIP, or the Duke DUHP (13). In a comparison of sensitivity to change in a study of hip replacement patients, the ranking of five instruments depended on whether the overall scores were used or the physical or psychological scores (19, Table 4). Using the overall scores, SF-36 was more sensitive to change than the SIP but less so than the Arthritis Impact Measurement Scales or the Functional Status Questionnaire. The physical score of the SF-36 was more sensitive than all but one of the other measures, but the psychological score was the least sensitive to change. The SF-36 manual presents confidence intervals and estimates of the sample sizes required to detect differences of various sizes under a variety of statistical designs for each SF-36 scale (6, Tables 7.4–7.9).

Alternative Forms

The standard version of the SF-36 refers to problems in the past four weeks, while an acute version refers to the past week. The questions are otherwise identical. A condition-specific variant of the SF-36 has been described for use with knee replacement patients, in which patients were asked to report only limitations in function due to their knee condition (16). A comparison of the condition-specific and generic versions indicated that some of the condition-specific scales (e.g., pain, role limitations) were more sensitive to the effects of treatment than were the equivalent generic scales, which reflected the combined effect of the knee condition and comorbidities (16, pMS248).

A British-English version has been prepared (14, 17). This alters the phrasing of six items; for example, "block" was standardized to "100 yards" and "feeling blue" was changed to "feeling low." Through an International Quality of Life Assessment Project, the SF-36 is being translated and adapted for use in other languages, including Swedish (22), German, Spanish, French, Italian, Danish, Dutch, and Japanese (6, p12:7; 23; 24, p381).

An alternative form of the five-item mental health scale has been validated; this is useful in studies requiring repeated administrations of the scale over short time periods (25).

The Rand Corporation has presented an alternative version of the SF-36 that differs in detail of the wording of two questions and in the scoring method (11).

Reference Standards

Norms for the general U.S. population are presented for seven age groups and by gender in the SF-36 manual, as are norms for 13 different medical conditions (6, Chapter 10; 7). Norms from a large British sample show mean scores by age, gender, socioeconomic class, and by the presence of chronic conditions (14, Table III). Other British norms are also available (26, 27). Table 9.4 shows summary population norms for the SF-36, derived from several studies. The Rand figures were based on 2,471 responses from the MOS and use the Rand scoring approach described earlier.

An indication of effect sizes can be derived from the comparison of patients with different types of chronic disease. McHorney et al. noted that a difference of 23 points on the physical functioning scale reflects the impact of a complicated chronic medical condition, while a difference of 27 points on the mental health scale is equivalent to the impact of serious depressive symptoms (18, p261).

Table 9.4   Population Norms for SF-36 Scales

Note: Figures show means (standard deviations in parentheses).

Scale	Rand study (11)	Elderly males (8)	U.S. general population (6)
Physical functioning	70.6 (27.4)	52.0 (30.7)	84.2 (23.3)
Role limitations (physical problems)	53.0 (40.8)	—	81.0 (34.0)
Pain	70.8 (25.5)	—	75.2 (23.7)
Social functioning	78.8 (25.4)	66.2 (35.6)	83.3 (22.7)
Mental health	70.4 (22.0)	—	74.7 (18.1)
Role limitations (emotional problems)	65.8 (40.7)	—	81.3 (33.0)
Vitality	52.2 (22.4)	—	60.9 (21.0)
General health perceptions	57.0 (21.1)	—	72.0 (20.3)

Commentary

The SF-36 has shown a meteoric rise to prominence; the New England Health Institute estimated that by 1992 a million forms were being administered each year, even though comparatively little evidence on reliability or validity was then available. The instrument has clearly met a need and has also been carefully promoted; there are several advantages in this. Attention is being paid to ensuring its standard administration. This is facilitated through the Medical Outcomes Trust, a nonprofit organization created to support the development and distribution of standardized outcome measures. Permission to use the SF-36 should be obtained from the Trust, which provides updates on its administration, scoring, and interpretation. We recommend contacting the Trust, as it is assembling a database from studies that have used the SF-36 and from which more detailed norms will be drawn. The SF-36 is in the public domain, and no royalties are required for using it.

The history of the SF-36 reflects the challenges inherent in designing any general health measurement. An instrument should be broad in scope but not unwieldy; a tradeoff has to be made between covering many topics superficially and achieving detailed coverage of a few; this translates into comprehensiveness versus precision. In this vein, the first abbreviation of the MOS instruments, the SF-20, was soon criticized as being too narrow. There ensued an explosion of rival abbreviations: Wu proposed a 30-item short form (28); subsequently, 36-, 38-, and 56-item versions were proposed (29). The SF-36 should now replace these; time will tell whether the SF-20 survives.

As with any abbreviated instrument, it remains possible to criticize the scope of the SF-36, and some have commented on the absence of cognitive function or distress (29). The physical activity items focus on gross activities such as walking, bending, and kneeling; coordinated actions that may be captured by items such as shopping or cooking are not covered (24, p380). Floor effects have been reported for the role scales in a study of hemodialysis (9) and other conditions (24, p379), suggesting that these scales might not detect further deterioration in the condition of patients. McHorney discussed ceiling and floor effects, suggesting that the two role scales may not be broad enough in scope, but her analyses were based on people with chronic conditions, and may have to be reexamined in analyses of healthy groups (10, p53). As a measure of relatively well people, however, the SF-36 identified minor levels of discomfort missed by the Nottingham Health Profile (14).

The core descriptions of the reliability and validity of the SF-36 are exemplary (10, 18). The manual is excellent, giving a complete and balanced view of the instrument; attention to detail is outstanding. For example, 15 internal consistency checks are programmed into the SF-36 scoring to identify respondents who may be making internally inconsistent responses (6, p7:16). A guide to the physical and mental component summary measures provides validity results and references standards (30). Given the quality of the instrument and the strength of the team that is developing the SF-36, it will surely become one of the standard measures.

Addresses

Technical Information
SF-36 Health Survey, The Health Institute, New England Medical Center Hospitals, Box 345, 750 Washington Street, Boston, Massachusetts, USA 02111

Computerized Scoring System
Response Technologies, Inc., 3399 South County Trail, East Greenwich, Rhode Island, USA 02818

SF-36 Forms
The Medical Outcomes Trust, PO Box 1917, Boston, Massachusetts, USA 02205

REFERENCES

(1) Ware JE, Sherbourne CD. The MOS 36-item Short-Form Health Survey (SF-36). I. Conceptual framework and item selection. Med Care 1992;30:473–483.

(2) Lohr KN, Brook RH, Kamberg CJ, et al. Use of medical care in the Rand Health Insurance Experiment. Diagnosis- and service-specific analyses in a randomized controlled trial. Med Care 1986; 24(suppl):S1–S87.

(3) Stewart AL, Greenfield S, Hays RD, et al. Functional status and well-being of patients with chronic conditions. JAMA 1989; 262:907–913.

(4) Tarlov AR, Ware JE Jr, Greenfield S, et al. The Medical Outcomes Study: an application of methods for monitoring the results of medical care. JAMA 1989;262:925–930.

(5) Bindman AB, Keane D, Lurie N. Measuring health changes among severely ill patients: the floor phenomenon. Med Care 1990;28:1142–1152.

(6) Ware JE Jr, Snow KK, Kosinski M, et al. SF-36 Health Survey: manual and interpretation guide. Boston, Massachusetts: The Health Institute, New England Medical Center, 1993.

(7) McHorney CA, Kosinski M, Ware JE Jr. Comparisons of the costs and quality of norms for the SF-36 health survey collected by mail versus telephone interview: results from a national survey. Med Care 1994;32:551–567.

(8) Weinberger M, Samsa GP, Hanlon JT, et al. An evaluation of a brief health status measure in elderly veterans. J Am Geriatr Soc 1991;39:691–694.

(9) Kurtin PS, Davies AR, Meyer KB, et al. Patient-based health status measures in outpatient dialysis: early experiences in developing an outcomes assessment program. Med Care 1992;30(suppl):MS136–MS149.

(10) McHorney CA, Ware JE Jr, Lu JFR, et al. The MOS 36-item Short-Form Health Survey (SF-36): III. Tests of data quality, scaling assumptions, and reliability across diverse patient groups. Med Care 1994; 32:40–66.

(11) Rand Health Sciences Program. Rand 36-item Health Survey 1.0. Santa Monica, California: Rand Corporation, 1992.

(12) Medical Outcomes Trust. How to score the SF-36 Short-Form Health Survey. Boston, Massachusetts: The Medical Outcomes Trust, 1992.

(13) Beaton DE, Bombardier C, Hogg-Johnson S. Choose your tool: a comparison of the psychometric properties of five generic health status instruments in workers with soft tissue injuries. Qual Life Res 1994;3:50–56.

(14) Brazier JE, Harper R, Jones NMB, et al. Validating the SF-36 Health Survey questionnaire: new outcome measure for primary care. Br Med J 1992;305:160–164.

(15) Nerenz DR, Repasky DP, Whitehouse FW, et al. Ongoing assessment of health status in patients with diabetes mellitus. Med Care 1992;30(suppl):MS112–MS123.

(16) Kantz ME, Harris WJ, Levitsky K, et al. Methods for assessing condition-specific and generic functional status outcomes after total knee replacement. Med Care 1992;30(suppl):MS240–MS252.

(17) Jenkinson C, Wright L, Coulter A. Criterion validity and reliability of the SF-36 in a population sample. Qual Life Res 1994;3:7–12.

(18) McHorney CA, Ware JE Jr, Raczek AE. The MOS 36-item Short-Form Health Survey (SF-36): II. Psychometric and clinical tests of validity in measuring physical and mental health constructs. Med Care 1993;31:247–263.

(19) Katz JN, Larson MG, Phillips CB, et al. Comparative measurement sensitivity of short and longer health status instruments. Med Care 1992;30:917–925.

(20) Fryback DG, Dasbach ED, Klein R, et al. Health assessment by SF-36, Quality of Well-Being Index, and time tradeoffs: predicting one measure from another. Med Decision Making 1992;12:348.

(21) Brazier J, Jones N, Kind P. Testing the validity of the Euroqol and comparing it with the SF-36 Health Survey questionnaire. Qual Life Res 1993;2:169–180.

(22) Sullivan M, Karlsson J, Bengtsson C, et al. Health-related quality of life in Swedish populations: validation of the SF-36 Health Survey. Qual Life Res 1994;3:95.

(23) Aaronson NK, Acquadro C, Alonso J, et al. International quality of life assessment (IQOLA) Project. Qual Life Res 1992;1:349–351.

(24) Anderson RT, Aaronson NK, Wilkin D. Critical review of the international assessments of health-related quality of life. Qual Life Res 1993;2:369–395.

(25) McHorney CA, Ware JE Jr. Construction and validation of an alternate form general mental health scale for the Medical Outcomes Study Short-Form 36-item Health Survey. Med Care 1995;33:15–28.

(26) Jenkinson C, Coulter A, Wright L. Short

Form 36 (SF-36) Health Survey questionnaire: normative data from a large random sample of working age adults. Br Med J 1993;306:1437–1440.

(27) Jenkinson C, Wright L, Coulter A. Quality of life measurement in health care: a review of measures and population norms for the UK SF-36. Oxford: Health Services Research Unit, University of Oxford, 1993.

(28) Wu AW, Rubin HR, Matthews WC. A health status questionnaire using 30 items from the Medical Outcomes Study: preliminary validation in persons with early HIV infection. Med Care 1991;29:786.

(29) Hays RD, Shapiro MF. An overview of generic health-related quality of life measures for HIV research. Qual Life Res 1992;1:91–97.

(30) Ware JE Jr, Kosinski M, Keller SD. SF-36 physical and mental health summary scores: a user's manual. Boston, Massachusetts: The Health Institute, New England Medical Center, 1994.

THE SHORT-FORM-20 HEALTH SURVEY
(Anita L. Stewart, 1988)

Purpose

This 20-item abbreviation of the Rand Medical Outcomes Study (MOS) instrument is designed as a general outcome measure in clinical studies and as a health status measure in population studies (1). It covers physical, social, and role functioning as well as mental health, pain, and health perceptions.

Conceptual Basis

The shortened forms of the MOS measures responded to the common need to severely limit the length of questionnaires while retaining broad coverage. The instrument was to cover only the most important health concepts and "to reduce respondent burden while achieving minimum standards of precision for purposes of group comparisons" (2, p277). The physical, social, and role function scales cover the behavioral effects of health problems. The mental health, pain, and health perceptions scales "reflect more subjective components

of health and general well-being. These six health concepts were selected to be comprehensive in terms of those aspects of health considered most important to patients." (3, p909)

Description

Eighteen items were taken from Rand scales, including the Mental Health Inventory reviewed in Chapter 5 (4). The social functioning and pain items were written for this instrument. The 20 questions, shown in Exhibit 9.15, form six scales. Questions 2a to 2f form the physical functioning scale, while role functioning includes questions 4 and 5, and question 6 indicates social functioning. A mental health scale is formed from questions 7 through 11. The health perceptions scale is based on questions 1 and 12a to 12d. Pain is measured by item 3. The instrument is self-administered and takes three to four minutes (1, p725), although an average of 16 minutes was required for elderly subjects in one study (5, p254).

In scoring the instrument, the response scales for items 1, 8, 10, 12b, and 12c are reversed so that higher scores indicate better health (1, p727). Question 1 is rescored to more adequately indicate the unequal intervals in the ordinal response scale: $1 = 5$, $2 = 4.36$, $3 = 3.43$, $4 = 1.99$, and $5 = 1$. For each of the six scales, item scores are added, and the resulting sum is transformed to a 0-to-100 scale in which 100 represents the best possible functioning on each scale except for pain, where a high score indicates more pain. Stewart et al. recommend how to handle missing answers (1, p727). Note that in some studies, raw scores are presented, without converting to 0-to-100 scales (2).

Cutting points for defining "poor health" were developed for each of the scales, based mainly on the scores of the lowest 20% of the population sample in the MOS (1, Table 2). Poor physical and role functioning are defined as one or more limitations; poor social functioning as limi-

Exhibit 9.15   The Short-Form-20 Health Survey

1. In general, would you say your health is:

   1 ☐ Excellent
   2 ☐ Very Good
   3 ☐ Good
   4 ☐ Fair
   5 ☐ Poor

2. For how long (if at all) has your health limited you in each of the following activities?
   (Check One Box on Each Line)

	Limited for more than 3 months	Limited for 3 months or less	Not limited at all
	1	2	3
a. The kinds or amounts of vigorous activities you can do, like lifting heavy objects, running or participating in strenuous sports	☐	☐	☐
b. The kinds or amounts of moderate activities you can do, like moving a table, carrying groceries or bowling	☐	☐	☐
c. Walking uphill or climbing a few flights of stairs	☐	☐	☐
d. Bending, lifting, or stooping	☐	☐	☐
e. Walking one block	☐	☐	☐
f. Eating, dressing, bathing, or using the toilet	☐	☐	☐

3. How much bodily pain have you had during the past 4 weeks?

   1 ☐ None
   2 ☐ Very Mild
   3 ☐ Mild
   4 ☐ Moderate
   5 ☐ Severe
   6 ☐ Very Severe

4. Does your health keep you from working at a job, doing work around the house or going to school?

   1 ☐ Yes, for more than 3 months
   2 ☐ Yes, for 3 months or less
   3 ☐ No

5. Have you been unable to do certain kinds or amounts of work, housework or schoolwork because of your health?

   1 ☐ Yes, for more than 3 months
   2 ☐ Yes, for 3 months or less
   3 ☐ No

For each of the following questions, please check the box for the one answer that comes closest to the way you have been feeling during the past month.
   (Check One Box on Each Line)

Exhibit 9.15   *(Continued)*

Exhibit 9.15 *(Continued)*

	All of the Time	Most of the Time	A Good Bit of the Time	Some of the Time	A Little of the Time	None of the Time
	1	2	3	4	5	6
6. How much of the time, during the past month, has your health limited your social activities (like visiting with friends or close relatives)?	☐	☐	☐	☐	☐	☐
7. How much of the time, during the past month, have you been a very nervous person?	☐	☐	☐	☐	☐	☐
8. During the past month, how much of the time have you felt calm and peaceful?	☐	☐	☐	☐	☐	☐
9. How much of the time, during the past month, have you felt downhearted and blue?	☐	☐	☐	☐	☐	☐
10. During the past month, how much of the time have you been a happy person?	☐	☐	☐	☐	☐	☐
11. How often, during the past month, have you felt so down in the dumps that nothing could cheer you up?	☐	☐	☐	☐	☐	☐

12. Please check the box that best describes whether each of the following statements is true or false for you. (Check One Box on Each Line)

	Definitely True	Mostly True	Not Sure	Mostly False	Definitely False
	1	2	3	4	5
a. I am somewhat ill	☐	☐	☐	☐	☐
b. I am as healthy as anybody I know	☐	☐	☐	☐	☐
c. My health is excellent	☐	☐	☐	☐	☐
d. I have been feeling bad lately	☐	☐	☐	☐	☐

Adapted from Stewart AL, Hays RD, Ware JE Jr. The MOS Short-Form General Health Survey: reliability and validity in a patient population. Med Care 1988;26:733-735. With permission.

tations "a good bit of the time" or more frequently; poor mental health as a score of 67 or lower; poor health perceptions as a score of 70 or lower; while for pain the cutting point lies between mild and moderate pain.

The main reliability and validity analyses were based on a sample of 11,186 adults in the MOS who made an outpatient health care consultation during a nine-month period in one of three study sites. The mean age was 47, and 38% were male (1, p725).

Additional testing was carried out on a general population sample (6).

Reliability

Internal consistency coefficients for the four multi-item scales were 0.81 (role functioning), 0.86 (physical), 0.87 (health perceptions), and 0.88 (mental health) (1, Table 3). Slightly higher figures were found in a longitudinal study of 414 patients (7); slightly lower figures were quoted by Ware et al. (although it is not clear whether identical questions were used) (2). The alpha reliability of the pain and social measures were estimated at 0.76 and 0.67, respectively (3). Results were consistent across diagnostic, age, and educational groups. These reliability figures are only moderately lower than those of the full-length measures from which the SF-20 scales were derived.

Guttman analyses were also undertaken; the coefficient of reproducibility for the role functioning scale was 0.97; that for the physical functioning items was 0.89 (2, p281). Item-scale correlations ranged from 0.41 to 0.74 for the physical functioning scale and from 0.54 to 0.65 for mental health (2, p282). Using Mokken Scale Analysis (a method for identifying unidimensional and cumulative scales), two satisfactory scales were identified: mental health (items 7–11) and health perceptions (items 1, 6, 12a to 12d) (8, Tables 1, 2).

Validity

Convergent and discriminant validity were tested in a multitrait analysis. The patterns of correlations indicate that physical and role functioning scales correlated highly; the health perceptions score correlated substantially with each of the other scales while the mental health and pain scales showed lower associations with the others (1, Table 3).

Patients were significantly more likely ($p < 0.001$) to be rated in poor health on all scales than people in the general population (1, p729; 3, Table 4). Scores were associated with sociodemographic characteristics in a manner consistent with other studies (1, p729).

Nelson et al. compared the SF-20 with the Dartmouth COOP Charts using a multitrait–multimethod analysis. Convergent correlations ranged from 0.45 to 0.78; the average convergent correlations in two samples were 0.62 and 0.46 (9, Table 1). The average divergent correlation were 0.39 and 0.32 (9, p1117). Regression analyses compared the sensitivity of the COOP Charts and SF-20 scales in reflecting the

impact of selected chronic conditions on functioning. The variance explained by the physical function scale was slightly superior for the COOP Chart, whereas for the emotional, role, and overall scales, the SF-20 scales were better (markedly so for the emotional questions: $R^2 = 0.29$ for the COOP Charts versus 0.52 for the Rand questions) (9, Table 3). A study of elderly patients compared the validity of COOP and SF-20 scores in predicting future health status; both provided significant and almost identical predictions of nursing-home placement and hospitalization (5). Siu et al. compared the convergent and divergent validity of *change* scores on the COOP and SF-20. The average convergent validity correlation was 0.37, and the average divergent correlation was 0.18 (10, p1096). Moderate to strong convergent correlations were observed only for pain, social, and mental scores. The SF-20 function score showed significant association with deterioration over time recorded by performance-based measures of gait and balance (10, Table 5); the SF-20 was superior to the COOP Chart and the Katz ADL scale using this indicator of sensitivity to change.

Reference Standards

Stewart et al. present mean scores for the six components for a general population sample (N = 2,008), for patients with no chronic conditions (N = 2,595), and for several groups of patients with chronic conditions (3, Table 4). These offer some interpretation of scores: "For example . . . a 9-point difference in physical functioning is equivalent to the effect of having arthritis or back problems. . . . A 13-point difference in health perceptions is equivalent to the effect of having diabetes or congestive heart failure" (3, p911).

Commentary

The Short-Form-20 was based on the extensively tested MOS measures. The items are well written; the instrument was carefully developed and has been tested in large population studies. The SF-36 (see previous review) was designed in response to criticisms that the 20-item version was too limited in scope. As the shorter cousin of the SF-36, it may nonetheless find a place as a brief general health rating of patients in primary care settings or in population surveys. One study of primary care patients compared the SF-20 unfavorably to the 17-item DUKE instrument; patients found the DUKE easier to understand, faster to complete, and preferable (11). This conclusion was, however, reached by the group that developed the DUKE instrument.

While the available data suggest validity in population surveys, the SF-20 requires further testing as a measure of change before it can be recommended as an outcome indicator in clinical trials. It may not be able to discriminate among more severe levels of disability (7). This was especially notable on the single-item pain and social dimensions and prevented the instrument from indicating further deterioration which was implied by responses to other questions. "The floor in the response range leads to an instrument bias against documenting a decline in the health of severely ill patients, the group in which it may be most important to detect it" (7, p1148).

Stewart et al. summarize the advantages of generic health status instruments:

They are useful for monitoring patients with more than one condition. They can be used to compare patients who have different conditions by providing a common yardstick. . . . Finally, the same measures can be appropriately applied to both general and patient populations with the advantage of comparing patient groups against the "healthy" standard of a general population. (3, p912)

The reader is advised also to examine the SF-36 when considering applying the SF-20.

REFERENCES

(1) Stewart AL, Hays RD, Ware JE Jr. The MOS Short-Form General Health Survey: reliability and validity in a patient population. Med Care 1988;26:724–735.

(2) Ware JE Jr, Sherbourne CD, Davies AR. Developing and testing the MOS 20-item Short-Form Health Survey: a general population application. In: Stewart AL, Ware JE Jr, eds. Measuring functioning and well-being: the Medical Outcomes Study approach. Durham, North Carolina: Duke University Press, 1992:277–290.

(3) Stewart AL, Greenfield S, Hays RD, et al. Functional status and well-being of patients with chronic conditions. JAMA 1989; 262:907–913.

(4) Brook RH, Ware JE Jr, Davies-Avery A. Overview of adult health status measures fielded in Rand's Health Insurance Study. Med Care 1979;17(suppl):1–131.

(5) Siu AL, Reuben DB, Ouslander JG, et al. Using multidimensional health measures in older persons to identify risk of hospitalization and skilled nursing placement. Qual Life Res 1993;2:253–261.

(6) Ware JE Jr, Sherbourne CD, Davies AR. A short-form general health survey. Santa Monica, California: Rand Corporation, 1988. (Publication P-7444).

(7) Bindman AB, Keane D, Lurie N. Measuring health changes among severely ill patients: the floor phenomenon. Med Care 1990;28:1142–1152.

(8) Moorer P, Suurmeijer TP. A study of the unidimensionality and cumulativeness of the MOS Short-form General Health Survey. Psychol Rep 1994;74:467–470.

(9) Nelson EC, Landgraf JM, Hays RD, et al. The functional status of patients. How can it be measured in physicians' offices? Med Care 1990;28:1111–1126.

(10) Siu AL, Ouslander JG, Osterweil D, et al. Change in self-reported functioning in older persons entering a residential care facility. J Clin Epidemiol 1993;46:1093–1101.

(11) Chen AL-T, Broadhead WE, Doe EA, et al. Patient acceptance of two health status measures: the Medical Outcomes Study Short-Form General Health Survey and the Duke Health Profile. Fam Med 1993; 25:536–539.

THE SELF-EVALUATION OF LIFE FUNCTION SCALE
(Margaret W. Linn and Bernard S. Linn, 1984)

Purpose

The Self-Evaluation of Life Function (SELF) Scale was designed as a comprehensive measurement of the physical, psychological, and social functioning of people aged 60 years or older. The objective was to develop a short multidimensional scale that the elderly could complete themselves.

Conceptual Basis

No information is available.

Description

A pool of 130 items was derived from existing scales. On the basis of factor analysis, the items were reduced to 54 loading on six factors: ADL and physical disability (13 items), symptoms of aging (13 items), self-esteem (seven items), social satisfaction (six items), depression (11 items), and personal control (four items). Other questions cover diagnoses, medications, sick days, and pain. Questions refer to the past month or current health; four-point response scales are used for all questions except diagnoses and medications. Factor scores are then used to weight each question in forming section scores, and these are used in analysis. The scale, too long to reproduce here, is shown in Linn and Linn's 1984 article (1).

The SELF was tested on 548 people who were 60 years of age or older and who were of at least moderate cognitive functioning (with scores above 20 on the Mini-Mental State Examination).

Reliability

Test–retest intraclass correlations were calculated for 101 elderly people after three to five days. Results ranged from 0.99 to 0.36 for items, while section scores ranged from 0.96 for physical disability to 0.59 for self-esteem (1, p609, Table 2).

Validity

The six factors show modest intercorrelations, with one third exceeding 0.40 (1, Table 2). The scale was tested on four groups (institutionalized patients, mental health outpatients, those receiving counseling, and community residents), and all factors discriminated significantly among groups, in the expected direction (1, Table 3). Physical disability was the best discrimi-

nator. The SELF showed agreement with rating of improvement made by health care providers ($p < 0.007$). Predictive validity after one year was assessed for a variety of outcomes (1, Table 5). The factor scores predicted the number of weeks in institutions ($R^2 = 0.37$) and visits to the physician ($R^2 = 0.28$). The most frequent predictors of outcome were physical disability and symptoms of aging (1, p611). Hawkins et al. obtained a canonical correlation of 0.75 between the subscales and a set of variables covering health practices and demographic data (such as exercise, sleeping, education, and age) (2). In contrast to studies that use a single question, Hawkins et al. found an association between self-reported health practices and health status variables for the elderly.

Alternative Forms

A 16-item version was adapted for telephone administration and used with patients after surgery for aneurysm (3).

Commentary

The SELF is a self-report multidimensional scale that appears to be acceptable to respondents. Although the SELF was based on established scales and shows promise, it needs further testing. The scoring system is complicated and it would be interesting to see how well a simpler scoring method agrees. Linn and Linn conclude that the SELF scale is useful for research and screening when a short, comprehensive, inexpensive, self-report measure of the overall function of the elderly is needed.

REFERENCES

(1) Linn MW, Linn BS. Self-Evaluation of Life Function (SELF) Scale: a short, comprehensive self-report of health for elderly adults. J Gerontol 1984;39:603–612.
(2) Hawkins WE, Duncan DF, McDermott RJ. A health assessment of older Americans: some multidimensional measures. Prev Med 1988;17:344–356.
(3) Rohrer MJ, Cutler BS, Wheeler HB. Long-term survival and quality of life following ruptured abdominal aortic aneurysm. Arch Surg 1988;123:1213–1217.

THE MULTILEVEL ASSESSMENT INSTRUMENT
(M. Powell Lawton, 1982)

Purpose

The Multilevel Assessment Instrument (MAI) was designed to measure the overall well-being of elderly persons living in the community. It covers health problems, activities of daily living (ADL) skills, psychological well-being, environment, and social interaction.

Conceptual Basis

Lawton argued that to assess the quality of life, of an elderly person, ratings must be made on four dimensions: behavioral competence, psychological well-being, perceived quality of life, and objective quality of the environment (1). A fuller discussion of Lawton's approach to defining quality of life among elderly people is given in his 1983 article (2). Reflecting this framework, the MAI built on existing measurement instruments, notably the OARS Multidimensional Functional Assessment Questionnaire (OMFAQ). Lawton argued that the MAI incorporated, but went beyond, existing instruments by considering environmental factors, by separating social interaction from personal pursuits such as hobbies, and by separating cognitive ability from psychological well-being (1).

The functional abilities section of the MAI was based on the theme of "behavioral competence," which Lawton viewed in terms of a hierarchy of increasingly complex activities ranging from the basic biological functions required for life maintenance, through perception and cognition, followed by skills for physical self-maintenance, up to exploratory behavior and complex social interactions (3). Within each of these dimensions, a further hierarchy of competence is identified; thus, for example, the social behavior dimension ranges from sensory contact through intimacy, to nurturance, and eventually to creative leadership (2, Figure 1). The term "multilevel assessment" is used to imply assessment on each of the levels of this hierarchy.

Description

This is one of several measurement scales developed at the Philadelphia Geriatric Center. Others that are reviewed in this book include the Physical Self-Maintenance Scale and the Philadelphia Geriatric Center Morale Scale. The MAI comprises seven dimensions with 147 items; a further 81 items cover medical and demographic data, but these are not considered in this review. Items were taken from a wide variety of established indices (1), and the MAI incorporates the ADL and IADL questions from the OMFAQ. The psychological domain includes questions on morale and psychiatric symptoms, and the environmental dimension covers housing quality and personal security (1). Space does not permit listing all the MAI questions, but the seven dimensions are shown in Exhibit 9.16 (note: this describes a revised questionnaire). Most of the dimensions are divided into subscales—there are 14 in all (e.g., perceived environment includes housing quality, neighborhood quality, and personal security). Each subscale contains between three and 24 items.

The instrument is administered in a home interview that takes an average of 50 minutes to complete. Some of the information must be obtained from the elderly person, but much can be obtained from the spouse or other informant. Scores are based on the numbers of items checked in each section; these may be added to give scores for each of the seven dimensions. Unweighted scores were found to correlate well with more complicated scoring methods (1).

Reliability

Lawton reported several studies of the agreement between two independent raters. Intraclass correlations between ratings on the seven dimensions ranged from 0.88 (for the IADL scale) to a low of 0.58 (for the social interaction scale) (1, p95).

Exhibit 9.16   The Scope of the Multilevel Assessment
Instrument, Showing Numbers of Items in Each Subscale

	Number of items
1. Physical health:	
Self-rated health	4
Use of health services	3
Health conditions	26
Mobility	3
Use of aids, prostheses, etc.	13
2. Cognition:	
Mental status	6
Cognitive symptoms	4
3. Activities of daily living:	
IADL Scale	10
Personal Self-Maintenance Activities	6
4. Time use:	
Social activities, sports, hobbies	18
5. Social relations and interactions:	
Family	12
Friends	5
6. Personal adjustment:	
Morale	9
Psychiatric symptoms	3
7. Perceived environment:	
Housing quality	9
Neighborhood quality	12
Personal security	4
	147

Adapted from Lawton MP, Moss M, Fulcomer M, Kleban MH. A research
and service oriented Multi-level Assessment Instrument. J Gerontol 1982;37:96,
Table 2.

Agreement between two interviewers lay within a one-point discrepancy for 95% of the ratings on the summary scales for a sample of 484 (1). Alpha internal consistency results for 590 respondents ranged from 0.69 for the cognitive and psychiatric symptom scales to 0.93 for ADL. Two coefficients, for health behavior and personal security, were lower at 0.39 and 0.57. Three-week test–retest reliabilities for 22 respondents ranged from 0.55 to 0.99 with the exception of ADL, which had a correlation of 0.35 (3, Table 2).

Validity

The MAI showed a weak ability to distinguish respondents living independently in the community from those in institutional care. Correlations for the seven dimension scores fell between 0.05 and 0.54 (1, Table 2).

Correlation with a psychologist's independent rating of 590 individuals was 0.23 for the cognition dimension of the MAI although, curiously, agreement between the psychologist's rating of other dimensions and the MAI scores was higher, ranging from 0.56 to 0.69. Agreement with ratings made by a housing administrator on 180 respondents for the seven dimensions ranged from 0.12 (for social interaction) to 0.59 (for ADL). The interviewers who applied the MAI made their own summary ratings of each dimension, and these were correlated against scores on the MAI. Coefficients ranged from 0.36 to 0.87 (1, Table 2). Lawton and Brody reported correlations between the IADL section and the

Physical Self-Maintenance Scale and a variety of other measurements. The correlations ranged from 0.36 to 0.62 (3, Table 6).

Commentary

The MAI was based on a clearly enunciated conceptual framework and on existing measurements. The reliability findings are promising, and yet the scale could clearly benefit from further testing and refinement. The validity results show quite low correlations between the method and independent assessments. Those scales showing low validity coefficients also showed low reliability scores, and Lawton noted that the psychometric properties of the social interaction and time use scales require improvement. The developers of the MAI also experienced some problems in selecting the most appropriate questions for the environmental scales. The low validity agreement between the psychologist's rating of cognition, and the corresponding MAI score is a cause for concern; it may be that the cognition measure discriminates only at very low levels of cognitive functioning. Lawton discussed the strengths and weaknesses of the MAI and argued in favor of a simple scoring system and against abbreviating the scale. He noted that scale norms based on representative population samples are not yet available, and the social and environmental domains show particular need for further research and development. He concluded that the physical health, the cognition, and the ADL dimensions of the MAI are the most robust.

This scale shows potential but lacks adequate documentation and validity analysis. The MAI needs to be refined but fills a potential niche for a scale to assess the well-being of the elderly living in the community.

Address

M. Powell Lawton, PhD, Philadelphia Geriatric Center, 5301 Old York Road, Philadelphia, Pennsylvania, USA 19141

REFERENCES

(1) Lawton MP, Moss M, Fulcomer M, Kleban MH. A research and service oriented Multilevel Assessment Instrument. J Gerontol 1982;37:91–99.
(2) Lawton MP. Environment and other determinants of well-being in older people. Gerontologist 1983;23:349–357.
(3) Lawton MP, Brody EM. Assessment of older people: Self-Maintaining and Instrumental Activities of Daily Living. Gerontologist 1969;9:179–186.

THE OARS MULTIDIMENSIONAL FUNCTIONAL ASSESSMENT QUESTIONNAIRE
(Older Americans Resources and Services, Duke University, 1975, Revised 1988)

Purpose

The OARS Multidimensional Functional Assessment Questionnaire (OMFAQ) was designed to assess the overall personal functional status and service use of adults, and in particular of the elderly (1, p1). It can be used as a screening instrument, to evaluate outcomes, and in modeling the cost-effectiveness of alternative approaches to providing care.

Conceptual Basis

The Older Americans Resources and Services (OARS) Program forms the clinical facet of the Duke University Center for the Study of Aging and Human Development. The eight-year program began in 1972 as a study of alternatives to institutional care for frail elderly people with a view to maintaining their independence in the least restrictive environment (1). The program invested a major effort in developing an information system that included the OMFAQ as a broad-ranging patient assessment, along with evaluation procedures to help ensure that services are tailored to needs (2). The OARS assessment model considered three elements: personal functional status; a method for classifying services into their generic elements and counting the use of each category of service; and a transition matrix to assess the impact of service packages for people according to functional level (1, p54). The transition matrix describes the proportions of people in each functional class who progress to higher or lower functional classes over time, with the provision of various types of support service. Parts A and B of the OMFAQ cover the first two of these elements; the transition matrices are being developed empirically (3).

Description

The OMFAQ is a structured questionnaire that is divided into part A, the Multidimensional Functional Assessment Questionnaire, and part B, the Services Assessment Questionnaire. Part A includes five sections, covering social and economic resources, mental and physical health, and activities of daily living. Sixty-six questions are asked of the respondent and a further ten questions record judgments made by an informant. Many of the questions have subparts, making a total of 120 items. In addition, the interviewer makes five summary ratings, one for each of the sections, based on information collected in the interview. The Services Assessment Questionnaire covers 24 categories of services received and needed; full definitions of each service are provided (1, pp39–44). The two questionnaires can be used separately, but when the entire instrument is used, some of the service use items are interleaved among the functional assessment sections to improve the flow of the interview (1, p3).

The OMFAQ evolved from revisions to an Intake Form, developed for an outpatient clinic population, that was later modified into a Community Survey Questionnaire for assessing people at home (4). While these instruments were designed for the elderly, items were later added to the OMFAQ to make it suitable for people aged 18 years and over. Questions were drawn from existing instruments and the

source of each is given in the manual. For example, it includes the Short Psychiatric Evaluation Schedule, and the Short Portable Mental Status Questionnaire (SPMSQ) that we review in Chapter 7. Over time, the original questions were clarified and their answer categories updated for the questions on economic matters (such as the amount of rent paid); these revisions were published in 1988 (1, Chapter 8).

The OMFAQ is administered by a trained interviewer. Two-day interviewer training courses are available from the Duke University Center for Aging; further details on administering the scale are given in the manual (2, p133) and in Fillenbaum's book (1, Chapter 7). The method was designed as a single interview schedule to be used in its entirety—the originators advise against extracting particular sections (5). Part A takes about 30 minutes to complete and the whole interview takes about 45 minutes (2). The entire scale is too long to present here; the earlier version is shown in the OARS manuals (2, 5) and the revised version in Fillenbaum's book (1, pp125–172). The contents of the OMFAQ are summarized in Exhibit 9.17; a rationale for the topics included is given by Pfeiffer. To illustrate the actual questions, Exhibit 9.18 shows the ADL and IADL sections.

The OMFAQ may be scored either as a rating scale or using computer-assigned scores. The first allows raters a measure of subjectivity in interpreting responses in the manner of a clinical rating; the computer rating seeks to avoid possible discrepancies between raters (3). In the first mode, a rater reads the answers to each item and summarizes the level of function for that section on a six-point scale: 1, outstanding functioning; 2, good functioning; 3, mild impairment; 4, moderate impairment; 5, severe impairment; and 6, complete impairment. The computer scoring system seeks to replicate clinical judgment in weighting each question and is summarized in the form of computer code that calculates scores for each section (1, Tables 7–11).

Exhibit 9.17 Contents of the OARS Multidimensional Functional Assessment Questionnaire

Note: In addition to basic demographic and interview specific information, the OMFAQ includes two sections: Part A, Assessment of Individual Functioning, and Part B, Assessment of Services Utilization.

Part A: Assessment of individual functioning

Part A is divided into seven major sections. These sections, in order, with a listing of the number of primary questions (some questions include several items) and a description of their content, are:

Section	No. of questions	Content
Basic demographic	11	Address; date; interviewer; informant; place of interview; duration; sex; race; age; education; telephone number.
Social resources	9	Marital status; resident companions; extent and type of contact with others; availability of confidante; perception of loneliness; availability, duration, and source of help.
Economic resources	15	Employment status; major occupation of self (and of spouse, if married); source and amount of income; number of dependents; home ownership or rental, and cost; source and adequacy of financial resources; health insurance; subjectively assessed adequacy of income.
Mental health	6	Short Portable Mental Status Questionnaire (SPMSQ), a ten-item test of organicity; extent of worry, satisfaction, and interest in life; assessment of present mental status and change in the past five years; fifteen-item Short Psychiatric Evaluation Schedule.
Physical health	16	Physician visits, days sick, in hospital and/or nursing home in past six months; medications in past month; current illnesses and their extent of interference; physical, visual, and hearing disabilities; alcoholism; participation in vigorous exercise; self-assessment of health.
Activities of daily living	15	Extent of capacity to: telephone, travel, shop, cook, do housework, take medicine, handle money, feed self, dress, groom, walk, transfer, bathe, and control bladder and bowels. Also, presence of another to help with ADL tasks.
Informant assessments	10	Information on the focal person's level of functioning on each of the five dimensions is sought from a knowledgeable informant. Specifically: Social: Capacity to get along with others; availability, duration, and source of help in time of need. Economic: Extent to which income meets basic self-maintenance requirements. Mental: Ability to make sound judgments, cope; interest in life; comparison with peers; change in past five years. Physical: Assessment of health; extent of interference of health problems.
Interviewer section (a) interview specific	4	Sources of information; reliability of responses.
(b) interview assessments	15	Social: Availability and duration of help when needed; adequacy of social relationships. Economic: Assessed adequacy of income; presence of reserves; extent to which basic needs are met. Mental: Ability to make sound judgments, cope; interest in life; behavior during interview. Physical: Whether obese or malnourished. Rating scales: Five six-point scales, one for each dimension.

Part B: Services assessment

For each of the twenty-four nonoverlapping services named below, enquiry is made into (a) utilization in the past six months, (b) intensity of present utilization (e.g., frequency), (c) service provider (e.g., self, family and friends, agency), and (d) perceived current need for service.

1. Transportation	13. Physical therapy
2. Social/recreational	14. Continuous supervision
3. Employment	15. Checking
4. Sheltered employment	16. Relocation and placement
5. Educational services, employment related	17. Homemaker-household
6. Remedial training	18. Meal preparation
7. Mental health	19. Administrative, legal, and protective
8. Psychotropic drugs	20. Systematic multidimensional evaluation
9. Personal care	21. Financial assistance
10. Nursing care	22. Food, groceries
11. Medical services	23. Living quarters (housing)
12. Supportive services and prostheses	24. Coordination, information, and referral

Reproduced from Multidimensional functional assessment: the OARS methodology. A manual. 2nd ed. Durham, North Carolina: Duke University, Center for the Study of Aging and Human Development. 1978:13–15. Copyright Duke University Center for the Study of Aging and Human Development. With permission. Permission required to use.

Fillenbaum also gives regression equations that indicate which questions contribute most to each section score (1, Table 12).

However they are derived, the section scores can be presented in several ways (1, pp46–49). First, the five section scores may be presented as a profile (2), or second, they may be added to form a Cumulative Impairment Score (CIS) ranging from 5 (excellent function in all areas) to 30 (totally impaired). The CIS gives equal weighting to each of the five section scores. Scores below 10 suggest excellent functioning; those over 18 indicate significant impairment in several areas (2). Third, each of the five scores may be dichotomized into not impaired or impaired, giving 2^5, or 32 permutations, and the respondent can be classified into one of these (1, p47). The cutting point for each section is left to the user and is chosen according to the purpose of the classification. Fillenbaum suggests grouping ratings 1 and 2 versus 3 through 6 if the purpose is to compare those with unimpaired function against all others; if the focus is on more severe levels of disability, ratings 1 through 4 may be compared against 5 and 6 (1, p47). The OARS manual, by contrast, mentions grouping ratings 1 to 3 as unimpaired and 4 to 6 as impaired (2). Finally, instead of the profile, a simple

count of the number of sections on which a patient shows significant impairment (typically, scores of 4 or more) may be used.

Reliability

Some reliability testing has been carried out on part A of the OMFAQ and on the Community Service Questionnaire from which it was derived (2, 5). Because section scores on the OMFAQ are typically assigned by raters who review the questionnaire responses, the assessment of inter-rater agreement is pertinent. Fillenbaum and Smyer reported inter-rater agreement for the OMFAQ for 11 raters who evaluated 30 patients. Intraclass correlations were 0.66 for physical health, 0.78 for economic resources, 0.80 for mental health, 0.82 for social resources, and 0.87 for self-care. Raters were in complete agreement for 74% of the ratings (1, p19).

Other reliability data refer to the Community Service Questionnaire, giving inter-rater Kendall coefficients of concordance between 0.70 and 0.93, with 11 out of 25 coefficients being 0.85 or above (2, p32). Ratings of the same questionnaires made 12 to 18 months apart gave correlations between 0.47 and 1.00, with only six of 35 coefficients lying below 0.80 (2, p32).

Activities of daily living

Now I'd like to ask you about some of the activities of daily living, things that we all need to do as a part of our daily lives. I would like to know if you can do these activities without any help at all, or if you need some help to do them, or if you can't do them at all.

[*Be sure to read all answer choices if applicable in questions 56 through 69 to respondent.*]

Instrumental ADL

56. Can you use the telephone . . .
     2 without help, including looking up numbers and dialing,
     1 with some help (can answer phone or dial operator in an emergency, but need a special phone or help in getting the number or dialing),
     0 or are you completely unable to use the telephone?
     — Not answered

57. Can you get to places out of walking distance . . .
     2 without help (can travel alone on buses, taxis, or drive your own car),
     1 with some help (need someone to help you or go with you when traveling) or
     0 are you unable to travel unless emergency arrangements are made for a specialized vehicle like an ambulance?
     — Not answered

58. Can you go shopping for groceries or clothes [assuming subject has transportation] . . .
     2 without help (taking care of all shoping needs yourself, assuming you had transportation),
     1 with some help (need someone to go with you on all shopping trips),
     0 or are you completely unable to do any shopping?
     — Not answered

59. Can you prepare your own meals . . .
     2 without help (plan and cook full meals yourself),
     1 with some help (can prepare some things but unable to cook full meals yourself),
     0 or are you completely unable to prepare any meals?
     — Not answered

60. Can you do your housework . . .
     2 without help (can you scrub floors, etc.),
     1 with some help (can do light housework but need help with heavy work),
     0 or are you completely unable to do any housework?
     — Not answered

61. Can you take your own medicine . . .
     2 without help (in the right doses at the right time),
     1 with some help (able to take medicine if someone prepares it for you and/or reminds you to take it),
     0 or are you completely unable to take your medicines?
     — Not answered

62. Can you handle your own money . . .
     2 without help (write checks, pay bills, etc.),
     1 with some help (manage day-to-day buying but need help with managing your checkbook and paying your bills),
     0 or are you completely unable to handle money?
     — Not answered

63. Can you eat . . .
     2 without help (able to feed yourself completely),
     1 with some help (need help with cutting, etc.),
     0 or are you completely unable to feed yourself?
     — Not answered

64. Can you dress and undress yourself . . .
     2 without help (able to pick out clothes, dress and undress yourself),
     1 with some help,
     0 or are you completely unable to dress and undress yourself?
     — Not answered

65. Can you take care of your own appearance, for example combing your hair and (for men) shaving . . .
    2 without help,
    1 with some help,
    0 or are you completely unable to maintain your appearance yourself?
    – Not answered

66. Can you walk . . .
    2 without help (except for a cane),
    1 with some help from a person or with the use of a walker, or crutches, etc.,
    0 or are you completely unable to walk?
    – Not answered

67. Can you get in and out of bed . . .
    2 without any help or aids,
    1 with some help (either from a person or with the aid of some device),
    0 or are you totally dependent on someone else to lift you?
    – Not answered

68. Can you take a bath or shower . . .
    2 without help,
    1 with some help (need help getting in and out of the tub, or need special attachments on the tub),
    0 or are you completely unable to bathe yourself?
    – Not answered

69. Do you ever have trouble getting to the bathroom on time?
    2 No
    0 Yes
    1 Have a catheter or colostomy
    – Not answered
    [If "Yes" ask a.]
    a. How often do you wet or soil yourself (either day or night)?
       1 Once or twice a week
       0 Three times a week or more
       – Not answered

70. Is there someone who helps you with such things as shopping, housework, bathing, dressing, and getting around?
    1 Yes
    0 No
    – Not answered
    [If "Yes" ask a. and b.]
    a. Who is your major helper?
       Name _____   Relationship _____
    b. Who else helps you?
       Name _____   Relationship _____

Five-week test–retest correlations for 30 elderly subjects were 0.82 for the physical ADL questions, 0.71 for the IADL questions, and 0.79 for those on economic resources. The test–retest correlation for the objective questions on social resources was 0.71 and that for the subjective questions was 0.53. Coefficients for life satisfaction and mental health were lower: 0.42 and 0.32, respectively (2, p30).

Validity

Fillenbaum and Smyer presented criterion validity results for the OMFAQ on 33 family medicine patients, using separate criterion ratings for each section in the questionnaire (4). Spearman correlations between the OMFAQ and these ratings were 0.68 for the economic section, 0.67 for mental health, 0.82 for physical health, and 0.89 for self-care capacity (1, Table 3; 4, Table 3).

Several validity results are available for the Intake Form and the Community Survey Questionnaire, the earlier versions of the OMFAQ. Scores on physical and mental health from the questionnaire were compared with ratings made by psychiatrists and physicians' assistants for 82 patients. The Spearman correlation for mental health was 0.62 and for physical health it was 0.70 ($p < 0.001$) (2, p27). OMFAQ scores have been compared to health care expenditures, showing an increase in expenditures by a factor of 13 as the OMFAQ scores rose from the lowest to the highest level of impairment (2). Scores from three contrasting populations (985 community residents, 78 patients, and 76 institutionalized elderly) showed clearly differing profiles on the instrument (6, Figure 1).

While each section on the OMFAQ receives a single, overall score, it was recognized that the sections cover different themes. Several studies have examined the factor structure of the scales. Fillenbaum ran factor analyses on each section separately and identified three factors in the social resources section, one in the economic section, four in the mental health section, and one each in the physical health, ADL, and IADL (1, Table 6). The reliability of the 11 factor scales ranged from alpha 0.52 to 0.87 (1, p25). Factor analyses of the physical function questions shown in Exhibit 9.18 broadly confirmed the appropriateness of their classification into ADL and IADL sections (7, Table 2). Analysis of the OMFAQ mental health items suggested that they represent four dimensions: life satisfaction, psychosomatic symptoms, alienation, and cognitive deficit; items on affect were lacking (8). Liang et al. argued that for screening purposes the first three of these could be combined into a single score, but that the SPMSQ cognitive rating should be treated separately (8, pP136).

Five of the IADL items formed a Guttman scale and scores on this were found to predict mental and physical health status one year later (correlations between 0.48 and 0.51, according to age). IADL scores also predicted mortality rates; for example, those unable to perform any activities showed a 5.4 times higher death rate than the sample as a whole (7, p704).

Alternative Forms

Pfeiffer et al. developed an abbreviated version of the OMFAQ called the Functional Assessment Inventory (FAI) (9). Note that this is completely distinct from the instrument with the same name developed by Crewe and Athelstan and reviewed in this chapter. The two instruments were developed at the same time and were published in different locations, preventing the duplication of names from being detected. Pfeiffer et al.'s FAI omits most of the questions on medical services from part B of the OMFAQ, reduces the number of answer categories for some items, uses a modified coding scheme, and includes questions on life satisfaction and self-esteem not found in the OMFAQ. Five scores are produced: ADL impairment, physical health, mental health, economic resources, and social resources. The mean administration time for the FAI was 30.6 minutes in the home setting, compared to 44.6 for the OMFAQ (10, Table 6). A separate study found that the FAI required an average of 40 minutes to administer (11, p244). Four-week test–retest reliability by intraclass correlation was 0.81 for the cognitive score, 0.71 for the ADL section, 0.55 for mental health, and 0.51 for physical health. Reliability for the social and economic resources sections was lower, at 0.47 and 0.16. Inter-rater agreement ranged from 0.56 to 0.83 (10, Table 4). The correlation between FAI and OMFAQ section scores was 0.77 for cognitive and ADL sections, 0.59 for physical health, and 0.50 for mental health (10, Table 5). A small validity study of the FAI showed close agreement between FAI scores and independent clinical ratings of the same dimensions (12, p853). The FAI is able to distinguish between contrasting patient groups (11).

A Brazilian version of the 15-item Short Psychiatric Evaluation Schedule included in the OMFAQ has been described; it had a sensitivity of 61% at a specificity of 89% (13, p689).

Reference Standards

Norms from three U.S. random samples of people aged 60 and over, from the community, from adult day care, and from an institution, are given by Fillenbaum (1, Chapter 9). The mean CIS summary score for community residents aged 65 or over in Durham, North Carolina, was 12.2, while that for institutional residents was 20.7 (1, p47).

Reference standards for the seven IADL questions shown in Exhibit 9.18 were drawn from three large studies and are available by sex and age (7, Table 1).

Commentary

The development work for the OARS was thoroughly carried out over a long period by a large, multidisciplinary team. The OMFAQ has been cited as influential in the design of several subsequent scales, including the CARE developed by Gurland et al. The instrument is being used in a number of settings, reflecting the emphasis on developing a multipurpose instrument (3). Fillenbaum proposed five of the IADL items as a brief screening instrument that showed good correlations with physical and mental health; these items could identify people for whom a more extensive assessment is warranted (7). In its design, the OMFAQ combines elements of the clinical rating scale approach with the structured questionnaire. It uses set question wording but allows scope for interpretation by the rater; it also offers flexibility in scoring responses and in selecting cutting points suited to the purpose at the time: "the same basic set of data can be analyzed in several different ways to meet the needs of its many different users" (2, p68). This flexibility is also seen in the way that information from family members or other informants can be used to supplement the picture obtained during the interview. Documentation is excellent, as is the provision of training opportunities. The manuals provide clear details of the development, administration, and quality of the instrument. The Data Archive at the Center at Duke University holds a number of data sets that include the OARS instruments; these are available to the public. The archive also keeps a register of OARS users with descriptions of their projects and a bibliography of publications.

Much of the reliability testing refers to earlier versions of the instrument and relies on small samples. The results suggest, rather than prove, that the current version can be applied and scored in a consistent manner. The ADL and IADL sections show good validity and reliability, suggesting they are superior to many of the purpose-built instruments reviewed in Chapter 3. While the OARS team counsels against applying these separately, they have commonly been used as separate scales. It would be advantageous to see reliability and validity studies based on larger samples, and it would also be useful to derive reference standards from some of the larger studies in which the OMFAQ has been used. Despite these concerns, we have little hesitation in recommending the OMFAQ as a valuable instrument for providing a comprehensive profile of personal functioning and service use.

Address

George L. Maddox, PhD, Chairman, University Council on Aging and Human Development, Center for the Study of Aging and Human Development, Duke University Medical Center, Durham, North Carolina, USA 27710

REFERENCES

(1) Fillenbaum GG. Multidimensional functional assessment of older adults: the Duke Older Americans Resources and Services procedures. Hillsdale, New Jersey: Lawrence Erlbaum Associates, 1988.

(2) Multidimensional functional assessment: the OARS methodology. A manual. 2nd ed. Durham, North Carolina: Duke University Center for the Study of Aging and Human Development, 1978.

(3) George LK, Fillenbaum GG. OARS methodology: a decade of experience in geriatric assessment. J Am Geriatr Soc 1985; 33:607–615.

(4) Fillenbaum GG, Smyer MA. The development, validity, and reliability of the OARS Multidimensional Functional Assessment Questionnaire. J Gerontol 1981;36:428–434.

(5) Fillenbaum G. Reliability and validity of the OARS Multidimensional Functional Assessment Questionnaire. In: Pfeiffer E, ed. Multidimensional Functional Assessment: the OARS methodology. A manual. Durham, North Carolina: Duke University Center for the Study of Aging and Human Development, 1975.

(6) Maddox GL. Assessment of functional status in a programme evaluation and resource allocation model. In: Holland WW, Ipsen J, Kostrzewski J, eds. Measurement of levels of health. Copenhagen: World Health Organization 1979:353–366. (WHO Regional Publications European Series No. 7).

(7) Fillenbaum GG. Screening the elderly: a brief instrumental activities of daily living measure. J Am Geriatr Soc 1985;33:698–706.

(8) Liang J, Levin JS, Krause NM. Dimensions of the OARS mental health measures. J Gerontol 1989;44:P127–P138.

(9) Pfeiffer E, Johnson TM, Chiofolo RC. Functional assessment of elderly subjects in four service settings. J Am Geriatr Soc 1981;29:433–437.

(10) Cairl RE, Pfeiffer E, Keller DM, et al. An evaluation of the reliability and validity of the Functional Assessment Inventory. J Am Geriatr Soc 1983;31:607–612.

(11) Pfeiffer BA, McClelland T, Lawson J. Use of the Functional Assessment Inventory to distinguish among the rural elderly in five service settings. J Am Geriatr Soc 1989; 37:243–248.

(12) Robinson BE, Lund CA, Keller D, et al. Validation of the Functional Assessment Inventory against a multidisciplinary home care team. J Am Geriatr Soc 1986; 34:851–854.

(13) Blay SL, Ramos LR, Mari JJ. Validity of a Brazilian version of the Older Americans Resources and Services (OARS) mental health screening questionnaire. J Am Geriatr Soc 1988;36:687–692.

THE COMPREHENSIVE ASSESSMENT AND REFERRAL EVALUATION
(Barry Gurland, 1977, Revised 1983)

Purpose

The Comprehensive Assessment and Referral Evaluation (CARE) is a semi-structured interview that evaluates the health and social problems of people aged 65 years and over (1, 2). It covers psychiatric, medical, nutritional, economic, and social problems and was intended to assess the individual's need for care and preventive services and to indicate the likely prognosis.

Conceptual Basis

The main feature of the CARE is its broad scope. There are several reasons for this. In assessing people living in the community, the interpretation of symptoms may be more complex than among hospitalized patients:

The situation is very different with regard to persons who have been randomly selected from the community based population. It cannot be assumed that their symptoms (if any) have clinical significance, nor, if they do have significance, to which disciplinary domain they might pertain. For example, weight loss which may indicate depression in a hospitalized psychiatric patient may, in a community resident, just as well be normal (e.g., the person is on a reducing diet), due to a medical condition (e.g., a wasting disease), or due to a social condition (e.g., poverty, or lack of help in preparing food). (1, p18)

Gurland et al. also noted that most elderly people suffer from more than one health or social problem, and each must be distinguished in order to determine appropriate treatment (2). Treatment will depend on the combination of problems encountered and may require continual monitoring of all of them.

The conceptual model on which the CARE is based identifies a causal sequence of health problems in the elderly. The sequence begins with age, race, and social circumstances; these influence medical condition and cognitive states and thereby influence functional capacity. Functional capacity in turn may cause the person to seek care and may also lead to demoralization and family inconvenience (3).

Description

Gurland described the CARE as follows:

The CARE is a new assessment technique which is intended to reliably elicit, record, grade and classify information on the health and social problems of the older person. The CARE is basically a semi-structured interview guide and an inventory of defined ratings. It is designated *comprehensive* because it covers psychiatric, medical, nutritional, economic and social problems rather than the interests of only one professional discipline. The style, scope and scoring of the CARE makes it suitable for use with both patients and non-patients, and a potentially useful aid in determining whether an elderly person should be *referred*, and to whom, for a health or social service. The CARE can also be employed in *evaluating* the effectiveness of that service if given. (1, p10)

The items included in the CARE were drawn from existing instruments, including Wing's Present State Examination, Gurland's SSIAM, the OMFAQ, the Mental Status Questionnaire, and various ADL scales (1). Developmental tests of the CARE were carried out in London and in New York.

The original version of the CARE contained 1,500 items and was administered in an interview lasting about 90 minutes (2). Shortened versions have subsequently been derived (2): the CORE-CARE (329 items; see Exhibit 9.19) and the SHORT-CARE (143 items).

Interviewers receive detailed training (2). The interview is not completely standard, permitting the interviewer to alter the order of questions to suit each respondent. A manual gives questions that the interviewer is trained to partly memorize to enhance the flow of the interview (1). To clarify the meaning of questions to a respondent who does not understand, the guide contains standard alternative question phrasings.

Some years after the initial development of the CORE-CARE, a scoring system was

Exhibit 9.19   22 Indicator Scales of the CORE-CARE

	Number of items
Psychiatric problems	
1. Cognitive impairment	10
2. Depression/demoralization	29
3. Subjective memory problems	9
	48
Physical problems	
4. Somatic symptoms	34
5. Heart disorder	15
6. Stroke effects	9
7. Cancer	6
8. Respiratory symptoms	6
9. Arthritis	9
10. Leg problems	9
11. Sleep disorder	8
12. Hearing disorder	14
13. Vision disorder	11
14. Hypertension	4
15. Ambulation problems	27
16. Activity limitation	39
	191
Service needs	
17. Service utilization	15
	15
Environmental social problems	
18. Financial hardship	8
19. Dissatisfaction with neigh-borhood	8
20. Fear of crime	18
21. Social isolation	34
22. Retirement dissatisfaction	7
	75
	329

Adapted from Golden RR, Teresi JA, Gurland BJ. Development of indicator scales for the Comprehensive Assessment and Referral Evaluation (CARE) interview schedule. J Gerontol 1984;39:141–145, Tables 1, 2.

proposed that provided summary scores for 22 "indicator scales" covering psychiatric and medical problems, service needs, and social conditions. These scales were formed by selecting items from the original interview schedule on the basis of expert judgment of face validity and importance and using empirical data on internal consistency collected from 445 randomly selected elderly residents in New York and 396 in London (4). Exhibit 9.19 summarizes the 22 indicator scales. Exhibit 9.20 gives an

Exhibit 9.20   An Example of an Indicator Scale from the CORE-CARE

Cognitive impairment
1. Doesn't know his age
2. Doesn't know the year of his birth
3. Doesn't know the number of years in neighborhood
4. Doesn't know his address
5. Doesn't know the rater's name, first try
6. Can't recall the President's name, current or previous
7. Doesn't know the month
8. Doesn't know the year
9. Doesn't know the rater's name, second try
10. Failed knee-hand-ear test

Adapted from Golden RR, Teresi JA, Gurland BJ. Development of indicator scales for the Comprehensive Assessment and Referral Evaluation (CARE) interview schedule. J Gerontol 1984;39:141–144, Table 1.

example of one of the scales. Copies of the questionnaire are available from Dr. Gurland; scoring instructions may be obtained from the National Technical Information Service (see Address section).

The SHORT-CARE is intended as a simpler instrument focusing on psychiatric impairment and physical disability. It contains 143 items drawn from six of the CORE-CARE scales: depression/demoralization, dementia, memory problems, sleep, somatic symptoms, and activity limitation. The interview is in two parts. The first, taking about 30 minutes to complete, contains 143 items; the second part, containing additional items on depression and dementia, identifies the need for clinical intervention (5).

Reliability

Alpha internal consistency scores for the 22 CORE-CARE indicator scales were high, ranging from 0.72 for retirement dissatisfaction to 0.95 for activity limitation (3, Tables 1-5; 1, Table 2). Intercorrelations among the indicator scales were reported by Golden (4).

The agreement between two raters for 30 interviews on the CORE-CARE gave kappas ranging from 0.70 to 0.80 (4, p145). For the original CARE instrument, the intraclass correlation was used to measure agreement among four raters in applying the scale to videotaped interviews with eight older women. Agreement was close for the psychiatric dimensions with correlations between 0.82 and 0.97 (1, Table 3). Agreement was lower for the medical and physical dimensions, and ranged widely, reflecting the specialty of the rater (1). Correlations ranged from 0.01 to 0.83. Agreement for the social dimensions was intermediate, with correlations ranging from 0.48 to 0.92 (1, Table 3).

Inter-rater reliability for the SHORT-CARE was 0.76 for dementia, 0.94 for depression, and 0.91 for disability (5, p167). Equivalent figures in a second study ranged from 0.66 to 0.96 (6, p1016). Coefficient alphas for the same scales, calculated on a population sample of 283 elderly people, were 0.64, 0.75, and 0.84.

Validity

Validity of the SHORT-CARE was reported by Gurland et al. (5). The convergent validity was 0.33 for the depression scale, 0.51 for cognitive impairment, and 0.70 for disability (3, Table 5). For 26 respondents, classified as psychiatric cases or normal by psychiatrists, the sensitivity of the combined SHORT-CARE psychiatric scales was 100%; the specificity was 71%. Predictive validity results were impressive in that the "diagnosed pervasive dementias had one year outcomes consistent with that expected of dementia (e.g., death, institutional admission, deterioration) in all cases" (5, p167). Those diagnosed as demented at initial interview had a mortality of 27% compared with 6% for an age-matched sample drawn from the remaining interviewees. Those who were diagnosed as depressed at initial interview had a higher use of psychotropic medication than others. Gurland et al. assessed how well the depression and dementia scales could discriminate between the two conditions. Using multivariate analyses, only three of 138 cases were misclassified; using a simpler approach of setting cutting points on each scale, 22 cases (16%) were misclassified (7, p123).

The extensive validity results for the complete CARE instrument are presented under three headings: construct, criterion, and predictive validity.

Construct Validity. Teresi et al. reported the construct validity of the CARE, using multitrait–multimethod matrices and path analyses. They provided extensive details of the correlations between the CARE scales and data provided by family informants and from global diagnostic ratings (3). The results provided strong evidence for the validity of the measures of functional capacity (correlations ranging from 0.51 to 0.70). The validity coefficients for the medical scales ranged from 0.47 to 0.59. Validity of the service utilization scale was somewhat lower, although adequate, with correlations falling between 0.40 and 0.75. The correlations for service needs were lower, ranging from 0.29 to 0.54 (3, p150). Correlations between CARE scales and the judgments made by other informants were highest for the scales that assess behavior or are more objective (activity limitation, medical conditions, service use), with correlations falling in the range 0.47 to 0.70 (3, Table 5). Agreement over the more subjective ratings (depression, service needs) ranged from 0.30 to 0.60.

Criterion Validity. The CARE depression and cognitive impairment scales were compared with clinicians' ratings of 26 cases, 16 of whom had some form of psychiatric impairment. Kappa coefficients were 0.76 and 0.78 for the two CARE scales, giving sensitivity results of 93% and 67% (3, p154). The CARE was compared with two criterion scales that assessed family inconvenience and the extent to which the family had made plans to institutionalize the elderly relative. Sensitivity and specificity analyses yielded overall correct classification rates for the CARE activity limitation scale ranging from 60% to 89% (8, Tables 1, 2). Equivalent figures for the cognitive impairment scale ranged from 0.44 to 0.85, according to the cutting point used (8, Table 3).

Predictive Validity. The predictive ability of 21 of the indicator scales to identify people who subsequently died was examined; discrimination was significant for seven scales ($p < 0.01$), with odds ratios as high as 3.1 (8, Table 5). Logistic regression was used to test the ability of several CARE scales to predict death, a diagnosis of dementia or depression, activity restriction, and service utilization. The results, presented in terms of odds ratios attaching to each indicator scale, suggest that the likelihood of the outcomes, given a high score on the CARE, are as much as five to ten times greater than for those with low scores.

Alternative Forms

Other forms of the CARE include the IN-CARE for people in institutions (9), the MERGE-CARE, and GLOBAL-CARE (2).

An Italian version of the depression and dementia indicator scales showed high reliability and validity (10). Inter-rater reliability (kappa coefficient) was 0.83 and 0.96, respectively; sensitivity for the dementia scale was 77% at a specificity of 96%; sensitivity and specificity for the depression scale were 95% and 92% (10, pp509–510). A Spanish version of the CARE was produced in California (11).

Commentary

The validity testing of the CARE is extensive and the available results are impressive; the CARE scales continue to be developed and refined. As a broad-ranging assessment it is valuable for assessing elderly people living in the community, although it has been used in other settings with reliable results. The original long form is normally replaced by one of the abbreviated versions which do not require such detailed training of interviewers. The validity of the SHORT-CARE is such that it can be used by psychiatrists or non-psychiatrists as an accurate screening tool for depression and dementia.

The purpose of the CARE instruments is similar to that of the Multilevel Assessment

Instrument (MAI) and the OARS Multidimensional Functional Assessment Questionnaire (OMFAQ) also reviewed in this chapter. Of the three, the MAI is perhaps the least well tested. The other two scales show similar levels of reliability and validity; the OMFAQ has the advantage of an extensive user's manual and documentation, while the CARE has the advantage of being available in several shortened versions.

Address

Barry J. Gurland, MRCP (London), FRC Psych, Columbia University Center for Geriatrics, 100 Haven Avenue, Tower 3–29F, New York, New York, USA 10032

Scoring instructions may be obtained from the National Technical Information Service, U.S. Department of Commerce, Springfield, Virginia, USA 22151

REFERENCES

(1) Gurland B, Kuriansky J, Sharpe L, et al. The Comprehensive Assessment and Referral Evaluation (CARE)—rationale, development and reliability. Int J Aging Hum Dev 1977;8:9–42.
(2) Gurland BJ, Wilder DE. The CARE interview revisited: development of an efficient, systematic clinical assessment. J Gerontol 1984;39:129–137.
(3) Teresi JA, Golden RR, Gurland BJ, et al. Construct validity of indicator-scales developed from the Comprehensive Assessment and Referral Evaluation interview schedule. J Gerontol 1984;39:147–157.
(4) Golden RR, Teresi JA, Gurland BJ. Development of indicator scales for the Comprehensive Assessment and Referral Evaluation (CARE) interview schedule. J Gerontol 1984;39:138–146.
(5) Gurland B, Golden RR, Teresi JA, et al. The SHORT-CARE: an efficient instrument for the assessment of depression, dementia and disability. J Gerontol 1984;39:166–169.
(6) Gurland BJ, Teresi J, Smith WM, et al. Effects of treatment for isolated systolic hypertension on cognitive status and depression in the elderly. J Am Geriatr Soc 1988;36:1015–1022.
(7) Gurland B, Golden R, Challop J. Unidimensional and multidimensional approaches to the differentiation of depression and dementia in the elderly. In: Corkin S, Crowdon JH, Davis KL, Usdin E, eds. Alzheimer's disease: a report of progress. New York: Raven Press, 1982:119–125.
(8) Teresi JA, Golden RR, Gurland BJ. Concurrent and predictive validity of indicator scales developed for the Comprehensive Assessment and Referral Evaluation interview schedule. J Gerontol 1984;39:158–165.
(9) Gurland B, Cross P, Defiguerido J, et al. A cross-national comparison of the institutionalized elderly in the cities of New York and London. Psychol Med 1979;9:781–788.
(10) Spagnoli A, Foresti G, MacDonald A, et al. Italian version of the organic brain syndrome and the depression scales from the CARE: evaluation of their performance in geriatric institutions. Psychol Med 1987;17:507–513.
(11) Lopez-Aqueres W, Kemp B, Plopper M, et al. Health needs of the Hispanic elderly. J Am Geriatr Soc 1984;32:191–198.

THE DISABILITY AND DISTRESS SCALE
(Rachel M. Rosser, 1978)

Purpose

Rosser's Disability and Distress Scale provides a numerical summary index of health status that can be used in estimating quality-adjusted life years (QALYs). The scale is designed for evaluation, planning, and allocation of health service resources; by permitting comparisons across treatments and medical conditions, it is intended to measure the performance of a health service as a whole (1, 2).

Conceptual Basis

The Disability and Distress Scale originated in a program to measure hospital output. A hospital was viewed as a system which organizes resources (such as staff and equipment) to change the state of patients between admission and discharge. The output of the system is recorded in terms of the difference between utilities assigned to the states of health on admission and discharge; the effect of death is incorporated by adding the difference in utilities for death and residual morbidity among survivors (1, pp134–135; 3). Utilities are not seen as absolute but are expected to vary according to the patient's morbidity state, attributes (such as age, occupation, and marital status), and also by the characteristics of the raters.

Description

This is a rating scale administered by a clinician. Two dimensions are rated: disability, which includes eight categories ranging from no disability to unconscious; and subjective distress, with four categories (see Exhibit 9.21). The disability rating covers mobility and social function and includes elements that a sample of physicians considered when judging severity (1, p136). Patients in the first seven disability categories are also rated on the distress scale, giving 28 possible combinations, to which unconscious is added, making 29 categories. As unconscious people are assumed not to be actively suffering, they are classified as being free of distress (4, p56).

Exact questions are not specified, but the patient is classified on the basis of observation, interview, chart review, or other health status measurements. Clinicians familiar with the patient can make the rating in about ten seconds; patient acceptability is not an issue as no questions need be asked. Rosser warns against using ratings by non-clinicians, who may be unduly influenced by factors such as patient denial (2, p141).

Several approaches to calculating values for the 29 states were tested, including an

---

Exhibit 9.21 The Disability and Distress Scale: Descriptions of States of Illness

Note: The Disability rating describes the extent to which a patient is judged to be unable to pursue the activities of a normal person at the time at which the classification is made. Patients in Class 2 are slightly disabled, but performance in their normal work is not limited. This degree of disablement affects social activities and personal relations. It includes such conditions as mild cosmetic defects, slight injuries and diseases which may interfere with hobbies but not with essential activities, and some of the less severe psychiatric states which cause some social disablement.
The *Distress* rating describes the patient's pain, mental suffering in relation to disablement, anxiety and depression.

Disability

8 Unconscious

7 Not in 8 but confined to bed

6 Not in 7 but confined to chair or wheelchair or able to move around in the home only with support from an assistant

5 Not in 6 but unable to undertake any paid employment. Unable to continue any education. Old people confined to home except for escorted outings and short walks and unable to do shopping. Housewives only able to perform a few simple tasks

4 Not in 5 but choice of work or performance at work very severely limited. Housewives and old people able to do light housework only, but able to go out shopping

3 Not in 4 but severe social disability and/or slight impairment of performance at work. Able to do all housework except very heavy tasks

2 Not in 3 but slight social disability

1 No disability

Distress

Pain and mental suffering

D Severe

C Moderate

B Mild

A None

Adapted from Rosser RM. A health index and output measure. In: Walker SR, Rosser RM, eds. Quality of life: assessment and application. Lancaster: MTP Press, 1987:Table 7.1.

analysis of the monetary value of court awards for injury compensation (3). The weights normally used were derived from a magnitude estimation scaling task, setting optimum health at 1.0 and death at 0.0, providing an interval scale (5). This approach does not assume that death is the worst possible state, and states judged worse than death can receive negative valuations. Rosser argued that phenomena such as suicide, withdrawal of life support, and living wills indicate that death should not be the worst state on the scale (2). The original weights were based on judgments made by a mixed group of 70 doctors, nurses, patients, and health volunteers (6). They are shown in Exhibit 9.22.

Reliability

Test–retest reliability of the scaling procedure was estimated for 50 volunteers and the percentage agreement was 97.2%; internal consistency of the ratings was estimated for ten raters and nine of the ten were internally consistent (6, p351).

Validity

Rosser has paid considerable attention to the validity of the scale weights derived from the magnitude estimation procedure. The extent to which this provided a true ratio scale was tested by plotting the pre-

sumed ratio values against values calculated under a simpler, ordinal assumption; the results showed that the expected log-linear relationship was obtained (1, p140). Rosser also showed that when the data were processed as a paired comparisons exercise, the resulting interval scale could be transformed into a ratio scale with a close fit ($r = 0.93$) (7, p63). These results offered some evidence that the ratio scale was, in fact, achieved. Scale weights were calculated for subsets of the original 70 judges, and there was no difference according to the age, social class, or other characteristics of the judges (6). Comparing scale weights derived from different types of patient suggested that psychiatric patients made more severe valuations of the health states than medical patients (1, Figure 2; 5). However, of 14 such comparisons made, only two reached statistical significance (6, Table 4). The assignment of weights therefore appears relatively robust.

An external validation of the scale values was obtained from comparisons with levels of compensation awarded to patients with varying types of disability as a result of injury (7, p63). The correlation was 0.81; the main discrepancy lay in the more severe states, where the psychometric valuations were much more severe (1, Figure 7.3; 5).

Alternative Forms

The distress rating has been used in most of Rosser's work but has recently been extended to distinguish five levels of pain and five levels of emotional distress (1, p137). This gives 175 possible states in the Index of Health-Related Quality of Life (IHQL) (8; 9, pp147–148). The hierarchical structure of the index divides global health-related quality of life into disability, discomfort, and distress dimensions. The disability dimension is further divided into dependence and dysfunction attributes; the discomfort dimension includes pain and symptoms, while the distress dimension is divided into dysphoria, disharmony and fulfilment attributes (9, p150). Three questionnaires have been designed for the

Exhibit 9.22   The Disability and Distress Scale: Valuation Matrix for Health States

Disability rating	Distress rating			
	A	B	C	D
1	1.000	0.995	0.990	0.967
2	0.990	0.986	0.973	0.932
3	0.980	0.972	0.956	0.912
4	0.964	0.956	0.942	0.870
5	0.946	0.935	0.900	0.700
6	0.875	0.845	0.680	0.000
7	0.677	0.564	0.000	−1.486
8	−1.028			

Adapted from Rosser RM. A health index and output measure. In: Walker SR, Rosser RM, eds. Quality of life: assessment and application. Lancaster: MTP Press, 1987:Table 7.2.

IHQL, including a self-completed version, a version used by a trained observer and a version completed by a relative (9, p82). Work on this instrument was in progress at the time of writing, and data on reliability and validity of these questionnaires were not available; a scaling study was under way (9, p86).

A self-completed questionnaire version has been proposed by the Health Economics group at York University (10, 11). This is called the Health Measurement Questionnaire and covers mobility, self-care, usual activities, social relationships, and feelings (11, p87). These permit classification into the 29 states, and Rosser's utility weights are then applied. Scores correlated −0.43 with the General Health Questionnaire; correlations with section scores on the Nottingham Health Profile ranged from −0.23 to −0.62 (11, pp88–89).

Commentary

Along with the Quality of Well-Being Scale (QWB), this index is one of the leading statistical methods with which outcomes may be compared across various forms of treatment. Rosser's scale is briefer and simpler to administer and deliberately combines ratings of function with subjective distress. Rosser's scale has not been as fully examined for validity; we know little about how it compares to the QWB or to other scales. The QWB is likely to be more sensitive to minor deviations from well-being owing to its inclusion of mild symptoms. Because the Rosser classification contains no positive health items, it is unlikely to discriminate among minor levels of disability, and so is unlikely to be suitable for community health surveys. In one representative population sample, 74.6% of people reported no disability and 54.6% reported no distress on the scale (11, Table 3).

While it is primarily intended as a research tool for policy formation, the scale can also be used in individual case studies. Applied at admission and discharge it can be used, for example, to describe the output of hospital services; Rosser gives a telling illustration of the use of the scale in peer review, drawing comparisons of the output of medical and surgical specialties in a teaching hospital and comparing the progress made by patients seen by different clinicians within each specialty (1). She notes that the scale "seems to be yielding information and insights which cannot be obtained from routinely-available data and which are relevant to clinical practice and Health Service management and policy" (1, p151). The scale offers a direct comparison of the progress made by patients under different teams and highlights differences in criteria for admission, length of stay, and discharge. As originally formulated, however, the method is not expected to be sufficiently sensitive to serve as an outcome indicator for clinical trials; instead, its intent is more to compare results across trials (1, p158). Time will tell whether the modified Index of Health-Related Quality of Life offers a more sensitive scale.

REFERENCES

(1) Rosser RM. A health index and output measure. In: Walker SR, Rosser RM, eds. Quality of life: assessment and application. Lancaster, England: MTP Press, 1987:133–160.

(2) Rosser RM. Recent studies using a global approach to measuring illness. Med Care 1976;14(suppl):138–147.

(3) Rosser RM, Watts VC. The measurement of hospital output. Int J Epidemiol 1972;1:361–368.

(4) Rosser R. A history of the development of health indicators. In: Teeling-Smith G, ed. Measuring the social benefits of medicine. London: Office of Health Economics, 1983:50–62.

(5) Kind P, Rosser R, Williams A. Valuation of quality of life: some psychometric evidence. In: Jones-Lee MW, ed. The value of life and safety. Amsterdam: Elsevier North-Holland, 1982:159–170.

(6) Rosser R, Kind P. A scale of valuations of states of illness: is there a social consensus? Int J Epidemiol 1978;7:347–358.

(7) Rosser R. Issues of measurement in the design of health indicators: a review. In: Culyer AJ, ed. Health indicators. Amsterdam: North Holland Biomedical Press, 1983:36–81.

(8) Rosser R. The history of health related quality of life in 10½ paragraphs. J R Soc Med 1993;86:315–318.

(9) Rosser R, Cottee M, Rabin R, et al. Index of Health-Related Quality of Life. In: Hopkins A, ed. Measures of the quality of life and the uses to which such measures may be put. London: Royal College of Physicians of London, 1992:81–89,147–153.

(10) Williams A. Applications in management. In: Teeling-Smith G, ed. Measuring health: a practical approach. Chichester, England: John Wiley, 1988:225–243.

(11) Kind P, Gudex CM. Measuring health status in the community: a comparison of methods. J Epidemiol Community Health 1994;48:86–91.

THE EUROQOL QUALITY OF LIFE SCALE
(The EuroQol Group, 1990, Revised 1993)

Purpose

The European Quality of Life (EuroQol) measure expresses health status in a single index score; it is intended for use in evaluative studies and policy research (1). It is a generic scale intended to form one component of a measurement battery supplemented, for example, by disease-specific questions.

Conceptual Basis

The European Quality of Life Group brought researchers from five countries together in 1987 to address the growing diversity of quality of life outcome measures. While accepting that no measurement method can suit every application, they noted that "there are a great number of rival approaches aiming to do very similar things, with little or no attempt at systematic comparison of their respective strengths and weaknesses either at a conceptual or at an empirical level" (2, p200). The EuroQol Group therefore resolved to define a core set of generic health related quality of life items. These would be supplemented in particular studies but would permit cross-national comparisons and would encourage methodological standardization.

The design of the EuroQol balanced the desire to cover all topics that might be relevant against producing an instrument brief enough to be practical. The measure was designed as a self-completed questionnaire that would be acceptable for use in postal surveys and that would provide a single index value for each health state (2, p202).

Description

The EuroQol covers five dimensions of health: mobility, self-care, role (or main) activity, family and leisure activities, pain and mood (see Exhibit 9.23). Within each dimension, the respondent chooses one of three items that best describes him. Note that an earlier version of the EuroQol included six dimensions (1, pp178–179); role activities and family leisure were merged, and the number of items in each dimension was standardized. Unfortunately, most of the available validity and reliability results refer to the earlier version. Our exhibit shows pages 2 and 3 of the instrument; in addition there is a second section that includes a valuation task. In normal use, the thermometer shown in the exhibit is drawn 20 cms long.

Weights are used in scoring the responses. The weights may either use the respondent's own expressed preferences using a 0-to-100 scale that indicates her overall valuation of her current state of health, or established scale values may be used. Valuations for the 15 responses are being derived from studies in several countries. As an illustration, values obtained in a study in Britain are shown in Table 9.5. The values came from 3,000 interviews of a nationally representative community sample. The figures were derived from regressions using individual data points which are equivalent to mean figures; other values (not shown) are based on medians. As with the Quality of Well-Being Scale, the values are expressed as negative weights that are subtracted from the maximum score of 1.0, representing well-being. In addition to subtracting the values shown in the table, the constant of 0.081 is subtracted if one or more items is scored as 2 or 3. If one or more items is scored 3, a further constant, shown at the foot of the table, is subtracted. Thus, for example, a response pattern of someone with extreme anxiety 11113 scores $1.0 - 0.081 - 0.236$

Exhibit 9.23 The EuroQol Quality of Life Scale

By placing a tick (thus √) in at least one box in each group below, please indicate which statements best describe your own health state today.

Mobility

1. I have no problems in walking about ☐
2. I have some problems in walking about ☐
3. I am confined to bed ☐

Self-care

1. I have no problems with self-care ☐
2. I have some problems with self-care ☐
3. I am unable to wash or dress myself ☐

Usual activities

1. I have no problems with performing my main activity (e.g. work, study, housework, family or leisure activities) ☐
2. I have some problems with performing my usual activities ☐
3. I am unable to perform my usual activities ☐

Pain/discomfort

1. I have no pain or discomfort ☐
2. I have moderate pain or discomfort ☐
3. I have extreme pain or discomfort ☐

Anxiety/Depression

1. I am not anxious or depressed ☐
2. I am moderately anxious or depressed ☐
3. I am extremely anxious or depressed ☐

Visual analogue scale

To help people say how good or bad a health state is, we have drawn a scale (rather like a thermometer) on which the best state you can imagine is marked by 100 and the worst state is marked by 0.

We would like you to indicate on this scale how good or bad is your own health today, in your opinion. Please do this by drawing a line from the box below to whichever point on the scale indicates how good or bad your health state is.

Best imaginable health state

100

90

80

70

60

50

40

30

20

10

0

Your own health today

Worst imaginable health state

Adapted from an original provided by Dr. A Williams. With permission.

Table 9.5 Dimensions and Weights for the EuroQol

Note: The weights indicated are subtracted from 1.00.

Dimensions	Item weights		
	1	2	3
Mobility	− 0.0	− .069	− .314
Self-care	− 0.0	− .104	− .214
Usual activity	− 0.0	− .036	− .094
Pain/discomfort	− 0.0	− .123	− .386
Anxiety/depression	− 0.0	− .071	− .236
constants	− 0.0	− .081	− .269

Figures supplied by Prof. A Williams. With permission.

− 0.269 = 0.414 and a pattern of 11222 scores $1.0 - 0.081 - 0.036 - 0.123 - 0.071 = 0.689$. Alternatively, a score can be based on the respondent's own valuation derived from the 0-to-100 rating of "how good or bad your health is today." In this case, part one of the questionnaire merely provides descriptive information.

Reliability

A secondary source reported test–retest reliability for the dimensions in the original version of the EuroQol as ranging from 0.69 to 0.94 (3, Table 1). Test–retest reliability for the current version has been reported: 0.86 for group level coefficients calculated for each state and averaged over health states and 0.90 for a coefficient derived from individual correlations considering all health states simultaneously (4, p1543).

Validity

Evidence for construct validity of the preliminary version of the EuroQol has been drawn from the pattern of responses across age, gender, and socioeconomic groups and between those who had recently used health care services and those who had not (1, Table 2). The instrument identified significant contrasts in the anticipated direction for most of these comparisons across most of the six dimensions.

Correlations between the preliminary version of the EuroQol scores and three subscores on the Health Assessment Questionnaire ranged from 0.46 to 0.76 on two testing occasions for patients with rheumatoid arthritis (5, Table III). The EuroQol correlated 0.51 with depression scores and 0.44 with anxiety scores from the Hospital Anxiety and Depression scale. Correlations between the EuroQol and the visual analogue scale were 0.37 and 0.54 on two testing occasions (5, Table III).

The EuroQol and the SF-36 were applied in a general population survey which revealed a ceiling effect of the EuroQol. Those achieving the maximum score on each EuroQol dimension were divided into two groups according to their SF-36 scores and, in each instance, there were significant differences between the groups in terms of medical care consultation rates and selected demographic variables (1, Tables 6A and 6B). Hence, the SF-36 appeared sensitive to relevant differences that were missed by the EuroQol. It remains to be seen whether this result persists with the new EuroQol classification.

Alternative Forms

The EuroQol was developed simultaneously in Dutch, English, Finnish, Norwegian, and Swedish. Translations into other European languages are also available (see Address section).

Reference Standards

Brazier, Jones, and Kind indicate the proportions of people reporting a problem in each dimension of the EuroQol by age group, sex, and socioeconomic class from a survey in Sheffield, England (1, Table 2). Further population norms will be published from the surveys used to establish valuations, such as the British study of 3,000 adults described earlier.

Commentary

This is a very recently developed health index, and we only have preliminary evidence for its validity. Since the new version of the EuroQol is being used in several studies, results should soon be available. The EuroQol was developed through an international collaborative program, a worthy goal in a field that has suffered too much parochialism and fragmentation of effort. It provides a single valuation of health, as does Kaplan's Quality of Well-Being Scale and Rosser's Disability and Distress Scale. Compared to the Kaplan and Rosser scales, however, the EuroQol is a simpler instrument with fewer scale levels, a brief time referent, and no coverage of symptoms.

A concern with the EuroQol lies in the coarseness of its categories. While the new EuroQol generates 243 theoretically possible permutations of the 15 items (plus unconscious and dead), this is only a mathematical possibility, and many of the permutations seem implausible (e.g., confined to bed and yet able to perform usual role activities). Whereas Rosser's index includes distress and Kaplan's includes symptoms to give finer discrimination, the EuroQol includes only the core functional status questions. It is not surprising, therefore, that it appears insensitive to variations in well-being at the upper ends of the health continuum. The EuroQol is well suited to measuring the health in populations with major morbidity (6, p382), but early results from the newer version appear to improve its applicability in general population studies. In three postal surveys only 59%, 66%, and 60% of the questionnaires that were returned were fully usable (2, pp205–206).

As the EuroQol is in the early stages of its testing and seems promising, we do not have definitive evidence for its quality. Where a single, numerical index summary of health is required, users will have to choose carefully among the EuroQol, Rosser, and Kaplan scales.

Address

Further information on the EuroQol can be obtained from

Dr. Frank de Charro, EuroQol Group Business Manager, Centre for Health Policy and Law, Sanders Institute, Erasmus University Rotterdam, PO Box 1738, 3000 DR Rotterdam, The Netherlands

REFERENCES

(1) Brazier J, Jones N, Kind P. Testing the validity of the Euroqol and comparing it with the SF-36 Health Survey questionnaire. Qual Life Res 1993;2:169–180.
(2) EuroQol Group. EuroQol: a new facility for the measurement of health-related quality of life. Health Policy 1990;16:199–208.
(3) Uyl-de Groot CA, Rutten FFH, Bonsel GJ. Measurement and valuation of quality of life in economic appraisal of cancer treatment. Eur J Cancer 1994;30A:111–117.
(4) Van Agt HME, Essinck-Bot M-L, Krabbe PFM, et al. Test–retest reliability of health state valuations collected with the EuroQol questionnaire. Soc Sci Med 1994; 39:1537–1544.
(5) Hurst NP, Jobanputra P, Hunter M, et al. Validity of Euroqol—a generic health status instrument—in patients with rheumatoid arthritis. Br J Rheumatol 1994;33:655–662.
(6) Anderson RT, Aaronson NK, Wilkin D. Critical review of the international assessments of health-related quality of life. Qual Life Res 1993;2:369–395.

THE QUALITY OF WELL-BEING SCALE (Formerly the Index of Well-Being) (J.W. Bush and R.M. Kaplan, 1973, Revised 1976, 1994)

Purpose

The Quality of Well-Being Scale (QWB) is a health index that summarizes a person's current symptoms and disability in a single number that represents a judgment of the social undesirability of the problem and expresses it in terms of quality-adjusted life years. This value can be adjusted to reflect the likely prognosis of any existing medical condition. The QWB is intended for use as an outcome indicator and in estimating present and future need for care (1, 2). It can be applied to individuals and to populations and can be used with any type of disease.

Conceptual Basis

The QWB is part of a General Health Policy Model which defines an approach to quantifying the output of a health care system (3–6). To compare treatments for different types of disease, the model requires an index to quantify health status that combines mortality with estimates of the quality of life among survivors. This is the purpose of the QWB, which

quantifies the health output of any treatment in terms of the years of life, adjusted for their diminished quality, that it produces or saves. Thus, a "Well-Year" can be defined conceptually as the equivalent of a year of completely well life. . . . A disease that reduces the health-related quality of life by one-half, for example, will take away .500 Well-Years over the course of one year. If it affects two people, it will take away 1.0 Well-Year (= 2×.500). . . . Dividing the cost of a program by the number of Well-Years gives its relative efficiency or "cost-effectiveness." (7, p64)

In the years since the QWB was developed, the concept of Quality-Adjusted Life Years (QALYs, see page 23) has come to be used as an alternative to cost-benefit analysis for allocating health care resources; well-years form the units through which QALYs can be measured. "Quality-adjusted life years integrate mortality and morbidity to express health status in terms of equivalents of well-years of life" (8, p66).

The General Health Policy Model and the QWB Scale are based on a three-component model of health (4). The assessment of health begins with an objective appraisal of current functional status, based on performance. Second, a value reflecting the relative desirability or utility is associated with each functional level (1, 9). These values are anchored at zero, which represents death. Otherwise, if mortality were ignored, the death of a disabled patient would appear to improve the net population estimate of health status (10). Third, health implies a consideration not only of present state but also of the future prognosis for any illness present. This per-

mits a distinction to be drawn, for example, between two people with similar current functional levels, one of whom has a malignancy: information crucial in assessing future need for health care. The prognostic component can also reflect the notion of positive health (3).

Description

Originally called the Health Status Index (1), the scale was renamed the Index of Well-Being (10) and later the Quality of Well-Being Scale to stress its focus on quality of life (7). Various modifications have been made to the QWB over the years; the 1994 version is described.

The procedure for classifying an individual may be described in three stages, corresponding to the three components of the model just described.

Assessing Functional Status. A structured interview is used to record symptoms and medical problems experienced on each of the previous eight days and to classify the respondent's level of functioning. The questions were derived from the Health Interview Survey and from the Social Security Administration Survey of the disabled. The interview is structured so that screening questions lead to more detailed investigation of problems that are identified. According to the respondent's level of health, the current, abbreviated interview takes seven minutes or more; the earlier version took ten to 30 minutes (11; 12, p963). The questions on function cover performance rather than capacity; self-reports are used rather than observation. Questions cover three dimensions of functioning: mobility and confinement (e.g., in hospital or institution); physical activity, especially ambulation; and social activity, which includes work, housekeeping, and self-care. As shown in Exhibit 9.24, there are three categories on the mobility and physical activity scales and five on the social activity scale. Note that this is an abbreviation of the earlier version of the QWB described in the first edition of this book. The social activity

Exhibit 9.24   Dimensions, Function Levels, and Weights of the Quality of Well-Being Scale

Step	Step definition	Weight
	Mobility Scale (MOB)	
5	No limitations for health reasons	−.000
4	Did not drive a car, health related; did not ride in a car as usual for age (younger than 15 yr), health related, *and/or* did not use public transportation, health related; *or* had or would have used more help than usual for age to use public transportation, health related	−.062
2	In hospital, health related	−.090
	Physical Activity Scale (PAC)	
4	No limitations for health reasons	−.000
3	In wheelchair, moved or controlled movement of wheelchair without help from someone else; *or* had trouble or did not try to lift, stoop, bend over, or use stairs or inclines, health related; *and/or* had any other physical limitation in walking, or did not try to walk as far as or as fast as others the same age are able, health related	−.060
1	In wheelchair, did not move or control the movement of wheelchair without help from someone else, *or* in bed, chair, or couch for most or all of the day, health related	−.077
	Social Activity Scale (SAC)	
5	No limitations for health reasons	−.000
4	Limited in other (e.g. recreational) role activity, health related	−.061
3	Limited in major (primary) role activity, health related	−.061
2	Performed no major role activity, health related, but did perform self-care activities	−.061
1	Performed no major role activity, health related, *and* did not perform or had more help than usual in performance of one or more self-care activities, health related	−.106

Reproduced from an original supplied by Dr. Kaplan. With permission.

scale retains five categories as these are needed to derive QWB scores from other survey instruments. The respondent is placed into one level of each scale, giving $3 \times 3 \times 5$, or 45 possible combinations plus death, making 46 function levels.

The interview also records the presence of symptoms or problem complexes, or "CPX." Note that these refer to problems on the previous day, so the past tense is used. By recording symptoms, even where these are not sufficient to cause a restriction in activity levels, the QWB is sensitive to minor deviations from complete well-being. There are currently 27 symptom or problem complexes, as shown in Exhibit 9.25, increased from 23 in previous versions of the QWB by the addition of four mental health symptoms. The interview takes about 18 minutes, slightly less than the Sickness Impact Profile (SIP) (13, Table 2).

Copies of the interview schedule, too long to reproduce here, and a 30-page interviewer manual can be ordered at cost from Dr. Kaplan. An interview format is generally used since early tests showed that a self-administered version identified only 45% of disabilities compared with 89% for the interviewer version (14, p466). Kappa coefficients of agreement between the two versions ranged from 0.48 to 0.58 for the three sections (15, p134). Anderson et al. concluded that the additional cost of the interviewer version is warranted (15, p134). However, further attention has been paid to developing a self-administered version which may soon be available from Dr. Kaplan.

Scaling the Responses. Preference weights for each function level were derived originally from an equal-appearing interval scal-

Exhibit 9.25   Symptom and Problem Complexes (CPX) for the Quality of Well-Being Scale

CPX No.	CPX description	Weight
1	Death [not on respondent's card]	−.727
2	Loss of consciousness such as seizure (fits), fainting, or coma (out cold or knocked out)	−.407
3	Burn over large areas of face, body, arms, or legs	−.387
4	Pain, bleeding, itching, or discharge (drainage) from sexual organs—does not include normal menstrual bleeding	−.349
5	Trouble learning, remembering, or thinking clearly	−.340
6	Any combination of one or more hands, feet, arms, or legs either missing, deformed (crooked), paralyzed (unable to move), or broken—includes wearing artificial limbs or braces	−.333
7	Pain, stiffness, weakness, numbness, or other discomfort in chest, stomach (including hernia or rupture), side, neck, back, hips, or any joints or hands, feet, arms, or legs	−.299
8	Pain, burning, bleeding, itching, or other difficulty with rectum, bowel movements, or urination (passing water)	−.292
9	Sick or upset stomach, vomiting or loose bowel movement, with or without chills, or aching all over	−.290
10	General tiredness, weakness, or weight loss	−.259
11	Cough, wheezing or shortness of breath, *with* or *without* fever, chills, or aching all over	−.257
12	Spells of feeling upset, being depressed, or of crying	−.257
13	Headache, or dizziness, or ringing in ears, or spells of feeling hot, nervous or shaky	−.244
14	Burning or itching rash on large areas of face, body, arms, or legs	−.240
15	Trouble talking, such as lisp, stuttering, hoarseness, or being unable to speak	−.237
16	Pain or discomfort in one or both eyes (such as burning or itching) or any trouble seeing after correction	−.230
17	Overweight for age and height or skin defect of face, body, arms, or legs, such as scars, pimples, warts, bruises or changes in color	−.188
18	Pain in ear, tooth, jaw, throat, lips, tongue; several missing or crooked permanent teeth—includes wearing bridges or false teeth	−.170
19	Took medication or stayed on a prescribed diet for health reasons	−.144
20	Wore eyeglasses or contact lenses	−.101
21	Breathing smog or unpleasant air	−.101
22	No symptoms or problems [not on respondent's card]	−.000
23	Standard symptom/problem	−.257
24	Trouble sleeping	−.257
25	Intoxication	−.257
26	Problems with sexual interest or performance	−.257
27	Excessive worry or anxiety	−.257

Reproduced from an original supplied by Dr. Kaplan. With permission.

ing task involving 867 raters (10). The weights reflect social preferences or judgments of the relative importance that members of society associate with each function level (10, 16); they do not consider the patient's diagnosis. Bush et al. emphasized that preference ratings should be collected empirically rather than be based on the assumptions or clinical experience of the researchers (17). Category weighting was considered more appropriate than a magnitude estimation approach which did not yield a true ratio scale and gave values that were counter-intuitive (16); further validation of the scaling procedure has been reported by Kaplan and Ernst (18). Similarly, weights were derived for the symptom and problem complexes, as described in various articles (16, 19–21).

The overall QWB score ranges from 1 (complete well-being) to 0 (death), although the scoring does permit values below 0, to represent a state "worse than death," such as a prolonged vegetative existence (7). The general scoring approach is that the QWB score, known as $W = 1 -$ (MOB step $\times$ MOB weight) $-$ (PAC step $\times$ PAC weight) $-$ (SAC step $\times$ SAC weight) $-$ (symptoms or problems $\times$ CPX weight). Weights for the functional categories and symptoms or problem complexes are negative, indicating the reduction in well-being implied by each functional category or CPX. The CPX weights range from -0.0 (no problems) to -0.727 (death), as shown in Exhibit 9.25. Readers should be aware that there are inconsistencies in the weights quoted in different articles describing the QWB; the weights listed in Exhibit 9.25 are the correct ones. Where there are multiple problems, the one considered most undesirable is scored (16); where a problem complex is present but is unknown, a value of -0.257 is used. A person who has died receives a CPX score of -0.727, and the lowest score on the three functional scales, giving an overall score of 0.

W represents a person's well-being at a point in time. To indicate QALYs, W is multiplied by the time spent in that state, and this calculation repeated and summed as the person's symptoms or functional level change over the time period being considered. Kaplan gives the example of a person who is well for 65.2 years, then experiences disability for 4.5 years ($W = 0.59$), followed by bed disability for 1.9 years ($W = 0.34$). While the person has lived a total of 71.6 years, the QWB indicates that this is equivalent to ($65.2 \times 1.0 + 4.5 \times 0.59 + 1.9 \times 0.34$), or 68.5 years of healthy life (3, p41). This calcula-

tion can be extended to groups of patients and used as a program output indicator (10, p493; 8, Table 1).

Indicating Prognosis. W can be adjusted to reflect prognoses. The prognostic adjustment reflects an estimate of the time spent at each level of disability for patients with a given medical condition, based on empirical studies of patients' progress. These durations are expressed in terms of the probabilities of future transitions to worse or better levels of function and well-being within a fixed time (1, 16). The "Well-Life Expectancy" (E) weights W by the expected duration of stay in each functional level, summed across levels of disability (10, p484). This gives an estimate only, adequate for use with groups of patients rather than with individuals. At present, transition weights are only available for certain diseases, such as the likelihood of developing mental retardation following various forms of phenylketonuria (22).

Reliability

Considerable attention has been paid to the stability of estimates of preference weights. The reliability coefficient obtained when judges reassessed scale values for the function levels was 0.90 (7, 20). The preference weights obtained from different judges at different times showed small, although systematic, variations (11). A replication of the original preference rating exercise, using 288 patients with rheumatoid arthritis, again indicated that raters achieved high levels of consistency in their ratings, and agreed closely with the original weights. QWB scores for 132 patient scenarios based on the original weights correlated 0.94 with scores using the weights provided by the patients with arthritis (23, p978).

Kaplan and Bush noted that in applying the scale in assessing over 50,000 person-days, the classification accuracy exceeded 96% (7, p70). Stability of the W statistic was studied by correlating the rating of the first day with the mean of ratings made on eight subsequent days. Correlations in excess of 0.93 were obtained (11).

Validity

Arguments for the content validity of the QWB note its broad scope and that it is the only instrument to consider mortality, symptoms, and problems as well as functional levels—all of which are central components of the concept of health (10, 24).

Kaplan et al. reported correlations of −0.75 between QWB scores and the number of reported symptoms and of −0.96 between the QWB and the number of chronic health problems (10, pp497–498). The correlation with the number of physician contacts in the preceding eight days was −0.55. Read et al. obtained the much lower correlation of −0.48 with number of self-reported symptoms (13, p15S).

Because the functional scales of the QWB offer relatively coarse indicators, sensitivity to change has been widely reviewed. It has been demonstrated that the QWB is capable of showing significant treatment effects—in a study of chronic obstructive pulmonary disease (25), in a trial of AZT for AIDS (26), and in a trial of dietary and exercise interventions for diabetic patients (27). In a trial of auranofin the QWB proved a slightly more sensitive outcome indicator than the physical and pain scores of the Arthritis Impact Measurement Scales (AIMS) (26, Table 6; 28, Table 7). Correlations between the QWB and the AIMS were −0.57 for the AIMS physical score, −0.40 for the pain score, and −0.17 for the AIMS psychological score (26, Table 4). Liang et al. compared the sensitivity of five health measures to change and found that the QWB was ranked in the middle of the five for most comparisons (29, Table 2).

The QWB has been evaluated in several studies of respiratory conditions. For 44 patients with cystic fibrosis, QWB scores correlated significantly with pulmonary function tests: 0.55 with forced expiratory volume (FEV_1) and 0.58 with peak oxygen consumption (Vo_2max) (26, pS38; 30, Table 3). In a study of chronic obstructive

pulmonary disease, QWB scores correlated 0.51 with FEV_1 and 0.41 with a treadmill test of exercise tolerance (25, Tables 4, 5). In the study by Read et al., the QWB scores correlated 0.32 with time achieved on treadmill and 0.32 with forced expiratory capacity; the variance in QWB scores explained (R^2) was 0.35 (13, p15S). These correlations were lower than equivalent results for the Sickness Impact Profile, for which the R^2 was 0.62.

The QWB correlated 0.46 with a modified version of Jette's Functional Status Index; omitting the QWB symptom component raised this association to 0.57. This was explained because the symptom component appeared to capture variation toward the well end of the scale that was missed by Jette's scale (12, pp962–963). The QWB correlated 0.55 with the SIP and 0.57 with a ten-point rating of health over the past six days (13, p14S). The QWB correlated −0.58 with the AIMS physical scale and −0.41 with the AIMS pain scale (the negative correlations reflect the opposite scoring of the scales) (28, Table 5).

As the QWB does not contain items on psychological functioning its sensitivity to psychological distress is of interest. Correlations with the Center for Epidemiologic Studies Depression Scale were −0.31 (28, Table 5), and a correlation of 0.33 with a mental health scale has been reported (13, p15S). Interestingly, changes in QWB scores before and after treatment for arthritis correlated more highly with changes in the AIMS psychological score than in the AIMS physical score (28, Table 6), suggesting that as an outcome measure, the QWB does identify changes in emotional well-being. Perhaps because of its emphasis on role functioning, the QWB correlated 0.40 with employment status (13, p15S).

Alternative Forms

Reynolds, Rushing, and Miles have suggested a simplified scoring procedure for their version of the index called the Function Status Index (FSI) (24). They also recorded behavior on the previous day rather than the previous eight days, and separated the social activity scale and self-care scales. From a sample of 8,036 respondents in Alabama, a correlation of −0.61 was obtained between the FSI and the number of chronic health problems reported (24, Table 2). A gamma coefficient of −0.53 was obtained with the number of physician contacts (24, Table 3). Reynolds et al. also reported a correlation of −0.48 with a health worry scale (24, pp279, 281). Harkey et al. applied the FSI in a study (N = 16,569) of the relationship between social class and functional status (31).

A version of the QWB for children has shown good validity results (4, 32). A self-administered version of the QWB is currently under development; this will provide both an overall index score and section scores in the manner of the health profile measures. It will also include more categories of symptoms and problems.

Reference Standards

Some data on QWB norms for the general U.S. population are presented by Erickson et al. (33); unfortunately they only cover three broad age categories.

Commentary

The QWB was one of the earliest of the broad-spectrum numerical indices of health and the first to confront the conceptual and methodological issues of combining length and quality of life in a single score. The metric of the QWB, evaluating an intervention in terms of the well-year equivalents gained, is powerful and seems valuable in guiding patient decision-making (34). The QWB has also exerted a major influence on the design of other measures. It has been used in numerous cost-effectiveness studies (1, 4, 9, 22, 35), and the Kaplan and Bush summary tables comparing the cost-effectiveness of screening programs per well-year gained set an example that has since been followed in other fields (7). The prognostic dimension remains innovative, allowing the QWB to be applied equally to acute and chronic states,

whereas other scales cannot adequately compare the two, because of their different implications for the future need for care. The task of deriving the required transition probabilities for all diseases is daunting (36), although it may be feasible to estimate these for particular conditions; for example, the progression of physical medicine patients is being described by groups working with the Functional Independence Measure (see, for example, reference 37).

The QWB is also distinctive in its inclusion of symptoms; this seems to improve its sensitivity to minor deviations from complete well-being. It may therefore be ideal for evaluating policies in well populations with minor levels of morbidity. Used as a survey instrument, the QWB classifies a higher proportion of the population as unwell than do other measures. For example, Erickson et al. compared QWB scores with estimates of population health status based on an indicator of activity limitation, showing that only about 5% of the population aged 45 to 64 had no functional limitation on the QWB, compared to 75% when activity limitation was used as the criterion (33, Figure 1). They argued that activity limitation measures overestimate health status; the converse argument is that the QWB may be identifying trivial deviations from well-being.

Criticisms of any health measurement focus on two concerns: the items included and the scoring method. The coverage of the QWB is oriented strongly toward physical problems: the mobility dimension concentrates on ability to get around or transport oneself; the social activity dimension taps role functioning and self-care; and few of the symptom and problem complexes are explicitly oriented toward emotional distress. The criticism has therefore been made that the QWB underrepresents mental health (38, p94). Kaplan, however, responds that the division into mental and physical health is artificial, since the two affect each other (3, p45; 4). The significant correlations with measures of mental well-being seem to bear this out.

Criticisms of the QWB scoring focus on the scale weights. Concern was raised over apparent anomalies, whereby certain more disabled states appear preferable to less disabled ones (39). Bush et al. responded to this criticism, pointing out that desirability may differ between acute and chronic conditions. In acute conditions, for example, "being in a wheelchair is sometimes more comfortable (and therefore more desirable) than struggling to walk with limitations (e.g., with crutches)" (17). Haig and others criticized the use of category rating to derive weights, rather than magnitude estimation (40). They argued that anchoring the scale at 0, for death, caused a distortion and precluded the measurement of states worse than death. They proposed an alternative scaling procedure, although this correlated highly (-0.81) with the values produced by Kaplan et al. (40, Table 8).

Other commentaries on the QWB have noted the relative complexity of interviewer training (1 or 2 weeks), although once training is complete, the scale does not appear unduly difficult to administer (13). The new self-administered version will overcome this criticism.

As economic pressures on medical care increase, indices such as the QWB will take an increasingly important place in evaluation. Of the scales that provide estimates of QALYs, the QWB is the most widely used. Its advantages lie in its clear conceptual approach, attention to scaling, and widespread use.

Address

Interview Schedule and Manual: R.M. Kaplan, PhD, Professor and Chief, Division of Health Care Sciences 0622, School of Medicine, University of California, San Diego, La Jolla, California, USA 92093–0622

REFERENCES

(1) Fanshel S, Bush JW. A Health-Status Index and its application to health-services outcomes. Operations Res 1970;18:1021–1065.

(2) Chen MM, Bush JW, Patrick DL. Social indicators for health planning and policy analysis. Policy Sci 1975;6:71–89.

(3) Kaplan RM. New health promotion indicators: the General Health Policy Model. Health Prom 1988;3:35–49.

(4) Kaplan RM, Anderson JP. A General Health Policy Model: update and applications. Health Serv Res 1988;23:203–235.

(5) Kaplan RM, Anderson JP, Ganiats TG. The Quality of Well-Being Scale: rationale for a single quality of life index. In: Walker SR, Rosser RM, eds. Quality of life assessment: key issues in the 1990s. Dordrecht, Netherlands: Kluwer Academic Publishers, 1993:65–94.

(6) Kaplan RM. Application of a General Health Policy Model in the American health care crisis. J R Soc Med 1993; 86:277–281.

(7) Kaplan RM, Bush JW. Health-related quality of life measurement for evaluation research and policy analysis. Health Psychol 1982;1:61–80.

(8) Kaplan RM. Health-related quality of life with applications in nutrition research and practice. Clin Nutr 1988;7:64–70.

(9) Bush JW, Fanshel S, Chen MM. Analysis of a tuberculin testing program using a Health Status Index. Socio Econ Plan Sci 1972;6:49–68.

(10) Kaplan RM, Bush JW, Berry CC. Health status: types of validity and the Index of Well-Being. Health Serv Res 1976; 11:478–507.

(11) Kaplan RM, Bush JW, Berry CC. The reliability, stability, and generalizability of a Health Status Index. Proceedings of the Social Statistics Section, American Statistical Association, 1978:704–709.

(12) Ganiats TG, Palinkas LA, Kaplan RM. Comparison of Quality of Well-Being Scale and Functional Status Index in patients with artial fibrillation. Med Care 1992; 30:958–964.

(13) Read JL, Quinn RJ, Hoefer MA. Measuring overall health: an evaluation of three important approaches. J Chronic Dis 1987;40(suppl 1):S7–S21.

(14) Anderson JP, Bush JW, Berry CC. Classifying function for health outcome and quality-of-life evaluation: self-versus interviewer modes. Med Care 1986;24:454–470.

(15) Anderson JP, Bush JW, Berry CC. Internal consistency analysis: a method for studying the accuracy of function assessment for health outcome and quality of life evalu-

ation. J Clin Epidemiol 1988;41:127–137.

(16) Kaplan RM, Bush JW, Berry CC. Health Status Index: category rating versus magnitude estimation for measuring levels of well-being. Med Care 1979;17:501–523.

(17) Bush JW, Anderson JP, Kaplan RM, et al. "Counterintuitive" preferences in health-related quality-of-life measurement. Med Care 1982;20:516–525.

(18) Kaplan RM, Ernst JA. Do category rating scales produce biased preference weights for a health index? Med Care 1983;21:193–207.

(19) Patrick DL, Bush JW, Chen MM. Toward an operational definition of health. J Health Soc Behav 1973;14:6–23.

(20) Patrick DL, Bush JW, Chen MM. Methods for measuring levels of well-being for a Health Status Index. Health Serv Res 1973;8:228–245.

(21) Blischke WR, Bush JW, Kaplan RM. Successive intervals analysis of preference measures in a Health Status Index. Health Serv Res 1975;10:181–198.

(22) Bush JW, Chen MM, Patrick DL. Health Status Index in cost effectiveness: analysis of PKU program. In: Berg RL, ed. Health status indexes. Chicago: Hospital Research and Educational Trust, 1973:172–209.

(23) Balaban DJ, Sagi PC, Goldfarb NI, et al. Weights for scoring the Quality of Well-Being instrument among rheumatoid arthritics: a comparison to general population weights. Med Care 1986;24:973–980.

(24) Reynolds WJ, Rushing WA, Miles DL. The validation of a Function Status Index. J Health Soc Behav 1974;15:271–288.

(25) Kaplan RM, Atkins CJ, Timms R. Validity of a Quality of Well-Being Scale as an outcome measure in chronic obstructive pulmonary disease. J Chronic Dis 1984;37:85–95.

(26) Kaplan RM, Anderson JP, Wu AW, et al. The Quality of Well-Being Scale: applications in AIDS, cystic fibrosis, and arthritis. Med Care 1989;27(suppl):S27–S43.

(27) Kaplan RM, Hartwell SL, Wilson DK, et al. Effects of diet and exercise interventions on control and quality of life in non-insulin-dependent diabetes mellitus. J Gen Intern Med 1987;2:220–228.

(28) Kaplan RM, Kozin F, Anderson JP. Measuring quality of life in arthritis patients (including discussion of a general health-decision model). Qual Life Cardiovasc Care 1988;Autumn:131–139.

(29) Liang MH, Fossel AH, Larson MG. Comparisons of five health status instruments for orthopedic evaluation. Med Care 1990;28:632–642.

(30) Orenstein DM, Nixon PA, Ross EA, et al. The quality of well-being in cystic fibrosis. Chest 1989;95:344–347.

(31) Harkey J, Miles DL, Rushing WA. The relation between social class and functional status: a new look at the drift hypothesis. J Health Soc Behav 1976;17:194–204.

(32) Bradlyn AS, Harris CV, Warner JE, et al. An investigation of the validity of the quality of Well-Being Scale with pediatric oncology patients. Health Psychol 1993;12:246–250.

(33) Erickson P, Kendall EA, Anderson JP, et al. Using composite health status measures to assess the nation's health. Med Care 1989;27(suppl):S66–S76.

(34) Kaplan RM, Atkins CJ. The well-year of life as a basis for patient decision-making. Patient Educ Counseling 1989;13:281–295.

(35) Weinstein MC, Stason WB. Foundations of cost-effectiveness analysis for health and medical practices. N Engl J Med 1977;296:716–721.

(36) Chen MM, Bush JW, Zaremba J. Effectiveness measures. In: Shuman L, Speas R, Young J, eds. Operations research in health care—a critical analysis. Baltimore, Maryland: Johns Hopkins University Press, 1975:276–301.

(37) Long WB, Sacco WJ, Coombes SS, et al. Determining normative standards for Functional Independence Measure transitions in rehabilitation. Arch Phys Med Rehabil 1994;75:144–148.

(38) Hays RD, Shapiro MF. An overview of generic health-related quality of life measures for HIV research. Qual Life Res 1992;1:91–97.

(39) Anderson GM. A comment on the Index of Well-Being. Med Care 1982;20:513–515.

(40) Haig THB, Scott DA, Wickett LI. The rational zero point for an illness index with ratio properties. Med Care 1986;24:113–124.

CONCLUSION

This chapter reviews some of the most recently developed measurement scales; they are in many ways the showpiece of current health measurement technology. Most have avoided the pitfalls illustrated by other instruments reviewed in the book: lack of conceptual formulation, poor reliability and validity, and a tendency toward the haphazard development of alternative versions that are not strictly comparable. They also represent the major research instruments that are being used in evaluative studies to measure physical well-being: they are frequently selected in preference to those reviewed in Chapter 3.

Some reservations should be raised, however. Despite the high standard of many quality of life scales, health-related quality of life is still not a rigorously defined concept. There is little agreement over the content for such indices, or over how quality of life measurements relate to themes such as life satisfaction. During the 1980s, hastily constructed scales proliferated, and no health index seemed safe from being labeled a quality of life indicator. In exasperation, Spitzer pleaded:

We are now hopefully at the peak of an epidemic of quality of life measurement schemes. This embarrassment of riches bewilders clinicians and even investigators. It does not favor in-depth work dedicated to validation, and it militates against understanding and acceptance of these types of measures for clinical research and clinical practice. . . . I believe that most of what needs to be done in health services research can be accomplished with three or at most four or five thoughtfully developed and carefully validated measures of health status. (1, p469)

We agree, and argue that the term "quality of life" should be reserved for measurements that are very broad in scope. The term "general health measurements" should be applied to scales that cover physical, mental, and social functioning, while "quality of life" should be reserved for scales that are yet broader in scope, providing, in addition, overall ratings of environmental quality, subjective well-being, and life satisfaction. The emphasis in the coming years should be less on developing new measurements of these themes than on agreeing upon definitions and then on analyzing which of the existing indices best reflect those concepts. Only when a definite gap in the coverage of existing indices is identified should we attempt to develop new quality of life measurements.

Among the many scales that we have not included in this chapter we may mention the quality of life instrument currently under development by the World Health Organization (2, 3). It is premature to provide a separate review of the WHOQOL, but the preliminary work seems thorough and it may prove to be a valuable instrument. The WHOQOL represents a commendably broad approach to quality of life that reflects our previous comments. It covers six domains: physical, social, and psychological (which, in addition to the normal themes, includes positive feelings, self-esteem, and body image), plus level of independence (which includes dependency on medications, drugs, and medical aids), environment (which covers the physical environment plus level of freedom, work satisfaction, accessibility of care, and other themes), and spirituality. The instrument is being concurrently developed in countries on six continents and will be produced in long and short versions; it is intended for use in clinical trials and policy research (2, 3).

REFERENCES

(1) Spitzer WO. State of science 1986: quality of life and functional status as target variables for research. J Chronic Dis 1987;40:465–471.

(2) Kuyken W, Orley J. The development of the World Health Organization quality of life assessment instrument (the WHOQOL). In: Orley J, Kuyken W, eds. Quality of life assessment: international perspectives. Berlin: Springer-Verlag, 1994:41–57.

(3) WHOQOL Group. Study protocol for the World Health Organization project to develop a quality of life assessment instrument (WHOQOL). Qual Life Res 1993; 2:153–159.

10

Recommendations and Conclusions

THE CURRENT STATUS
OF HEALTH MEASUREMENT

There is considerable variation in the quality and sophistication of the health measurements we review. This may reflect the relative newness of the field: the development of health indices is a recent endeavor compared with measuring intelligence or public opinion. Certainly, health measurement has benefited from the theoretical and technical advances in test construction already achieved in the social sciences, but the application of this knowledge to health measurements has been uneven. In our first edition we noted that pain scales were the most successful in exploiting the more sophisticated scaling techniques and that physical disability measures were for the most part unsophisticated. Over the intervening years measurements of physical disability have begun to catch up, although there is still a need to refine and further test existing instruments rather than develop new methods. We are also pleased at the marked increase in comparisions between measurement instruments: for most scales we have now been able to report correlations with rival scales. Recent years have also seen growing attention to scoring

health measures. It is becoming less acceptable merely to score responses 1, 2, or 3, and more and more measures are using formal scaling methods for assigning numerical weights to response options. Rasch analysis has seen increased use, as have econometric scaling methods. While the economic and psychometric approaches come from different academic traditions, their meeting in the health measurement field appears to be encouraging some melding of the two. Kaplan et al., for example, review the criticisms made of each side by the other and suggest that the two traditions may now be finding common ground (1). All in all, things are moving, and in the right direction. We continue to hope that the comments contained in reviews such as this book will encourage the fuller development of the less adequate methods.

We have repeatedly mentioned the desirability of a conceptual definition of the topic being measured. This is intended to stress the role of measurement in scientific discovery: as science ultimately tests theories we must know what theoretical orientation each health index represents. This goal has been quite well achieved in the fields of pain measurement and emotional well-being, and to a limited extent in quality of life measures. Many of the measurements of functional disability, however, pay little more than lip service to the idea of a conceptual approach to the topic: the WHO definition may be given passing mention, or the distinction between disability and handicap. Although a useful start, this could be refined to indicate more closely what questions should be included and why.

While we may complain about the weakness and lack of coordinated development work in certain areas of health measurement, it is also true that the universal, perfect index can never exist. It is quite wrong to imagine one set of questions suited to all diseases, all individuals, and all applications. Such an instrument would have to make so many compromises it would probably not be suitable for any particular application. Fundamentally different scales will be required for policy analysis and for individual patient evaluation; we will continue to have generic and disease-specific scales, health indexes, and health profiles, and subjective and objective measures. Each has its place, although certain quality-control procedures can be followed in developing health indices of any type. Given some successes and some areas of weakness, what should be done to strengthen this field?

GUIDELINES FOR DEVELOPING HEALTH MEASUREMENTS

Gradually, we seem to be witnessing an effort to foster a science of health measurement, equivalent to psychometrics or econometrics. This is important, as decisions affecting the welfare of patients and the expenditure of public funds are based on the results of health measurements; and pressure to monitor the outcomes of treatment is virtually universal. In the first edition of this book, we argued strongly for a responsible attitude toward ensuring the quality of health measurements. We also regretted that an ethic of quality control

was sometimes lacking. An improvement is now visible, and efforts toward quality control are seen in several areas. For example, some medical disciplines have now published measurement standards (2–4). More measures now include administration manuals; several are very good (5). Sophisticated analytic procedures, such as item response theory, are being imported into this field to examine the adequacy of measurement scales (6–9). There is also a laudable tendency to concentrate on further testing the leading methods, in place of developing new scales.

While we now have recommendations on how to develop, test, and present a measurement in certain fields (2, 3), we need generally applicable technical standards for the broader discipline. Following the example of the American Psychological Association's handbook (10), this might be sponsored by a body such as the Agency for Health Care Policy and Research or the International Epidemiological Association.

Guidelines must tackle three shortcomings in health indices: inadequate development and testing of the instrument, inadequately detailed published descriptions of it, and a lack of leadership in ensuring continued development and promotion of the method. The latter may require responding to eventual criticisms and sometimes modifying the scale to improve it. It is always hard to describe a measurement in sufficient detail within the constraints of a journal article, a problem that emphasizes the need also to produce a manual describing the method and its administration. If a measurement has been adequately tested, it is certainly worth the additional effort of preparing a manual to describe it. Several pertinent suggestions on preparing manuals are included in the APA standards (10), which guided the following comments.

1. Published articles or a manual should provide a full description of the purpose of the method, specifying the population for which it is designed,

the populations on which it has been tested, and the intended use for the data collected.

2. The definitive version of the instrument must be made readily available to users, perhaps by having it formally printed and distributing it at cost. It is our earnest desire that this field will avoid the tendency, prevalent among psychological publishing houses, of copyrighting scales and erecting needless barriers to their use. The argument that scales can only be interpreted by a qualified expert does not apply in the field of general health measurement: these are not diagnostic instruments. Furthermore, most scales were developed using public money, so the ethics of copyrighting them are questionable. A copy of the scale should be included in the manual; this helps avoid confusion over precisely which version is the definitive one. The otherwise excellent manual for the General Health Questionnaire can be faulted for its omission of a copy of the scale itself (curious, since it had already been published in previous reports).

3. Measures should be given a name that accurately describes their content; some ADL scales were never named, making it difficult for subsequent users to indicate which scale they have used. If a scale has been revised or abbreviated, it is helpful to indicate this by a modification of the title. At the same time, authors of instruments should delay presenting revised versions until there is a very clear advantage in doing so. The credibility of authors who argue that they have developed a superior scale is diminished when they publish revisions on an almost annual basis. The description of the method should also outline pitfalls in its administration and interpretation and should show how high and low scores are to be interpreted (see the Commentary on the Health Opinion Survey in

Chapter 5). Authors should also be cautious over making exaggerated claims of the applicability of their scales; a lot of confusion was caused, for example, when it was asserted that the Nottingham Health Profile could serve as a survey instrument—a claim that later had to be withdrawn.

4. A rationale should be given for the design of the instrument; what conceptual definition of the topic of measurement does it reflect? As an example, the presentation of an anxiety measurement should outline which theoretical approach it takes to the concept. Specification in this detail has been achieved for relatively few of the indices that we review; the scales of Bradburn, of Bush, and of Melzack provide examples of adequate conceptual formulations.

5. The way in which questions were selected should be indicated: where did they come from and how were they sampled? The manual should describe the procedures used to develop the instrument; good illustrations of this are contained in descriptions of the General Health Questionnaire, of the SF-36, and of the Sickness Impact Profile. The content of most of the successful questionnaires has been set by a team of clinicians, measurement experts, and patients.

6. Revisions to the method should be clearly explained and data on the reliability and validity of the latest version should be presented. Academic pressures encourage the publication of preliminary versions; the danger is that users continue to use outdated versions of a measurement. The cautionary tale of the Health Opinion Survey should be heeded; many validation studies were wasted because they did not test comparable versions of the method— the Life Satisfaction Index has also suffered in this way. Many users have a tendency to abbreviate the published

measurement, a problem that Goldberg successfully forestalled by recommending standard abbreviations for the General Health Questionnaire. It is also helpful to compare the various abbreviations of a scale, indicating the sacrifices in accuracy that arise from using the abbreviated versions.

7. Instructions must be clear enough to ensure standard administration and scoring of the method. Criticisms of the Mini-Mental State Examination illustrate this issue. Responses can be very sensitive to the way in which a measure is presented, and even for a self-administered questionnaire the precise instructions for the respondent should be shown. Likewise, the setting in which the method was administered during the validation studies must be described. A good example of attention to detail of this type is given in the Structured and Scaled Interview to Assess Maladjustment. Published descriptions should provide details of how missing data should be handled, of how change scores should be calculated (e.g., as absolute changes or as a percentage of the initial score?) When there are alternative scoring methods, the advantages of each need to be given and their intercorrelation should be stated; Melzack has done this for the McGill Pain Questionnaire.

8. All measures should include reference scores from several populations. Ideally, these should include a population sample of healthy people and samples from various patient groups, to provide yardsticks against which to interpret the results of subsequent studies. This has been done for the SF-36 (5), while standards of improvement with treatment have been described for some diagnoses using the Functional Independence Measure (11, 12). Unfortunately, several measures have been applied in large studies that would permit the derivation of reference standards, but these have not been published. Secondary analyses of this type might provide material for student theses.

9. The validity and reliability testing should examine both the internal structure of the method (its internal consistency and factor structure) and also its relation to alternative measurements of the same concept. In criterion validation, the rationale for the selection of the criterion scores must be given, and attention must be paid to *their* validity. The expected level of correlation should be specified before the study is undertaken; good examples include the work of McHorney et al. on the SF-36 (13). All too often authors present a list of miscellaneous coefficients from which they conclude, magically, that the results demonstrate the construct validity of the method. This seems capricious and logically inadequate, and it precludes refutation of validity. Construct validity should include tests of discriminant and of convergent validity, always with an advance indication of how much discrimination is expected. More formal testing requires the construction of a multitrait–multimethod matrix and the specification of patterns of correlations within the various sectors of the matrix.

10. While there has been a recent increase in the numbers of studies that compare rival measurement methods, there is still a tendency to avoid head-to-head comparisons of scales. Ultimately, this is what users need to guide their choice among alternative methods. Furthermore, when measures are compared, a correlation coefficient is not sufficient to indicate the agreement between them. Statistics that show agreement, rather than association, are required (see Chapter 2); the way in which the two measures classify respondents at the extremes of the scale should also be compared.

11. Each measurement method should be

tested by users other than the original authors, indicating that it holds a wide appeal and that it can be used successfully by others to provide consistent results. It is almost a law of health measurement that the original authors achieve higher validity figures than subsequent users.

12. The most successful instruments are those for which the authors take long-term responsibility for the further refinement of the method. Few, if any, measures are perfect when first published: most of the leading scales have undergone revisions. Some scales (the Hamilton Rating Scale for Depression is an example) clearly filled a need and were of good quality; no one, however, took responsibility for continuing the development effort. Commonly, shortcomings are found in measures and possible improvements are proposed. Where there is no coordination of responses, users tend to make piecemeal changes in an uncoordinated fashion and rival versions proliferate, making comparisons between studies uncertain. This is unfortunate, as the desire to improve a method attests to its basic soundness (for otherwise it would be abandoned) and to the demand for it. Like children, health measures require care through adolescence, and those who develop measurements should recognize the need to remain in charge of their methods over the long term; while this poses funding difficulties, several teams have managed and examples may be found in every chapter in this book.

FINAL REMARKS

We repeat our awareness that these guidelines are exacting and represent an ideal that few scales have achieved. And yet the difficulty of the task should not condone inferior work. Why should health be measured any less accurately than other fields such as educational attainment?

There are several possible avenues along which health measurement may proceed. First, many methodological advances simply have not been applied, making health indices less good than their potential. Our tabular summaries of the strengths and weaknesses of existing measurements are intended to give an initial stimulus to further work in consolidating the field, and the guidelines just given suggest how this may be done. Second, more formal channels of recognition for the field are required: the development of a journal of health measurement analogous to *Psychometrika* would help to avoid the continuing diversity of outlets in which such articles are published. Methodological conferences on health indices are becoming more common, and university courses in measurement and evaluation indicate the depth of interest. A recognized body could be asked to take on a coordinating role in formalizing guidelines, making recommendations on choices among rival methods and possibly developing a journal.

As authors we may look forward (with some trepidation, it must be admitted) to the time when a new edition of this book is required, for this would imply further advances in the field and the establishment of new methods that are superior to many of the ones we have included. At such a time we would also attempt to expand the work to include some of the other topics such as patient satisfaction scales, measurements of sensory problems and health promotion that were originally planned, but for which space in this book and in our schedules proved insufficient.

REFERENCES

(1) Kaplan RM, Feeny D, Revicki DA. Methods for assessing relative importance in preference based outcome measures. Qual Life Res 1993;2:467–475.
(2) Task Force on Standards for Measurement in Physical Therapy. Standards for tests and measurements in physical therapy. Phys Ther 1991;71:589–622.
(3) Johnston MV, Keith RA, Hinderer SR.

Measurement standards for interdisciplinary medical rehabilitation. Arch Phys Med Rehabil 1992;73(suppl):S3–S23.

(4) Kraemer HC. Evaluating medical tests: qualitative and objective guidelines. Newbury Park, California: Sage, 1992.

(5) Ware JE Jr, Snow KK, Kosinski M, et al. SF-36 Health Survey: manual and interpretation guide. Boston, Massachusetts: The Health Institute, New England Medical Center, 1993.

(6) Fisher AG. The assessment of IADL motor skills: an application of many-faceted Rasch analysis. Am J Occup Ther 1993; 47:319–329.

(7) Chambon O, Cialdella P, Kiss L, et al. Study of the unidimensionality of the Bech-Rafaelsen Melancholia Scale using Rasch analysis in a French sample of major depressive disorders. Pharmacopsychiatry 1990;23:243–245.

(8) McArthur DL, Cohen MJ, Schandler SL. Rasch analysis of functional assessment scales: an example using pain behaviors.

Arch Phys Med Rehabil 1991;72:296–304.

(9) Granger CV, Hamilton BB, Linacre JM, et al. Performance profiles of the Functional Independence Measure. Am J Phys Med Rehabil 1993;72:84–89.

(10) American Psychological Association. Standards for educational and psychological testing. Washington, DC: American Psychological Association, 1985.

(11) Granger CV, Hamilton BB. The Uniform Data System for Medical Rehabilitation report of first admissions for 1991. Am J Phys Med Rehabil 1993;72:33–38.

(12) Long WB, Sacco WJ, Coombes SS, et al. Determining normative standards for Functional Independence Measure transitions in rehabilitation. Arch Phys Med Rehabil 1994;75:144–148.

(13) McHorney CA, Ware JE Jr, Raczek AE. The MOS 36-Item Short-Form Health Survey (SF-36): II. Psychometric and clinical tests of validity in measuring physical and mental health constructs. Med Care 1993; 31:247–263.

Glossary of Technical Terms

Alpha   Cronbach's alpha is a generalized formula used to express the internal consistency reliability of a test.

Category Scaling   See Scaling.

Coefficient of Concordance   While a rank order correlation shows the agreement between two sets of rankings, Kendall's coefficient of concordance provides a measure of the relationship among several rankings of objects or individuals. It is the nonparametric equivalent of the intraclass correlation.

Concurrent Validity   Validity indicated by comparing scores on a measurement with those obtained by applying alternative, equivalent measurements at the same time.

Construct Validity   Used when there is no criterion against which to evaluate the validity of a measurement. Validity assessed by comparing the results of several contrasting tests of validity (including concurrent, convergent, and divergent validation studies) with predictions from a theoretical model.

Convergent Validity   The extent to which two or more instruments that purport to be measuring the same topic agree with each other.

Content Validity   The extent to which a measurement covers all aspects of the topic it purports to measure.

Correlation   A measure of association that indicates the degree to which two or more sets of observations fit a linear relationship. There are various formulae for estimating the strength of the correlation; in each case the range lies between -1 and $+1$. A correlation close to zero indicates no association between the observations; as correlations rise, it becomes more possible to predict the value of the second observation from a knowledge of the first. The formula most commonly encountered is Pearson's r, suited to data measured at an interval or ratio scale level. Kendall's tau and Spearman's rho correlation formulae may be used to indicate the association between variables measured at the ordinal level, and are termed "rank order correlations."

Criterion Validity   Validity indicated by comparing the results obtained using a measurement scale with a "gold standard" or indicator of the true situation.

Discriminant Analysis   A multivariate statistical procedure that indicates how adequately a set of variables (here, typically, the replies to questions in a health measurement) differentiate between two or more groups of people who are known to differ on some characteristic (here, typically being sick or well). The analysis selects the set of questions that shows the most marked contrast in the pattern of replies between the groups, i.e., the most discriminative questions.

Discriminant Validity   The extent to which scores on a measurement distinguish between individuals or populations that would be expected to differ (e.g., people with or without a disease).

Equal-Appearing Interval Scales   See Scaling.

Factor Analysis   A mathematical technique that, like principal components analysis, reduces a large number of interrelated observations to a smaller number of common dimensions or factors. A factor is a cluster of variables (here, items on a health measurement instrument) that are highly related to each other. As an example, a factor analysis of questions asked to assess intelligence might identify discrete groups of questions that assess verbal ability, numerical ability, and visual–spatial judgments. The factors are composed of measurements or variables that intercorrelate but that are distinct from variables on other factors.

Goal Attainment Scaling   An evaluation method that assesses the efficacy of a program in attaining predetermined goals.

Guttman Scaling   See Scalogram Analysis.

Internal Consistency   See Reliability.

Inter-Rater Reliability   The extent to which results obtained by different raters or interviewers using the same measurement method will agree. The agreement is appropriately calculated using the intraclass correlation when the measurement provides interval-level data.

Interval Scale   See Scales of Measurement.

Intraclass Correlation   In testing the reliability of a measurement, correlation coefficients such as Pearson's r may be used to compare the ratings of a number of patients made by two raters. The intraclass correlation generalizes this procedure and expresses the agreement among more than two raters. Unlike the Pearson correlation, however, the intraclass correlation is a measure of agreement that records the average similarity of raters' actual scores on the ratings being compared.

Item The term "item" is used to refer to individual questions or response phrases in any health measurement. It replaces the more obvious term "question" simply because not all response categories are actually phrased as questions: some use rating scales and others use agree/disagree statements.

Item-Total Correlation The correlation between each item or question in a health measurement and the total score; used as an indication of the internal consistency or homogeneity of the scale, suggesting how far each question contributes to the overall theme being measured.

Kappa As a coefficient of agreement between two raters, kappa expresses the level of agreement that is observed beyond the level that would be expected by chance alone. A typical formula is

$$\kappa = (p_o - p_c)/(1 - p_c),$$

where p_o is the observed proportion of agreement and p_c is the proportion of agreement expected by chance alone. Chance agreement may be thought of as the agreement that would occur if one rater merely guessed or flipped a coin to make his ratings. The p_c is assessed as follows:

$$p_c = p_1p_2 + (1 - p_1)(1 - p_2),$$

where p_1 is the probability of rater 1 diagnosing a case, and p_2 is the equivalent probability for the second rater. Although in theory the range of kappa is from 0 to 1, in practice its upper value is limited by the sensitivity and specificity of the test. (See Grave WM et al. *Arch Gen Psychiatry* 1981;38:408–413.)

Kendall's Tau See Correlation.

Latent Trait The unobservable continuum (e.g., pain or health) that items in a test are intended to measure. Latent trait analysis evaluates how consistently the items measure a single trait.

Likelihood Ratio This is an approach to summarizing the results of sensitivity and specificity analyses for various cutting points on diagnostic or screening tests. Each cutting point produces a value for the true-positive ratio (i.e., sensitivity) and the false-positive ratio (i.e., $1 -$ specificity). The ratio of true to false positives is the likelihood ratio for each cutting point. These values are plotted on a graph whose axes show true- and false-positive values; the curve that results is known as a receiver operating characteristic (ROC) curve. This way of presenting validity data may aid in selecting the optimal cutting point, as described by McNeil BJ et al. *N Engl J Med* 1975;293:211–215. See also Sensitivity, Specificity.

Magnitude Estimation See Scaling.

Multitrait–Multimethod Matrix A format for presenting validity and reliability correlations in which the agreement among several measurement methods (multimethod) as applied to several traits (multitrait) is shown in a manner that simplifies the interpretation of construct validity. It is assumed, for example, that the correlations between different measurement methods will be higher when applied to the same topic of measurement than when applied to different topics. (A clear example of the approach and the underlying assumptions is given by Campbell DT, Fiske DW. Convergent and discriminant validation by the multitrait-multimethod matrix. *Psychol Bull* 1959;56:81-105).

Ordinal Scale   See Scales of Measurement.

Path Analysis   A procedure for testing causal hypotheses that indicates the extent to which a hypothesized causal pattern fits empirical data. Path analysis could, for example, be used in analyzing a set of data to calculate the relative strength of the causal influence exerted by smoking, obesity, sedentary living, and cholesterol levels in predicting cardiovascular disease. The strength of the causal influence is indicated by path coefficients which are derived from standardized regression coefficients.

Pearson Correlation   See Correlation.

Positive Predictive Value   The proportion of all people who were identified by a measurement or screening test as apparently having the disease who actually do have it.

Predictive Validity   The accuracy with which a measurement predicts some future event, such as mortality (see Chapter 2, page 31).

Rank Order Correlation   See Correlation.

Receiver Operating Characteristic Curve (ROC)   An analysis of validity of a screening test that combines indicators of sensitivity and specificity. The true positive rate (sensitivity) is plotted graphically against the false positive rate (1 − specificity) for all possible cutting scores on the screening test. A statistical description of the overall performance of the test is given by calculating the area under the ROC curve (AUC); this statistic runs from 0.5, indicating prediction no better than chance, to 1.0 (perfect accuracy). See also Likelihood Ratio.

Reliability   The proportion of variance in a measurement that is not error variance (see page 37). Reliability can be assessed in many ways, each of which differs in the definition it implies of error variance. Commonly, reliability refers to the stability of a measurement: how far it will give the same results on separate occasions. This is influenced by the internal consistency of the method: how far the questions it contains all measure the same theme.

Rho   See Correlation.

Ridit   Used in presenting the results of several health indices, a ridit is a way of expressing the observed score relative to an identified population (hence "ridit"). The average ridit calculated for the group of interest shows the probability that a member of that group is "worse off" than someone in the identified, reference population distribution. As an example, if the average ridit for a subgroup is 0.625, then 62.5% of the people in the reference population have a better score (e.g., are less sick) than the average individual in the subgroup.

Scalability Coefficient   See Scalogram Analysis.

Scales of Measurement   The mathematical qualities of numerical measurement scales vary and are of four main types.

1. Nominal scales. Numbers are assigned arbitrarily with no implication of an inherent order to their categories, as in telephone numbers. Such scales may only be used as classifications; no statistical analyses may be carried out that use the numerical characteristics of the scale.
2. Ordinal scales. Classification into a scale that implies a distinct order among the categories (such as house numbers on a street), but where there is no natural assumption concerning the relative distance between adjacent values. Statistical methods such as rank order correlations may be used.
3. Interval scales. Interval scales are so named because the distance between adjacent numbers in one region of the scale is assumed to be equal to the distance between adjacent numbers at another region of the scale (as in Fahrenheit or Celsius scales). Addition and subtraction are permissible, but not multiplication or division of such scales; statistical analyses such as the Pearson correlation, factor analysis, or discriminant analysis may be used with interval scales.
4. Ratio scales. A ratio scale is an interval scale with a true zero point, so ratios between values are meaningfully defined. Examples include weight, height, and income, as in each case it is meaningful to speak of one value being so many times greater or less than another value. All arithmetical operations, including multiplication and division, may be applied, and all types of statistical analysis may be used.

Scaling   A set of procedures used to assign numerical weights to replies to health questions to reflect the severity of disability implied. Weights may be used in scoring the answer categories to individual questions. (For example, mild pain might be scored 1; severe pain, 6.) Weights can also be used in rating the relative severity of different questions, typically giving more weight to more serious disabilities in forming an overall score. Scaling methods are of two broad types—category scaling (such as Thurstone's "equal-appearing interval" procedure), which produces weights at an interval scale level, and magnitude estimation, which provides a ratio scale. An index that uses category scaling is the Sickness Impact Profile (Chapter 9); the Pain Perception Profile is an example of a scale using magnitude estimation (Chapter 8). By no means do all health indices use scaling to derive numerical weights for scoring responses: many simply add up the scores for each individual question, thus providing an ordinal scale or count of numbers of areas of disability. Several scales described in this book have shown similar results with weighted and unweighted scoring systems; the PAMIE scale, the Multilevel Assessment Instrument, and the Health Opinion Survey are examples.

Scalogram Analysis   Also known as Guttman Scaling, this method of analysis is used to select questions that lie in a hierarchical order such that agreeing to an item at one end of the scale implies a positive answer to all other items on the scale. For example, a scale of functional ability may ask about walking ability using items like, "I can walk a block or more," "I can walk 100 yards," "I can walk to my front door," and "I can move around in my room." Statistical techniques developed by Guttman and others analyze the pattern of responses to such items and show how closely they lie in a consistent hierarchy of severity: are there respondents who said, "I can walk a block or more" but said they could not walk 100 yards? If so, the intention of the scale to measure varying levels of a single dimension may not have been met, perhaps because some respondents do not understand 100 yards, or because they feel that a "block or more" may be less than 100 yards. Whatever the reason, the items may be reworded during the test development process. The hierarchical consistency is evaluated by coefficients of scalability and of reproducibility that range from 0.0 to 1.0. The coefficient of scalability indicates how far the questions form a cumulative scale, and should exceed 0.6 if the scale is truly unidimensional. The coefficient of reproducibility shows how accurately the scale score indicates a person's entire pattern of responses. In a valid scale the coefficient of reproducibility will fall above 0.9.

Sensitivity   The ability of a measurement method or screening test to identify those who have a condition, calculated as the percentage of all cases with the condition who are judged by the test to have the condition. As a mnemonic, the complement of *sensitivity* is the false *negative* rate (i.e., the number of cases with a disease who are falsely classified as not having the disease).

Spearman Correlation   See Correlation.

Specificity   The ability of a measurement to correctly identify those who do *not* have the condition in question. As a mnemonic, the complement of *specificity* is the false *positive* rate: the number of people the test falsely classifies as having the disease. The word "specificity" refers to how narrowly a test is targeted: does it only identify people with a specific type of disease? A flashlight with a narrow beam is specific; one with a broad beam is more sensitive and consequently less specific.

Tau   See Correlation.

Test–Retest Reliability   The stability or repeatability of a measurement is evaluated in terms of the agreement between a measurement applied to a sample of people and the same measurement repeated later (typically one or two weeks afterward). Assuming that the state being measured has not changed, any change in scores can be regarded as error variance, and hence the level of agreement is used as an indicator of reliability.

Validity   Narrowly, the extent to which a measurement method measures what it is intended to. More generally, the range of interpretations that can be appropriately placed on a measure. For example, socioeconomic status may serve as a valid indicator of risk of premature mortality, even though it was not collected for that purpose. A fuller discussion of validity is given on pages 29–37.

Visual Analogue Scale   A broadly applicable format for a measurement scale in which the respondent places a mark at a point on a 10-cm line that indicates the intensity of his response. Phrases are printed at the ends of the line (e.g., "no pain" and "pain as bad as you can imagine") to indicate the scope of the scale (see page 341).

Yule's Q   A correlation formula used for estimating the association between two binary variables.

Index